Clinical Atlas of Anterior Segment OCT

Optical Coherence Tomography

Clinical Atlas of Anterior Segment OCT

Optical Coherence Tomography

Brett Levinson, MD
Specialized Eye Care
Greater Baltimore Medical Center
Baltimore, Maryland
United States

Fasika Woreta, MD, MPH
Eugene de Juan, MD, Professor of Ophthalmic Education
Associate Professor of Ophthalmology
Residency Program Director
Director, Eye Trauma Center
Wilmer Eye Institute
Johns Hopkins University School of Medicine
Baltimore, Maryland
United States

Kamran M. Riaz, MD
Clinical Professor
Director of Medical Student Research
Department of Ophthalmology
Dean McGee Eye Institute
University of Oklahoma
Oklahoma City, Oklahoma
United States

ELSEVIER

Elsevier
1600 John F. Kennedy Blvd.
Ste 1800
Philadelphia, PA 19103-2899

CLINICAL ATLAS OF ANTERIOR SEGMENT OPTICAL COHERENCE TOMOGRAPHY ISBN: 978-0-443-12046-6

Executive Content Strategist: Kayla Wolfe
Senior Content Development Specialist: Himanshi Chauhan
Publishing Services Manager: Shereen Jameel
Project Manager: Nandhini Thanga Alagu
Design Direction: Amy L. Buxton

Printed in India

Last digit is the print number: 9 8 7 6 5 4 3 2 1

Contributors

Aneesha Ahluwalia, MD
Department of Ophthalmology
Stanford University School of Medicine
Stanford, California
United States

Asim Ali, MD, FRCSC
Professor of Ophthalmology and Vision Sciences
University of Toronto
Ophthalmologist-in-Chief
Mira Godard Chair in Vision Research
Hospital for Sick Children
Toronto, Ontario
Canada

Diego Altamirano, MD
Centro de la Visión and Clínica
Santa María
Chile

Guillermo Amescua, MD
Professor of Clinical Ophthalmology
Medical Director, Ocular Microbiology Laboratory
Bascom Palmer Eye Institute
University of Miami Miller School of Medicine
Miami, Florida
United States

Abdelhalim Awidi, MD
Wilmer Eye Institute
Baltimore, Maryland
United States

J. Christian Berry, MD
Alamo City Eye Physicians
San Antonio, Texas
United States

Kraig Bower, MD
Associate Professor of Ophthalmology
Johns Hopkins University
Baltimore, Maryland
United States

Rachel Caywood, OD, FAAO
Department of Ophthalmology
Dean A. McGee Eye Institute
University of Oklahoma
Oklahoma City, Oklahoma
United States

Albert Y. Cheung, MD
Associate Professor
Department of Ophthalmology
Virginia Eye Consultants
Norfolk, Virginia
United States

Jessica Chow, MD
Associate Professor of Ophthalmology and Visual Science
Director, Cornea and External Disease
Residency Director
Vice Chair of Education, Ophthalmology and Visual Science
New Haven, Connecticut
United States

Zelia M. Correa, MD, PhD
Professor of Clinical Ophthalmology
Director, Ocular Oncology and Echography Service
Bascom Palmer Eye Institute
Co-Leader, Melanoma Site-Disease-Group
Sylvester Comprehensive Cancer Center
Miami, Florida
United States

Amanda Crum, OD, MS
Assistant Professor
Department of Ophthalmology
Wilmer Eye Institute
Baltimore, Maryland
United States

Yassine Daoud, MD
Chair of Ophthalmology
Howard County General Hospital
Associate Professor of Ophthalmology
Wilmer Eye Institute
Johns Hopkins University
Baltimore, Maryland
United States

Laura Di Meglio, OD, FAAO
Instructor of Ophthalmology
Wilmer Eye Institute
Baltimore, Maryland
United States

Allen Omid Eghrari, MD, MPH
Associate Professor of Ophthalmology
Wilmer Eye Institute
Baltimore, Maryland
United States

Dan Eisenberg, MD
Las Vegas, Nevada
United States

Helena Prior Filipe, MD, MMEd, FSACME, FAMEE, CPC(HC), FEACL
West Lisbon Hospitals Center (CHLO)
Hospital de Egas Moniz
Egas Moniz Center for Interdisciplinary Research (CiiEM)
Lisbon
Portugal

Michael Joseph Fliotsos, MD
Department of Ophthalmology and Visual Sciences
Yale University
New Haven, Connecticut
United States

Anat Galor, MD, MSPH
Staff Physician, Surgical Services
Miami Veterans Affairs Medical Center
Professor of Ophthalmology
Bascom Palmer Eye Institute
University of Miami Miller School of Medicine
Miami, Florida
United States

Samir Jabbour, MD
Department of Ophthalmology
Université de Montréal
Montréal, Quebec
Canada

Joseph H. Jeffrey, MD
Department of Ophthalmology
Brooke Army Medical Center
San Antonio, Texas
United States

Albert S. Jun, MD, PhD
Walter J. Stark, MD, Professor of Ophthalmology
Chief, Cornea, Cataract, and External Disease Division
Wilmer Eye Institute
Johns Hopkins Medical Institutions
Baltimore, Maryland
United States

Carol L. Karp, MD
Professor of Ophthalmology
Dr. Richard K. Forster Chair in Ophthalmology
Dr. Ronald and Alicia Lepke Professorship in Corneal Diseases
Bascom Palmer Eye Institute
University of Miami Miller School of Medicine
Miami, Florida
United States

Brett Levinson, MD
Specialized Eye Care
Greater Baltimore Medical Center
Baltimore, Maryland
United States

Monisha E. Nongpiur, MD, PhD
Associate Professor
Clinician-Scientist
Principal Investigator
Singapore National Eye Centre
Singapore

Kamran M. Riaz, MD
Clinical Professor
Cornea, Cataract, and Refractive Surgery
Department of Ophthalmology
Dean A. McGee Eye Institute
University of Oklahoma
Oklahoma City, Oklahoma
United States

Paula A. Sepulveda Beltran, MD
Bascom Palmer Eye Institute
Department of Ophthalmology
University of Miami Miller School of Medicine
Miami, Florida
United States

Nakul Shekhawat, MD, MPH
Assistant Professor of Ophthalmology
Cornea, Cataract, and External Disease
Wilmer Eye Institute
Johns Hopkins University School of Medicine
United States

Divya Srikumaran, MD
Vice Chair of Education
Associate Professor of Ophthalmology
Wilmer Eye Institute
Baltimore, Maryland
United States

Hursuong Vongsachang, MD, MPH
Department of Ophthalmology
Massachusetts Eye and Ear Infirmary
Boston, Massachusetts
United States

Sarah L. Wall, MD
Yale New Haven Hospital
New Haven, Connecticut
United States

Kendrick Wang, MD
Yale School of Medicine
New Haven, Connecticut
United States

Fasika Woreta, MD, MPH
Eugene de Juan, MD, Professor of Ophthalmic Education
Associate Professor of Ophthalmology
Residency Program Director
Director, Eye Trauma Center
Wilmer Eye Institute
Johns Hopkins University School of Medicine
Baltimore, Maryland
United States

Angela Y. Zhu, MD
Assistant Professor of Clinical Ophthalmology
Pediatric and Adult Cornea, Cataract, and External Diseases
Bascom Palmer Eye Institute
University of Miami Miller School of Medicine
Miami, Florida
United States

Foreword

I am often asked why I chose cornea and external disease among all the ophthalmic subspecialties. Although there are numerous reasons, including the elegance, precision, and overall excellent results of penetrating keratoplasty surgery (the main corneal surgery when I was a resident), a primary driver for me was the wide variety of corneal diseases one could encounter and diagnose based simply on a history and slit-lamp examination. As it turns out, I am very good at pattern recognition and really enjoyed making diagnoses after having seen a condition or even a few photographs of it in the past.

During my fellowship I began taking slit-lamp photographs of many of my patients both to document the state of their disease and also to accumulate a collection of the many different ways an entity can appear. I have continued this practice throughout my career and have used these images in subsequent publications and in teaching residents and fellows.

Slit-lamp examination, while invaluable in the evaluation and treatment of anterior segment disease, has its limitations. For one, it is difficult, if not impossible in many cases, to see what is going on deep to an area of opacification. If a corneal infiltrate or scar involves the front of the cornea, one cannot determine what is happening behind it, including the depth of the infiltrate/scar and whether there is posterior corneal thinning. In the same vein, in cases of severe corneal edema, a slit-lamp examination is unable to determine the status of the Descemet membrane or the iris or lens. Fortunately, advancements in all fields of medicine, including ophthalmology, have allowed us to image areas of the body we cannot see on the surface with better accuracy and safety.

Anterior segment optical coherence tomography (AS-OCT) is incredible, noninvasive technology that supplements the slit-lamp examination with high-resolution images of the cornea, iris, and anterior aspects of the lens and sclera. Accurate measurements of corneal dimensions (including thickness of the entire cornea or subsets of it, such as a LASIK flap) and pathologic entities such as corneal ulcers or iris cysts can be performed and monitored on subsequent examinations.

Dr. Levinson and his coauthors have compiled a superb clinical Atlas of AS-OCT. They begin with brief chapters on the history and basics of AS-OCT and quickly get into a wide range of clinical applications. Topics are addressed both anatomically and by disease state. Within the parts of the Atlas devoted to the cornea, there are separate chapters on anterior, stromal, and endothelial corneal abnormalities. Additionally, several chapters are devoted to surgery, including refractive surgery and corneal transplant surgery. They also cover pediatric conditions, infections, contact lenses, and trauma, among other topics. Many of the high-quality AS-OCT images throughout the text are paired with excellent corresponding slit-lamp photographs. One of my favorite aspects of the book is the "Clinical Pearls" in each chapter; these are bite-sized nuggets that emphasize important aspects of both diagnosis and treatment of anterior segment diseases.

I am extremely proud that Dr. Levinson, one of my former cornea fellows at Wills Eye Hospital, and his colleagues have put together such a timely, useful, and beautiful book. Each section is easily digestible and allows for wonderful pattern recognition of a wide range of AS-OCT images. It is a welcome addition for all of us treating patients with anterior segment conditions.

The more I see, the more I see there is to see.

John Sebastian

Christopher J. Rapuano, MD

Acknowledgments

I have a bookshelf full of medical textbooks, but I never gave a moment's thought to the work that is required to produce such a thing, until I sat down to write one myself.

Thank you to my friend and colleague Jon Slotkin, with whom I spent my undergraduate and medical school years, and who encouraged me to apply to the University of Maryland Medical School and showed me the "trick" to success – constant study, perseverance and repetition. And more repetition.

I owe a debt of gratitude to the late Milford "Mickey" Foxwell, the dean of admissions at the University of Maryland Medical school, for taking a chance on an out-of-state New York student. I still remember where I was when he called me on (my first) cell phone and told me that I was going to be a doctor.

I am immensely grateful to my mentor Allan Rutzen, who I met as medical student and we worked on the nascent field of endothelial transplantation before DESK and DMEK were even imagined, and who sat (and sat) with me in the operating room, always patient, and has continued to offer me advice on clinical practice, family and the delicate art of Ophthalmic surgery and of being a mensch.

Thank you to Sajeev Kathuria, who taught me the importance of precision in surgery, and in life.

I am thankful for the faculty at the University of Maryland for training me, and to Cornea Associates at Wills Eye Hospital for exposing me to the fascinating world of corneal medicine and surgery. I was lucky to study with luminaries in the Cornea world and bask in their years of experience, Peter Laibson, Brandon Ayres, Sadeer Hannush, Irv Raber, Elizabeth Cohen, and Kristen Hammersmith. I am especially grateful to Chris Rapuano, who sparked my interest in the intrinsic beauty of capturing images of the eye, and taught me the finer points of the epithelium and LASIK and of life, as well.

My heartfelt thanks goes out to my publisher, Elsevier, and our editor Kayla Wolfe. The draft of our Atlas was completed and we were awaiting further instructions when our publisher, with whom we had worked for half a decade, told us they were divesting their Ophthalmology publishing department, and we were adrift. Kayla and Elsevier threw us a lifeline and rescued our Atlas from sinking into publishing oblivion. Kayla and her team and the editorial and design team lead by Himanshi Chauhan and Nandhini "Nan" Thanga Alagu, performed the laborious task of getting our words, ideas and images onto the printed page (and digitally as well) and the more onerous task of keeping a gaggle of hard-working eye doctors on task and on deadline.

I could not have come close to completing this Atlas without my colleagues and friends, Fasika Woreta and Kamran Riaz. Fasika stepped in when I sitting at my desk, staring at outline and thinking the task was insurmountable. Fasika was able help provide structure, and more contributors, to complete the task. Kamran was the glue that brought this Atlas together, and he shares my passion for finding another awesome image for the book, (and he was able to put up with me always wanting to add another cool image or another section). I know that without him, this work would never have come to fruition.

From the bottom of my heart, a thank you to my colleagues from across the country and the world, who gave their time and expertise to this Atlas. A work like this is a collaboration, and I have loved working with everyone, and I am eternally grateful for the collegiality and friendship of the world of eye doctors.

My parents supported me through the years of college and medical school, internship, residency and fellowship. The confidence instilled in me from my mother and the passion for being an eye doctor and devotion to patient care I learned from my father has carried me to this point. My father recently (partially) retired from a 40-year career as an Optometrist and he would come home, often late, from the office and tell me that he loved his work because he could make people see better and feel better every day. He is a living reminder that the person who loves what he does, never works a day in his life. Thank you, Mom and Dad.

This Atlas would have never been possible without the efforts of my fantastic technical staff, who captured the images printed in the book. They (almost) never complained when I asked them to retake a fascinating image, and they were always quick to say "this is a good one for the Atlas!" Thank you to Jennifer, Natalie, and Kate for capturing these wonderful pictures and to Stacey for getting them scheduled. There would not be an Atlas without you.

My complete and all-encompassing gratitude is extending to my wife Sara. Sara has the dubious pleasure of being my office manager and she has to deal with my multiple, manifest flaws and foibles all day in the office, and at home as well. I really do not know how she puts up with me and all my talk about eyes, and other myriad nonsensical thoughts and non-sequiturs. You are the sun, and the moon and the stars, and I know that I could not have done any of this without you.

And thank you to Ruby and Ian, for allowing me to see the wonder and beauty of the world through youthful eyes.

Brett Levinson, MD

Acknowledgments

I am grateful to my friend and colleague Dr. Brett Levinson for his vision of creating an anterior segment optical coherence tomography (AS-OCT) Atlas and collecting beautiful images of his patients over the last decade. I am also thankful to Dr. Kamran Riaz and our many colleagues whose hard work contributed to the success of this Atlas. I am forever grateful to my numerous mentors at the Wilmer Eye Institute, Bascom Palmer Eye Institute, and other academic centers for their support and encouragement throughout my career. On a personal level, I would like to thank all my family—my loving parents, my sisters, my husband, and my two beautiful sons—for enabling me to pursue a career in academic ophthalmology and for the sacrifices they have made on my behalf. I am hopeful that this Atlas will be useful to our colleagues in learning how to use AS-OCT to take better care of our patients.

Fasika Woreta, MD, MPH

Acknowledgments

I am grateful to my family for their support and patience over these past 2 years working on this Atlas, especially my wife, Sanaa, and my three kids, Rabiyah, Nabeel, and Zaynab, for giving me the time, freedom, and encouragement (along with peace and quiet) to embark upon, continue, and finish this laborious project. I spent far too many evenings and weekends away from them to work on this book, and they graciously allowed me to work on this. Developing and naming the Rabiyah forceps, Nabeel forceps, and Zaynab scissors do not come close to showing how much I love the three of you.

I am also thankful to the numerous cornea and anterior segment mentors I have had. Specifically, I am very grateful to Surendra Basti, MD, R. Wayne Bowman, MD, and H. Dwight Cavanagh, MD, PhD. I should particularly acknowledge my very first mentor, Ali R. Djalilian, MD, who took me under his wing when I was a clueless medical student and helped me begin my journey as an ophthalmologist. I suppose I should also be thankful to several people in the world of academic ophthalmology who questioned my abilities and actively sought to hinder my career. Thank you for doubting me; I have channeled that into a relentless desire to work harder and realize that the best revenge is living well.

Finally, I dedicate this work to my mother, Fahmeeda Begum, MD, who initially matched into ophthalmology but decided she wanted something more challenging and had a brilliant career as an endocrinologist. You are the reason why I chose my career path so that someday I could be as fractionally good, as a clinician and as a person, as you.

Kamran M. Riaz, MD

Introduction

I love being an eye doctor. I really love everything about it.

When my patients ask me why I chose Ophthalmology, or if I am speaking to a medical student, I feel I sound more like a proselytizing missionary than an unbiased scientist and clinician. For the curious mind, Ophthalmology offers a smorgasbord of surgery and medicine. Our days in the office run the gamut from emergencies to longitudinal care, pediatrics to geriatrics, oncology, rheumatology, neurology, even obstetrics, and the mental challenge of physics and optics, (if that's your thing.) The surgical options vary from cataract removal, to lens and corneal based refractive surgery, to retina to cornea to glaucoma and plastics, sometimes even trauma and everything in-between, with new technologies, implants and devices becoming available seemingly every month.

But one of the most singular aspects of Ophthalmology and Optometry is that for the most part, we function as our own radiology departments. In my training, we were taught the importance of precision in performing A-scans to determine axial length for our pre-operative biometry and B scans in the trauma hospital to look for occult detached retinas. We even had a portable camera to image the fundus of newborns in the NICU.

I completed my cornea fellowship in 2007, and in these few years, the changes in our techniques to image the eye have evolved at warp speed. It is hard to believe now, but in my residency, we had a photography department that would take actual film out of an actual camera, and then develop this film in a dark room and put these images on slides so we could view the fluorescein angiographic images. In my training we had a GDx machine to image the optic nerve, and I put my hands on my first OCT, the Zeiss Stratus when I was started in clinical practice in 2007. I am now on third OCT machine, not including the software upgrades.

Multiple textbooks and articles are available to document the different optic nerve and retinal pathologies visible with OCT. But I quickly realized that no such volume existed for the most fascinating part of the eye – the cornea and the anterior segment. When I mentioned this paucity of published knowledge to my colleagues and co-workers, they all had the same response – "You should write your own Atlas!"

While I was (trying) to relax and defocus my mind and enjoy the calming waters of the Atlantic Ocean in Ocean City, Maryland on vacation in 2016, I sent out e-mails to medical publishers with my idea and to my great astonishment, someone said "Yes." Of course, that simple e-mail required me to put together all of my images, and the copious images of my colleagues as well, and now, 8 years later you are holding the fruits of our labor in your hands.

I have found the use of OCT to image the anterior segment of the eye to be a paradigm shift in my understanding of pathology. OCT has me helped to document disease states as well as change over time, and is also an aide to explain complex topics to patients as well. I also find that taking the images and looking at them, enhances my enjoyment of my chosen speciality of medicine and deepens my fascination for the incredible, magnificent evolved structure of the human eye.

Often when I have shown my colleagues some of my slit lamp images with the corresponding anterior segment OCT, the response has been "It would have never occurred to me to use the OCT in that case." We have found that the more we looked, the more we saw.

This Atlas is designed to be an answer to the question, "What can the anterior segment module of my OCT do for me?"

My publisher told me that this introduction should help the reader who is holding this book in their hands, decide if they want to add this seminal text to their personal library and give it an honored place on the shelf in their clinic office.

To those persons, contemplating our Atlas – firstly, I want to say thank you for reading this far. I don't think I have every read this much of an introduction to any book, ever. If you are reading this introduction at one of our yearly meetings, I am probably wandering around somewhere, mouth agape, looking at all the cool new stuff to buy and hearing new things to learn. Feel free to send me a text message and I'll tell you personally how great the Atlas is. Or, better yet, flip through the pages and be amazed at the awesome images we have collected. Our Atlas has been designed thematically, both by anatomy and pathology to allow you to quickly find multiple images of common and uncommon conditions. I am also very impressed with the wonderful layout and design created by our publishers at Elsevier. I find that this Atlas is just fun to flip through and I suspect that you will find new use for your anterior segment OCT in every chapter

The utilization of the Anterior Segment OCT in the operating room and the clinic has exploded and this work will hopefully be starting point to expand our knowledge and appreciation of this powerful imaging tool.

Collecting thousands of images and writing and editing the chapters and working with my colleagues to produce this volume over the past decade, has been a labor of love.

I truly hope that you enjoy reading this Atlas as much as we enjoyed putting it together.

Brett Levinson, MD
Baltimore
April 2024

Contents

SECTION 1 INTRODUCTION TO ANTERIOR SEGMENT OPTICAL COHERENCE TOMOGRAPHY

1 History of Anterior Segment Optical Coherence Tomography (AS-OCT), 2

2 Clinical Applications, 7

3 Quantitative Analysis of the Anterior Segment, 10

SECTION 2 CONJUNCTIVAL PATHOLOGIC CONDITIONS

4 Conjunctival Pathologic Conditions, 22

5 Pathology of the Corneal Epithelium and Subepithelium/Bowman's Layer, 33

SECTION 3 STROMAL AND ENDOTHELIAL DISORDERS

6 Stromal Dystrophies, Degenerations, and Depositions, 58

7 Corneal Ectasias, 81

8 Pathology of the Endothelium, 104

SECTION 4 IRIS, ANGLE AND LENS ABNORMALITIES

9 Abnormalities of the Iris, 118

10 Abnormalities of the Angle, 130

11 Abnormalities of the Crystalline Lens and Intra-Ocular Lens, 142

SECTION 5 SURGERY AND ASSOCIATED COMPLICATIONS

12 Refractive Surgery, 160

13 Use of Intraoperative AS-OCT in Corneal Transplant Surgery, 184

14 Use of Anterior Segment Optical Coherence Tomography (AS-OCT) in Postoperative Management of Full-Thickness Penetrating Keratoplasty and Lamellar Keratoplasty, 192

15 Use of AS-OCT in Postoperative Management of Endothelial Keratoplasty, 200

SECTION 6 PEDIATRICS, TRAUMA, CONTACT LENSES AND OTHER PATHOLOGIES

16 Pediatric Cornea and Anterior Segment Imaging, 214

17 Trauma, 223

18 Applications in Contact Lens Fitting, 235

19 Corneal Infections, 242

20 Ocular Inflammation, 274

Index, 299

SECTION 1

Introduction to Anterior Segment Optical Coherence Tomography

1 History of Anterior Segment Optical Coherence Tomography (AS-OCT)

J. Christian Berry | Kamran M. Riaz

I. INTRODUCTION

Among medical specialties, ophthalmology has significantly benefited from and increasingly relies upon advancements in imaging technology. New diagnostic imaging devices and resources have enhanced ophthalmologists' abilities to diagnose and treat the full spectrum of ocular pathologic conditions. As clinicians, we increasingly rely on these new imaging technologies to improve the care we provide to our patients daily.

This atlas aims to be the standard reference for normal and pathologic findings seen in anterior segment optical coherence tomography (AS-OCT) and how hese images can effectively diagnose and treat ophthalmic disease, including commonly seen and rare entities, and differences between the two. AS-OCT yields a noninvasive and increasingly precise method to visualize anterior segment structures ranging from the ocular surface to the crystalline lens. Compared with ultrasound biomicroscopy (UBM), AS-OCT offers a far more comprehensive view of the anterior segment and is an effective, efficient, and less invasive modality that clinicians and ancillary staff can quickly learn. We hope this text is a helpful resource and guidepost for practicing ophthalmologists, optometrists, trainees and technicians alike.

II. HISTORY OF OPTICAL COHERENCE TOMOGRAPHY DEVELOPMENT AND BRIEF REVIEW OF OPTICAL COHERENCE TOMOGRAPHY TECHNOLOGY

Optical coherence tomography (OCT) has become a standard imaging tool in ophthalmology, providing rapid, accurate, and noninvasive information on ocular anatomy and function. One major strength of OCT imaging is its ability to provide clinicians with a cross-sectional view that is accurate to the micrometer level. Clinicians can effectively use OCT imaging to diagnose disease, monitor progression, and observe long-term responses to therapy.

OCT was developed and first used as a technique in 1991 by Huang and colleagues, and the first in vivo retinal images were successfully captured in 1993 (Huang D, Swanson EA, Lin CP, 1991). Subsequent efforts were made to expand this technology to create standardized protocols for assessing glaucoma and macular pathology. In 1996 the first OCT machine came to market through Zeiss, although adoption was slow initially. It was in the early 2000s that OCT began gaining widespread use (Fujimoto J, Swanson E, 2016). Since then, advances have continued within this imaging technique, including novel ways to obtain a better resolution and overall imaging of the tissue in question.

Although a full review of each type of OCT technology is beyond this book's scope, we will briefly introduce this technology here. *Tomography* is an imaging technique that provides a real-time, accurate, and cross-sectional view of the imaged tissue. *Coherence* describes the ability of light waves (or two parts of the same light wave) to produce interference. Interference describes how light waves interact after passing through an aperture-type opening. If light waves align to create a more intensive light pattern, this is known as *constructive interference;* if these light waves align and create a less intensive light pattern, this is known as *destructive interference.* If two light waves can produce an interference pattern, they have demonstrated coherence.

There are two main types of coherence (Fig. 1.1). *Temporal coherence (points X and Z)* can be seen when two similar locations on two different light waves are separated by time. Temporal coherence is the basis for time-domain OCT (TD-OCT) imaging. *Spatial coherence (points X and Y)* occurs within the same light wave: two different points within the light wave that are equidistant from the center demonstrate spatial coherence, which is the basis for spectral-domain OCT (SD-OCT) imaging.

OCT uses low-coherence interferometry: long wavelength (near infrared) light is used to penetrate the scattering medium without collateral tissue damage. Tomographic images are generated by measuring the echo time delay of light backscattered from time structures (Ang M, Baskaran M, Werkmeister RM, 2018). Light is split into two arms of an interferometer: (1) a reference arm and (2) a sample/tissue arm. Given that the tissue scatters the light, it will recombine with the reference beam and provide a unique interference pattern, which is recorded in the detector. Interferometry is then used to collect reflected light from the tissue(s) of interest and to reject photons that have scattered multiple times ("background noise").

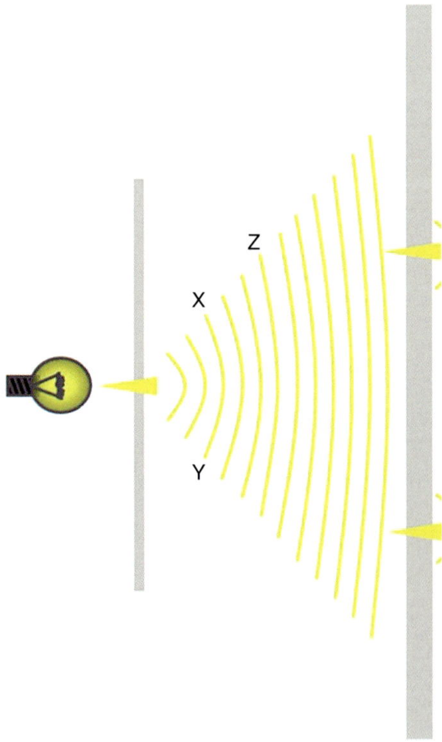

Fig. 1.1 Comparison of temporal coherence and spatial coherence.

OCT imaging systems have different approaches toward obtaining depth resolution, and they can be broadly divided into two types: TD-OCT and Fourier-domain OCT (FD-OCT).

With TD-OCT (comparing points X and Z [see Fig. 1.1]), time gating is used on the echo train of backscatter from the imaged tissue to generate an image by varying the path length of the reference arm in time (the reference mirror is translated longitudinally). A reflectivity profile (A-scan) of the sample can be obtained by scanning the mirror in the reference arm. The device's software combines multiple A-scans to generate a cross-sectional tomography image (B-scan). Approximately 400 A-scans per second can be generated using six radial slices oriented 30 degrees apart, yielding an accuracy down to the level of 10 to 15 microns (Yaqoob Z, Wu J, Yang C, 2005). TD-OCT devices provide images with high axial range and deeper tissue penetration with a resolution between 18 to 25 μm. However, because this technique relies on the movement of the reference mirror, image acquisition is slow. Eye movements during the scan may lead to unwanted artifacts in the acquired image. Commonly used devices that apply this technology include the Visante OCT (Carl Zeiss Meditec, Dublin, California, United States) and the Slit-Lamp OCT (SL-OCT; Heidelberg Engineering, Heidelberg, Germany).

With FD-OCT, the interference components are collected simultaneously without using a moving reference mirror to measure the target tissue at various depths. The most striking feature of FD-OCT is the sensitivity advantage that has increased acquisition speed by several orders of magnitude compared with TD-OCT without compromising image quality (de Boer JF, Leitgeb R, Wojtkowski M, 2017). FD-OCT includes both **spectral-domain OCT (SD-OCT)** and **swept-source OCT (SS-OCT)**. In both strategies, a sensor within the devices analyzes the beam intensity generated by interference (constructive, destructive, or partially constructive) of the reference arm beam and measuring arm beam.

SD-OCT systems use a spectrometer and a high-speed line scan camera to analyze the light; unlike TD-OCT, the SD-OCT reference mirror is static. With SD-OCT (comparing points X and Y [see Fig. 1.1]), information can be gathered by distributing the returning light waves (according to different optical frequencies) onto a detector stripe. This allows data of the full-depth scan to be acquired within a single exposure. SD-OCT takes approximately 20,000 to 40,000 A-scans per second to continuously image a 6-mm area of interest, yielding an accuracy down to the level of approximately 3 to 5 μm. Because SD-OCT devices use lower wavelength light sources (approximately 820–880 nm) with a greater number of A-scans, they provide images with excellent resolution compared with TD-OCT devices, although with limited tissue penetration (decreased depth). Commonly used devices employing this technology include the RTVue (Optovue, Fremont, California, United States) and Cirrus HD-OCT (Carl Zeiss Meditec).

SS-OCT measures the longer wavelength (1300-nm) dependent reflected light with a single detector. This narrow-band light source is then rapidly tuned over a large optical bandwidth. The wavelength is rapidly swept within the laser, allowing for the use of a point detector (Ang M, Baskaran M, Werkmeister RM, 2018). SS-OCT allows for several million A-scans per second using high-speed swept-source technology because of its ultrafast scanning system, greater depth range, and reduced motion sensitivity (Wieser W, Biedermann BR, Klein T, Eigenwillig CM, Huber R, 2010). Thus SS-OCT offers *deeper* tissue penetration (similar to TD-OCT devices) and *improved image details* (improving upon SD-OCT devices). Commonly used devices employing this technology include the Casia SS-1000 OCT (Tomey Corporation, Nagoya, Japan) and Triton SS-OCT (Topcon, Tokyo, Japan). As an aside, the SS-OCT imaging strategy can be used to measure the axial length of the eye and is used in devices such as the IOL Master700 (Carl Zeiss Meditec) and Anterion (Heidelberg Engineering) (Asam JS, Polzer M, Tafreshi A, Hirnschall N, Findl O, 2019).

Both SD-OCT and SS-OCT devices have their unique advantages and limitations. For example, SD-OCT imaging allows for *better axial resolution* than what is achieved by current SS-OCT systems. In addition, because SD-OCT uses wavelengths closer to visible light, it can provide *better image detail of anterior structures*, such as corneal layers, but has a *worse penetration into deeper ocular structures* than SS-OCT devices. Overall, the image acquisition rate is faster with SS-OCT devices. Furthermore, SD-OCT devices can more *effectively obtain maps of corneal epithelial thickness* compared with SS-OCT devices, given that the former imaging strategy has better axial resolution over a thin tissue area than the latter.

III. DEVELOPMENT OF ANTERIOR SEGMENT OPTICAL COHERENCE TOMOGRAPHY DEVICES

Soon after OCT was introduced, there were efforts to broaden its clinical application. In 1994, OCT was applied to the anterior segment of the eye (Izatt JA, Hee MR, Swanson EA, 1994). Initially, similar parameters to retinal OCT were used. Still, although shorter wavelengths of light provided optimal imaging of the retina, these wavelengths also resulted in suboptimal imaging for the anterior segment structures, given their limited penetration through connective tissue such as the sclera.

Researchers soon recognized that longer wavelengths of light (>1300 nm) were better suited for imaging the anterior segment. Using these wavelengths, better penetration and imaging of anterior segment tissues (e.g., scleral spur) were possible while minimizing the amount of light that reached the posterior segment.

Approved in the mid-2000s, the Zeiss Visante OCT (Carl Zeiss Meditec) and the Slit-Lamp OCT (SL-OCT, Heidelberg Engineering) were the first commercial AS-OCT machines. These devices employed TD-OCT technology and thus had limitations on both resolution (from 18–25 μm) and A-scan rates (2000/second with Visante OCT and 200/second with SL-OCT) (Ang M, Baskaran M, Werkmeister RM, 2018).

FD-OCT machines were introduced soon after, although they were designed for posterior segment imaging and had the limitation of smaller scanning areas. The first anterior segment SS-OCT was launched in 2008 (Casia SS OC, Tomey). This system has a much higher A-scan rate (30,000/second) and improved resolution (approximately 10 μm) (Wieser W, Biedermann BR, Klein T, Eigenwillig CM, Huber R, 2010).

With the newest devices that employ SS-OCT imaging, A-scan rates in the 100,000 per second range are possible, which has led to superior resolution of the target tissue(s). Higher image acquisition speeds also make acquired images less sensitive to motion artifacts, which are artifacts in the image due to the difficulty some patients have keeping their head still in the device

Table 1.1 provides a summary of commonly available AS-OCT devices. Fig. 1.2 compares the TD-OCT, SD-OCT, and SS-OCT imaging technologies.

Although this book primarily focuses on using AS-OCT in clinical practice, two other applications of AS-OCT technology may be of interest. First, OCT angiography (OCT-A) can be used to obtain information about ocular vessels by analyzing

TABLE 1.1 COMMONLY AVAILABLE ANTERIOR SEGMENT OPTICAL COHERENCE TOMOGRAPHY DEVICES[a]

Imaging Strategy and Technology	Device Name and Manufacturer	Features of Device
Time-domain	Visante OCT (Carl Zeiss Meditec, Dublin, CA, USA)	1310-nm wavelength provides a 2-dimensional view; 2000 A-scans/s
Time-domain	Slit-Lamp OCT (Heidelberg Engineering, Heidelberg, Germany)	1310-nm wavelength provides a 2-dimensional view; 200 A-scans/s
Fourier-domain (spectral-domain)	RTVue (Optovue, Fremont, CA, USA)	Provides limited 3-dimensional imaging of the cornea
Fourier-domain (spectral-domain)	Cirrus HD-OCT (Carl Zeiss Meditec)	1–3 mm scan uses 840-nm wavelength yielding shallower penetration than traditional devices
Fourier-domain (spectral-domain)	Anterior Segment Module (ASM) with SPECTRALIS SD-OCT device and Anterion (Heidelberg Engineering)	ASM is an add-on module for commonly used OCT for posterior segment imaging; it can provide single and raster-style scans
Fourier-domain (spectral-domain)	MS-39 (CSO, Florence, Italy)	850-nm wavelength allows for an axial resolution of 3–4 μm
Fourier-domain (swept-source)	Casia SS-100 OCT (Tomey Corporation, Nagoya, Japan)	3-dimensional scan uses 1300-nm wavelength; tissue resolution to approximately 10 microns
Fourier domain (swept-source)	Add-on lens module with Triton SS-OCT (Topcon, Tokyo, Japan)	1050-nm wavelength with a scan depth of 3 mm
Ultra-high-resolution OCT (deep range modification of swept-source AS-OCT)	Casia 2 (Tomey Corporation)	Scan depth of 13 mm allows for a single-shot view incorporating cornea and crystalline lens with a resolution of 1–4 μm

[a]Of note, some of these devices (such as the Anterion) are not available in the United States at the time of this writing (July 2021).

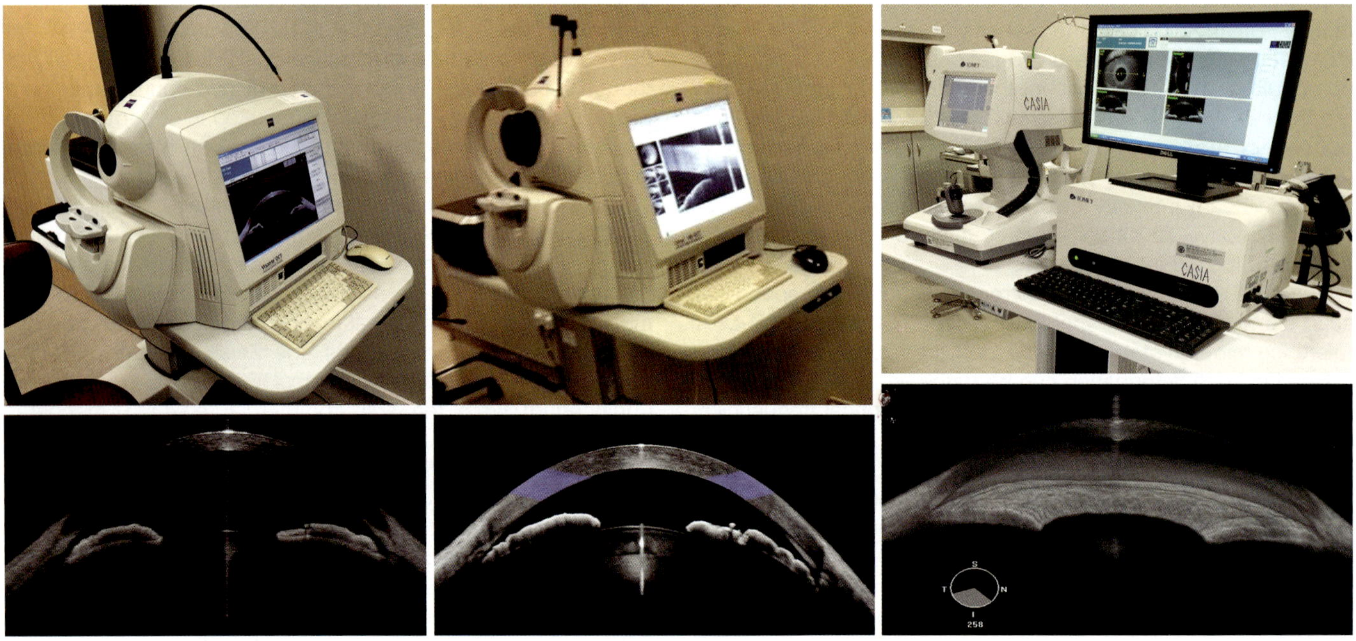

Time domain
1310 nm/10–20 microns
200–2,000 A-scan/sec

Spectral domain
840 nm/5 x 15 microns
26,000 A-scan/sec

Swept-source domain
1310 nm/<10 × <30 microns
30,000 A-scan/sec

Meridional (cross-sectional)

Circumferential (360 degree)

Fig. 1.2 Summary of time-domain OCT, spectral-domain OCT, and swept-source OCT. (Courtesy of Nikhil Gokhale, Gokhale Eye Hospial, Mumbai, India.)

variances of the OCT signal rapidly and without intravenous dyes. Although primarily used for posterior segment neovascularization, modifications of existing OCT-A devices can be used for anterior segment purposes, such as analysis of vascular conjunctival lesions, corneal vessels, and iris neovascularization. Second, intraoperative AS-OCT is used in many femtosecond laser–assisted cataract surgery devices. These devices use SD-OCT technology for intraoperative planning and visualization of laser-assisted corneal incisions, capsulotomy, and nuclear softening.

IV. FEATURES AND ADVANTAGES OF ANTERIOR SEGMENT OPTICAL COHERENCE TOMOGRAPHY

AS-OCT provides imaging of the entire anterior segment, including the ocular surface and tear film, conjunctiva, cornea, aqueous outflow system, iris, anterior chamber and angle, sclera, and the lenticular plane to image the natural crystalline lens and intra-ocular lenses (IOLs).

Commercially available devices have attachment lenses to better visualize the cornea and anterior segment as clinical presentation warrants (Fig. 1.3).

Historically, UBM served as the imaging modality of choice for the anterior segment (Binotti WW, Chiu S, Giaconi JA, Updated April 16, 2020). Although UBM still has essential clinical applications, AS-OCT provides several advantages over UBM and has become a preferred imaging modality in many clinical scenarios (Table 1.2) (Asam JS, Polzer M, Tafreshi A, Hirnschall N, Findl O, 2019).

First, AS-OCT is a noncontact test that can be performed with the patient seated upright, whereas UBM requires supine positioning with physical contact and immersive coupling. This may make AS-OCT a more feasible and preferred imaging technique for many patients because UBM requires additional resources and logistical efforts for optimized image acquisition. Additionally, AS-OCT provides higher resolution and scanning dimensions compared with UBM (Ishikawa H, 2007). UBM also requires an experienced technician to acquire the desired images, whereas most users can quickly learn AS-OCT.

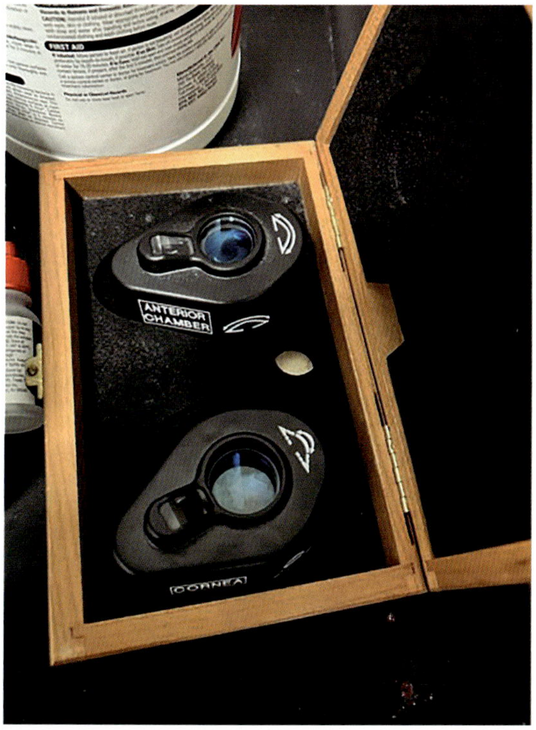

Fig. 1.3 Attachment lenses for anterior segment OCT devices. The anterior segment attachment lens can better image areas of interest in the iris-angle plane.

TABLE 1.2 COMPARISON OF ANTERIOR SEGMENT OPTICAL COHERENCE TOMOGRAPHY VERSUS ULTRASOUND BIOMICROSCOPY

	AS-OCT	UBM
Requires contact with eye	No	Yes
Quantitative	Yes	Yes
Imaging posterior to iris	Yes (but requires a special adaptive lens with limited resolution)	Yes
Resolution	15 μm	50 μm
Widest scan dimension	16 × 6 mm	5 × 5 mm
Real-time imaging	Yes	Yes

AS-OCT, Anterior segment optical coherence tomography; *UBM,* ultrasound biomicroscopy.
Modified from Radhakrishnan S, Aref AA, Patel AS, et al. Anterior segment optical coherence tomography. AAO EyeWiki website. Available at: https://eyewiki.aao.org/Anterior_Segment_Optical_Coherence_Tomography. Updated August 14, 2019. Accessed April 30, 2020.

Both modalities have applications when evaluating the angle and its structures. For example, even though gonioscopy is the gold standard for angle evaluation, it may not always be possible to perform this in certain patients. AS-OCT offers an excellent, noncontact method of obtaining objective clinical information about the anterior segment angle, especially for screening purposes. However, AS-OCT relies on a relatively clear cornea to accurately image the angle. For a cloudy cornea or suspected posterior pathologic condition (ciliary body cyst, effusion, lens issues, or plateau iris), UBM would be preferred (Maslin JS, Barkana Y, Dorairaj SK, 2015).

UBM remains the preferred and superior imaging technique (given the current state of AS-OCT technology) when considering structures behind the iris, such as the ciliary body, peripheral lens, and zonular complex. For example, for visualization of a dislocated or tilted IOL, UBM would be the preferred modality, especially given the depth of image acquisition with currently available AS-OCT devices. It is essential to recognize that the modalities are complementary, and the clinical course may warrant the singular or concurrent use of a given imaging modality. As the majority of clinicians have access to OCT technology, but not to UBM, the AS-OCT images, while more limited than UBM, can still be quite useful.

V. CLINICAL APPLICATIONS IN ANTERIOR SEGMENT PRACTICE

OCT imaging has revolutionized the field of ophthalmology. Although a thorough clinical examination is still vital and irreplaceable, OCT provides valuable information for the clinician, especially in subtle or difficult-to-appreciate ocular pathologic conditions. AS-OCT imaging is a relatively new diagnostic tool that has undergone much growth and improvement since its introduction.

Just as there was a historical lag between the advent of OCT and its widespread adoption in the diagnosis and treatment of posterior segment disease, it is likely that the application of AS-OCT will similarly expand in the future, especially in the detection and management of subtle anterior segment pathologic conditions.

The purpose of this book is to serve as a reference and consulting resource for clinicians as they use and apply AS-OCT imaging in their practices. The inclusion of numerous images of commonly encountered anterior segment pathologic findings, including variations and the spectrum-type presentation of a given disease, will hopefully serve as a visual atlas for the clinician on the value and applications of AS-OCT imaging in the workup, diagnosis, clinical decision-making, and surgical planning in practice. We hope the following chapters will encourage further use and development of this powerful imaging tool.

BIBLIOGRAPHY

Ang M, Baskaran M, Werkmeister RM, et al. Anterior segment optical coherence tomography. *Prog Retin Eye Res*. 2018;66:132-156.

Asam JS, Polzer M, Tafreshi A, Hirnschall N, Findl O. Anterior segment OCT. In: Bille J, eds. *High Resolution Imaging in Microscopy and Ophthalmology*. Springer, Cham; 2019. Available at: https://doi.org/10.1007/978-3-030-16638-0_13.

Binotti WW, Chiu S, Giaconi JA, et al. *Ultrasound Biomicroscopy*. AAO EyeWiki; Updated April 16, 2020. Available at: https://eyewiki.aao.org/Ultrasound_Biomicroscopy. Accessed April 30, 2020.

de Boer JF, Leitgeb R, Wojtkowski M. Twenty-five years of optical coherence tomography: the paradigm shift in sensitivity and speed

provided by Fourier domain OCT [Invited]. *Biomed Opt Express*. 2017;8(7):3248-3280.
Fujimoto J, Swanson E. The development, commercialization, and impact of optical coherence tomography. *Invest Ophthalmol Vis Sci*. 2016;57(9):OCT1-OCT13.
Huang D, Swanson EA, Lin CP, et al. Optical coherence tomography. *Science*. 1991;254(5035):1178-1181.
Ishikawa H. Anterior segment imaging for glaucoma: OCT or UBM? *Br J Ophthalmol*. 2007;91(11):1420-1421.
Izatt JA, Hee MR, Swanson EA, et al. Micrometer-scale resolution imaging of the anterior eye in vivo with optical coherence tomography. *Arch Ophthalmol*. 1994;112(12):1584-1589.
Maslin JS, Barkana Y, Dorairaj SK. Anterior segment imaging in glaucoma: an updated review. *Indian J Ophthalmol*. 2015;63(8):630-640.
Radhakrishnan S, Aref AA, Patel AS, et al. *Anterior Segment Optical Coherence Tomography*. AAO EyeWiki; Updated August 14, 2019. Available at: https://eyewiki.aao.org/Anterior_Segment_Optical_Coherence_Tomography. Accessed April 30, 2020.
Wieser W, Biedermann BR, Klein T, Eigenwillig CM, Huber R. Multi-megahertz OCT: high quality 3D imaging at 20 million A-scans and 4.5 GVoxels per second. *Opt Express*. 2010;18(14):14685-14704.
Yaqoob Z, Wu J, Yang C. Spectral domain optical coherence tomography: a better OCT imaging strategy. *Biotechniques*; 2005;39:S6-S13.

Clinical Applications

Jessica Chow | Aneesha Ahluwalia

2

INTRODUCTION

Anterior segment optical coherence tomography (AS-OCT) was first described in 1994 as a noninvasive imaging modality for detailed visualization of anterior structures of the eye. In comparison to ultrasound biomicroscopy (UBM), AS-OCT has higher resolution, faster acquisition, and a greater scan width and does not require an experienced operator. The noncontact nature of AS-OCT also increases patient comfort and is particularly useful in the anterior segment evaluation of children, who commonly require sedation for UBM. Additionally, in contrast to other anterior segment examination tools, such as slit-lamp biomicroscopy and in vivo corneal confocal microscopy, AS-OCT is neither restricted in its cellular resolution nor in its field of view. However, a major limitation of AS-OCT is its inability to visualize structures posterior to the iris, as the wavelength of light used to obtain images is blocked by pigment.

Since its introduction, technologic advancements have increased the imaging capabilities of AS-OCT, and numerous studies have demonstrated its potential utility in diagnosis, treatment planning, and disease monitoring. Because the imaging modality can be employed intraoperatively, it also has shown promise in guiding surgical decision-making. With a growing body of evidence demonstrating the potential use of AS-OCT in a variety of clinical contexts, it is more important than ever for ophthalmologists to be aware of the applications of this technology. This chapter will provide a brief overview of the clinical applications of AS-OCT.

DIAGNOSIS AND EVALUATION OF OCULAR PATHOLOGIES

Improvements in the acquisition speed and resolution of OCT images have facilitated the use of AS-OCT in evaluating pathologic changes in structures of the anterior segment, including the cornea, conjunctiva, sclera, anterior chamber (AC) angle, aqueous outflow system, and tear film. Ultra-high-resolution AS-OCT is particularly useful for distinguishing between similar-appearing malignant and benign conditions. For example, AS-OCT can aid in the differentiation of ocular surface squamous neoplasia, such as conjunctival or corneal intraepithelial neoplasia, from benign conjunctival changes such as pingueculae and pterygia. Additionally, AS-OCT can help distinguish melanoma from amelanotic conjunctival nevi through identification of cystic spaces that classically appear in the latter (Fig. 2.1). Finally,

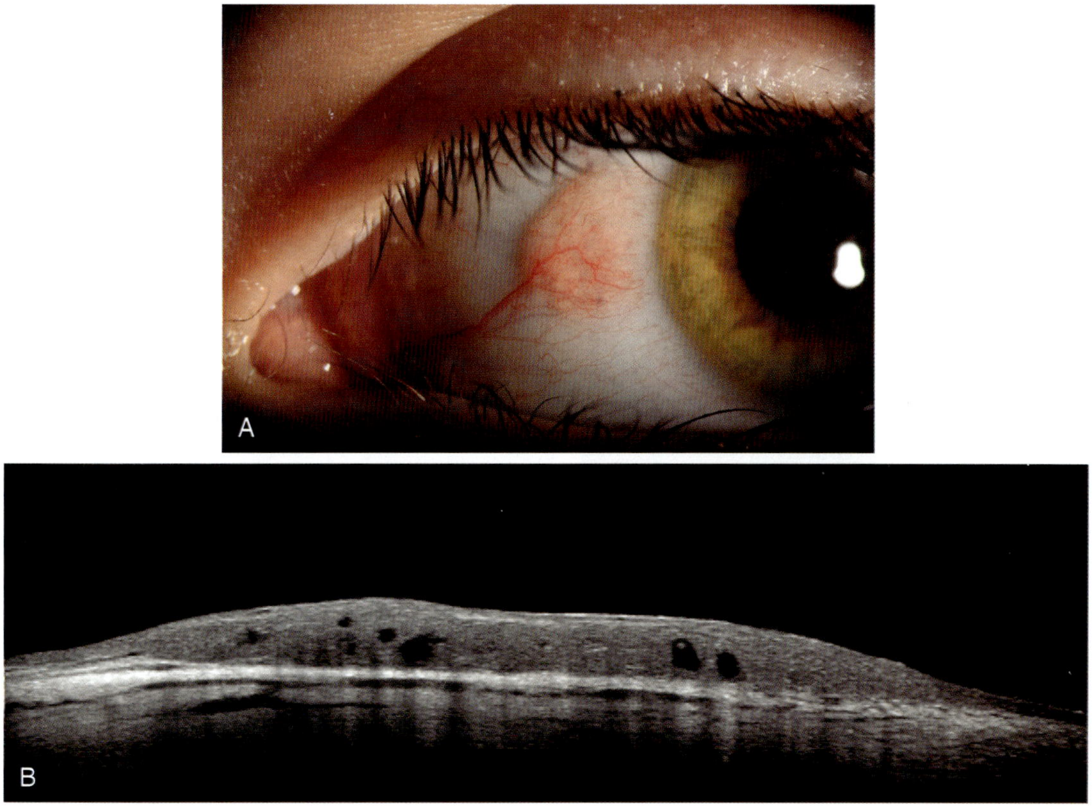

Fig. 2.1 (A) Slit-lamp photograph of conjunctival nevus. (B) AS-OCT of conjunctival lesion with cystic spaces. (Courtesy of Baltimore, MD, USA.)

hyperreflective lines in the corneal stroma and retrocorneal membranes can be imaged with AS-OCT to characterize cases of microbial keratitis.

CLINICAL PEARL

In an ideal cross-sectional image of the anterior segment, a bright line should be visible in the center of the image. This is a reflex saturation beam, which indicates perpendicularity of the eye to the scanning beam and minimal tilting of the image.

The use of AS-OCT also has been widely described in the diagnosis and evaluation of suspected angle-closure glaucoma. There are several advantages of AS-OCT in evaluating the AC angle. As a noncontact method, it can be useful when patient cooperativity with examination is limited or gonioscopy is not feasible because of an existing corneal pathologic condition. Furthermore, AS-OCT does not cause mechanical distortion of the angle and can be performed in the dark to verify cases of suspected angle closure (Figs. 2.2 and 2.3).

CLINICAL PEARL

Although AS-OCT can provide high-resolution imaging of the AC angle, it is not a replacement for gonioscopy. For example, the scleral spur is often difficult to identify in AS-OCT images, resulting in subjective and inaccurate quantification of the angle opening. Gonioscopy should be used as a primary tool, with the employment of AS-OCT for specific purposes, such as detailed characterization of the mechanism of angle closure.

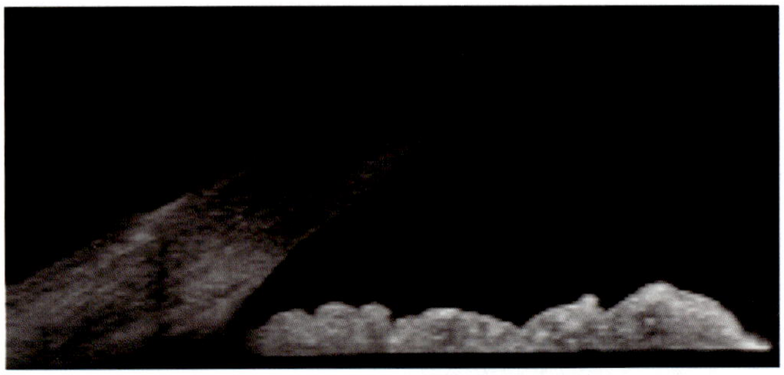

Fig. 2.2 Cross-section of an open anterior chamber angle. (Courtesy of Dr. Brett Levinson.)

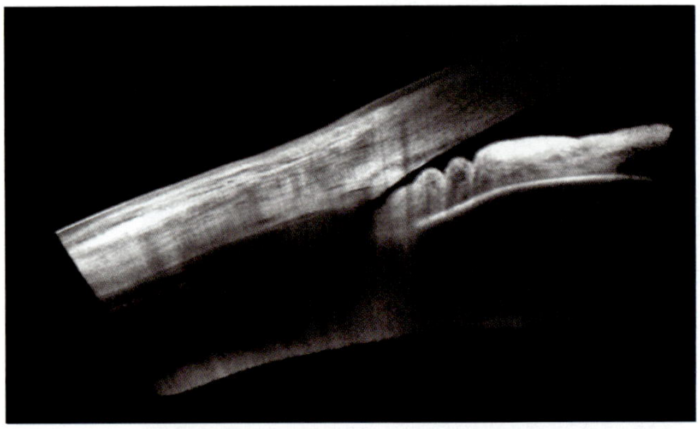

Fig. 2.3 Cross-section of an occluded anterior chamber angle. (Courtesy of Dr. Brett Levinson.)

MONITORING DISEASE PROGRESSION AND SEVERITY

The accuracy and reproducibility of AS-OCT in the measurement of various ocular parameters have also highlighted its potential utility in monitoring ocular disease progression. For example, AS-OCT can longitudinally characterize keratoconus severity and evaluate the risk of corneal hydrops by serial central corneal thickness and keratometry measurements. The imaging modality also has been used to monitor corneal thinning at the limbus in cases of peripheral ulcerative keratitis.

In the setting of dry eye disease, AS-OCT has enabled quantification of disease severity in terms of objective parameters. This is of particular interest given the challenge of correlating clinical signs and existing measures of severity, such as corneal staining and tear breakup time. For example, measurements of tear film thickness have been found to be significantly correlated with patients' subjective symptoms. AS-OCT also allows for the visualization and monitoring of pathologic changes throughout the anterior chamber, including the conjunctiva, layers of the cornea, anatomic angle, anterior chamber, iris, and natural cystaline lens and intraocular lenses.

PREOPERATIVE EVALUATION AND SURGICAL PLANNING

AS-OCT has numerous potential applications in the preoperative, intraoperative, and postoperative evaluation of surgical procedures, including corneal transplant, refractive, and glaucoma surgeries. AS-OCT is particularly advantageous in surgical planning when precise measurements are required. For example, in deep anterior lamellar keratoplasty (DALK), AS-OCT can evaluate the thickness of potential donor graft tissue and delineate between the corneal layers. The imaging modality also has utility in the preoperative stage of cataract surgery, including evaluating the anterior chamber and angle structures, considering the risk for complications, and aiding in the calculation of intraocular lens (IOL) power. Specifically, among patients with prior refractive surgery, IOL power calculations determined from AS-OCT have been shown to be equal to or superior to those obtained from standard measurements.

CLINICAL PEARL

AS-OCT can be a useful patient education tool, allowing patients to visualize their pathologic conditions and surgical procedures. For example, as many patients have difficulty understanding the concept of occludable angles, OCT images can be used to show the patient the narrow or closed angle, and better explain the risk of vision loss through pictures rather than words. Detailed imaging of corneal layers could also enhance understanding of keratoplasty procedures. Furthermore, it may be more useful and compelling for patients to see scans of their own eyes rather than stock diagrams or models.

INTRAOPERATIVE GUIDANCE

AS-OCT can be performed intraoperatively, either with a handheld OCT device or by coupling OCT to a microscope, which has potential implications for surgical decision-making and is discussed in detail in Chapter 13. Indeed, AS-OCT imaging of the cornea is routinely incorporated into many femtosecond cataract surgeries to guide placement of corneal incisions, visualize corneal wounds, and monitor the status of the posterior capsule. AS-OCT also can provide precise depth measurements of needle insertion in DALK, potentially increasing the likelihood of achieving a big bubble.

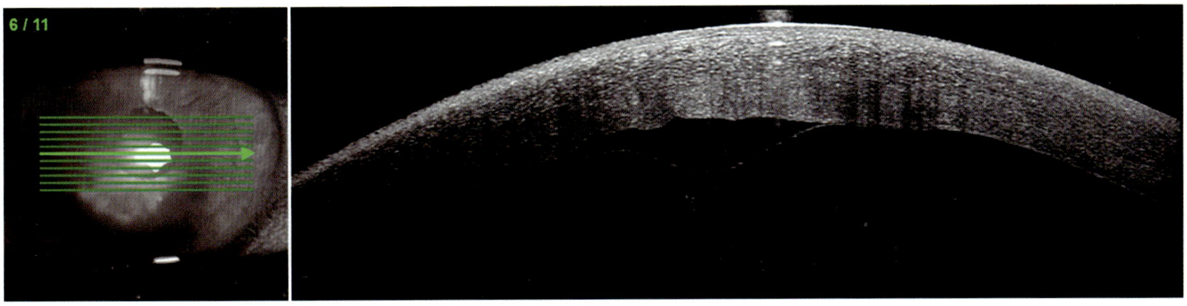

Fig. 2.4 Partial detachment of graft after DMEK. (Courtesy of Dr. Brett Levinson.)

Additionally, in Descemet stripping endothelial keratoplasty (DSEK), the technology could inform the need for further maneuvers by revealing persistent fluid or confirming graft apposition, with the goal of minimizing total surgical time and graft dislocations.

AS-OCT can be particularly advantageous in patients with preexisting risk factors for surgical complications. In DALK, AS-OCT can inform the initial trephination depth for cases with corneal scarring and thinning. AS-OCT may also provide enhanced visualization in challenging cases with poor visibility. For example, when performing Descemet membrane endothelial keratoplasty (DMEK) in patients with severe corneal edema or stromal scarring, AS-OCT can aid in determining graft apposition and graft orientation based on the direction of graft scrolling, particularly when ink markings are obscured.

POSTOPERATIVE MONITORING

Literature has also highlighted the utility of AS-OCT in postoperative evaluation and monitoring. In the early postkeratoplasty period, AS-OCT can detect complications such as graft detachment, pupillary block, and angle closure; it also has the potential to predict long-term graft failure (Fig. 2.4). After refractive surgeries, AS-OCT has been similarly employed to detect flap displacement, interface fluid collection, and corneal inflammation. In patients who have received laser-assisted in situ keratomileusis (LASIK), flap and residual stromal bed thickness can be measured to determine whether further treatment is appropriate.

Furthermore, AS-OCT–based quantification of additional postsurgical anatomic changes, including posterior cornea protrusion and changes in corneal power, have been reported after femtosecond-assisted laser refractive surgery and photorefractive keratectomy. After cataract surgery, AS-OCT has been used to evaluate corneal incisions, assess corneal epithelial remodeling, detect postoperative gape of small-incision cornea wounds, and evaluate the stability and location of the IOL. AS-OCT has also shown promise in evaluating the efficacy of other interventions, such as collagen cross linking for patients with keratoconus.

CONCLUSION

AS-OCT has the unique ability to rapidly acquire high-resolution images of the anterior segment in a noncontact manner. Since its introduction, this imaging modality has demonstrated potential utility in a wide range of ophthalmic clinical applications, including anatomic evaluation, diagnosis, operative planning, and monitoring. Later chapters will discuss specific applications of AS-OCT in more detail.

BIBLIOGRAPHY

Behrens A, Stark WJ, Pratzer KA, McDonnell PJ. Dynamics of small-incision clear cornea wounds after phacoemulsification surgery using optical coherence tomography in the early postoperative period. *J Refract Surg*. 2008;24(1):46-49.

Chan TC, Liu D, Yu M, Jhanji V. Longitudinal evaluation of posterior corneal elevation after laser refractive surgery using swept-source optical coherence tomography. *Ophthalmology*. 2015;122(4):687-692.

Ehlers JP, Goshe J, Dupps WJ, et al. Determination of feasibility and utility of microscope-integrated optical coherence tomography during ophthalmic surgery: the DISCOVER Study RESCAN Results. *JAMA Ophthalmol*. 2015;133(10):1124-1132.

Fujimoto H, Maeda N, Shintani A, et al. Quantitative evaluation of the natural progression of keratoconus using three-dimensional optical coherence tomography. *Invest Ophthalmol Vis Sci*. 2016;57(9):169-175.

Garg A, De Rojas J, Mathews P, et al. Using anterior segment optical coherence tomography to monitor disease progression in peripheral ulcerative keratitis. *Case Rep Ophthalmol Med*. 2018;2018:3705753.

Grewal DS, Schultz T, Basti S, Dick HB. Femtosecond laser-assisted cataract surgery: current status and future directions. *Surv Ophthalmol*. 2016;61(2):103-131.

Izatt JA, Hee MR, Swanson EA, et al. Micrometer-scale resolution imaging of the anterior eye in vivo with optical coherence tomography. *Arch Ophthalmol*. 1994;112(12):1584-1589.

Konstantopoulos A, Kuo J, Anderson D, Hossain P. Assessment of the use of anterior segment optical coherence tomography in microbial keratitis. *Am J Ophthalmol*. 2008;146(4):534-542.

Li Y, Netto MV, Shekhar R, Krueger RR, Huang D. A longitudinal study of LASIK flap and stromal thickness with high-speed optical coherence tomography. *Ophthalmology*. 2007;114(6):1124-1132.

Nanji AA, Sayyad FE, Galor A, Dubovy S, Karp CL. High-resolution optical coherence tomography as an adjunctive tool in the diagnosis of corneal and conjunctival pathology. *Ocul Surf*. 2015;13(3):226-235.

Rocha KM, Perez-Straziota CE, Stulting RD, Randleman JB. Epithelial and stromal remodeling after corneal collagen cross-linking evaluated by spectral-domain OCT. *J Refract Surg*. 2014;30(2):122-127.

Rosas Salaroli CH, Li Y, Huang D. High-resolution optical coherence tomography visualization of LASIK flap displacement. *J Cataract Refract Surg*. 2009;35(9):1640-1642.

Saad A, Sabatier P, Gatinel D. Graft orientation, optical coherence tomography, and endothelial keratoplasty. *Ophthalmology*. 2013;120(4):871-871.e3.

Shousha MA, Karp CL, Canto AP, et al. Diagnosis of ocular surface lesions using ultra-high-resolution optical coherence tomography. *Ophthalmology*. 2013;120(5):883-891.

Tang M, Wang L, Koch DD, Li Y, Huang D. Intraocular lens power calculation after previous myopic laser vision correction based on corneal power measured by Fourier-domain optical coherence tomography. *J Cataract Refract Surg*. 2012;38(4):589-594.

Yadav R, Lee KS, Rolland JP, Zavislan JM, Aquavella JV, Yoon G. Micrometer axial resolution OCT for corneal imaging. *Biomed Opt Express*. 2011;2(11):3037-3046.

Yeh RY, Quilendrino R, Musa FU, Liarakos VS, Dapena I, Melles GR. Predictive value of optical coherence tomography in graft attachment after Descemet's membrane endothelial keratoplasty. *Ophthalmology*. 2013;120(2):240-245.

Yoo YS, Whang WJ, Kim HS, Joo CK, Yoon G. Preoperative biometric measurements with anterior segment optical coherence tomography and prediction of postoperative intraocular lens position. *Medicine (Baltimore)*. 2019;98(50):e18026.

3 Quantitative Analysis of the Anterior Segment

Nakul Shekhawat | Kraig S. Bower

I. INTRODUCTION

Anterior segment optical coherence tomography (AS-OCT) is increasingly used for quantitative evaluation of anterior segment pathologic conditions for clinical care and research. AS-OCT offers the possibility of enabling more objective, precise, reproducible, and clinically relevant measurements of anterior segment anatomic and pathologic conditions. For fields such as cataract, cornea, external disease, and glaucoma that have historically relied on subjective grading of examination findings such as lesion size or angle width, this transition to more objective assessment represents an opportunity to produce a more rigorous evidence base guiding clinical and surgical decision-making. This chapter will provide a brief overview of several key measurements of different aspects of anterior segment anatomy. Details about each topic are provided in subsequent chapters.

II. CORNEA

Fig. 3.1 shows normal corneal anatomy on high-resolution AS-OCT. The tear film is a thin, bright hyperreflective line overlying the cornea and ocular surface. Where the corneal tear film comes into contact with the inferior eyelid margin, the tear meniscus also can be visualized. The epithelium typically measures 50 microns and appears darker than the overlying tear film or underlying collagen tissues such as the Bowman layer. Compared with the stroma, normal epithelium also tends to have more reflective homogeneity throughout. The Bowman layer appears as twin lines beneath the epithelium and measures 15 to 20 microns in thickness. The stroma is the thickest part of the cornea and has a regularly arranged pattern of hyperreflectivity and hyporeflectivity because of its arrangement of collagen fibers. In normal corneas, the Descemet membrane (DM) and endothelium often can be difficult to distinguish from one another on AS-OCT but appear as a slightly hyperreflective line posterior to the stroma.

A. Epithelium and Bowman Layer

Corneal epithelial thickness mapping by AS-OCT can provide novel insights into ocular surface diseases, such as dry eye and anterior basement membrane dystrophy, and improve detection of keratectasia development and progression. For example, in keratoconus, epithelial thickness mapping demonstrates a nonuniform pattern with a thinner epithelial layer at the apex and an annulus of thicker surrounding epithelium (Please see Chapter 5, Figures 5.1 and 5.2). These findings mirror observations made in earlier histopathologic studies of keratoconus, which showed that subclinical changes in the epithelium and Bowman layer are seen at a much earlier stage of disease than the classic signs noted on slit-lamp examination such as Fleischer iron ring, corneal curvature bowing, Munson sign, Vogt striae, Descemet tear, and hydrops. Epithelial thickness mapping is already available as a function in multiple commercially available AS-OCT platforms and is likely to become more widely available for clinical use over time.

B. Stroma

Fig. 3.2 shows an image obtained using the Cirrus machine with precise thickness measurements of the corneal epithelium, the LASIK flap, and the residual stromal bed. One of the most immediately useful functions of AS-OCT is precise measurement of corneal layer or lesion thickness, dimensions, and/or depth for clinical monitoring and procedural planning. Several machines, including the Cirrus, Visante, OptoVue, and Heidelberg Anterion, are equipped with caliper functions that allow precise measurement. The Heidelberg Spectralis anterior segment module can also perform manual measurements, although this feature is not cleared by the US Food and Drug Administration at the time of this writing. The Heidelberg Anterion's metrics application, available in Europe but not yet approved for clinical use in the United States, enables precise caliper measurements of stromal lesions and volumetric scans of different corneal layers such as the epithelium.

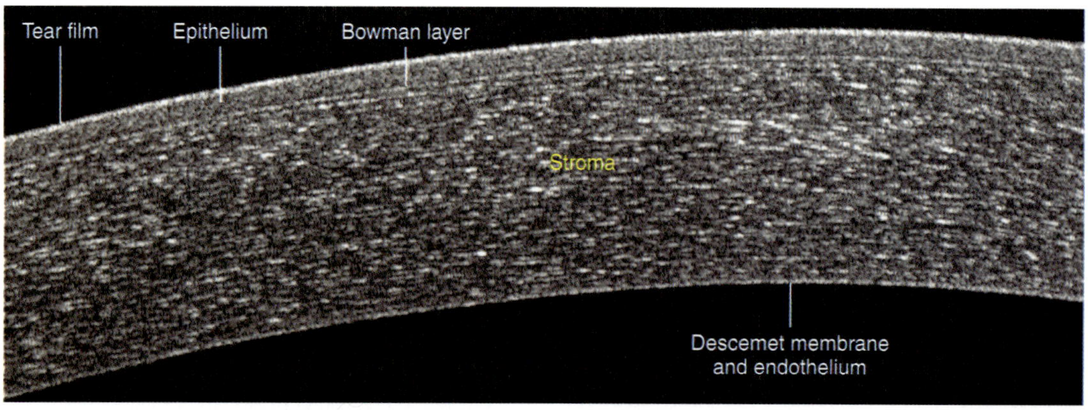

Fig. 3.1 Normal anatomy of the cornea. (Image courtesy Nikhil Gokhale.)

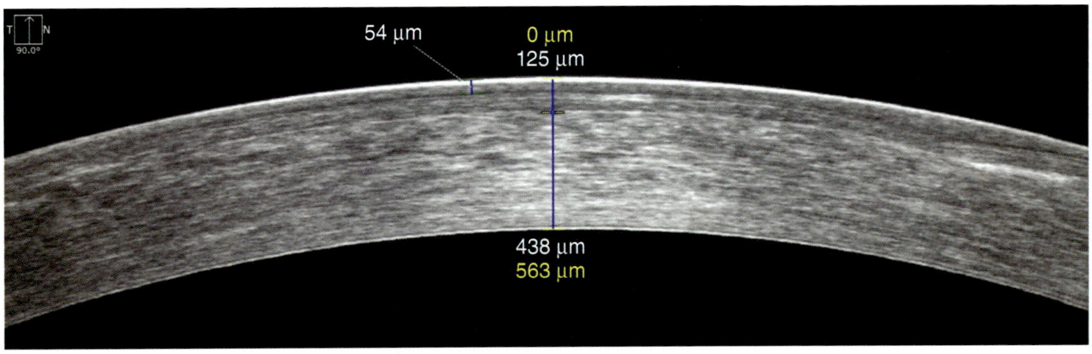

Fig. 3.2 Measurement of epithelium and LASIK flap thickness.

CLINICAL PEARL

When measuring the corneal thickness or lesion depth, caliper lines should be oriented perpendicular to the corneal surface to improve consistency and reproducibility of measurements. Similarly, when measuring corneal lesion width or length, we recommend orienting caliper lines parallel to the plane of stromal fibers or tangential to the normal corneal surface to improve measurement consistency. Other features that should be standardized to improve measurement reproducibility and comparability include image centration, eye fixation, and orientation of image cuts (radial vs. parallel raster images), and distance between image cuts.

AS-OCT can be immensely useful for preoperative surgical planning, intraoperative decision-making, and postoperative follow-up for surface ablation, lamellar keratectomy, and lamellar keratoplasty procedures that seek to treat stromal pathologic conditions. For subepithelial and anterior stromal lesions, phototherapeutic keratectomy (PTK) can be an excellent treatment option that obviates the need for keratoplasty. Preoperative AS-OCT can verify depth of stromal lesions and determine whether patients are good candidates for PTK or need more invasive procedures. Fig. 3.3 shows an AS-OCT image of corneal scarring after a partial-thickness traumatic laceration. In this patient, stromal scar depth was measured as part of the evaluation for PTK. Deep anterior lamellar keratoplasty (DALK) seeks to remove nearly all host stroma while sparing host DM. Preoperative AS-OCT can be used to measure the distance from the corneal surface to the DM, which can help plan intraoperative maneuvers such as lamellar dissection or big bubble formation. Intraoperative AS-OCT can provide live feedback during surgical dissection (Chapter 13). Postoperatively, AS-OCT imaging can quantify the depth of host stroma remaining after DALK (Chapter 14).

C. Descemet Membrane and Endothelium

Although measurement of DM thickness is not widely used in clinical practice at the time of this writing, promising developments in this regard may improve our understanding of endothelial disease and enable earlier detection of diseases such as Fuchs dystrophy and corneal graft rejection. For example, Abou Shousha and colleagues

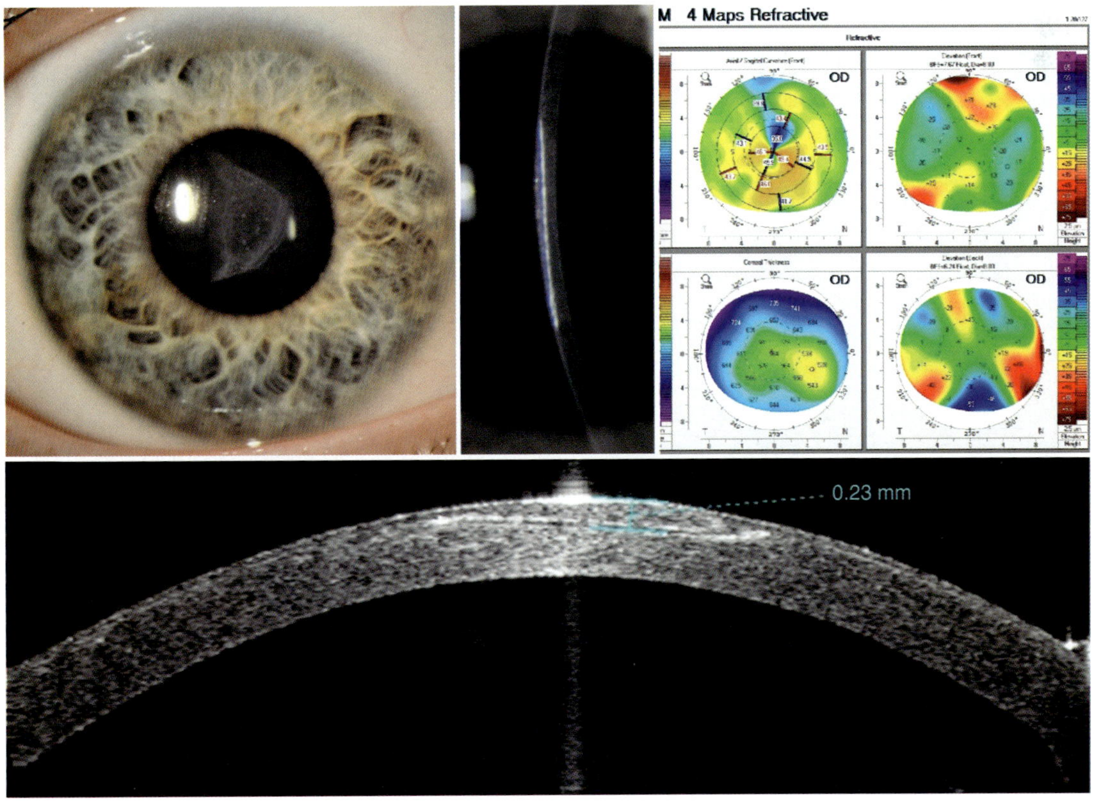

Fig. 3.3 Corneal scar depth measurement for PTK evaluation.

demonstrated that ultra-high-resolution AS-OCT can detect subclinical edema of endothelium/DM complex and that such changes may be a sensitive biomarker for early-stage graft rejection. AS-OCT also can be used to measure Descemet stripping endothelial keratoplasty lenticule thickness, both during graft preparation at the eye bank and after insertion of the graft. Increased stromal thickness within the lenticule as measured by AS-OCT can raise concern for graft rejection.

D. Corneal Curvature

AS-OCT can provide precise measurements of anterior and posterior corneal curvature to improve understanding and monitoring of corneal disease. For post-LASIK patients undergoing cataract surgery, AS-OCT mapping of posterior corneal curvature may improve accuracy of intraocular lens (IOL) formula calculations with specific formulas. For keratectasia screening, combining information from anterior curvature, posterior curvature, epithelial thickness mapping, and pachymetry mapping can improve detection of forme fruste keratoconus and improve risk prediction for development of post-refractive surgery ectasia.

III. CONJUNCTIVA

Fig. 3.4 shows the normal anatomy of the corneoscleral limbus and overlying conjunctiva. Compared with the homogeneous hyporeflective corneal epithelium, the limbal and conjunctival epithelium are slightly more hyperreflective. The underlying stroma has less regular reflectivity and is more hyperreflective than the conjunctiva.

As with corneal lesions, AS-OCT can be used to perform precise measurements of conjunctival lesion depth and dimensions. These can be used to differentiate lesions and monitor for changes over time, adding an objective and precise metric to what can otherwise be a subjective clinical evaluation. In some cases, AS-OCT can serve as a noninvasive means of measuring features that previously could be observed only on histopathologic specimens. For example, differences in ocular surface epithelial thickness can serve as a sensitive and specific biomarker differentiating pterygium from ocular surface squamous neoplasia. These differences are discussed in detail in Chapter 4.

IV. ANTERIOR CHAMBER, IRIS, AND IRIDOCORNEAL ANGLE

Fig. 3.5 shows an image of a phakic anterior chamber with normal iridocorneal angles. Several features of a good AS-OCT image are highlighted: a centered and well-aligned image, good corneal reflectance, good visualization of the transition zone between cornea and limbus, and a well-defined scleral spur.

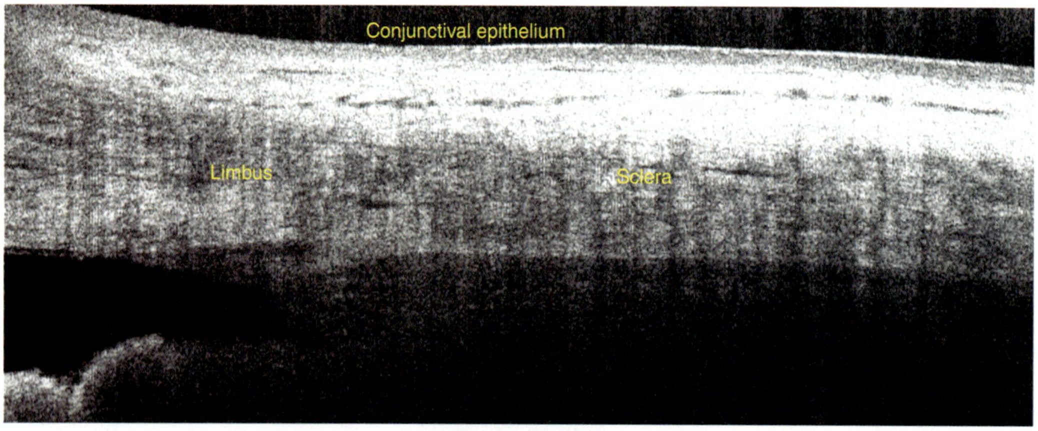

Fig. 3.4 Normal anatomy of the conjunctiva and sclera. (Image courtesy Nikhil Gokhale.)

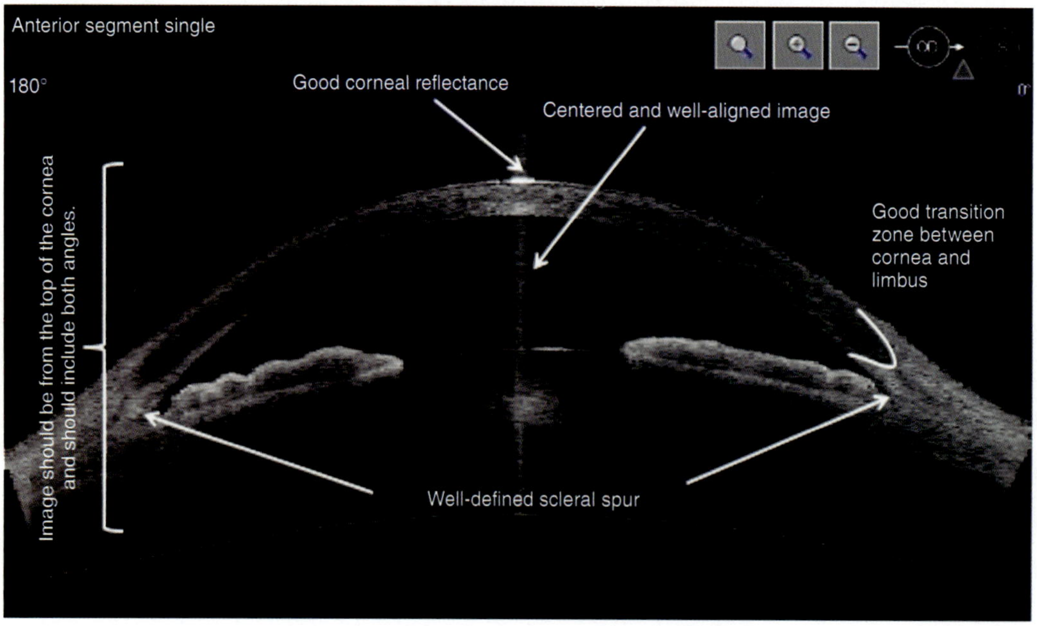

Fig. 3.5 Normal anatomy of the anterior chamber.

Fig. 3.6 shows examples of good versus poor visualization of the scleral spur on AS-OCT. When grading the angle and lens anatomy, ideally the image should include the corneal apex and both sides of the iridocorneal angle. With such images, it is possible to characterize iridolenticular touch, differences in iris contour under various light settings (Fig. 3.7), and changes in angle width and iris anatomy after laser peripheral iridotomy or cataract extraction (Fig. 3.8).

AS-OCT can provide precise measurement of anterior chamber depth, both via manual measurement tools and automated programs included in some commercially available platforms (Fig. 3.9). Commonly used biometric parameters of the anterior chamber include anterior chamber area, anterior chamber volume, and anterior chamber width. Anterior chamber depth measurements, when combined with measurements of keratometry and axial length, can then be used for phakic and pseudophakic IOL power selection formulas in a manner similar to those for optical biometry or ultrasonography. AS-OCT also can be used for objective measurement and grading of anterior chamber cell and flare in cases of intraocular inflammation.

AS-OCT can provide objective, precise, and reproducible measurements of the iris, iridocorneal angle, ciliary body, and associated anatomy (Chapter 10). Fig. 3.10 depicts measurement of anterior chamber depth, the iridocorneal angle, and phakic IOL vault after implantable collamer lens insertion. Commonly used biometric parameters of the iridocorneal angle and associated structures include the angle opening distance, angle recess area, trabecular-iris space area, iris thickness, iris curvature, iris area, and lens vault. These measurements can be used to screen for angle-closure glaucoma risk, evaluate for changes after laser peripheral iridotomy, and determine eligibility for glaucoma surgeries involving the angle. AS-OCT measurements of angle anatomy show great promise in surpassing measurements obtained by other modalities such as ultrasound biomicroscopy (UBM). For example, UBM depends on user expertise, requires direct contact with the eye, and can have suboptimal reproducibility of images across multiple sessions. Newer AS-OCT systems can bypass many of these limitations with noncontact imaging, greater ease of use, and increasingly reproducible images.

V. LENS

As with iridocorneal anatomy, newer AS-OCT systems, especially when used with special lens (Chapter 11), can image deeper aspects of lens anatomy in a manner that complements or may eventually obviate the need for UBM. Objective measurements of crystalline lens thickness, curvature, and tilt obtained by AS-OCT can help predict refractive outcomes after cataract surgery. For example, swept-source AS-OCT imaging has been used to demonstrate that preoperative crystalline lens tilt is predictive of postoperative IOL tilt within the capsular bag after cataract surgery. AS-OCT also can provide objective measurement of postoperative IOL position, whether within the capsular bag after routine cataract surgery or in alternative locations such as for anterior chamber IOLs or scleral-fixated IOLs. Several studies have used AS-OCT to evaluate postoperative IOL tilt and decentration after secondary IOL implantation. AS-OCT also can be used to evaluate the vault of phakic IOLs (see Fig. 3.10).

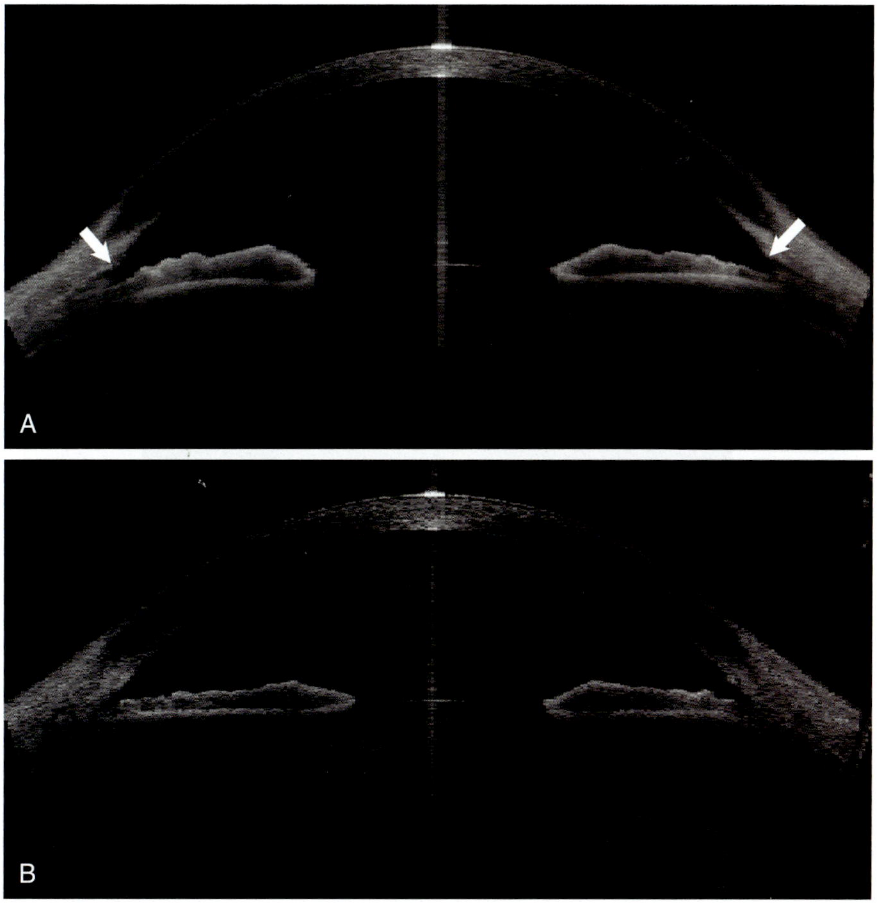

Fig. 3.6 Good versus poor visualization of scleral spur.

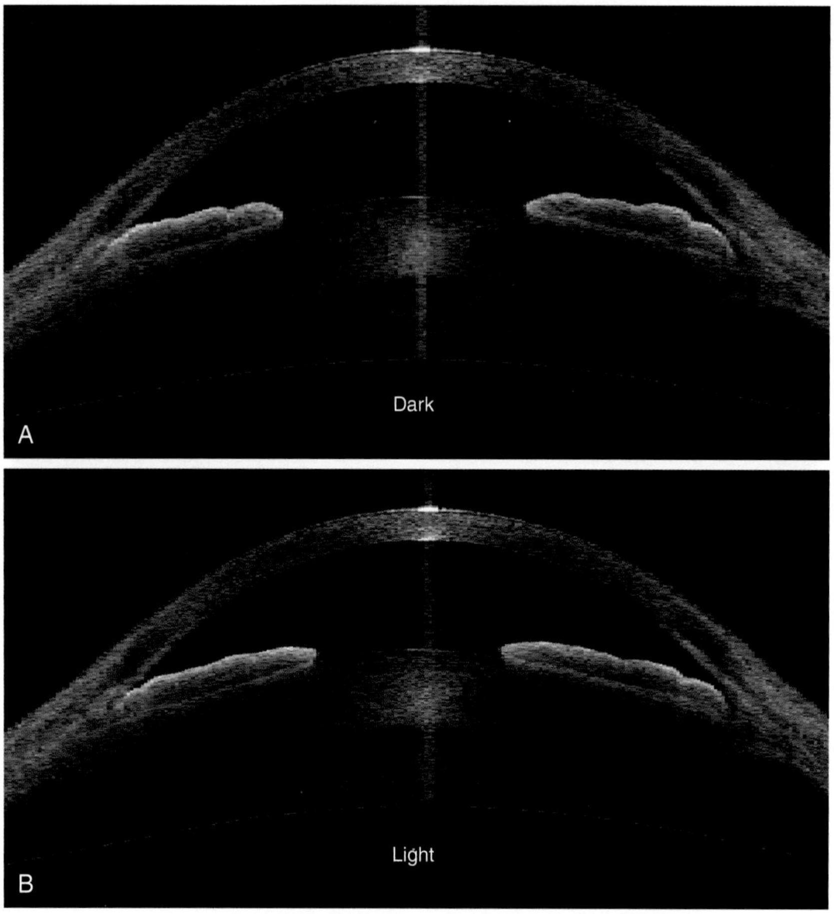

Fig. 3.7 Changes in iridolenticular touch in dark versus light settings.

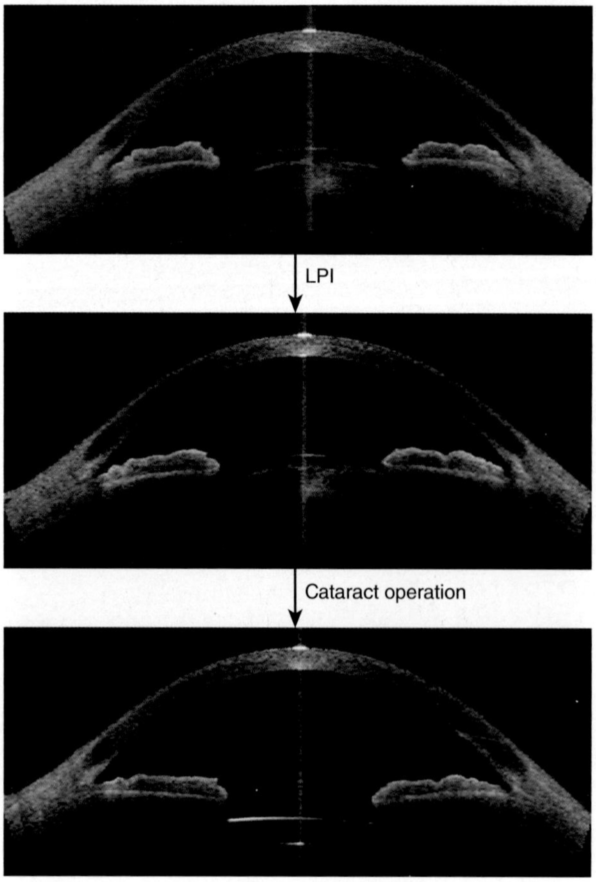

Fig. 3.8 Assessment of anterior chamber and angle anatomy by Visante and Casia machines. *LPI,* laser peripheral iridotomy.

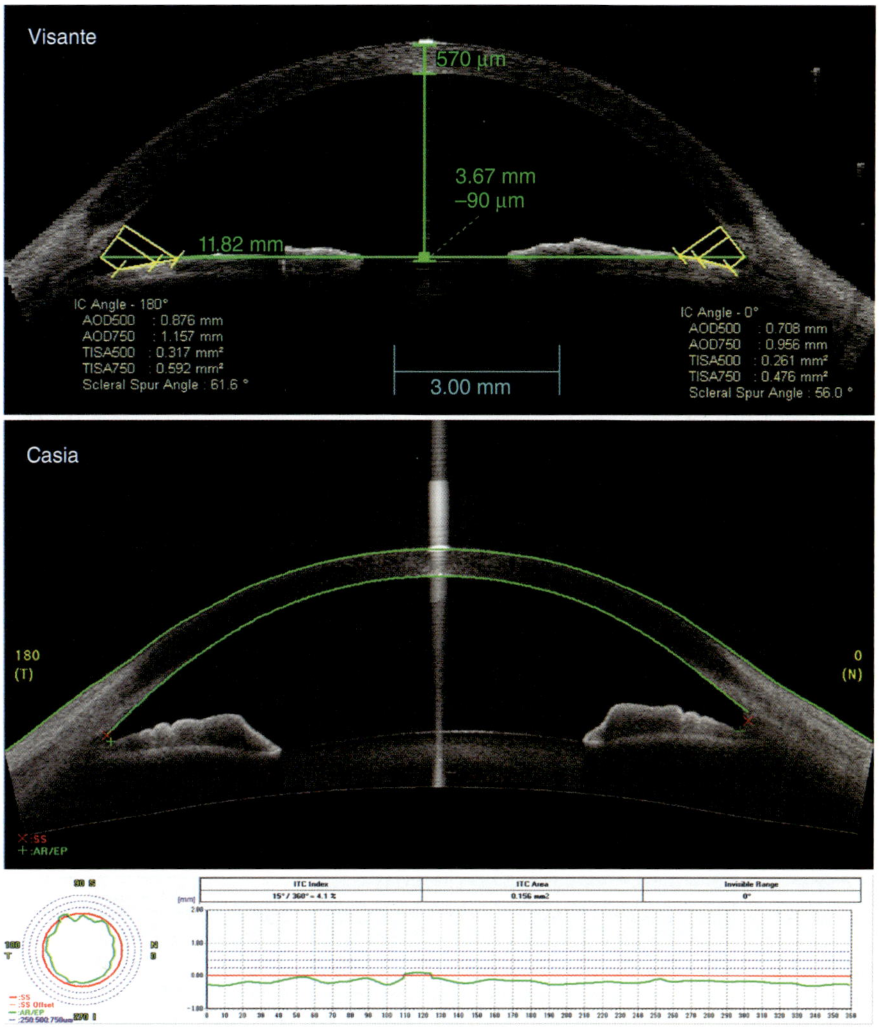

Fig. 3.9 Assessment of anterior chamber and angle anatomy by Visante and Casia machines.

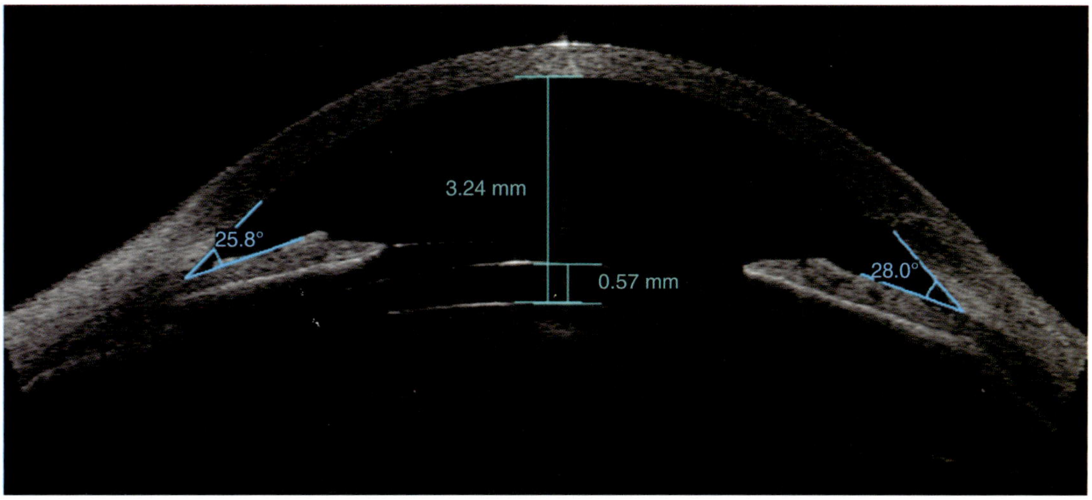

Fig. 3.10 Measurement of anterior chamber depth, iridocorneal angle, and IOL vault after implantable collamer lens insertion.

VI. TECHNIQUES

AS-OCT and the expanding options for scanning the anterior segment and analysis of the raw images allow for multiple different ways to view the front of the eye. Fig. 3.11 shows how to use the "5-line raster" protocol to view the anatomic angle. Fig. 3.12 shows how to use the "HD angle" function, and Fig. 3.13 shows how to adjust the image of the angle and different options for image capture on the Zeiss Cirrus 5000. Fig. 3.14 shows how to use the 5-line raster function to image the corneal layers, and Fig. 3.15 shows how to use the same function to push deeper into the eye to view the iris and anterior lens capsule and anterior lens structures.

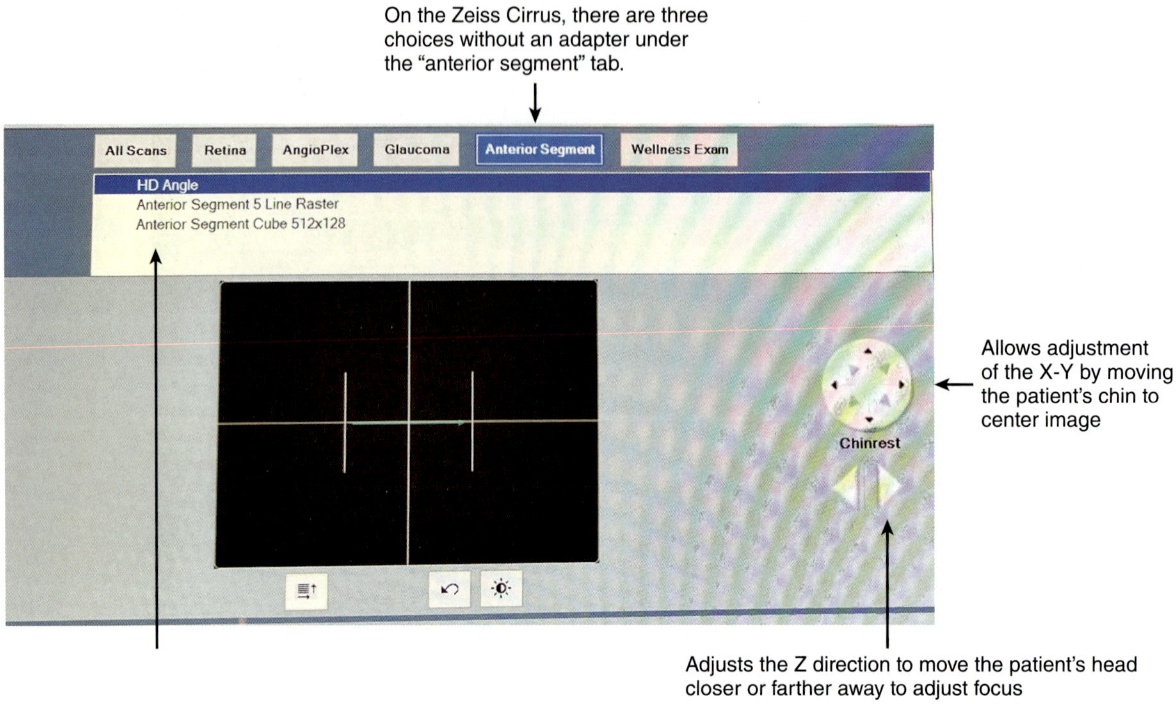

Fig. 3.11 Angle measurement.

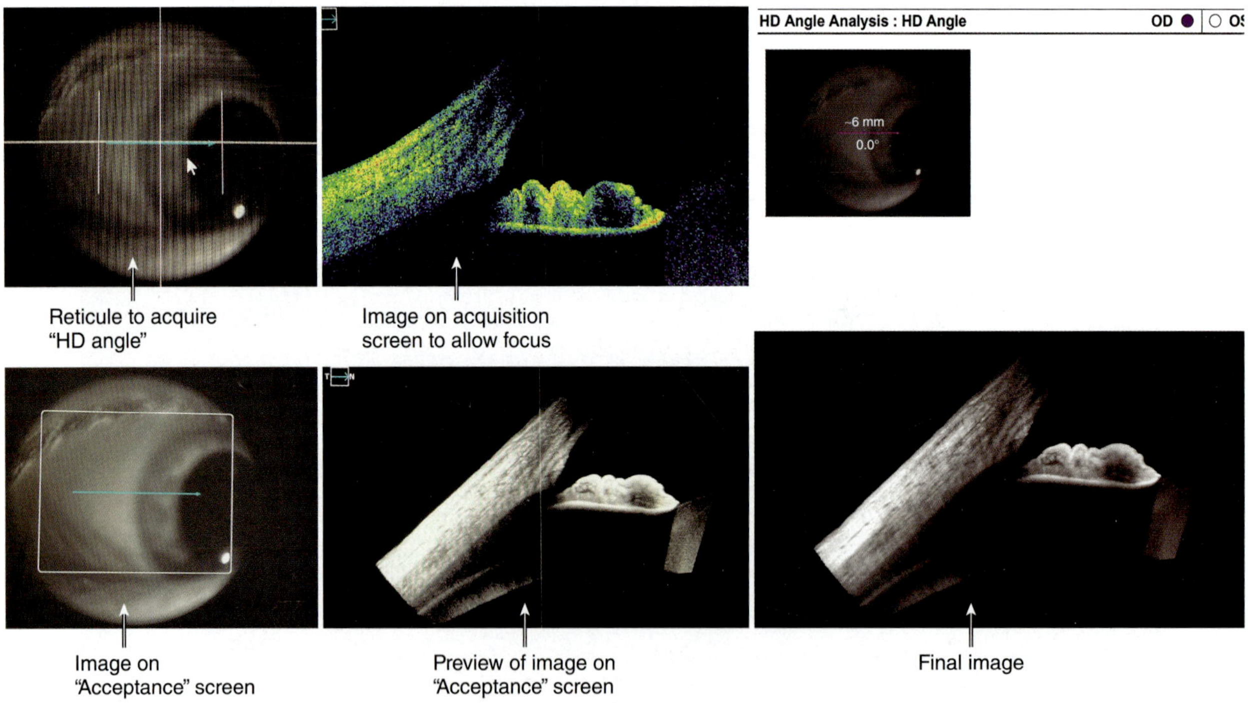

Fig. 3.12 Angle image capture.

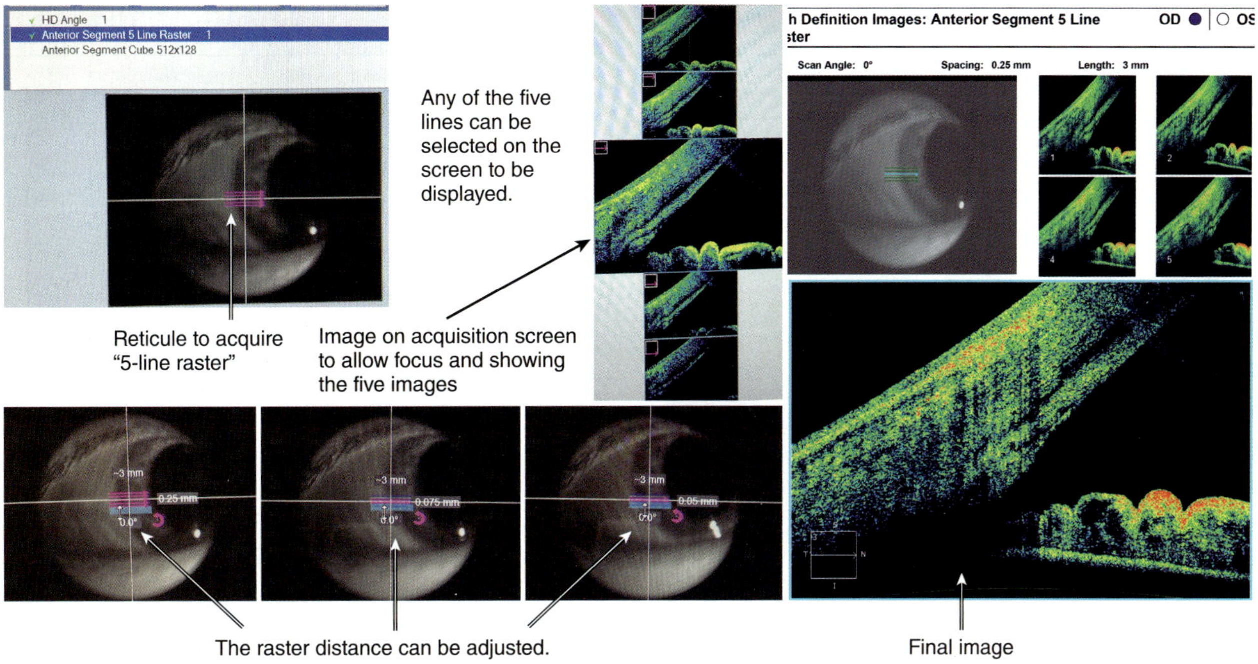

Fig. 3.13 Angle image adjustment.

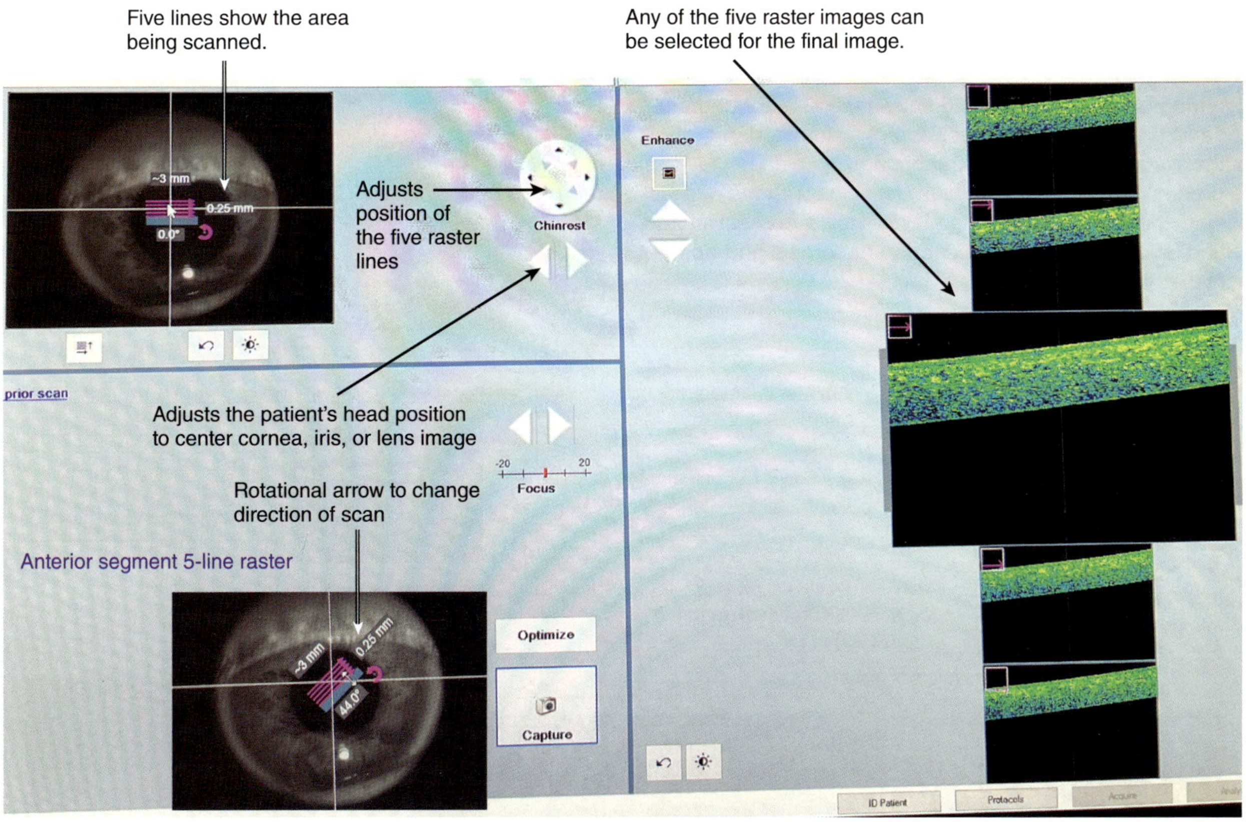

Fig. 3.14 5-Line raster image capture of cornea.

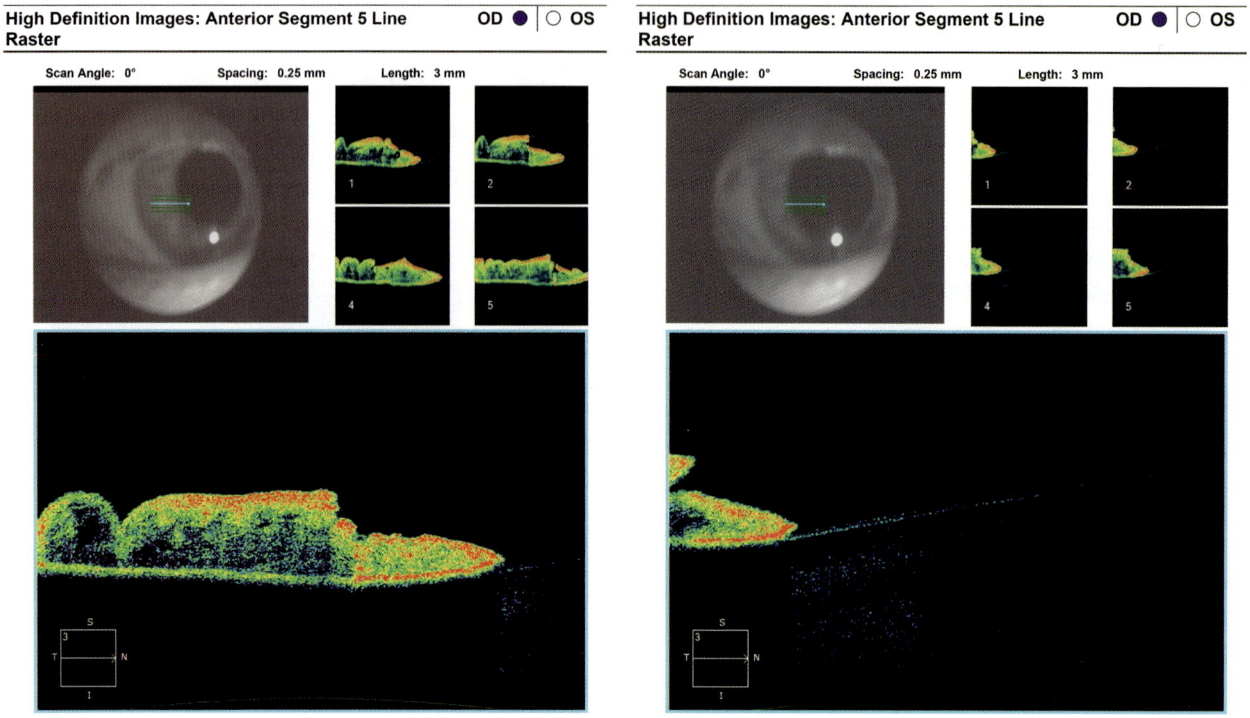

5-Line raster can be focused on the iris and anterior capsule/lens.

Fig. 3.15 5-Line raster image capture of iris and lens. 5-Line raster can be focused on the iris and anterior capsule/lens.

To adjust the focal distance of the OCT, which was originally designed to image the posterior segment, adapters are available. On the Zeiss Cirrus, Fig. 3.16 shows the anterior chamber adapter and the "anterior chamber analysis" function. Fig. 3.17 shows the "wide angle to angle" function.

The cornea can be imaged in high definition with the corneal adapter on the Zeiss Cirrus. Fig. 3.18 shows corneal image acquisition, and Fig. 3.19 shows capture of corneal and epithelial pachymetry.

CLINICAL PEARL

Each OCT device has different software and adapters, which are constantly being updated. Being familiar with the different scanning, analysis, and measurement options will make the use of the AS-OCT much more clinically valuable. Clinicians who have a firsthand knowledge of all of the options on their OCT device will allow for better training of staff members and better image quality and will greatly enhance the enjoyment and usefulness of this valuable tool. Taking images at different locations on the cornea of the same clinical entity or changing the image from color to black and white will enhance understanding. The more that one images with the AS-OCT, the more one will want to see.

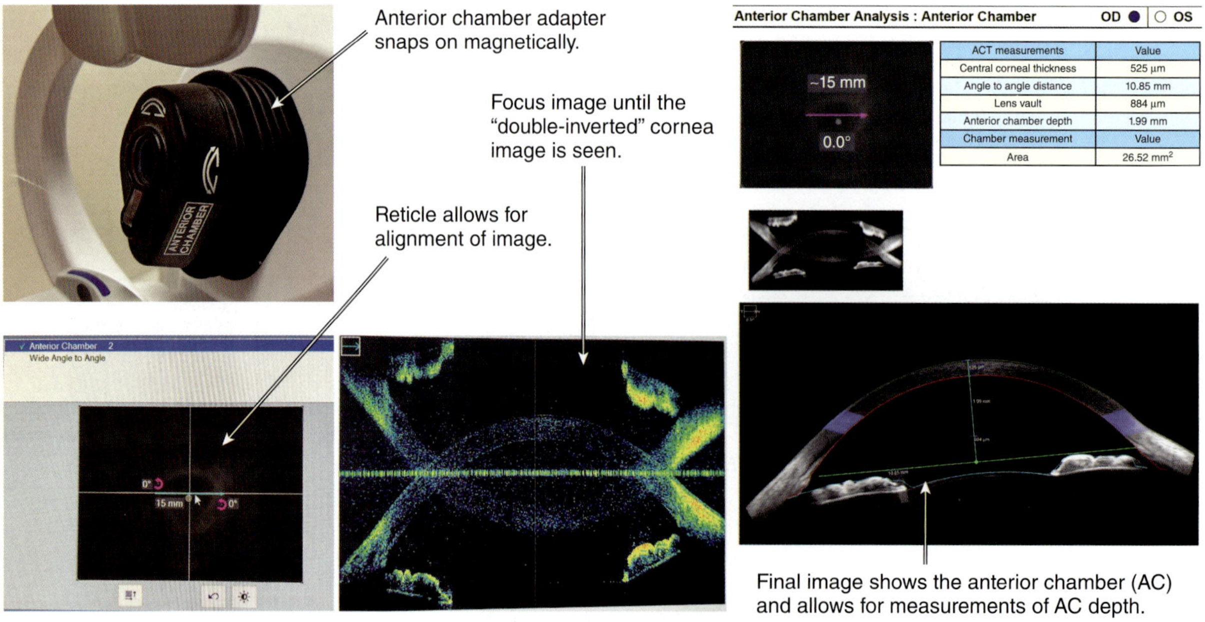

Fig. 3.16 Anterior chamber image capture.

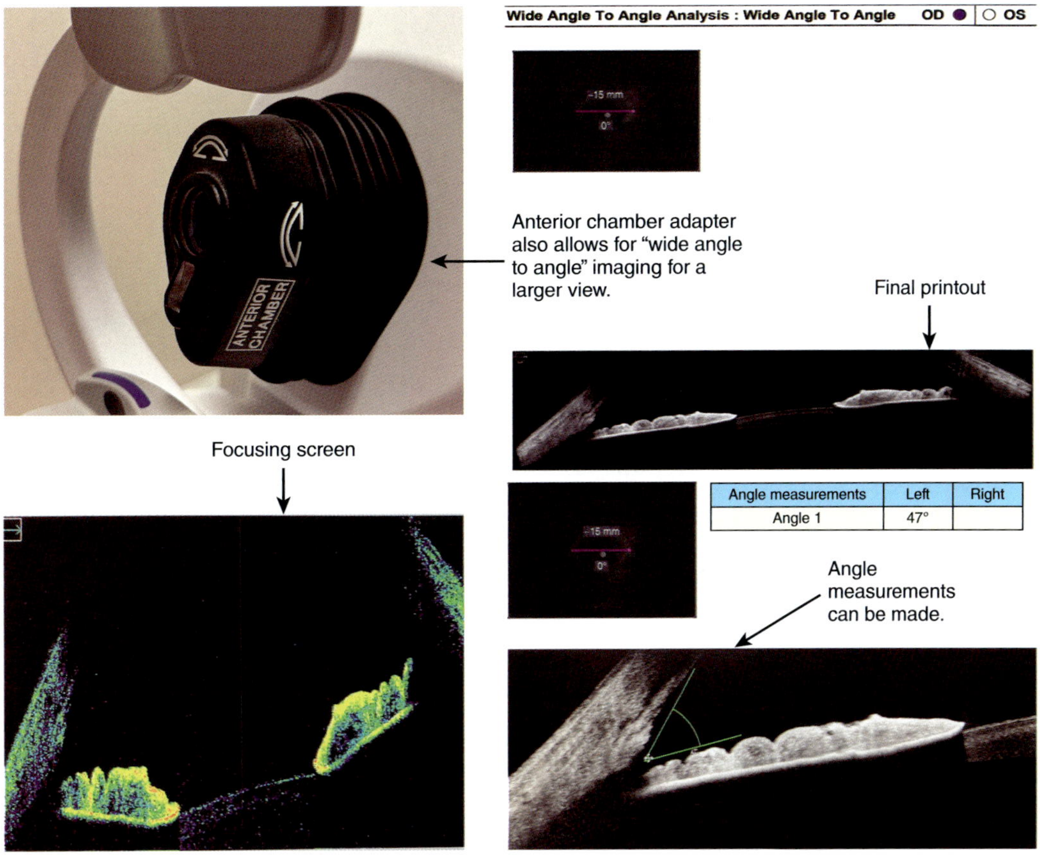

Fig. 3.17 **Anterior chamber image capture adjustment.**

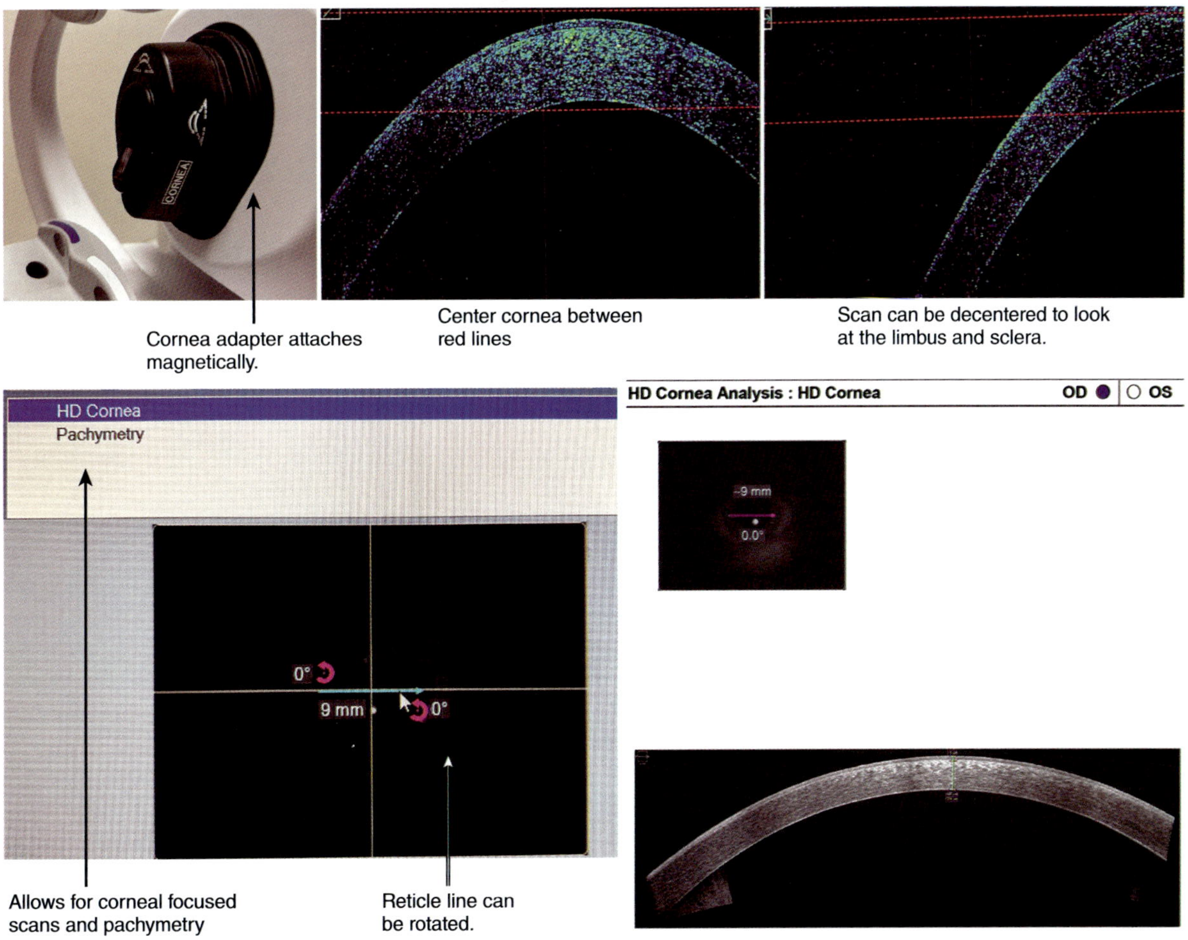

Fig. 3.18 **Cornea image capture.**

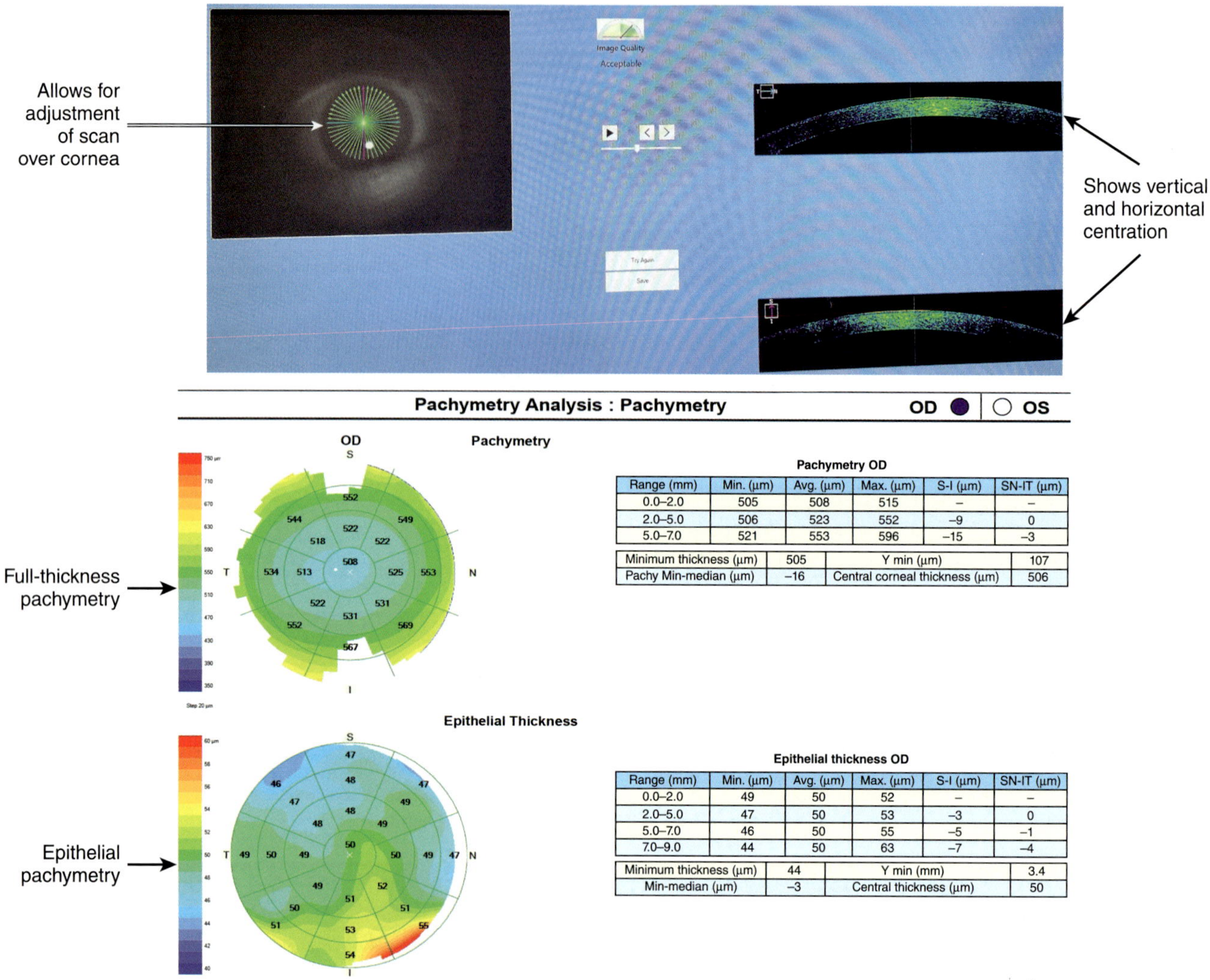

Fig. 3.19 Pachymetry image capture.

BIBLIOGRAPHY

Ang M, Baskaran M, Werkmeister RM, et al. Anterior segment optical coherence tomography. *Prog Retin Eye Res*. 2018;66:132-156.

Eleiwa TK, Cook JC, Elsawy AS, et al. Diagnostic performance of three-dimensional endothelium/descemet membrane complex thickness maps in active corneal graft rejection. *Am J Ophthalmol*. 2020;210:48-58.

Kanski J, Bowling B. *Cornea. Kanski's Clinical Ophthalmology: A Systematic Approach*. 8th ed. London, UK: Saunders Ltd; 2016:167-238.

Krachmer JH, Mannis MJ, Holland EJ. *Cornea: Fundamentals, Diagnosis and Management*. 3rd ed. Cincinnati, OH: Mosby Elsevier; 2011.

Venkateshwaran N, Galor A, Wang J, et al. Optical coherence tomography for ocular surface and corneal diseases: a review. *Eye Vis (Lond)*. 2018;5:13.

SECTION 2

Conjunctival Pathologic Conditions

4 Conjunctival Pathologic Conditions

Sarah L. Wall | Anat Galor | Carol L. Karp

I. BENIGN LESIONS

Common benign ocular surface lesions include pterygia and pinguecula from chronic sun exposure. A pinguecula will appear on anterior segment high-resolution optical coherence tomography (AS-OCT) as a subepithelial, well-demarcated, hyporeflective or hyperreflective mass that does not extend past the corneal limbus (Figs. 4.1 and 4.2).

> **CLINICAL PEARL**
>
> In evaluating an ocular surface lesion with HR-OCT, the first aim is to identify the normal hyporeflective epithelium. Next the lesion in question is identified. If the epithelium is abnormally thickened and hyperreflective, the differential diagnoses narrow to include ocular surface squamous neoplasia (OSSN), sebaceous cell carcinoma (SCC), papilloma, and granuloma. A lesion that is noted to be subepithelial entails a broader differential that can be narrowed by noting whether the lesion is hyporeflective or hyperreflective. A hyporeflective subepithelial mass is more likely to be a pinguecula or a lymphoma. A hyperreflective subepithelial mass is more likely to be a pterygium, nevus, amyloid, or melanoma. A pterygium has "stringy," fibrous-appearing hyperreflectivity; a nevus usually reveals cysts; amyloid shows hyperreflective "lines"; and melanoma demonstrates highly cellular hyperreflectivity. If there is no distinct lesion but linear hyperreflectivity of the basal epithelium is present, complexion-associated melanosis (CAM) or primary acquired melanosis (PAM) should be considered.

A pterygium will similarly appear on HR-OCT as a subepithelial mass but will be hyperreflective with fibrotic strands that often elevate the overlying epithelium. The epithelium overlying a pterygium is of normal thickness but may be variably hyperreflective because of actinic damage. Furthermore, pterygia typically extend past the corneal limbus and may involve the visual axis over time, in which case surgical excision may be considered with placement of an amniotic membrane or autologous conjunctival graft to minimize recurrence (Fig. 4.3).

Pterygia and OSSN share a common predisposing factor of ultraviolet light, and OSSN may be difficult to distinguish clinically from an underlying pterygium. In cases of an atypical lesion, HR-OCT can effectively rule out OSSN in the absence of a thickened and hyperreflective epithelium with an abrupt transition from normal to abnormal epithelium (for more information on OSSN see later discussion) (Fig. 4.4).

II. PIGMENTED LESIONS

Pigmented lesions entail a lengthy differential, ranging from benign cystic nevi to life-threatening melanomas. To further complicate the diagnosis, lesions that are classically pigmented may manifest as amelanotic disease. In such cases, HR-OCT can be used to look for benign features, such as cysts in a nevus, that may guide a more conservative approach, or to look for malignant features that would prompt a more aggressive treatment regimen.

Nevi may contain both epithelial and subepithelial components and often contain subepithelial cysts as an indicator of benign chronicity. It is not uncommon for a young child or adolescent to present with an amelanotic nevus with prominent feeder vessels that may concern the clinician for a potential malignancy. Visualization of cysts on HR-OCT can reassure the clinician that the lesion is a nevus and can be expected to darken and/or grow with hormonal changes of puberty or pregnancy (Figs. 4.5 to 4.7).

CAM is another commonly encountered benign ocular surface lesion, typically seen in patients with more darkly pigmented skin. CAM often manifests in both eyes asymmetrically, with multiple flat patches of pigment of a "cobble-stoned"

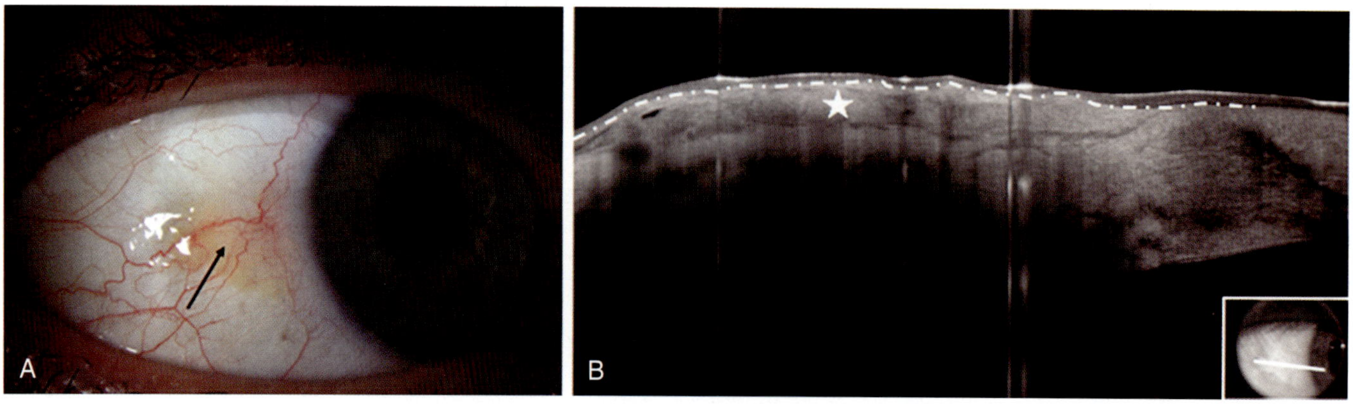

Fig. 4.1 Temporal pinguecula. (A) Slit-lamp photograph of the right eye in a 65-year-old White woman demonstrates an area of yellowing of the temporal conjunctiva *(arrow)*. (B) High-resolution optical coherence tomography (HR-OCT) reveals a subepithelial, hyperreflective, well-circumscribed mass *(star)* with overlying epithelium of normal thickness, characteristic of a pinguecula. The epithelial basement membrane is indicated with the *dotted line*. *Inset* shows scan location.

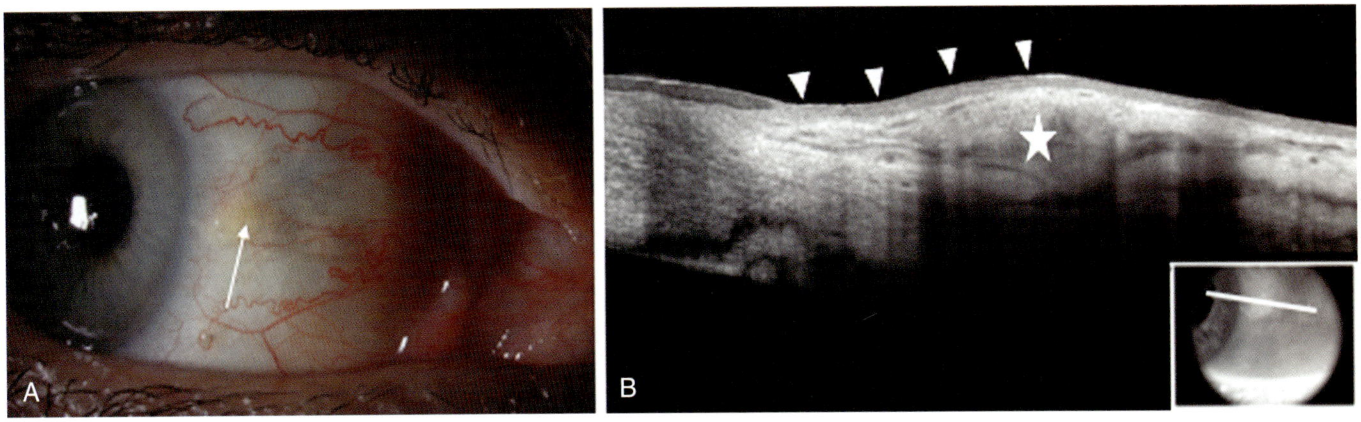

Fig. 4.2 Nasal pinguecula. (A) Slit-lamp photograph of the right eye in a 65-year-old White woman demonstrates an area of yellowing of the nasal conjunctiva *(arrow)*. (B) High-resolution optical coherence tomography (HR-OCT) reveals a subepithelial, hyperreflective, well-circumscribed mass *(star)* and normal-thickness overlying epithelium *(arrowheads)*, characteristic of a pinguecula. *Inset* shows scan location.

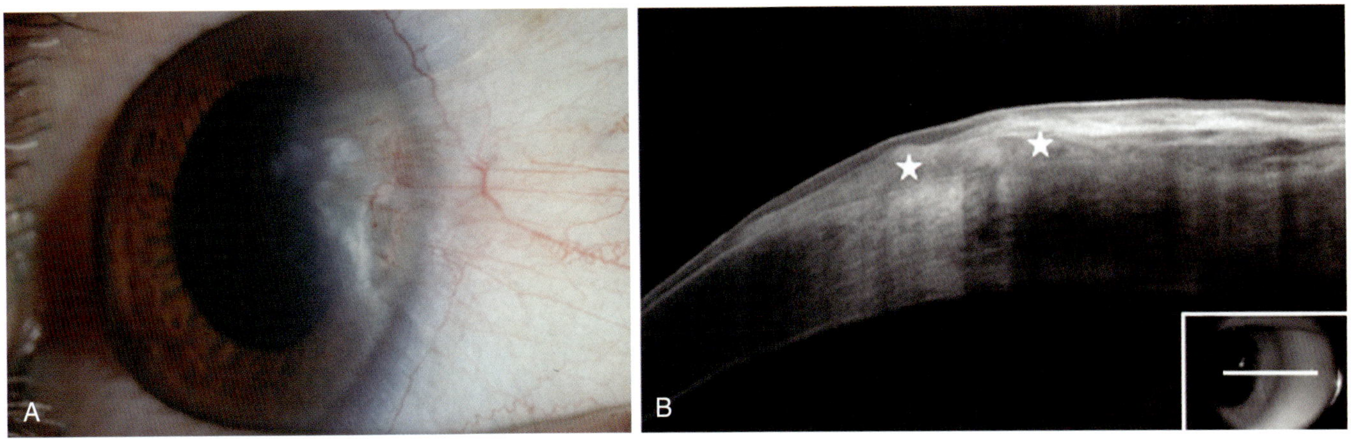

Fig. 4.3 Pterygium. (A) Slit-lamp photograph of the right eye in a 77-year-old Hispanic woman shows an elevated, gelatinous, "wing-shaped" growth extending from the nasal conjunctiva onto the cornea from two to four o'clock to involve the visual axis. The patient reported significant sun exposure. (B) High-resolution optical coherence tomography (HR-OCT) reveals a subepithelial, hyperreflective mass *(stars)* with overlying epithelium that is of normal thickness. The epithelium is hyporeflective in most areas but can be hyperreflective and nonthickened in areas to still be consistent with a pterygium. The lesion was surgically excised, and pathologic examination confirmed pterygium. *Inset* shows scan location.

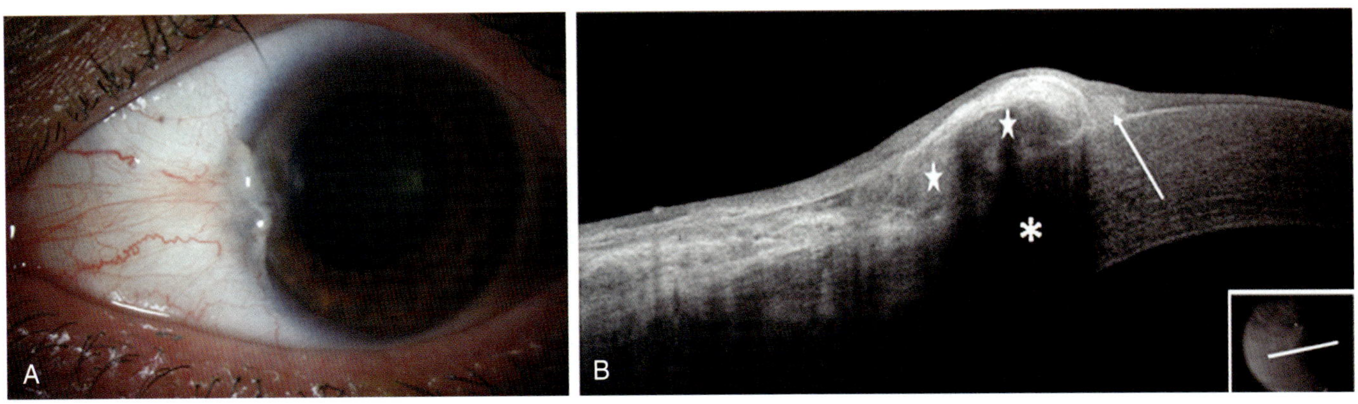

Fig. 4.4 Pterygium versus ocular surface squamous neoplasia (OSSN). (A) Slit-lamp photograph of the left eye in a 63-year-old Hispanic man shows an elevated gelatinous growth extending from the nasal conjunctiva onto the cornea from 8 to 10 o'clock. The patient reported significant sun exposure. Differential diagnoses included atypical pterygium versus OSSN. (B) High-resolution optical coherence tomography (HR-OCT) reveals a subepithelial, hyperreflective mass *(stars)* with posterior shadowing *(asterisk)* elevating the overlying normal-thickness epithelium, characteristic of a pterygium. Note the overlying epithelium is somewhat hyperreflective but otherwise thin and without an abrupt transition, effectively ruling out OSSN. *Arrow* indicates a hyperreflective, subepithelial corneal scar and should not be mistaken for an abrupt transition characteristic of OSSN because the overlying epithelium is normal. *Inset* shows scan location.

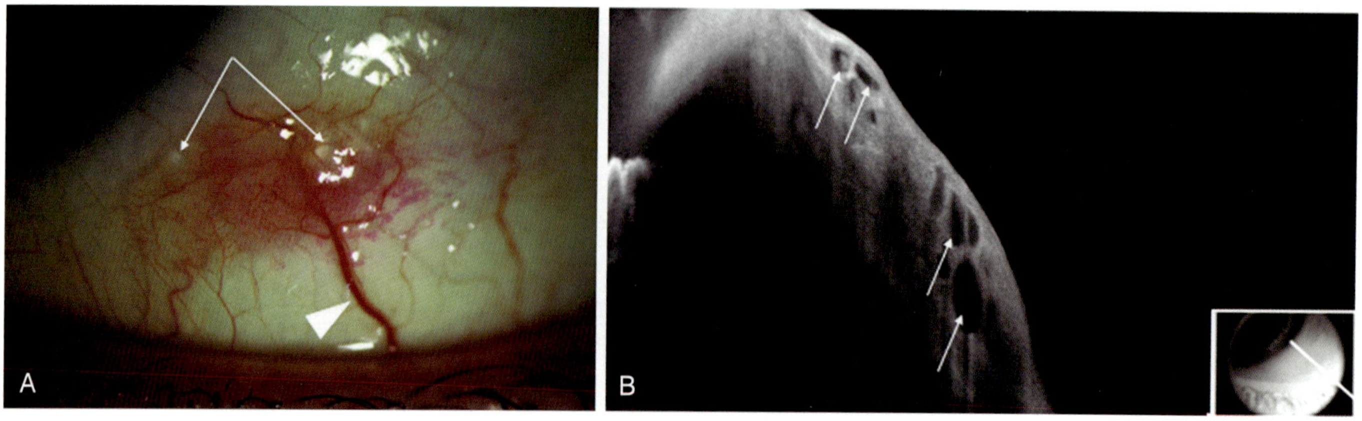

Fig. 4.5 Amelanotic cystic nevus. (A) Slit-lamp photograph of the left eye in a 20-year-old White man reveals a nonpigmented cystic *(arrows)* lesion located inferotemporally, with a prominent feeder blood vessel *(arrowhead)* and punctate staining with rose Bengal. (B) High-resolution optical coherence tomography (HR-OCT) reveals a subepithelial lesion with hyporeflective cystic spaces *(arrows)* and a normal overlying epithelium, characteristic of a cystic nevus. *Inset* shows scan location.

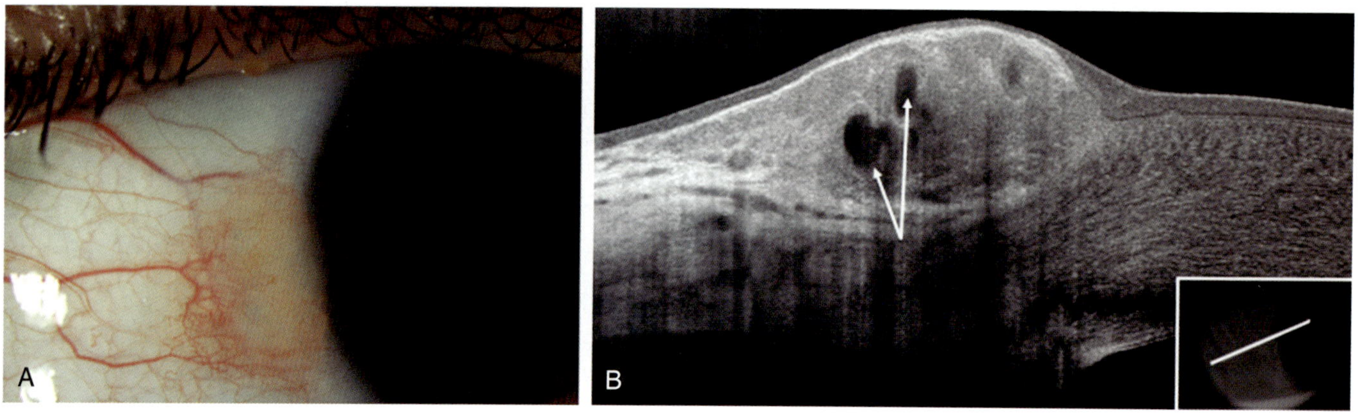

Fig. 4.6 Amelanotic cystic nevus. (A) Slit-lamp photograph of the right eye in a 10-year-old White girl shows a nonpigmented, elevated lesion of the temporal conjunctiva. Note blood vessels to the lesion. (B) High-resolution optical coherence tomography (HR-OCT) reveals a subepithelial mass containing hyporeflective cystic spaces *(arrows)* with no posterior shadowing and a normal overlying epithelium consistent with a cystic nevus. The HR-OCT was able to clearly display the clinically subtle cysts. *Inset* shows scan location.

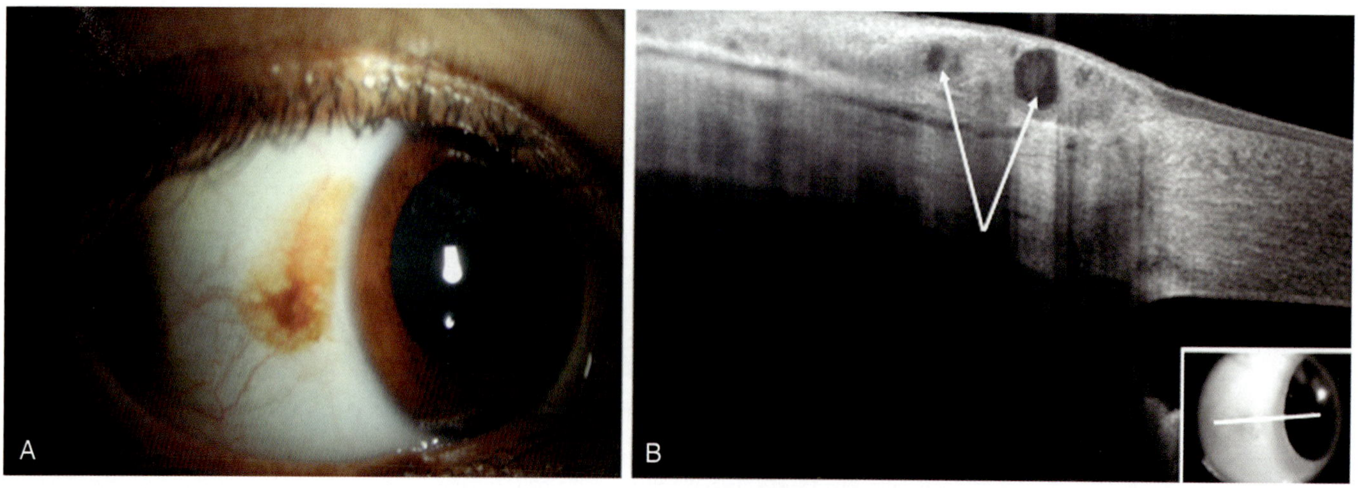

Fig. 4.7 Melanocytic nevus. (A) Slit-lamp photograph of the right eye of an 18-year-old White woman demonstrates a well-delineated patch of pigment on the temporal conjunctiva. The patient reported darkening of the lesion with puberty. (B) High-resolution optical coherence tomography (HR-OCT) reveals a subepithelial mass with hyporeflective cystic spaces *(arrows)* consistent with a nevus. *Inset* shows scan location.

or "microfold" appearance. HR-OCT typically reveals hyperreflectivity in the basal epithelium. CAM can be routinely followed because it has no known chance of malignant transformation (Figs. 4.8 and 4.9).

PAM differs from CAM in that PAM typically presents unilaterally in patients of lighter complexion as an isolated or diffuse patch of pigment. The lesion can be described as "peppery" and appears similar to CAM on HR-OCT with the visualization of hyperreflectivity of the basal epithelium. Because of limited cellular detail with the current resolution, HR-OCT is presently unable to identify the presence of atypia. Histopathologic analysis is currently required to determine the presence of atypia in PAM, which is the leading risk factor for conjunctival malignant melanoma (CMM) (Figs. 4.10 and 4.11).

CMM can often be suspected clinically in cases of melanocytic masses with abrupt onset and growth. However, in cases of atypical melanoma that lack pigmentation, the HR-OCT can be an instrumental diagnostic aid. Melanomas are classically visualized on HR-OCT as subepithelial, hyperreflective masses with significant posterior shadowing. Because melanoma can arise from PAM, nevi, or de novo, features of underlying PAM or nevi may be seen on HR-OCT (Figs. 4.12 to 4.14).

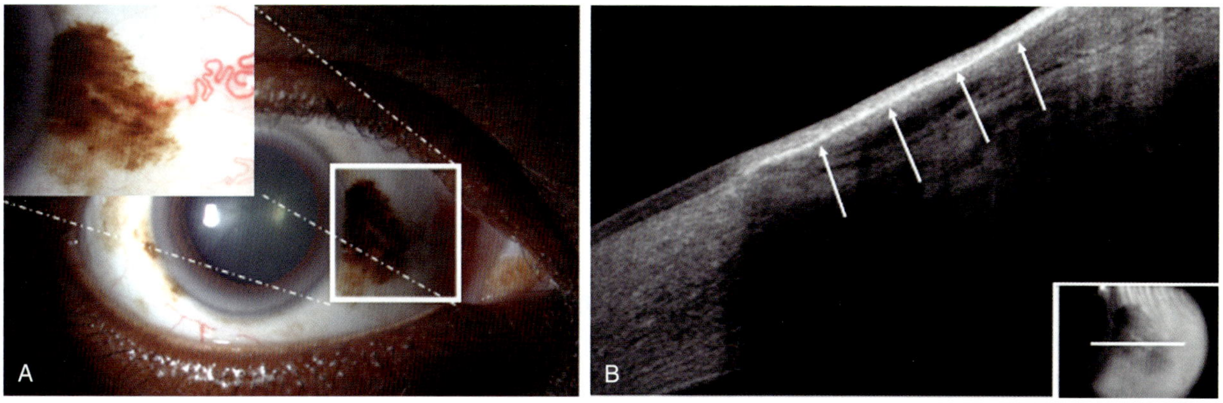

Fig. 4.8 Complexion-associated melanosis. (A) Slit-lamp photograph of the right eye in a 57-year-old Black woman demonstrates multiple perilimbal flat patches of pigmentation. *Inset* shows magnification of the largest patch of pigmentation. The patient had similar patches of pigment in the left eye and perilimbal in both eyes. The patient confirmed the long duration of the lesion. Note the darker complexion of the patient. (B) High-resolution optical coherence tomography (HR-OCT) reveals intraepithelial linear hyperreflectivity at the basal epithelium *(arrows),* with normal-thickness and somewhat hyperreflective epithelium. *Inset* shows location of scan.

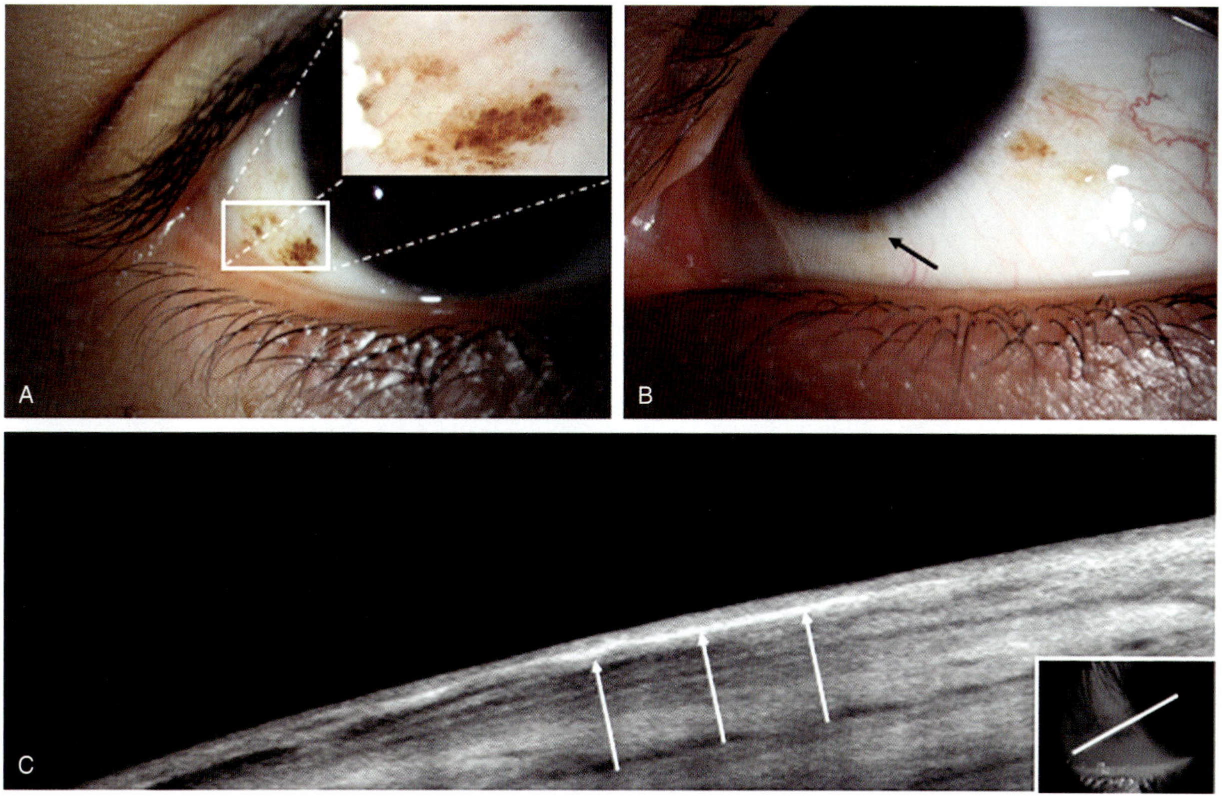

Fig. 4.9 Complexion-associated melanosis. (A) Slit-lamp photograph of the right eye in a 40-year-old Hispanic woman demonstrates flat, freely mobile melanosis of the conjunctiva. *Inset* shows magnification of the melanosis. (B) Slit-lamp photograph of the left eye of the same patient shows similar perilimbal patches of pigmentation with a microfold appearance *(black arrow).* (C) High-resolution optical coherence tomography (HR-OCT) reveals linear hyperreflectivity of the basal, normal-thickness epithelium, consistent with melanosis. *Inset* shows scan location.

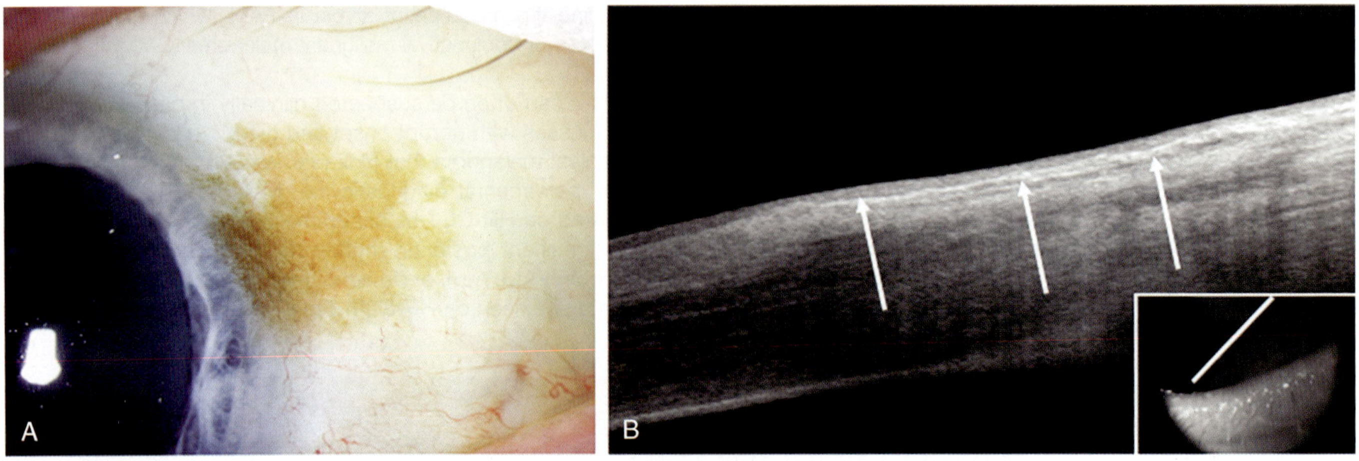

Fig. 4.10 Primary acquired melanosis. (A) Slit-lamp photograph of the left eye in a 77-year-old White man shows an isolated, flat patch of variable pigmentation adjacent to the corneal limbus from one to two o'clock. The patient reported significant sun exposure. Note the light complexion of the patient. (B) High-resolution optical coherence tomography (HR-OCT) demonstrates linear hyperreflectivity of the epithelial basement membrane *(arrows).* Note that primary acquired melanosis and complexion-associated melanosis appear similar on HR-OCT.

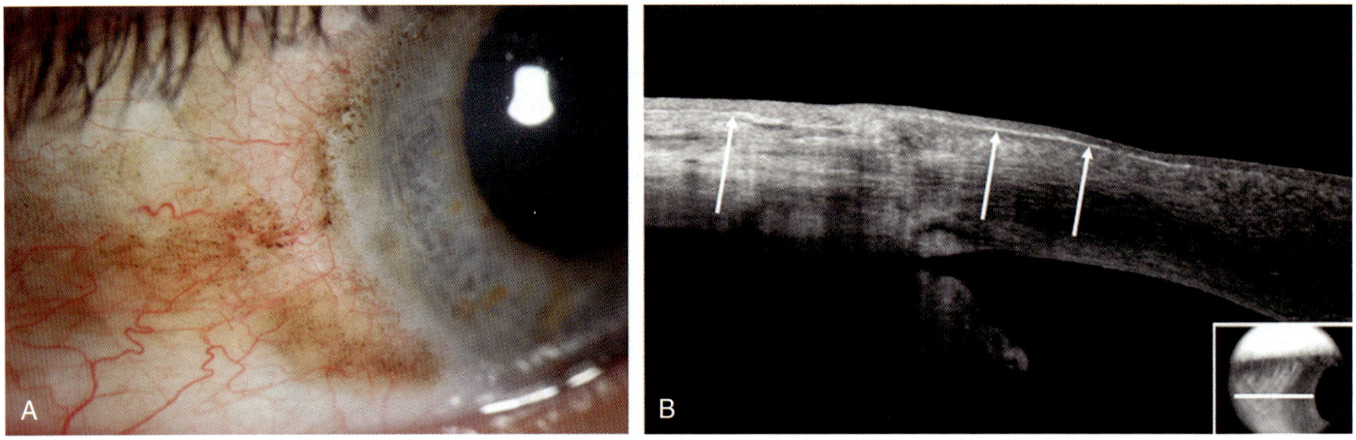

Fig. 4.11 Primary acquired melanosis. (A) Slit-lamp photograph of the right eye in a 54-year-old White man shows a flat patch of "peppery" pigmentation extending from the temporal conjunctiva toward the corneal limbus and extending onto the cornea from 9 to 11 o'clock. The patient reported significant sun exposure. Note the light complexion of the patient. (B) High-resolution optical coherence tomography (HR-OCT) demonstrates linear hyperreflectivity of the epithelial basement membrane *(arrows).*

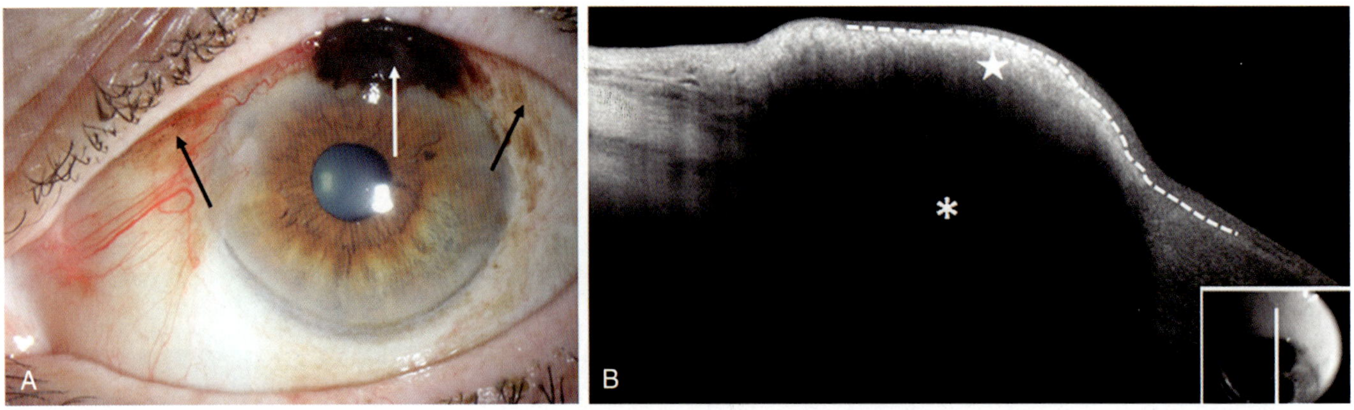

Fig. 4.12 Melanoma. (A) Slit-lamp photograph of the left eye in a 60-year-old Hispanic woman demonstrates an elevated, well-vascularized, densely pigmented lesion *(white arrow)* extending from the superior conjunctiva onto the cornea. Two areas of "peppery" pigmentation concerning for primary acquired melanosis are noted from 10 to 11 o'clock and from 1:30 to 3:00 *(black arrows).* The patient reported significant sun exposure. (B) High-resolution optical coherence tomography (HR-OCT) reveals a subepithelial, hyperreflective mass *(star)* with significant posterior shadowing *(asterisk)* consistent with a melanoma. *Dotted line* indicates basement membrane of epithelium. *Inset* shows scan location. The patient underwent excision of the lesion with cryotherapy/mitomycin-c/amniotic membrane transplant, and pathologic examination confirmed the presence of conjunctival malignant melanoma. Systemic workup was negative.

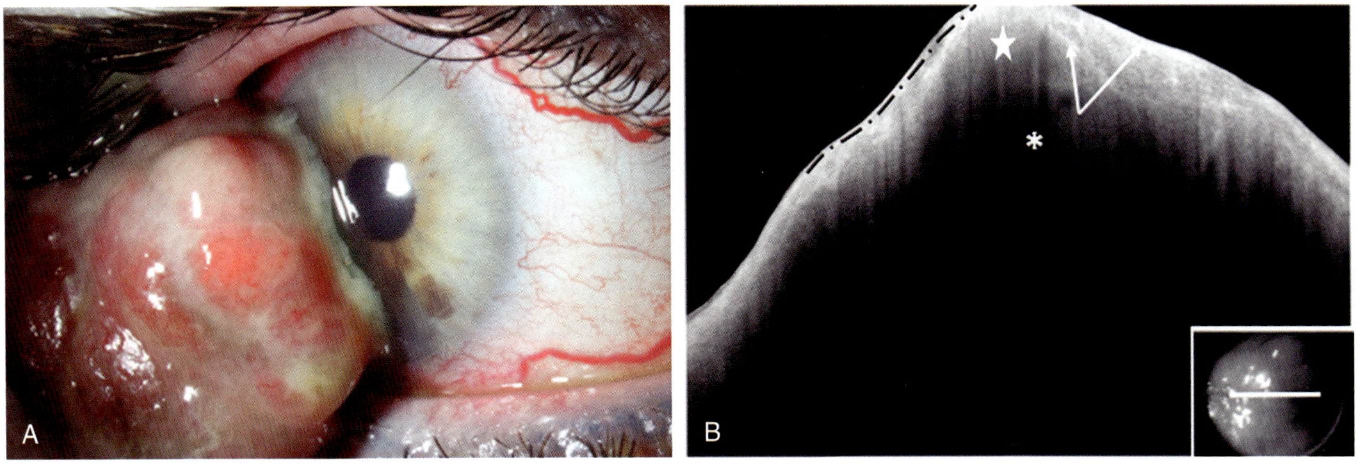

Fig. 4.13 Amelanotic melanoma. (A) Slit-lamp photograph of the right eye in a 60-year-old White woman demonstrates a large, amelanotic, well-vascularized mass of the temporal conjunctiva involving the corneal surface from 5 to 11 o'clock. (B) High-resolution optical coherence tomography (HR-OCT) reveals a subepithelial, hyperreflective mass *(star)* with significant posterior shadowing *(asterisk)* consistent with a melanoma. *Dotted line* indicates basement membrane of epithelium, with epithelial linear hyperreflectivity consistent with primary acquired melanosis (PAM) *(arrows). Inset* shows scan location. The patient underwent excision of the lesion with cryotherapy/mitomycin-c/amniotic membrane transplant, and pathologic examination confirmed the presence of conjunctival malignant melanoma arising from a PAM.

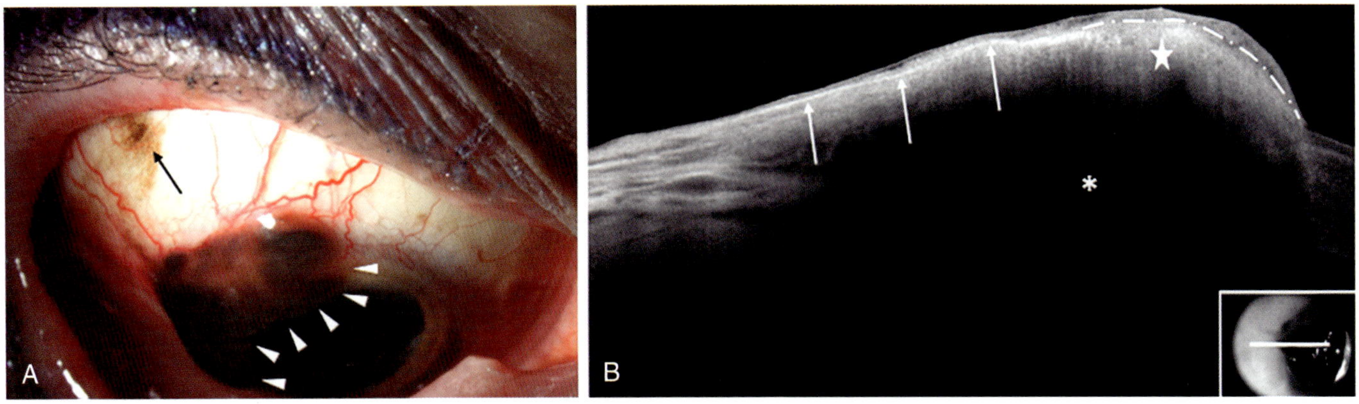

Fig. 4.14 Melanoma. (A) Slit-lamp photograph of the right eye in an 86-year-old White woman demonstrates a large, darkly pigmented lesion of the bulbar conjunctiva involving the corneal surface from 6 to 12 o'clock *(arrowheads)* with multiple feeder blood vessels and a region of primary acquired melanosis (PAM) *(black arrow).* (B) High-resolution optical coherence tomography (HR-OCT) reveals a subepithelial, hyperreflective mass *(star)* with significant posterior shadowing *(asterisk)* consistent with a melanoma. *Dotted line* indicates basement membrane of epithelium, with focal linear hyperreflectivity indicative of PAM *(arrows). Inset* shows scan location. The patient underwent excision of the lesion with cryotherapy/mitomycin-c/amniotic membrane transplant, and pathologic examination confirmed the presence of conjunctival malignant melanoma with extension to the cornea.

III. OCULAR SURFACE SQUAMOUS NEOPLASIA

The most common nonpigmented malignant tumor of the conjunctiva is OSSN, an umbrella term that encompasses all neoplasms of squamous cell origin ranging from mild dysplasia to invasive squamous cell carcinoma. The clinical picture of OSSN can be variable and includes leukoplakic, papillary, opalescent, and gelatinous manifestations. These lesions, although often classic, can sometimes be difficult to diagnose when small, when combined with an underlying pterygium, or when present amid other ocular surface diseases. HR-OCT can be a key diagnostic tool in detecting atypical presentations of OSSN through the identification of three highly specific features: a thickened epithelium, a hyperreflective epithelium, and an abrupt transition from normal to abnormal epithelium. The presence of such features enables the treating physician to diagnose OSSN and subsequently monitor the treatment response of OSSN to topical chemotherapy and ensure complete resolution before terminating medical therapy (Figs. 4.15 to 4.19).

CLINICAL PEARL

OSSN will exhibit three key characteristics on HR-OCT: a hyperreflective epithelium, a thickening of the epithelium, and an abrupt transition from normal to abnormal epithelium. The presence of epithelium measured to exceed 120 microns in thickness is highly specific and sensitive for OSSN.

CLINICAL PEARL

When evaluating a lesion suspicious for OSSN, the lack of a thickened, hyperreflective epithelium with an abrupt transition on HR-OCT should prompt consideration of other diagnoses. An opalescent Salzmann nodule can clinically masquerade as OSSN, but HR-OCT will reveal a subepithelial corneal lesion with overlying normal and thin epithelium, thus ruling out OSSN. See Chapter 5 for more information on Salzmann nodular degeneration.

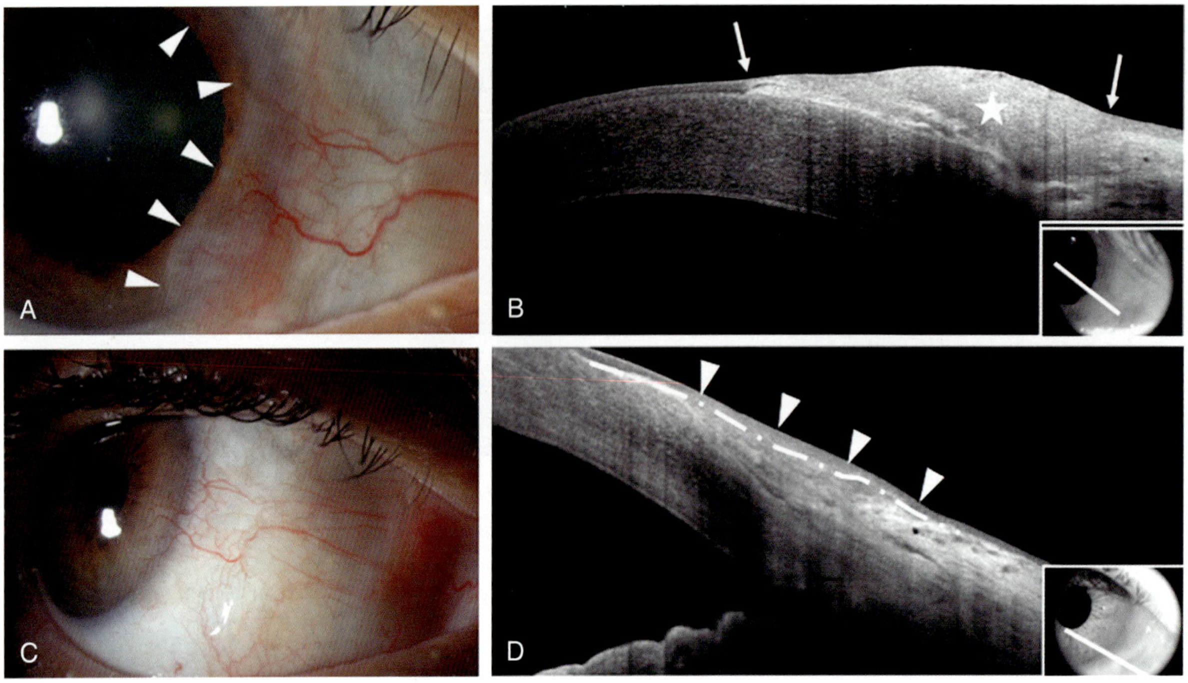

Fig. 4.15 Recurrent ocular surface squamous neoplasia (OSSN) responsive to 5-fluorouracil 1% (5-FU). (A) Slit-lamp photograph of the right eye in a 65-year-old Hispanic man shows an opalescent lesion *(arrowheads)* with smooth borders arising from the limbus and extending onto the cornea from one to five o'clock. The patient had undergone excisional biopsy for a similar lesion five years earlier, with pathologic examination confirming OSSN. The patient reported significant sun exposure. (B) High-resolution optical coherence tomography (HR-OCT) reveals a thickened and hyperreflective epithelium *(star)* with abrupt transitions *(arrows)* from normal to abnormal epithelium on either side of the lesion consistent with OSSN. *Inset* shows scan location. (C) Slit-lamp photograph of the same eye after the patient underwent two cycles of topical 5-FU four times daily for a week separated by a three-week drug holiday demonstrates significant resolution of the lesion. (D) HR-OCT after treatment reveals normalization of the epithelium *(arrowheads). Dotted line* indicates basement membrane of epithelium. *Inset* shows scan location. The patient continued treatment for a total of four cycles of 5-FU.

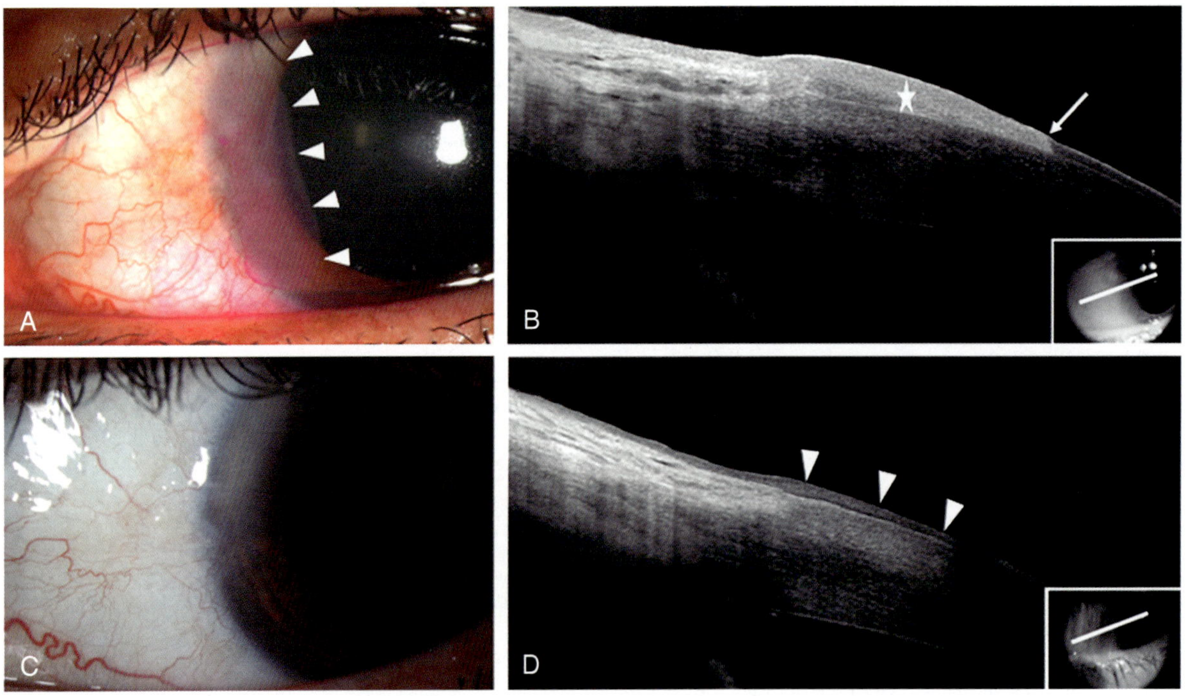

Fig. 4.16 Rose Bengal staining of ocular surface squamous neoplasia (OSSN). (A) Slit-lamp photograph of the left eye in a 60-year-old Hispanic woman demonstrates a well-circumscribed, opalescent lesion stained with rose Bengal arising from the nasal corneal limbus and extending onto the cornea from 8 to 10 o'clock *(arrowheads).* The patient reported significant sun exposure and smoking. (B) High-resolution optical coherence tomography (HR-OCT) reveals a hyperreflective and thickened epithelium *(star)* with an abrupt transition from normal to abnormal epithelium *(arrow),* concerning for OSSN. *Inset* shows scan location. (C) Slit-lamp photograph of the same eye after the patient underwent six cycles of topical 5-fluorouracil 1% four times daily for seven days with a three-week drug holiday for every week of treatment. The lesion is resolved, and there is no staining of the ocular surface with rose Bengal. (D) HR-OCT after treatment demonstrates normalization of the epithelium *(arrowheads). Inset* shows scan location.

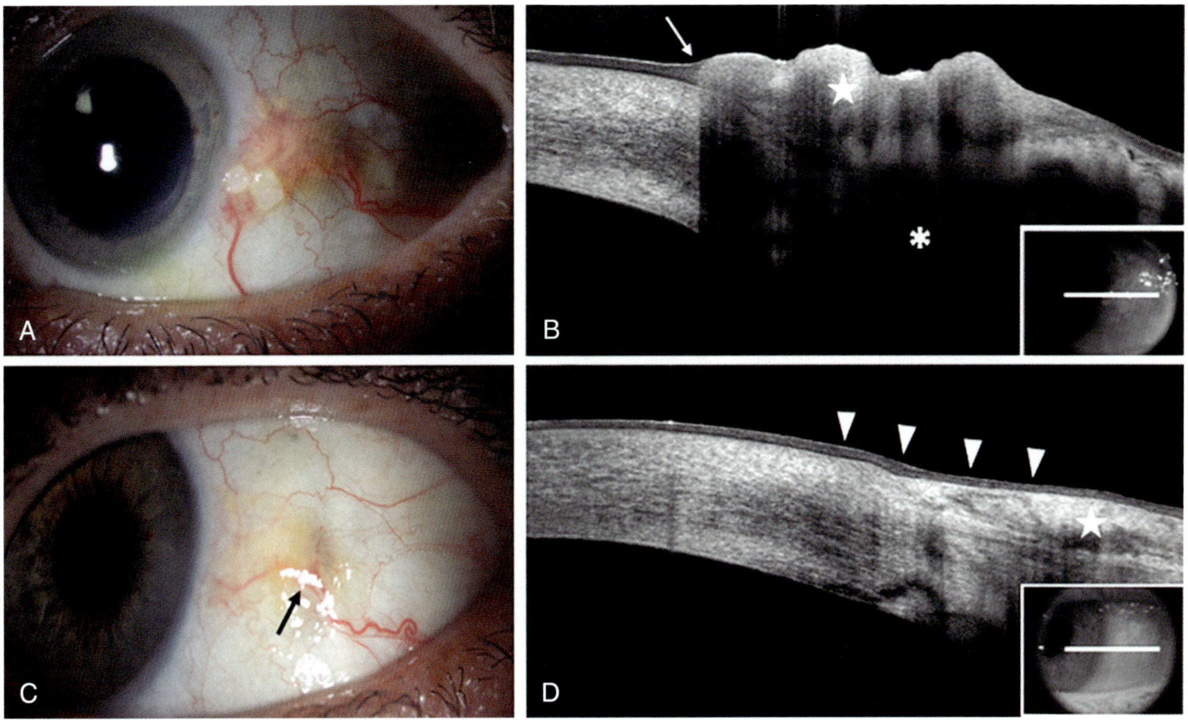

Fig. 4.17 Ocular surface squamous neoplasia (OSSN) responsive to mitomycin-c. (A) Slit-lamp photograph of the left eye in a 64-year-old White woman shows a gelatinous lesion with two elevated areas of leukoplakia with prominent feeder blood vessels. The patient reported significant sun exposure. (B) High-resolution optical coherence tomography (HR-OCT) reveals a thickened and hyperreflective epithelium *(star)* with an abrupt transition from normal to abnormal epithelium *(arrow)* with posterior shadowing *(asterisk)*, concerning for OSSN. *Inset* shows scan location. (C) Slit-lamp photograph of the same eye after the patient underwent three one-week cycles of topical mitomycin-c 0.04% after failing eight cycles of topical 5-fluorouracil 1%. The lesion is dramatically improved, with yellowing of the temporal conjunctiva *(arrow)* indicative of pinguecula. (D) HR-OCT after treatment shows resolution of the epithelium *(arrowheads)* with a subepithelial, well-demarcated, hyperreflective mass *(star)* consistent with pinguecula. *Inset* shows scan location.

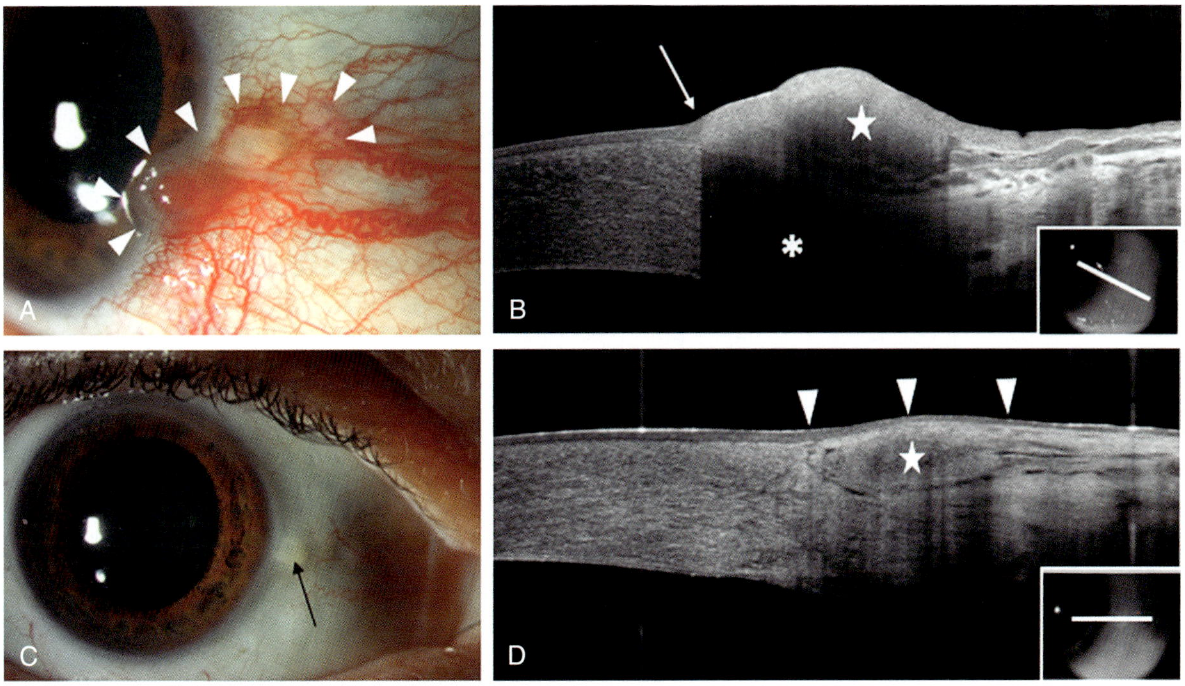

Fig. 4.18 OSSN responsive to interferon-α2b (IFN-α2b). (A) Slit-lamp photograph of the right eye in a 60-year-old Hispanic man demonstrates a vascularized, elevated, gelatinous lesion *(arrowheads)* of the nasal conjunctiva extending onto the cornea. The patient reported significant sun exposure, and the lesion had been present and slowly growing over the previous three years, unresponsive to topical prednisone. (B) High-resolution optical coherence tomography (HR-OCT) reveals a thickened and hyperreflective epithelium *(star)* with an abrupt transition from normal to abnormal epithelium *(arrow)* and significant posterior shadowing *(asterisk)* concerning for OSSN. *Inset* shows scan location. (C) Slit-lamp photograph of the same eye after the patient underwent six months of topical IFN-α2b (1 mIU/mL four times daily) shows dramatic resolution of the lesion. A small, slightly raised, yellowish lesion of the nasal conjunctiva is noted at the corneal limbus *(black arrow)*, representative of a pinguecula. (D) HR-OCT after treatment demonstrates normalization of the epithelium, now thin and dark *(arrowheads)*. A subepithelial, well-demarcated mass *(star)* consistent with a pinguecula is noted. *Inset* shows scan location.

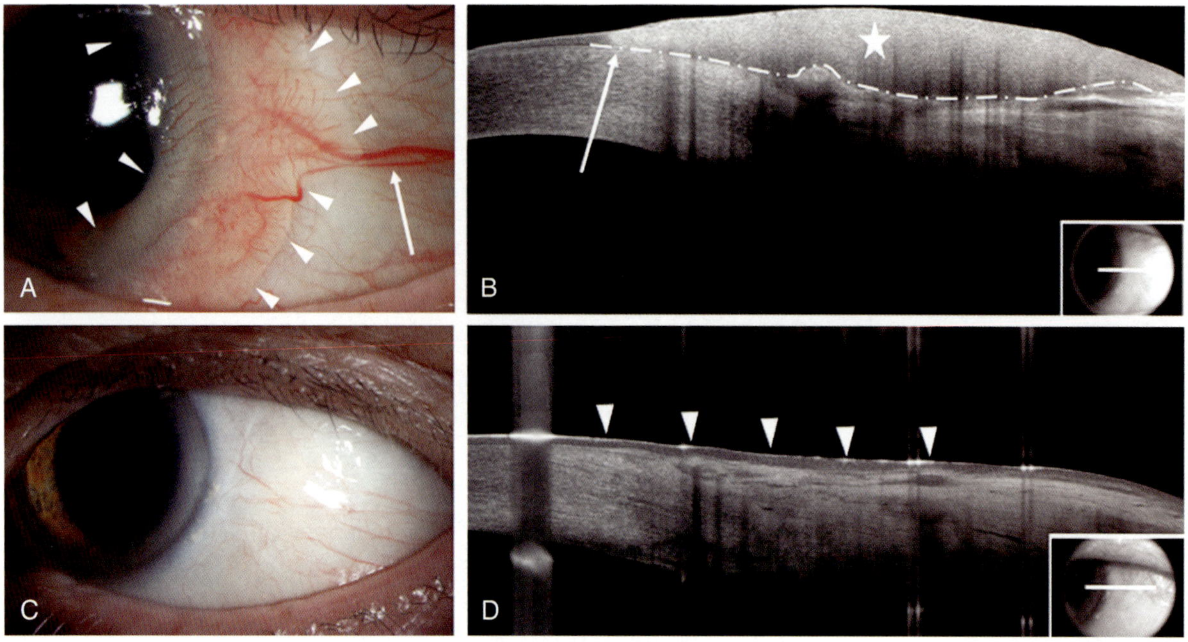

Fig. 4.19 OSSN resistant to 5-fluorouracil 1% (5-FU). (A) Slit-lamp photograph of the left eye in a 70-year-old White female demonstrates a temporal conjunctival gelatinous lesion extending onto the cornea *(arrowheads)* with vascularization and prominent feeder blood vessels *(arrow)*. The patient reported a family and personal history of malignant melanoma. (B) High-resolution optical coherence tomography (HR-OCT) reveals a thickened and hyperreflective epithelium *(star)* with an abrupt transition from normal to abnormal epithelium *(arrow)* consistent with OSSN. *Dotted line* indicates epithelial basement membrane. *Inset* shows scan location. (C) Slit-lamp photograph of the same eye with resolved tumor after the patient completed two months of topical interferon-α2b (1 mIU/mL four times daily) after failing 10 cycles of topical 5-FU four times daily with a three-week drug holiday for every week of treatment. (D) HR-OCT after treatment demonstrates normalization of the epithelium *(arrowheads)*, confirming resolution of the lesion. *Inset* shows scan location.

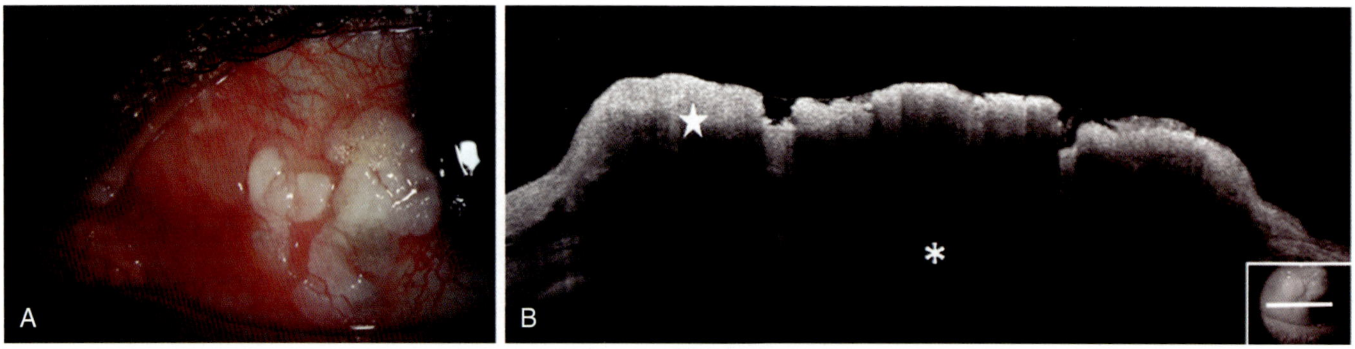

Fig. 4.20 Squamous cell carcinoma. (A) Slit-lamp photograph of the left eye in a 52-year-old Black man demonstrates extensive leukoplakic lesions of the nasal conjunctiva. The patient noticed the lesions two months before presentation, and medical history was significant for a double lung transplant for which the patient was taking immunosuppressant medications. (B) High-resolution optical coherence tomography (HR-OCT) reveals epithelial thickening and hyperreflectivity *(star)* and significant posterior shadowing *(asterisk)*. This is worrisome for subepithelial invasion because no deep border of the lesion can be visualized. *Inset* shows scan location. The lesion was treated with preoperative chemoreduction with 5-fluorouracil 1% (5-FU) and mitomycin-c (MMC), followed by wide surgical excision, cryotherapy, and MMC.

CLINICAL PEARL

OSSN may be successfully treated with topical agents such as interferon, mitomycin-c, or 5-fluorouracil. Topical 5-fluorouracil 1% (5-FU) is typically administered four times a day for one week, followed by a three-week drug holiday, for a minimum of four cycles. HR-OCT can enable the clinician to monitor the response of the tumor to the chemotherapy and ensure the resolution of the tumor before treatment is stopped. If no HR-OCT is available, the clinician should continue treatment with 5-FU for an additional two cycles after clinical resolution is achieved.

Squamous cell carcinoma (SCC) is the invasive form of OSSN. In addition to the findings of epithelial thickening and hyperreflectivity with an abrupt transition point characteristic of OSSN on HR-OCT, SCC will also exhibit subepithelial involvement indicative of invasion. SCC requires surgical excision with adjuvant medical therapy and/or placement of a radioactive plaque (Figs. 4.20 and 4.21).

IV. LYMPHOMA

Subepithelial conjunctival lesions are often a diagnostic challenge. Conjunctival lymphomas may manifest as a smooth "salmon-pink" mass, as subtle yellow-pink lesions, as conjunctival follicles, or as chronic chemosis. HR-OCT can be a key diagnostic aid in identifying classic features of conjunctival lymphoma, including a homogenous, hyporeflective, subepithelial mass with discrete borders, monomorphic dotlike infiltrates, and a normal overlying epithelium (Figs. 4.22 and 4.23).

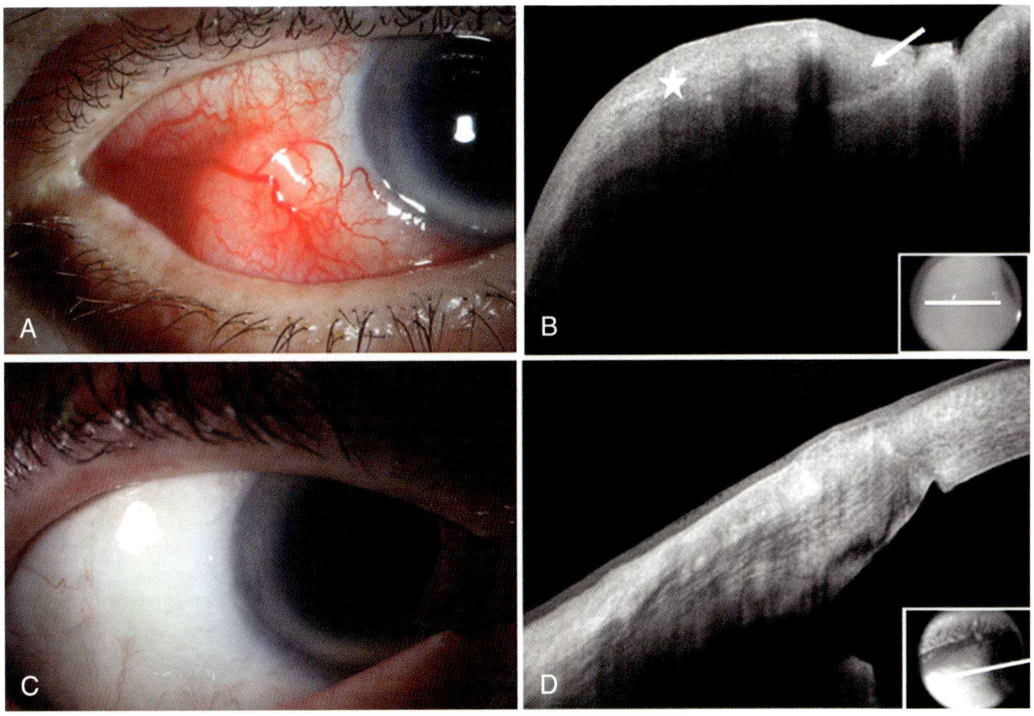

Fig. 4.21 Squamous cell carcinoma (SCC). (A) Slit-lamp photograph of the right eye in an 81-year-old Hispanic man demonstrates a temporal subconjunctival, immobile, elevated nodule with prominent feeder blood vessels. (B) High-resolution optical coherence tomography (HR-OCT) reveals a hyperreflective, thickened epithelium *(arrow)* over the surface of a hyperreflective subconjunctival lesion *(star)* with demonstration of subepithelial invasion. *Inset* shows scan location. The patient underwent excision of the lesion with cryotherapy/mitomycin-c/ethyl alcohol/amniotic membrane transplant. Pathologic examination confirmed invasive SCC with positive margins, requiring neoadjuvant topical chemotherapy and placement of a radioactive plaque. (C) Slit-lamp photograph of the same eye after treatment shows dramatic resolution of the lesion. (D) HR-OCT after treatment reveals normalization of the epithelium. *Inset* shows scan location.

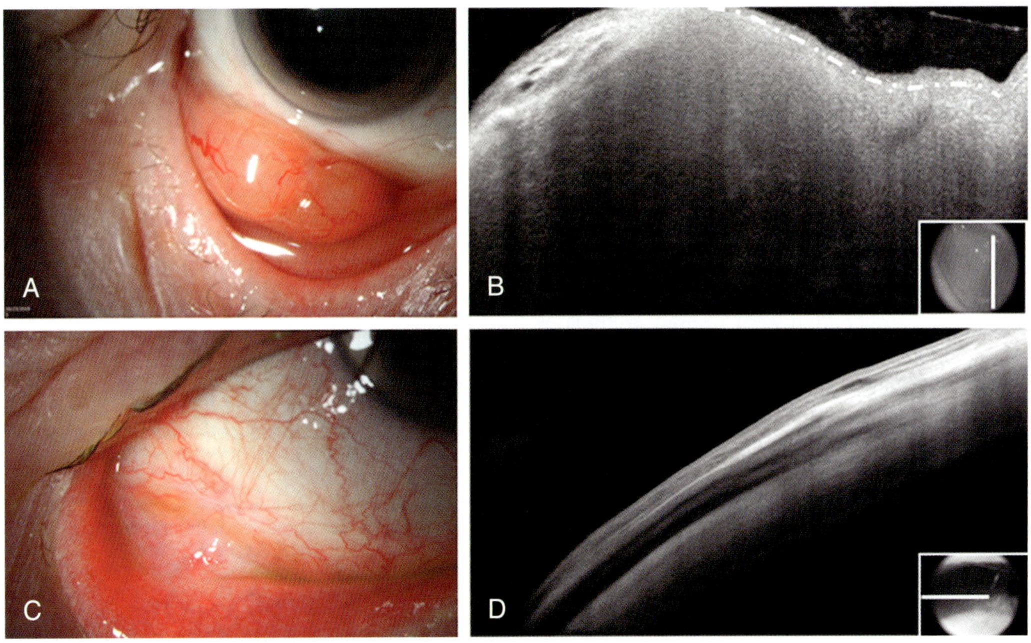

Fig. 4.22 Lymphoma. (A) Slit-lamp photograph of the right eye in a 68-year-old White man shows a multilobulated, subconjunctival, mobile, 10- × 5-mm pinkish mass located in the inferotemporal fornix with prolapse on eyelid retraction. The patient reported a foreign body sensation beginning four months before presentation. (B) High-resolution optical coherence tomography (HR-OCT) demonstrates a subepithelial, hyporeflective, homogenous lesion with monomorphic dotlike infiltrates. *Dotted line* indicates the epithelial basement membrane. *Inset* shows scan location. Pathologic examination confirmed mantle cell lymphoma of the conjunctiva. (C) Slit-lamp photograph of the same eye after the patient underwent 12 fractions of external beam radiation (total dose 24 Gy) shows resolution of the lesion. (D) HR-OCT after treatment demonstrates normalization of the subepithelial lesion. *Inset* shows scan location.

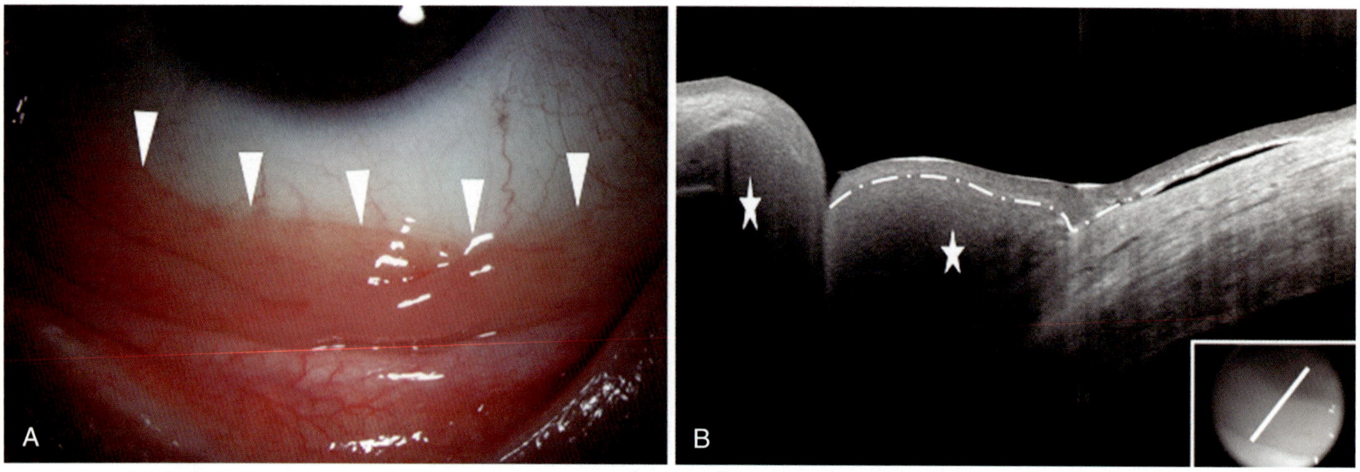

Fig. 4.23 Recurrent lymphoma. (A) Slit-lamp photograph of the left eye in a 67-year-old White man shows an elevated, salmon-appearing lesion *(arrowheads)* of the inferior fornix extending from the caruncle to lateral canthus. Three months before presentation, the patient reported new-onset night sweats. The patient had a history of non-Hodgkin mucosa-associated lymphoid tissue (MALT) lymphoma of the conjunctiva in the left eye eight years before presentation, treated with interferon eye drops and radiation therapy. (B) High-resolution optical coherence tomography (HR-OCT) demonstrates a subepithelial, hyporeflective, homogenous lesion *(stars)* with smooth borders. *Dotted line* indicates the epithelial basement membrane. *Inset* shows scan location. Pathologic examination confirmed a conjunctival MALT lymphoma.

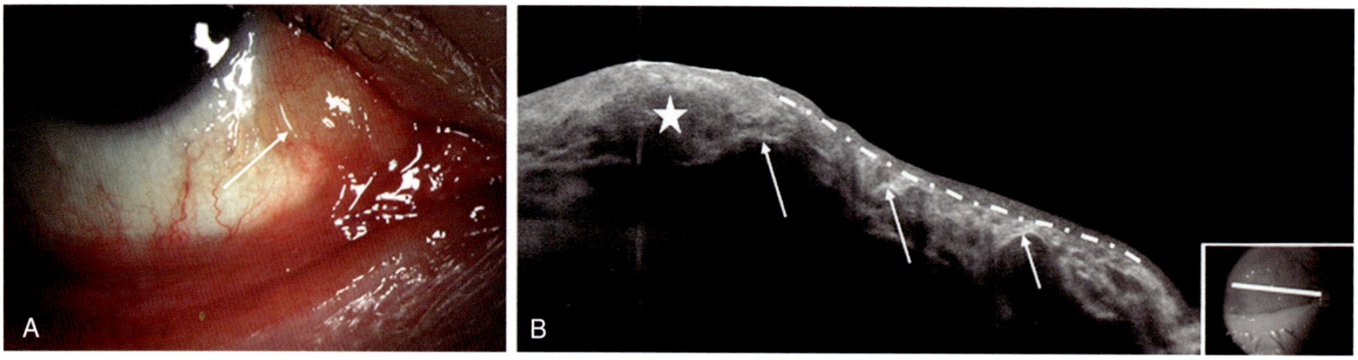

Fig. 4.24 Amyloidosis. (A) Slit-lamp photograph of the right eye in a 58-year-old White woman shows a gelatinous lesion *(arrow)* of the nasal conjunctiva measuring 5.5- × 6.5-mm that did not stain with lissamine green. (B) High-resolution optical coherence tomography (HR-OCT) demonstrates a subepithelial, hyperreflective, heterogeneous lesion *(star)* with linear deposits *(arrows)* consistent with amyloid. *Dotted line* indicates the epithelial basement membrane. *Inset* shows scan location. Pathologic examination confirmed amyloid deposition.

V. AMYLOIDOSIS

The rare presentation of conjunctival amyloidosis may closely resemble that of lymphoma, in which case HR-OCT can aid in diagnosis through the identification of a normal epithelium overlying a heterogeneous mass with irregular borders and hyperreflective linear deposits characteristic of conjunctival amyloidosis (Fig. 4.24). The authors report no relevant or related conflicts of interest. The authors alone are responsible for the content and writing of the paper.

BIBLIOGRAPHY

Alzahrani YA, Kumar S, Abdul Aziz H, Plesec T, Singh AD. Primary acquired melanosis: clinical, histopathologic and optical coherence tomographic correlation. *Ocul Oncol Pathol*. 2016;2(3):123-127.

Nanji AA, Sayyad FE, Galor A, Dubovy S, Karp CL. High-resolution optical coherence tomography as an adjunctive tool in the diagnosis of corneal and conjunctival pathology. *Ocul Surf*. 2015;13(3): 226-235.

Thomas BJ, Galor A, Nanji AA, et al. Ultra high-resolution anterior segment optical coherence tomography in the diagnosis and management of ocular surface squamous neoplasia. *Ocul Surf*. 2014;12(1):46-58.

Tran AQ, Venkateswaran N, Galor A, Karp CL. Utility of high-resolution anterior segment optical coherence tomography in the diagnosis and management of sub-clinical ocular surface squamous neoplasia. *Eye Vis (Lond)*. 2019;6:27.

Venkateswaran N, Galor A, Wang J, Karp CL. Optical coherence tomography for ocular surface and corneal diseases: a review. *Eye Vis (Lond)*. 2018;5:13.

Pathology of the Corneal Epithelium and Bowman's Layer

5

Brett Levinson

I. EPITHELIAL (ANTERIOR) BASEMENT MEMBRANE DYSTROPHY

Epithelial basement membrane dystrophy (EBMD) is also called anterior basement membrane dystrophy, map-dot-fingerprint dystrophy, or Cogan microcystic dystrophy, as the condition was first described in print by Dr. David G. Cogan in 1946.

The variable names of this condition reflect the variable nature of the clinical presentation. EBMD can appear like fine lines in the cornea, geographic maps, or the classic dots described by Cogan. Sometimes the condition is occult and cannot be seen with white light at the slit-lamp. Using sodium fluorescein (NaFl) or other vital dyes on the ocular surface, EBMD is often best seen with negative staining; the fluorescein pools in the relative depressions made by the irregular epithelium and the elevated areas have a lack of staining.

Although the original papers on EBMD described this as an uncommon condition, the prevalence of EBMD has been estimated at 2–3% of the population. However, it may be more common in reality because the signs can be subtle and easily overlooked. EBMD is a common cause of recurrent erosions—painful breakdowns in the epithelium, most commonly noted on awakening. Another frequent symptom of EBMD is decreased quality of vision as a result of optical blur and irregular astigmatism. EBMD in the central visual axis is a common cause of serially shifting refraction. One diagnostic test to determine whether the epithelium is the cause of decreased vision is overrefraction using a rigid gas-permeable (RGP) contact lens. Automated or manual topography and auto-refraction can also confirm distortions in the central mires. In a patient being screened for cataract surgery, a mismatch between the refractive and keratometric astigmatism (either in the power of the cylinder or the axis), or shifting or distorted keratometry should raise suspicion for EBMD (Figs. 5.1 and 5.2).

It can be difficult to photograph EBMD at the slit-lamp with white light, and photographs after instilling fluorescein can be much more illustrative (Fig. 5.3).

The use of anterior segment optical coherence tomography (AS-OCT) can be helpful to visualize and diagnose EBMD. Figs. 5.3 and 5.4 are images of the same patient. In some areas, thickening of the epithelium can be seen, whereas other sections show epithelial thinning. Although the fluorescein staining sometimes may appear dark green and can be confused with a frank epithelial defect, AS-OCT clearly shows that the epithelium is intact but irregular.

If a patient presents with a new epithelial defect, even in the setting of trauma, the clinician should have a high suspicion for underlying occult EBMD. Normal epithelium is quite adherent to Bowman's layer and is difficult to remove without an underlying pathologic condition. Some patients will find the idea that there is an underlying pathologic condition difficult to believe because it "makes sense" to patients that being poked in the eye would cause an epithelial defect. However, just as it is difficult to break the skin with digital trauma, the healthy epithelium is quite resistant to trauma. (Trying to manually debride healthy epithelium for photorefractive keratectomy (PRK) or collagen cross linking will demonstrate the difficulty of removing normal epithelium.) It is recommended to discuss with patients the risk for recurrent erosions resulting from underlying EBMD at some point during the treatment of the initial epithelial defect. Starting with conventional dry eye therapy, including punctal plugs, is a rational option, because the initial epithelial defect in patients with EBMD can be a harbinger of further epithelial pathologic conditions and increase the risk for infection. Dryness of the ocular surface can be a trigger for recurrent erosions in the setting of EBMD.

One illustrative AS-OCT finding of EBMD is loss or thinning of the epithelial tissue, with a thin layer of superficial overlying epithelium. This creates the classic pooling or negative staining pattern seen with fluorescein at the slit-lamp. However, reflective of the variable clinical appearance of EBMD, the AS-OCT findings can also show thickening of the epithelium, which forms the "maps", "dots", and "fingerprints" seen at the slit lamp (Fig. 5.4).

In another patient, the classic negative staining of fluorescein is noted and the corresponding changes are noted on the

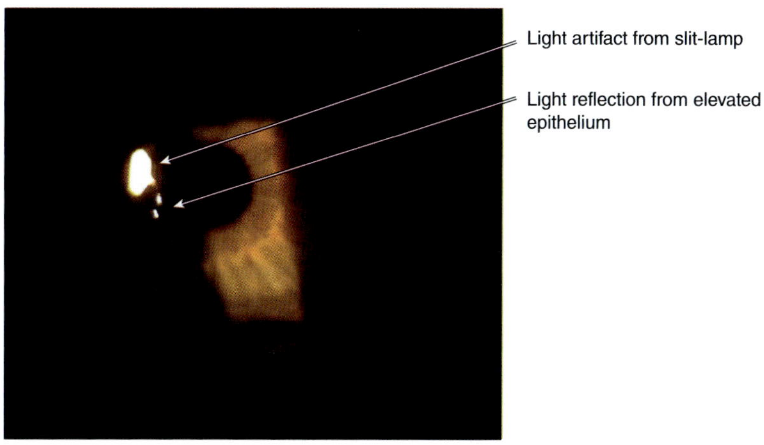

Fig. 5.1 White light reflection seen with EBMD at slit-lamp.

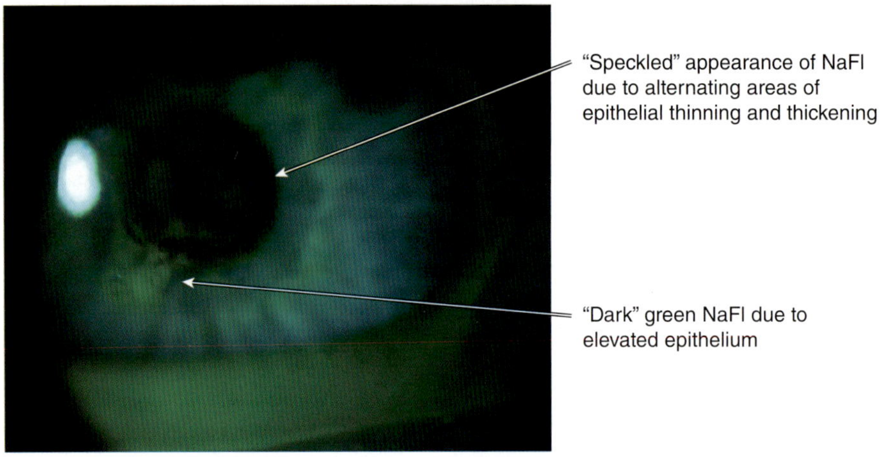

Fig. 5.2 EBMD at slit-lamp after fluorescein staining.

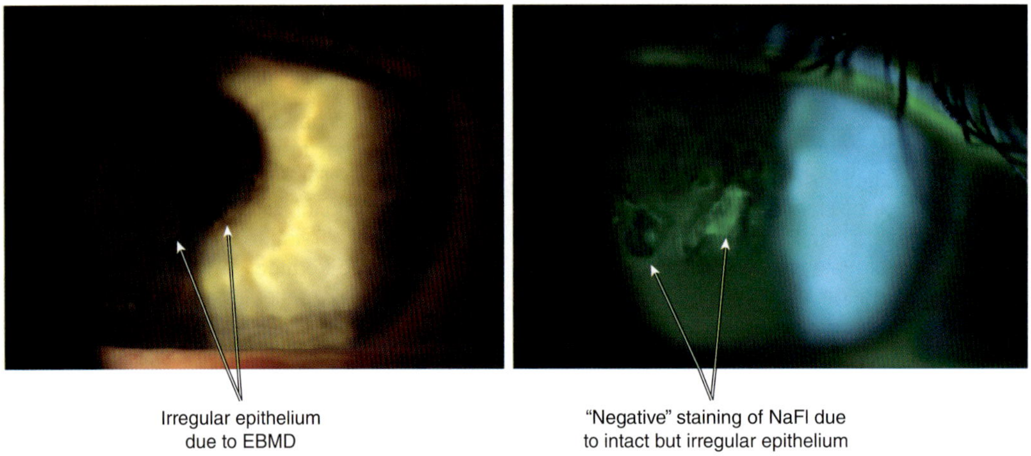

Fig. 5.3 Comparison of white light and fluorescein staining of EBMD.

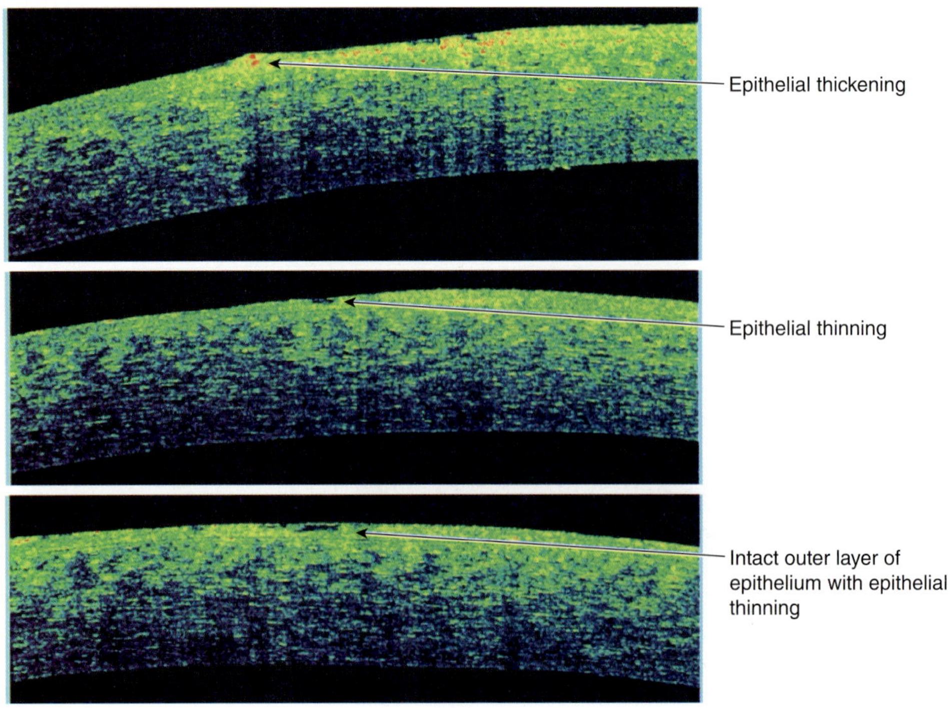

Fig. 5.4 Serial images of EBMD on AS-OCT. Areas of epithelial thickening and thinning can be readily appreciated in these images.

AS-OCT images. Alternating areas of thickening and thinning of the epithelium are classic findings in EBMD and can be seen clearly on the AS-OCT scans (Fig. 5.5).

Sometimes the epithelium is diffusely thickened and can be seen on both color and black-and-white images. In the color images, the abnormal epithelium appears red instead of the usual green of normal epithelium. Small areas of loss of the epithelium can be seen in the larger area of epithelial thickening.

Fig. 5.6 shows another example of almost complete loss of the epithelial layer, with a residual linear basement membrane and a thin superficial layer of epithelium. The hyperreflective outer layer of the epithelium provides a contrast to the regular, unaffected epithelium. The irregular, thickened epithelium is denser and appears whiter and hyperreflective, and the areas of epithelial loss are blacker and hyporeflective (see Fig. 5.6).

In this patient in Fig. 5.7, a large inferior-central area of irregular epithelium from EBMD can be seen with white light and with the cobalt blue filter after the instillation of fluorescein.

Because of the central elevation of the irregular epithelium, a "halo" effect can be seen with fluorescein. The central elevated area of epithelium will stain brightly with fluorescein, while the surrounding relatively thinner areas of epithelium will have a darker appearance as a result of pooling of the fluorescein-stained tear film. This also can be seen on the AS-OCT images (Figs. 5.8 and 5.9).

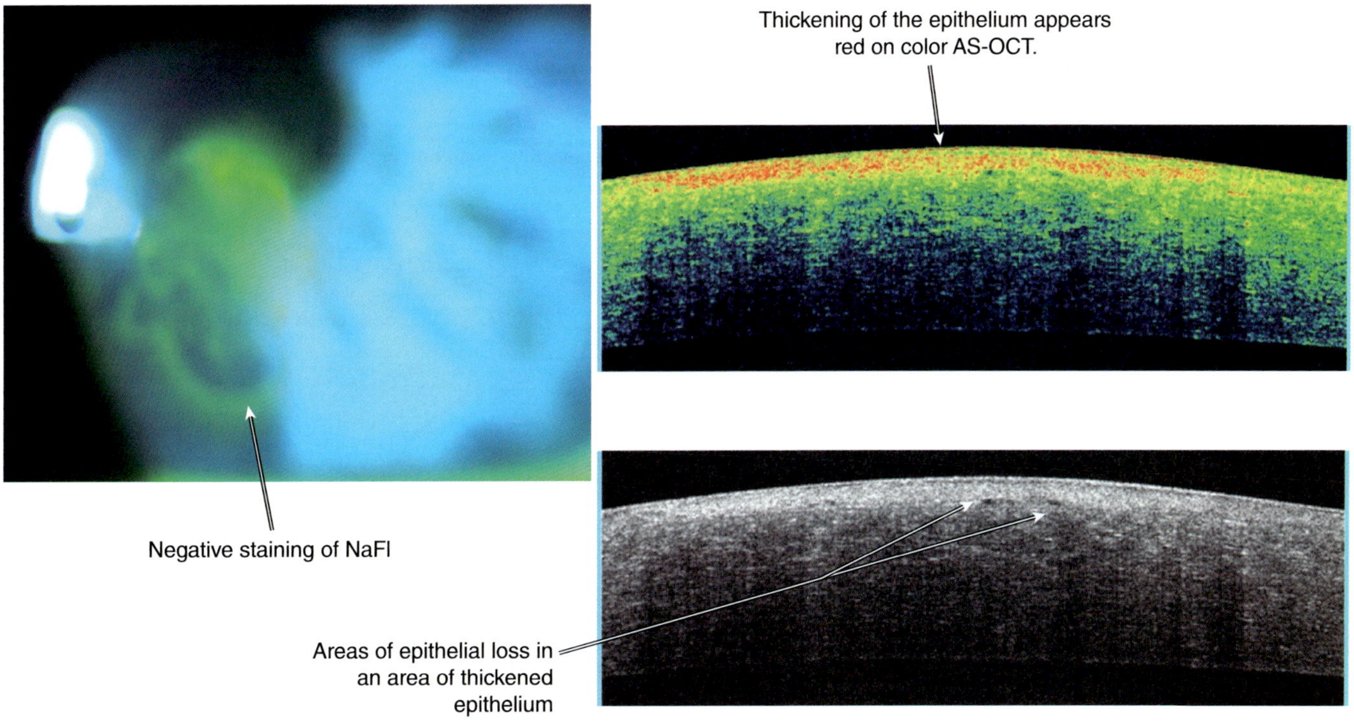

Fig. 5.5 Comparison of color and black and white AS-OCT images of EBMD. In the color AS-OCT images, abnormal epithelium appears red; in the black-and-white AS-OCT images, abnormal epithelium appears more hyperreflective than healthy epithelium. Areas of epithelial loss in both imaging schemes appear dark or hyporeflective.

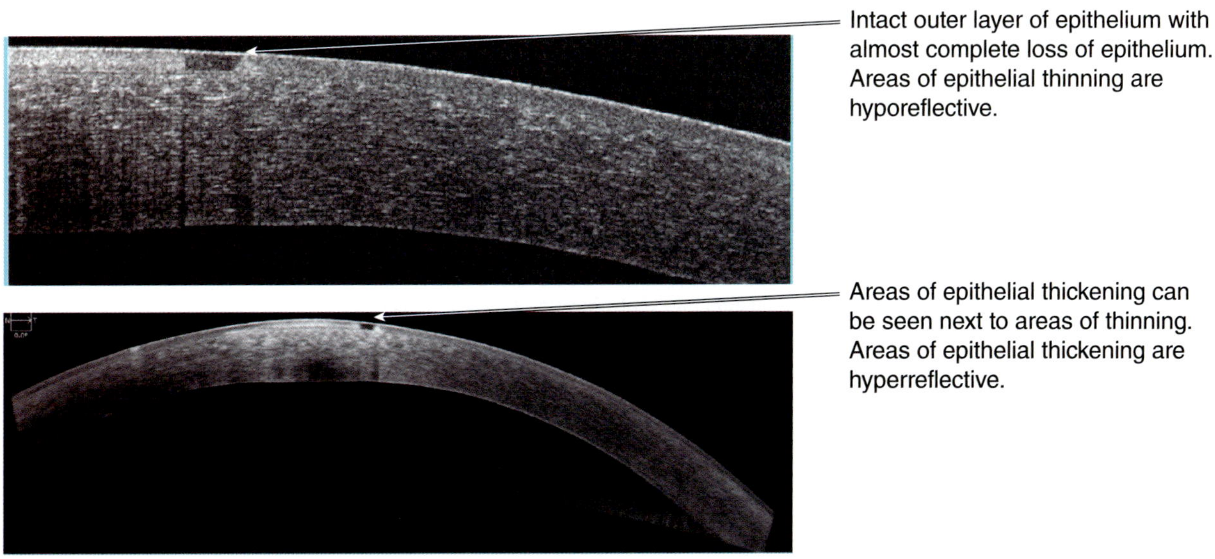

Fig. 5.6 Epithelial changes on AS-OCT in EBMD.

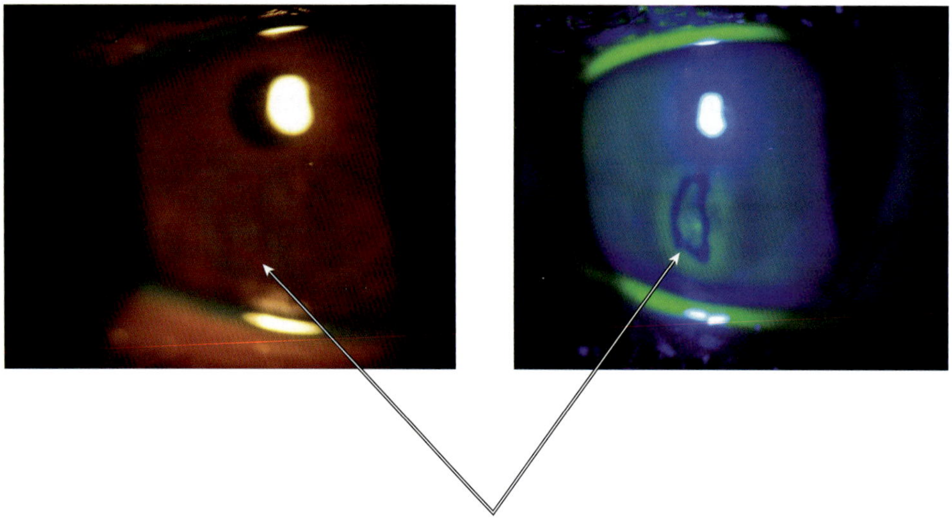

Fig. 5.7 Comparison of EBMD at slit-lamp after fluorescein with white and cobalt blue light.

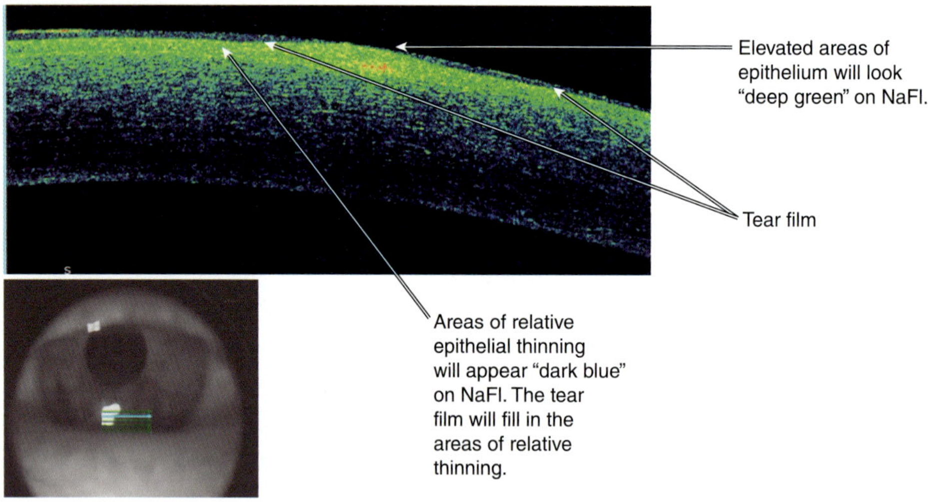

Fig. 5.8 Relative thickening and thinning of epithelium in EBMD with AS-OCT.

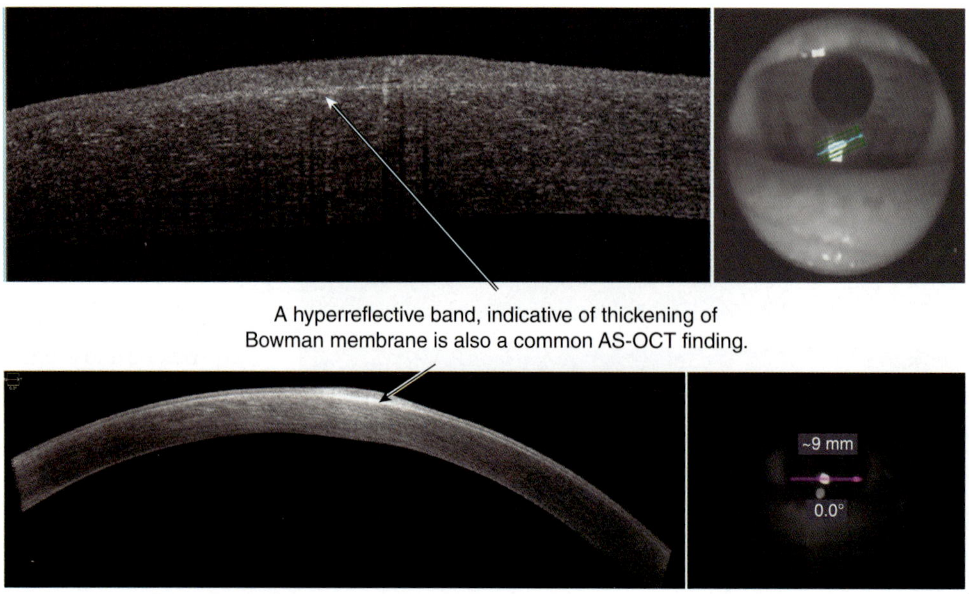

Fig. 5.9 Thickening of the Bowman membrane appears as a hyperreflective band on AS-OCT in EBMD.

CLINICAL PEARL

EBMD is a common reason for referral to corneal specialists. This is partially because of the many ways EBMD can manifest. At the slit-lamp, the irregularity of the epithelium can appear elevated, like a dendrite or pseudodendrite, or it can have areas of thinning with irregularity that look like maps or lines. Thickened areas of the epithelium can appear as dots. EBMD can be diffuse or localized to a small area of the cornea and can appear different on serial examinations, sometimes being difficult to visualize on white light and fluorescein staining on slit-lamp examination. Some patients will have a history of epithelial defects or difficulty finding the correct pair of glasses, whereas other patients will have no symptoms of EBMD at all. Although the clinical examination findings can be quite variable, the AS-OCT images can help make the diagnosis.

EBMD often can be peripheral, and the patient may have no symptoms, as seen in Fig. 5.10. The EBMD often has a "scalloped" appearance at the corneal periphery.

However, when the EBMD is centrally located, this can create visual distortion. In the slit-lamp photograph, the central epithelial irregularity is easily seen and bisects the visual axis. The AS-OCT images show the epithelium thickened to more than double its normal size.

Often, the EBMD will create an abnormality of the anterior refracting surface because of the irregularity of the epithelium (Fig. 5.11). While this irregularity may be subtle and easily missed on slit-lamp exam, AS-OCT can better highlight the areas of irregularity for both the patient and surgeon to determine the best course of management.

However, in the same patient, when the AS-OCT scan is taken slightly off-center to the area of the maximal epithelial thickening, the anterior refractive surface can look quite normal. A change in the composition and density of the epithelial cells is seen as hyperreflective areas on AS-OCT. Variable areas of thickening of the Bowman's Layer and sub-Bowman thickening also can be seen (Fig. 5.12).

The images in Fig. 5.13 show the same patient as in Fig. 5.12 at three weeks after a superficial keratectomy with diamond burr polishing of the anterior stroma. The epithelium is now more regular, and the thickening noted previously has resolved. Although the epithelium is not the same thickness throughout because of the thickening of the sub-Bowman's layer, the anterior refracting surface is normalized, and the patient had significantly improved vision.

In the patient in Fig. 5.14, who had prior LASIK and subsequent trauma, 2 small epithelial defects can be seen in areas of EBMD. Enhancement of the flap edge can also be seen because of inflammation of the epithelium secondary to the epithelial defect. The epithelium normalized five days later, but inflammation at the level of the LASIK flap can still be seen (Fig. 5.15).

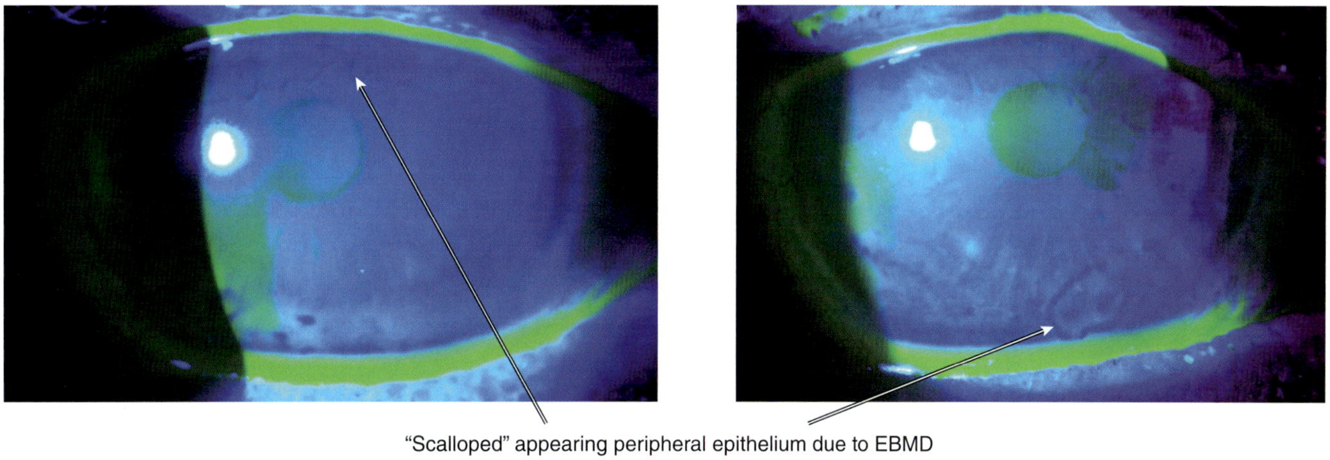

Fig. 5.10 Peripheral epithelial changes in EBMD seen at slit-lamp with fluorescein staining and cobalt blue filter.

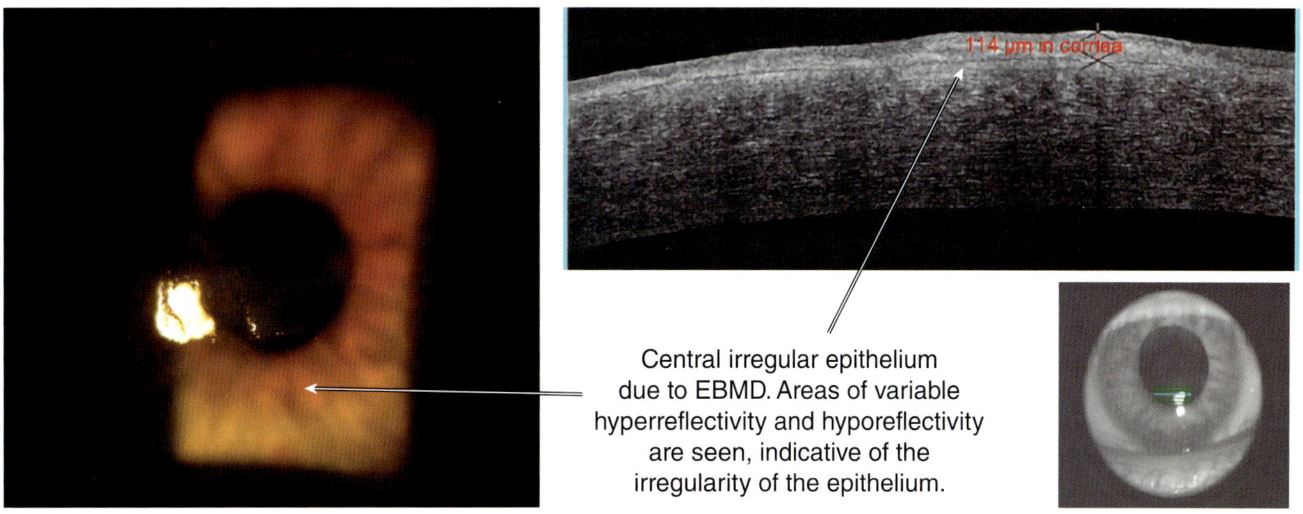

Fig. 5.11 Central epithelial changes seen at slit-lamp and AS-OCT in EBMD.

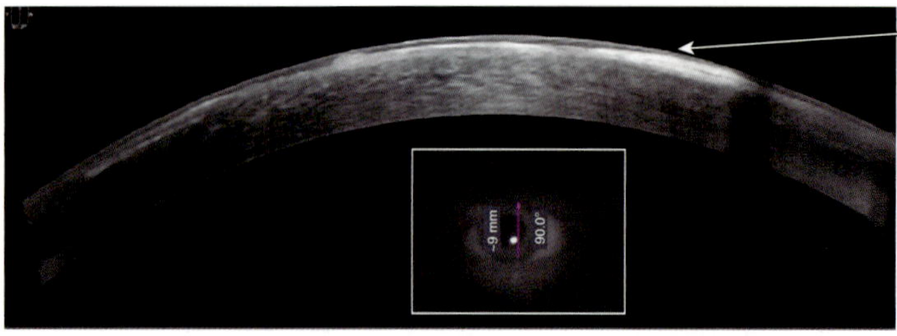

Fig. 5.12 Thickening of the Bowman membrane seen on AS-OCT in EBMD.

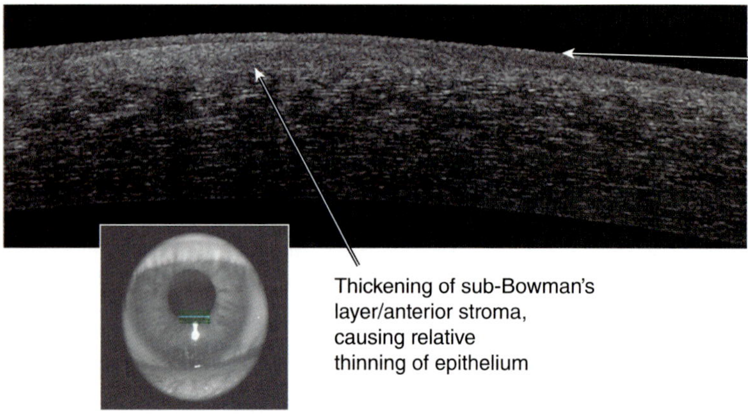

Fig. 5.13 Normal anterior refracting surface in paracentral cornea in EBMD.

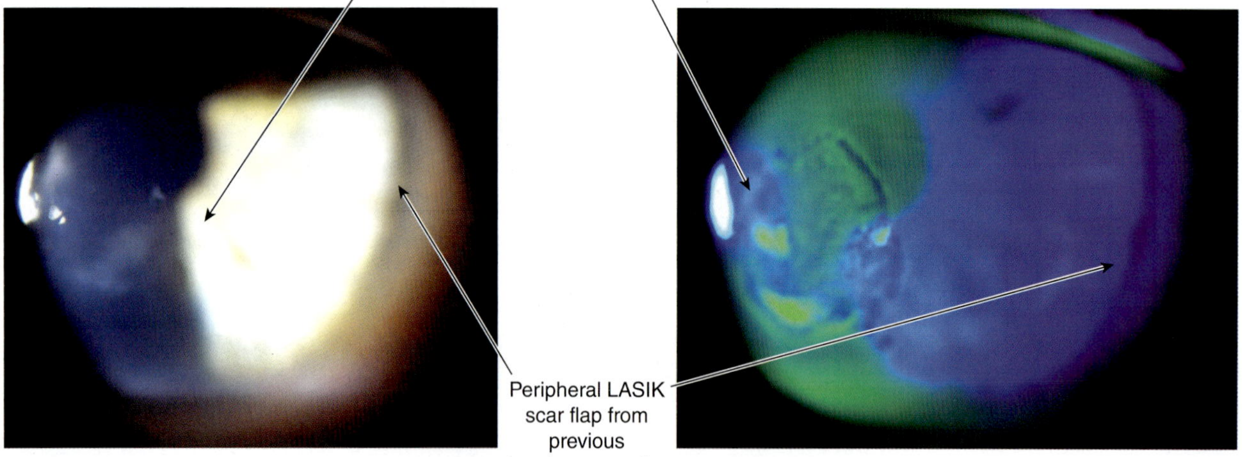

Fig. 5.14 EBMD in a post-LASIK patient at slit-lamp.

II. CALCIFIC BAND KERATOPATHY

Calcific band keratopathy, usually secondary to the deposition of calcium in the cornea, is a common finding in eyes with ophthalmic pathology, and often seen after multiple intraocular surgeries, especially silicone oil, or in eyes with a history of ocular trauma, persistent intraocular inflammation, or low vision. Sometimes, patients with chronic ocular surface disease will develop band keratopathy, which often develops at the limbus at three and nine o'clock in the interpalpebral regions of the cornea. Although many textbooks note that there can be a link with systemic conditions that can cause hypercalcemia (e.g., renal failure, hyperparathyroidism), a systemic workup is rarely indicated because band keratopathy is almost always noted clinically to be due to a primary corneal or ocular condition.

Band keratopathy can have a variable appearance—sometimes looking flat and sometimes elevated with a breakdown of the overlying epithelium and with a grayish to whitish color (Figs. 5.16 and 5.17).

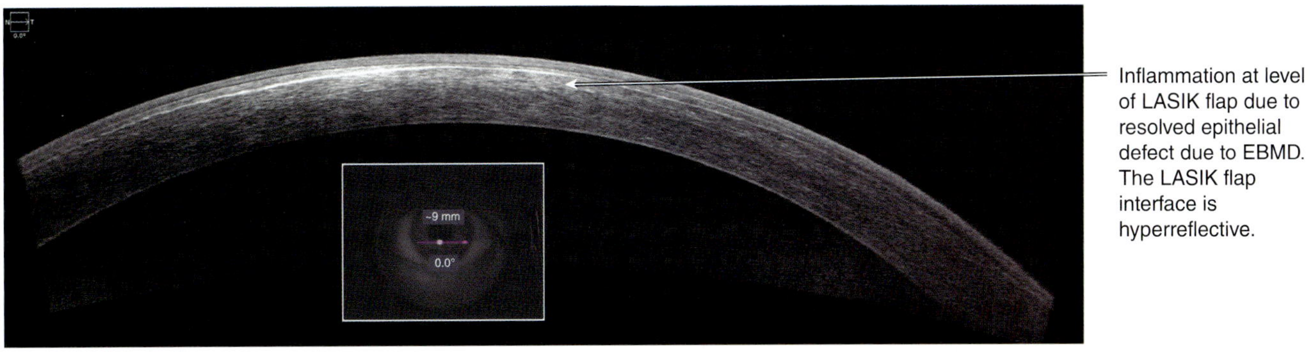

Fig. 5.15 Appearance of inflammation at the level of the LASIK flap (diffuse lamellar keratitis [DLK]) with EBMD in a post-LASIK patient on AS-OCT.

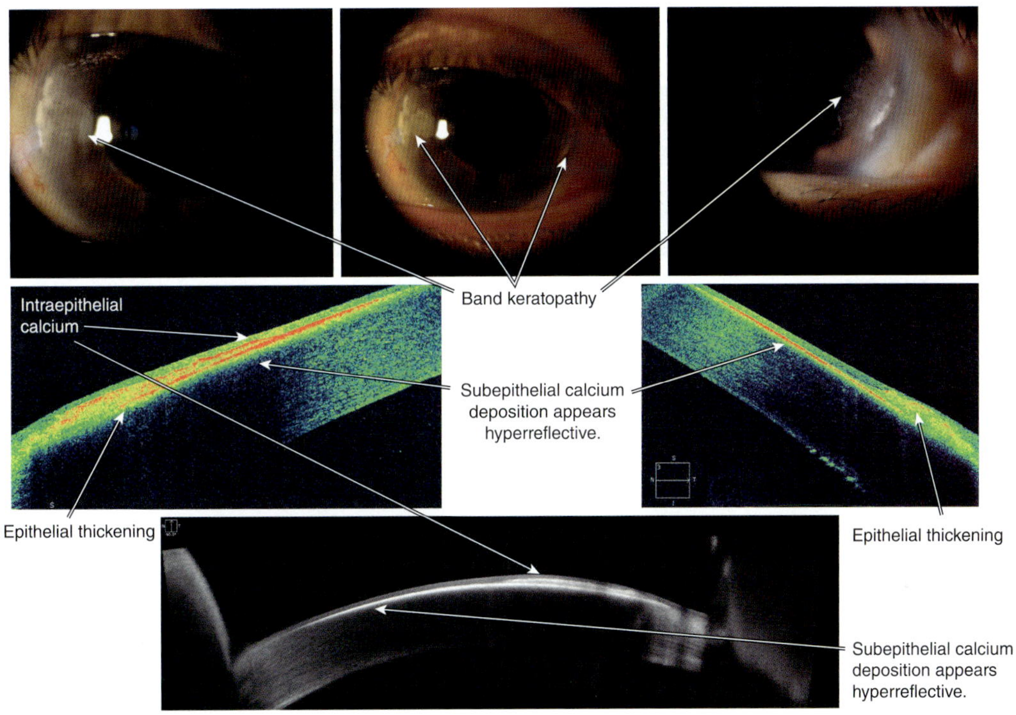

Fig. 5.16 Band keratopathy showing characteristic limbal appearance with intraepithelial and subepithelial calcium deposition.

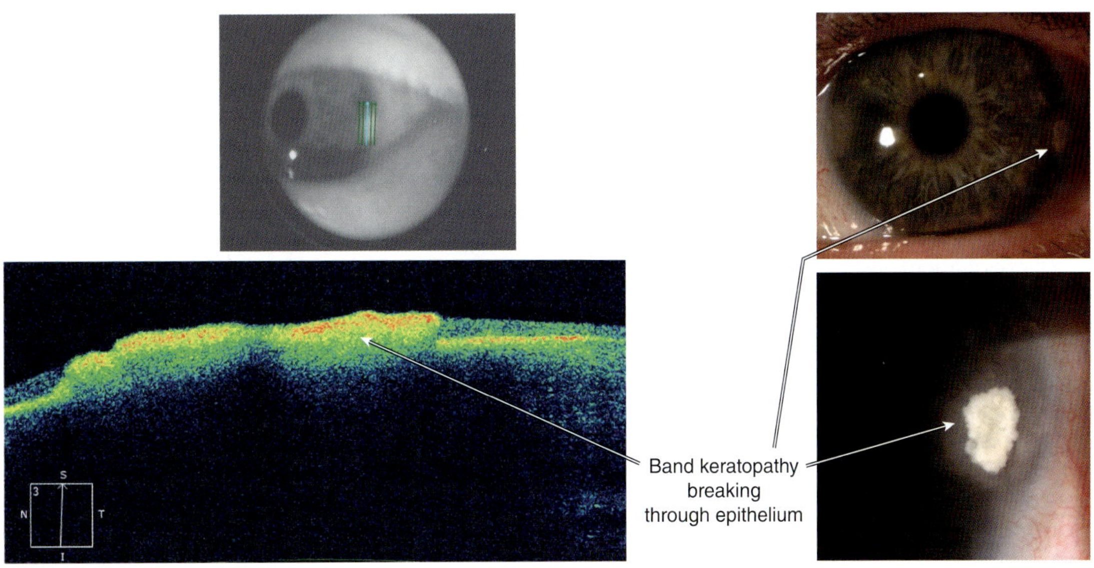

Fig. 5.17 Ba and keratopathy with breakdown of the overlying epithelium.

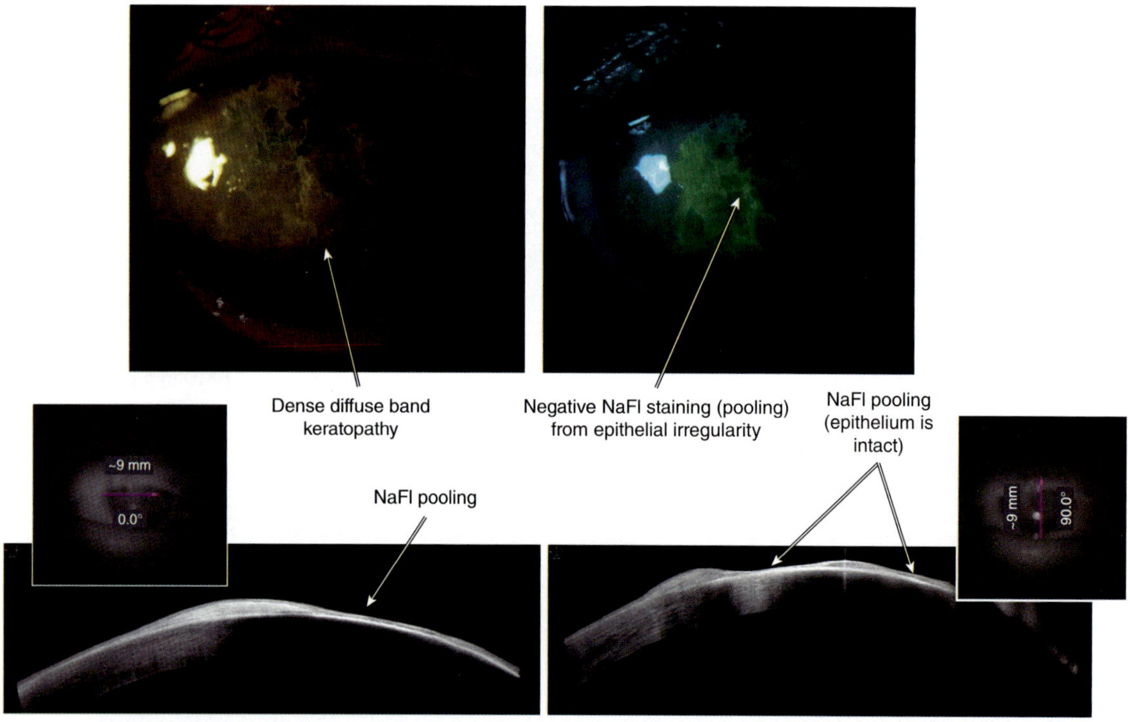

Fig. 5.18 Diffuse band keratopathy with negative staining of fluorescein and intact epithelium.

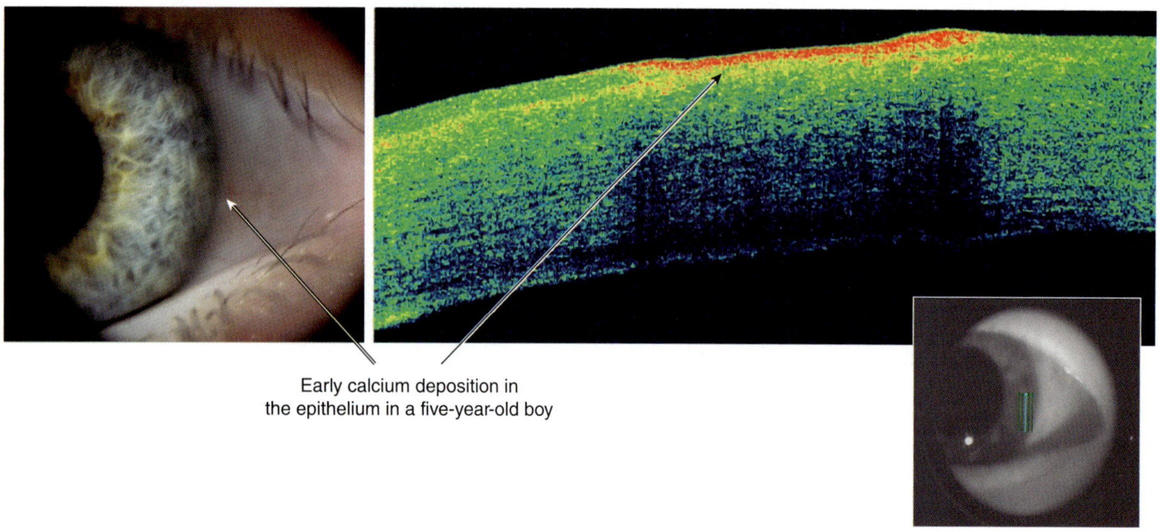

Fig. 5.19 Early band keratopathy. Note the epithelium appears red on AS-OCT due to the calcific changes.

Band keratopathy often is seen intrapalpebrally at the limbus in eyes with low vision or prior trauma; however, the band keratopathy can be quite diffuse and irregular. The patient in Fig. 5.18 had a history of trauma (BB gunshot to the eye) with a subsequent detached retina and low vision. Because the band keratopathy creates an irregular ocular surface, negative staining can be seen with fluorescein. Although the intense fluorescein uptake can be confused with an epithelial defect, AS-OCT clearly shows intact epithelium and confirms this to be fluorescein *pooling* rather than staining. In figure Fig. 5.19, the changes in the epithelium due to calcium deposition at the limbus can be seen in a 5 year-old boy. In the color image, the normal green healthy epithelium looks red due to the calcific changes.

The limbal girdle of Vogt can be considered on the spectrum of band keratopathy. Calcium deposition starts at the limbus nasally and temporally and spreads centrally. It can be seen in healthy eyes with no obvious cause (Fig. 5.20).

CLINICAL PEARL

Similar to many pathologic conditions causing irregularity of the epithelium, band keratopathy can cause confusion when looking at fluorescein staining patterns. AS-OCT can help differentiate between staining from a *true epithelial defect* versus *pooling* of fluorescein. In pooling, the epithelium is clearly seen to be intact on AS-OCT.

III. SALZMANN NODULAR DEGENERATION

Salzmann nodular degeneration (SND) consists of grayish or whitish elevations of the peripheral cornea, normally superior-temporally or superior-nasally. The cause is unknown, but SND is much more

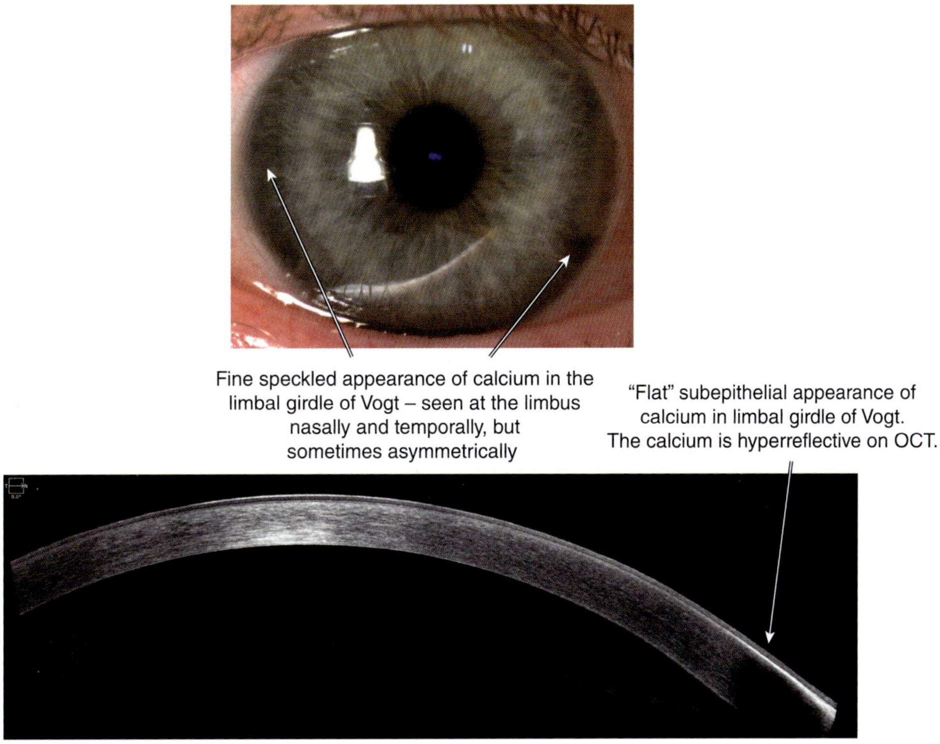

Fig. 5.20 Limbal girdle of Vogt. Limbal girdle of Vogt. Calcific changes appear as focal areas of hyperreflectivity limited to the periphery with a relatively normal appearance of the cornea on AS-OCT.

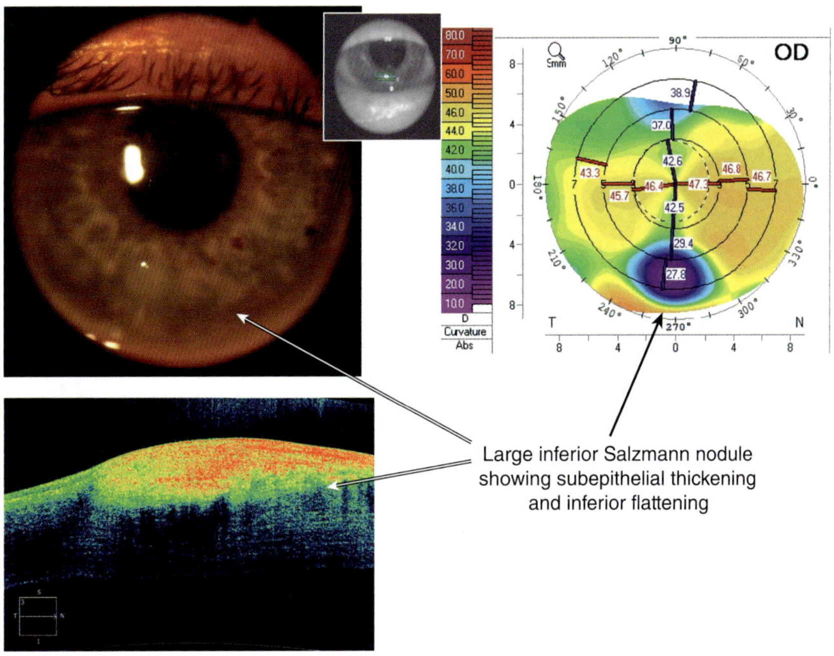

Fig. 5.21 Paracentral Salzmann nodule.

common clinically in women than men and is more common with advancing age. Ocular surface disease (dryness and meibomian gland dysfunction) and contact lens use are common comorbid conditions and are most likely exacerbating factors.

Often SND is asymptomatic and is a common referral to corneal specialists from ophthalmologists and optometrists who may be concerned about a possible ulcer in a new patient given the sometimes large whitish area in the cornea with an abnormal staining pattern. SND can be symptomatic and, when large, can exacerbate the symptoms of ocular surface disease. Patients can report a foreign body sensation, contact lens intolerance, and intermittent blurry vision. As SND enlarges and approaches the visual axis, it can cause irregular astigmatism, which is noted on topography normally with a flattening of the cornea at the site of the nodule and steepening 90 degrees. (Fig. 5.21.)

SND is commonly located superonasally and inferonasally. Normally, treatment consists of maximizing the quality of the ocular surface, as dryness of the cornea and meibomian gland dysfunction are presumed to increase the risk for SND. When not visually significant, surgical removal is not indicated.

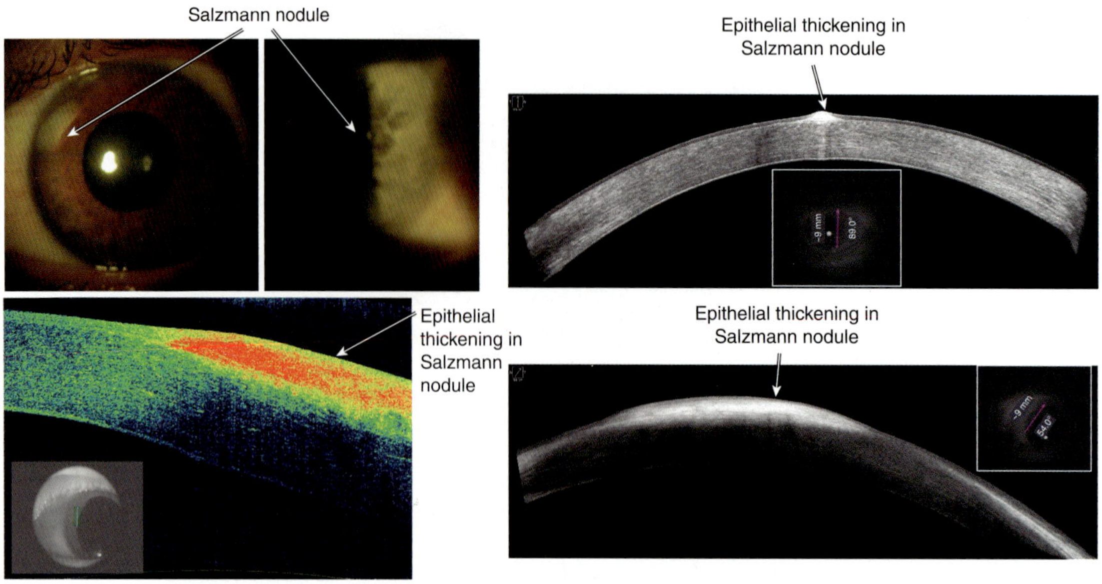

Fig. 5.22 Peripheral and central Salzmann nodules.

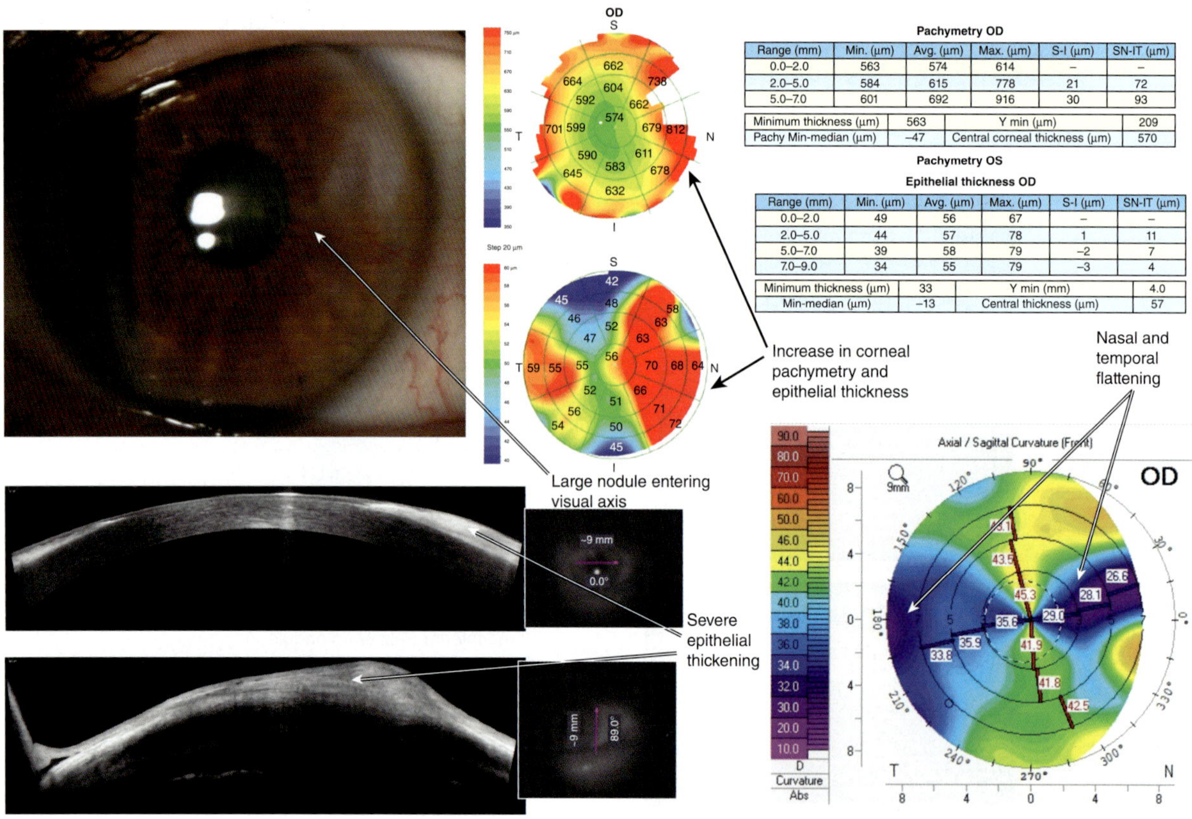

Pachymetry OD

Range (mm)	Min. (μm)	Avg. (μm)	Max. (μm)	S-I (μm)	SN-IT (μm)
0.0–2.0	563	574	614	–	–
2.0–5.0	584	615	778	21	72
5.0–7.0	601	692	916	30	93

Minimum thickness (μm)	563	Y min (μm)	209
Pachy Min-median (μm)	–47	Central corneal thickness (μm)	570

Pachymetry OS

Epithelial thickness OD

Range (mm)	Min. (μm)	Avg. (μm)	Max. (μm)	S-I (μm)	SN-IT (μm)
0.0–2.0	49	56	67	–	–
2.0–5.0	44	57	78	1	11
5.0–7.0	39	58	79	–2	7
7.0–9.0	34	55	79	–3	4

Minimum thickness (μm)	33	Y min (mm)	4.0
Min-median (μm)	–13	Central thickness (μm)	57

Fig. 5.23 Large peripheral Salzmann nodule entering visual axis.

SND also can occur centrally and can be due to contact lens overwear, especially tight RGP lenses. When these nodules appear centrally in contact lens wearers, they can cause discomfort and can be easily removed at the slit-lamp (Fig. 5.22).

When Salzmann nodules extend adjacent to or into the visual axis, vision can be distorted. Improvement in vision with RGP lenses is suggestive that the nodule is creating irregular astigmatism and is the cause of decreased vision. This is especially important to consider in patients with SND lesions with concurrent visually significant cataract. Nodules can be removed at the slit-lamp or in the operating room (Fig. 5.23).

At one week after removal of the nodule, the epithelium appears normalized (Fig. 5.24).

IV. REIS-BÜCKLERS DYSTROPHY

Reis-Bücklers dystrophy is not commonly seen clinically but is a well-described degeneration of the epithelium and Bowman membrane. Bowman's membrane develops idiopathic changes causing corneal cloudiness and recurrent erosions. Treatment

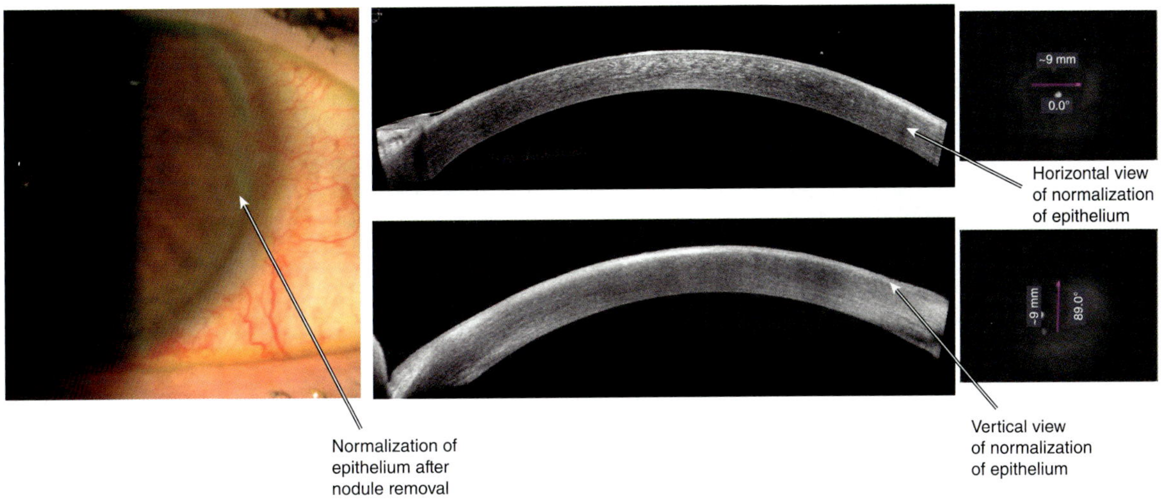

Fig. 5.24 After nodule removal.

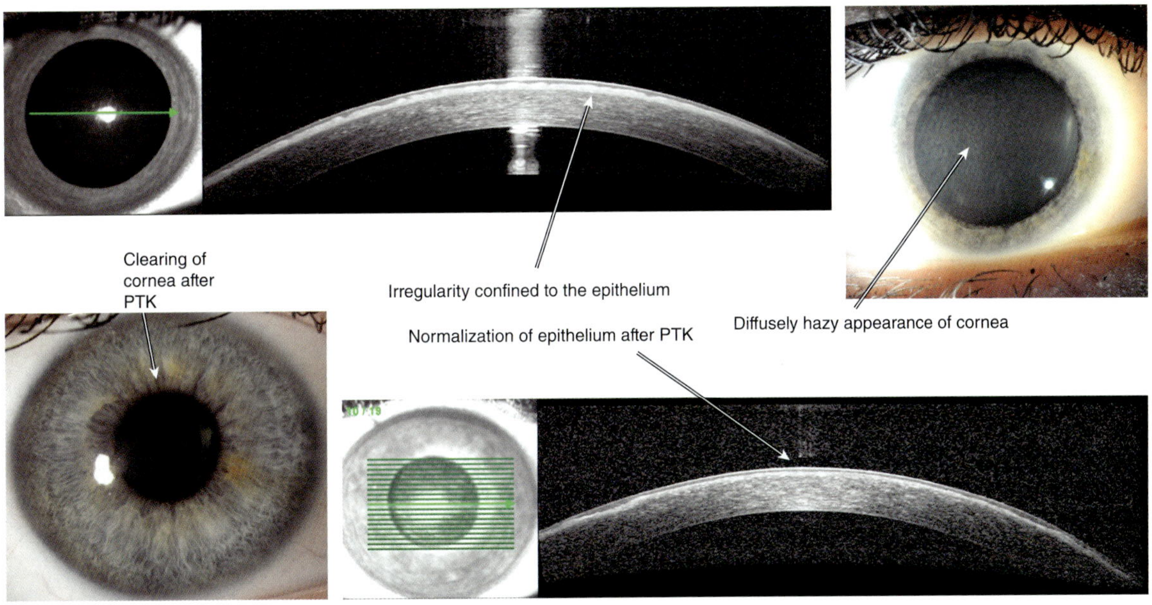

Fig. 5.25 Reis-Bücklers before and after phototherapeutic keratectomy (PTK).

includes superficial keratectomy or PTK. Reis-Bücklers exists along a spectrum of autosomal dominant corneal dystrophies caused by mutations in the transforming growth factor, β, (TGF-β_1) gene. PTK and superficial keratectomy at the slit-lamp with diamond burr polishing are both treatment options. (Fig. 5.25) shows the diffuse haziness of the cornea on slit lamp photography, and the AS-OCT demonstrates that the pathology is confined to the epithelium and Bowman's membrane. Normalization of the epithelium after PTK can be seen on the AS-OCT image.

V. PERIPHERAL ULCERATIVE KERATITIS

Peripheral ulcerative keratitis (PUK) is an inflammatory condition, sometimes with a systemic cause, such as an autoimmune condition PUK can be mild with minimal stromal thinning or can progress to advanced stromal thinning and, while rare, corneal perforation. Treatment includes topical anti-inflammatories, oral steroids, amniotic membrane transplantation, conjunctival resection, and, in cases of perforation, crescentic corneal transplantation (Fig. 5.26).

Amniotic membrane can be placed on the cornea in cases of PUK to decrease inflammation and enhance epithelialization (Fig. 5.27).

VI. STAPHYLOCOCCAL MARGINAL KERATITIS

Staphylococcal marginal keratitis (often called Staph marginal) is commonly seen in patients with meibomian gland dysfunction and causes stromal inflammation, typically appearing as an irregular whitish lesion near the limbus, often at the lid margins. Often the epithelium is intact but irregular, and negative staining of fluorescein is noted at the slit-lamp. Sometimes, there are small areas of complete epithelial defects. Staphylococcal marginal keratitis is not thought to be due primarily to an infectious cause but likely occurs as inflammation secondary to bacterial overgrowth of the eyelids in blepharitis. Treatment consists of therapy for meibomian gland dysfunction and topical combination steroid/antibiotic drops and ointments. While the appearance of staph marginal keratitis at the slit lamp can mimic a limbal corneal bacterial keratitis (corneal ulcer) with a frank epithelial defect, the AS-OCT can

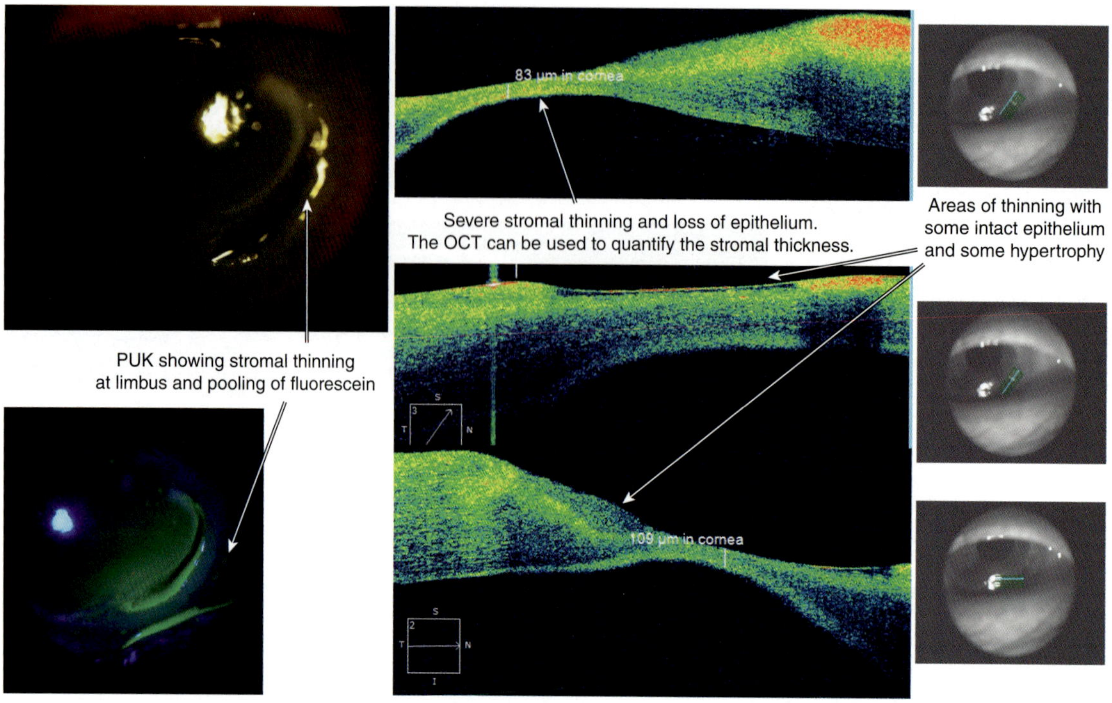

Fig. 5.26 Peripheral ulcerative keratitis.

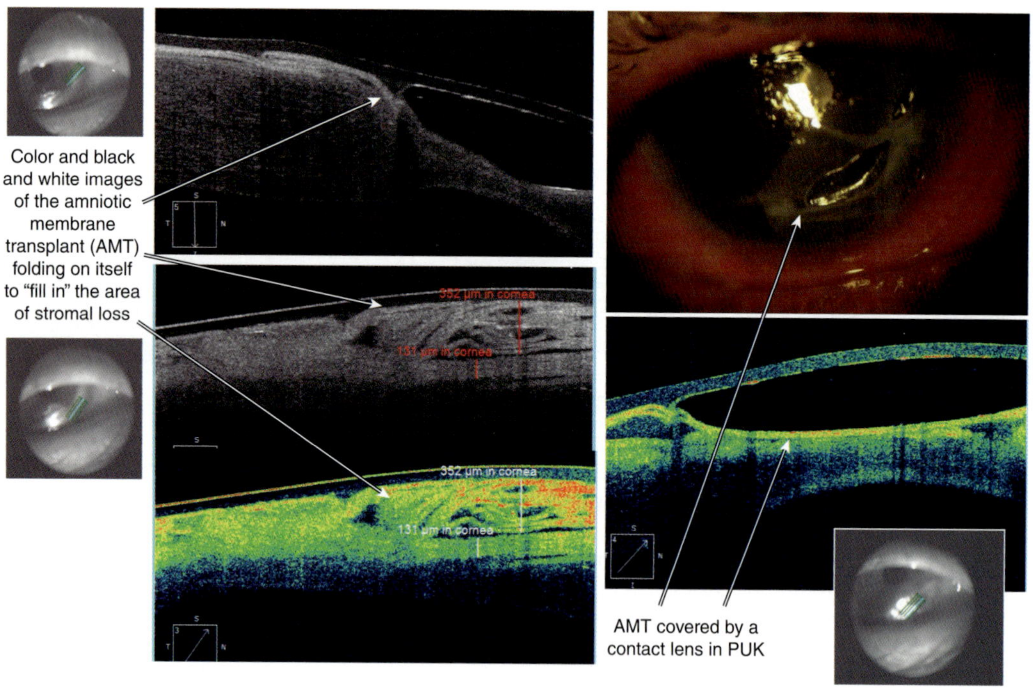

Fig. 5.27 PUK with amniotic membrane.

be used to image the area and verify often intact epithelium with stromal thickening (rather than thinning), allowing the clinician to differentiate the two entities (Fig. 5.28).

CLINICAL PEARL

AS-OCT can be very helpful in differentiating between infectious infiltrates with true epithelial defects and areas of stromal inflammation with mostly intact epithelium.

VII. EPITHELIAL HYPERTROPHY

After stromal loss, whether the result of trauma, infection, or inflammation, the corneal epithelium will often undergo hypertrophy to replace the lost corneal stroma. The patient in Fig. 5.29 had a corneal trauma years earlier, and the AS-OCT shows the extent of the epithelial hypertrophy. The epithelium can sometimes be better visualized in black and white than in color, as seen in the composite image.

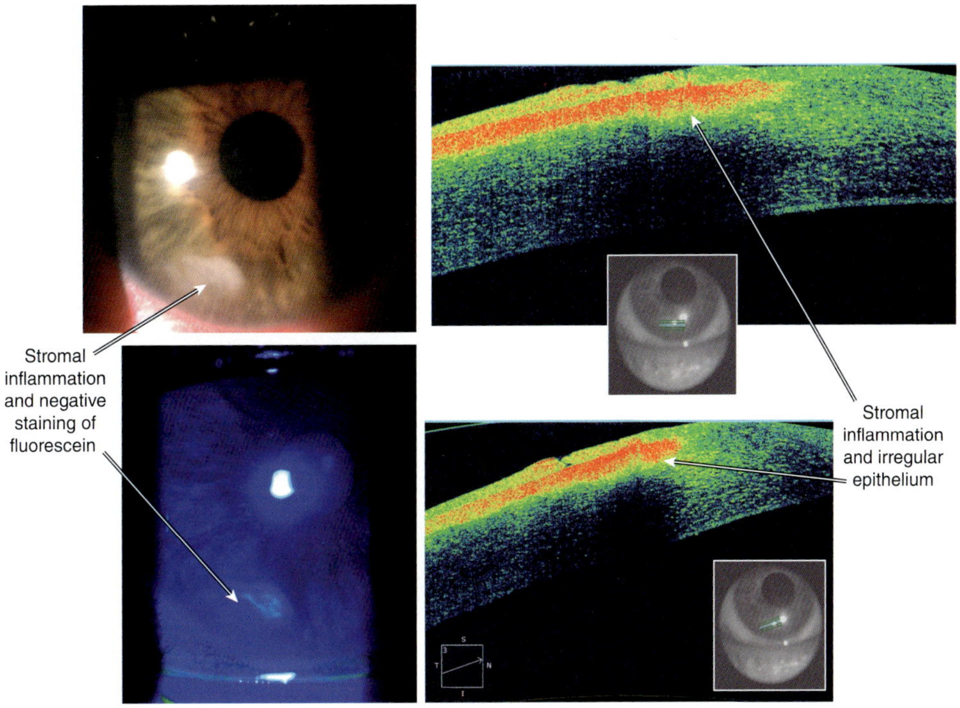

Fig. 5.28 Staphylococcal marginal keratitis.

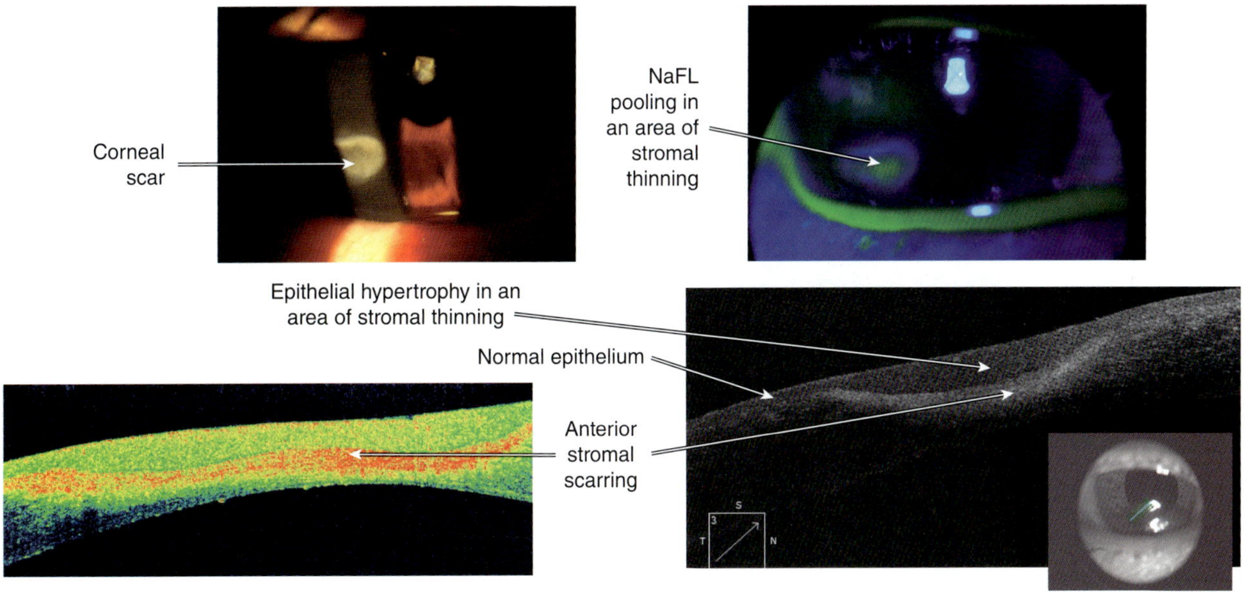

Fig. 5.29 Stromal scarring and epithelial hypertrophy after stromal loss.

VIII. SUPERFICIAL PUNCTATE KERATOPATHY OR PUNCTATE EPITHELIAL EROSIONS

Superficial punctate keratopathy (SPK) can be caused by any process that damages the epithelium. Ocular surface disease (dry eye) is certainly a common cause of SPK, but overuse of preserved medications and toxic injury to the ocular surface are also known causes. AS-OCT shows the partial loss of the central epithelium and intact superficial epithelium, which appears as the classic slit-lamp appearance of SPK with fluorescein (see Fig. 5.30).

IX. CONTACT LENS OVERWEAR, HYPOXIA, AND CONTACT LENS ASSOCIATED RED EYE (CLARE)

Contact lens use, either in standard hydrogel or silicone hydrogel material, especially in the setting of a dry ocular surface or overnight contact lens wear, can lead to corneal hypoxia and inflammation. The clinical appearance of contact lens overwear is typically located in the peripheral cornea near the limbus, is round and can be quite dense, and often has surrounding corneal inflammation. Often there can be an intense uptake of

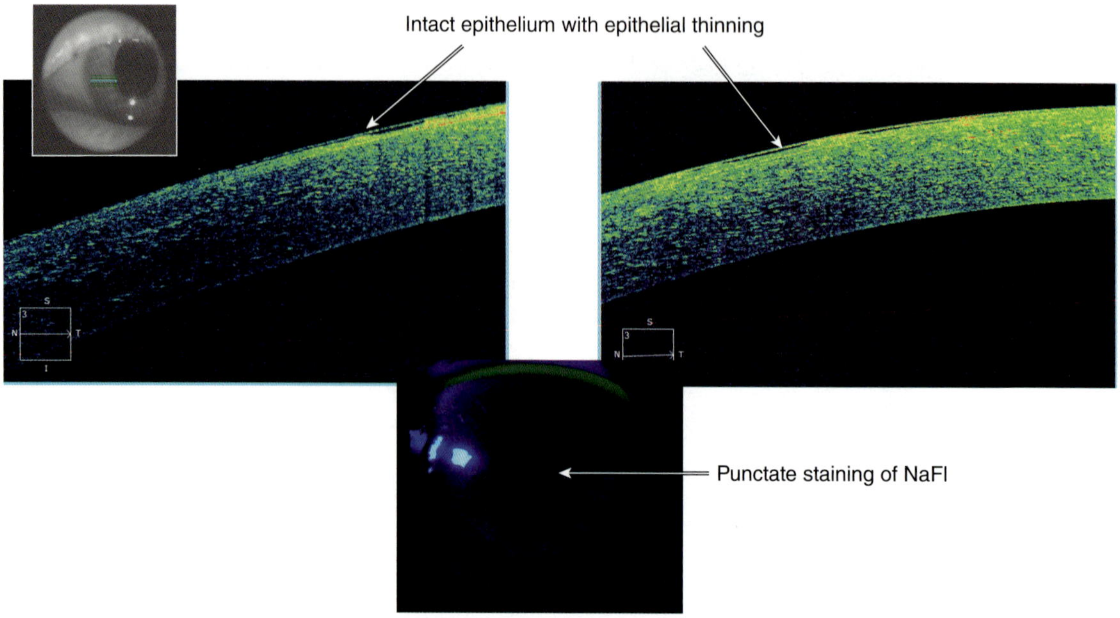

Fig. 5.30 Superficial punctate keratopathy.

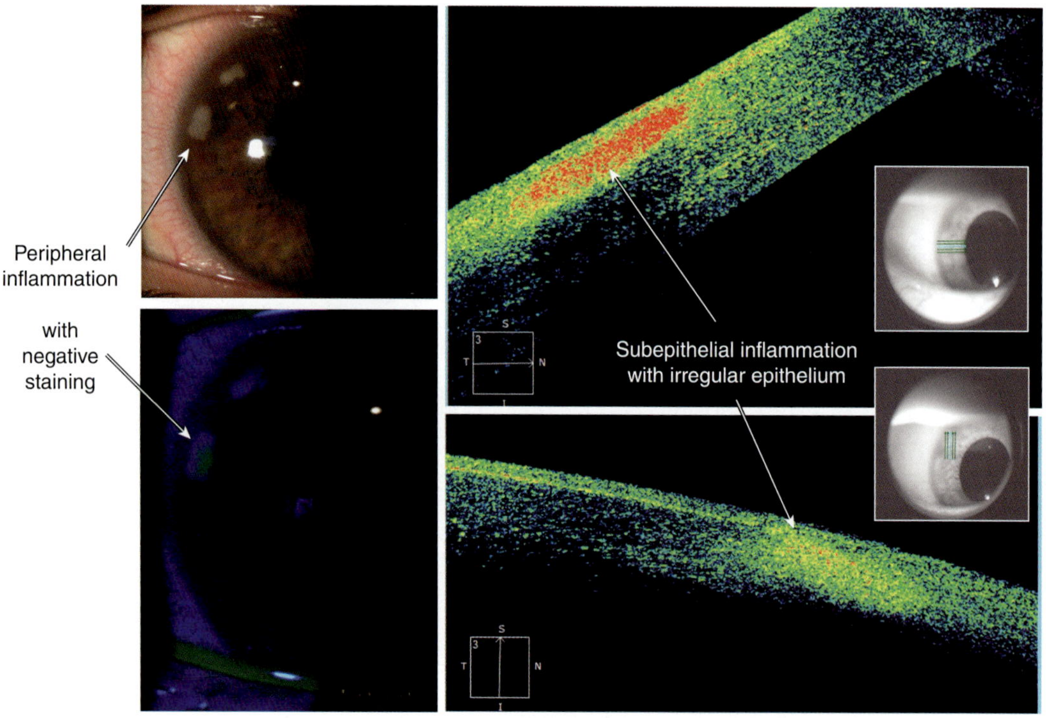

Fig. 5.31 Contact lens overwear.

fluorescein, but normally there is negative staining because of the presence of a mostly intact epithelium. Often, these patients will have small peripheral faint, round stromal scars indicative of prior episodes of contact lens overwear. AS-OCT is an excellent modality to differentiate between a true infectious keratitis, with a frank epithelial defect, as opposed to contact lens overwear, which will have a mostly intact epithelium (Fig. 5.31).

Sometimes, changing from the color image to black and white on AS-OCT can help delineate the contours of the epithelium in the setting of underlying inflammation (Fig. 5.32).

Hypoxia from contact lens use can also appear as small circular, clear areas of the epithelium with negative staining; these areas will have a bright punctate pattern with fluorescein. On AS-OCT, small areas of epithelial loss in an otherwise intact epithelium can be clearly seen in Fig. 5.32. The patient in Fig. 5.33 had an epithelial debridement for a Salzmann nodule and had been wearing a bandage soft contact lens for one week. The punctate pattern is common after extended contact lens use and is not clinically concerning.

In a patient with underlying dry eye and ocular surface disease, the epithelial changes induced by contact lens overwear are clearly seen on white light during slit lamp exam and fluoroscein staining. AS-OCT shows *hyperreflective areas* corresponding to inflammation of the epithelium and *hyporeflective*

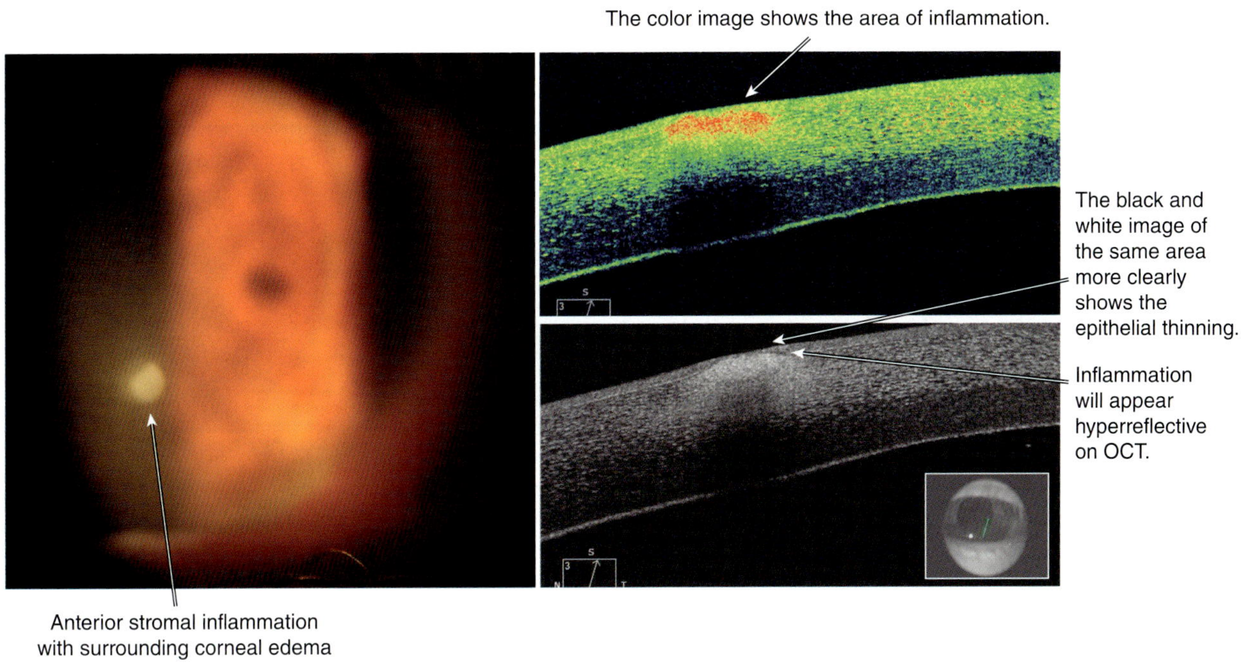

Fig. 5.32 Contact lens overwear with corneal edema.

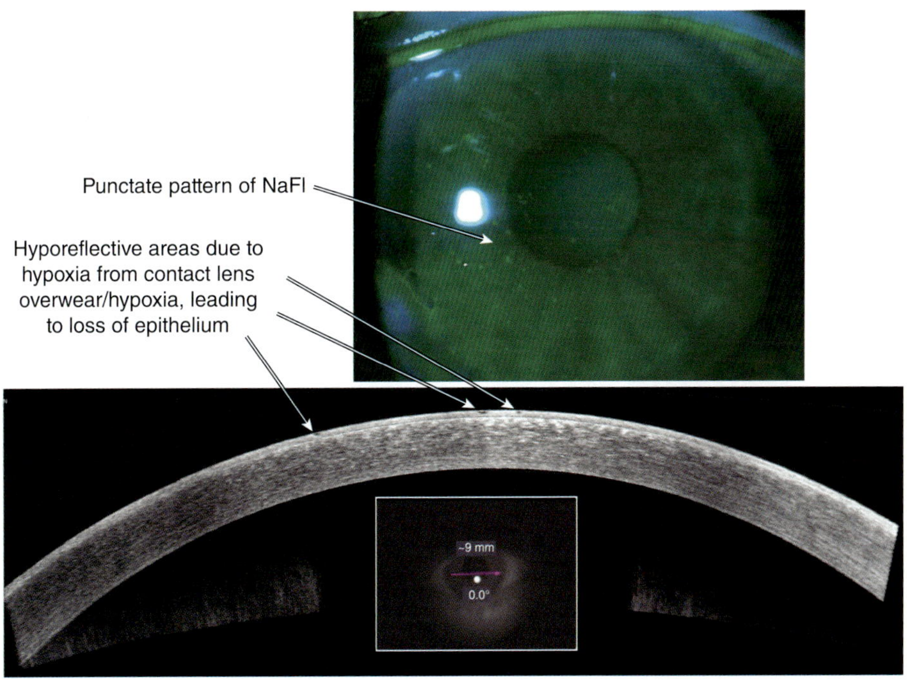

Fig. 5.33 Punctate staining from hypoxia from a bandage contact lens.

areas as a result of cell death/loss of the most superficial layers of the epithelium (Fig. 5.34).

CLINICAL PEARL

In the setting of contact lens–related corneal changes, bacterial keratitis is always on the differential diagnosis. AS-OCT can be helpful in the diagnosis of contact lens overwear versus infectious causes. In cases of inflammation due to contact lens overwear or hypoxia, stromal inflammation and intact epithelium will be seen on AS-OCT while loss of the epithelium (the corneal ulcer) and sometimes stromal loss can be seen in infectious keratitis, In the acute phase of infectious keratitis, the stromal loss can be difficult to appreciate due to corneal edema and inflammation.

X. DELLEN

Dellen are areas of depression in the peripheral corneal epithelium and stroma and are formed because of localized elevations of the surrounding ocular surface, such as conjunctival chemosis, subconjunctival hemorrhage, or a high-filter bleb. Relative dryness of the cornea as a result of the localized elevation of the surrounding conjunctiva causes dehydration of the stromal and thinning of the epithelium. The condensation of the stroma and the intact epithelium can be seen on AS-OCT. Although there can be significant fluorescein uptake, AS-OCT clearly shows that the epithelium is intact; this is pooling of fluorescein, rather than the staining seen in a true epithelial defect (Fig. 5.35).

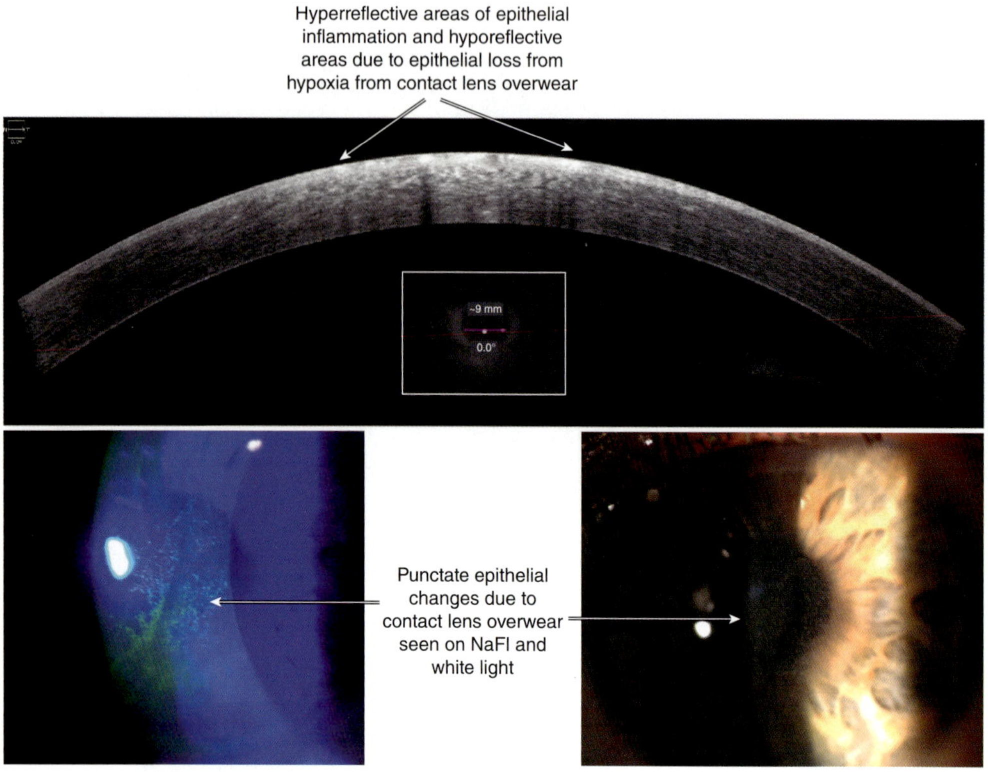

Fig. 5.34 Punctate staining from hypoxia from contact lens overwear.

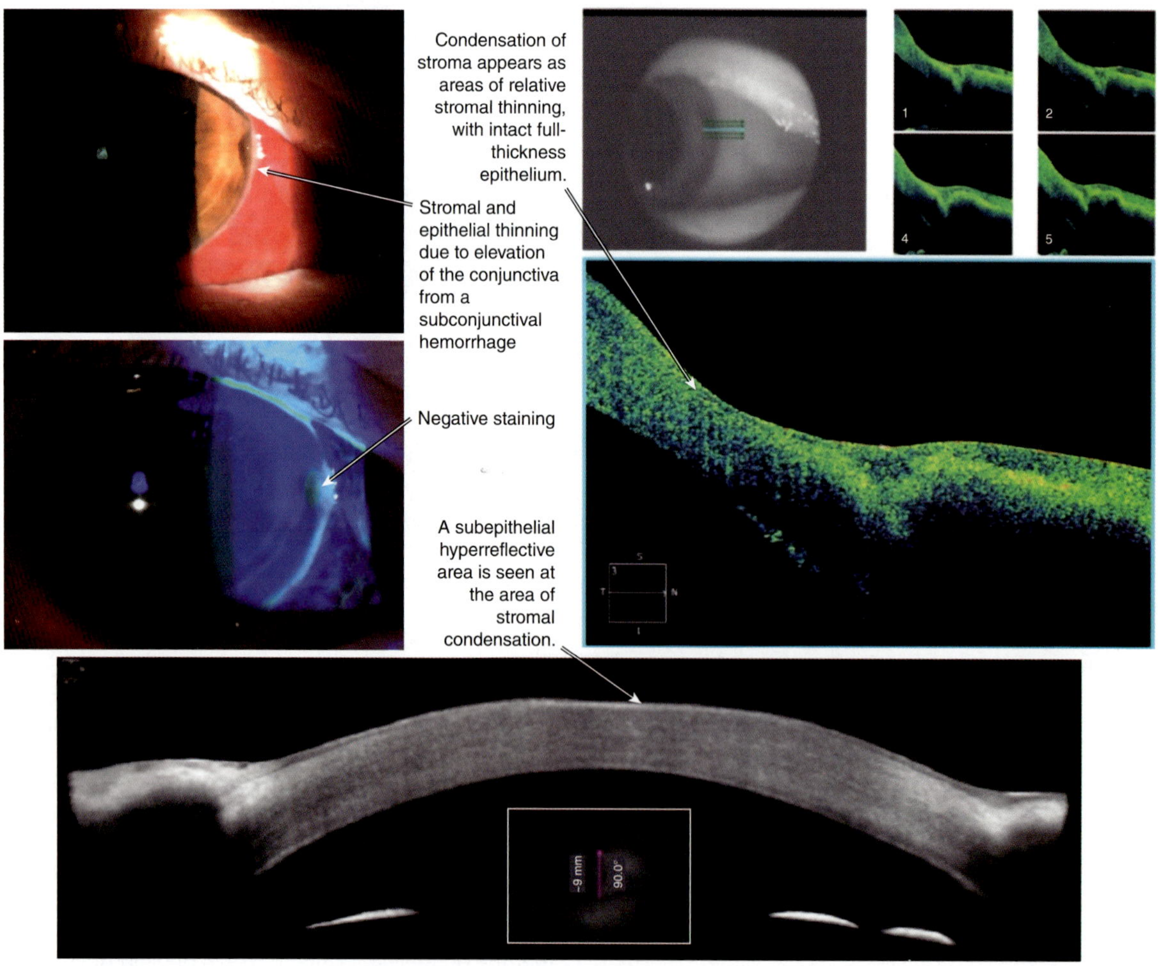

Fig. 5.35 Appearance of dellen on slit-lamp exam and AS-OCT. AS-OCT demonstrates that the overlying epithelium is intact.

XI. DENDRITES VERSUS PSEUDODENDRITES

One of the most common epithelial changes is due to herpes simplex virus keratitis HSV), and often classic corneal dendrites can be seen clinically while herpes zoster virus keratitis (HZV) sometimes can present with "pseudo-dendrites." HSV, when seen early, will cause very subtle epithelial changes, often in the classic branching, dendritic pattern. The patient in Figs. 5.36 and 5.39, is a contact lens wearer who reported discomfort, and epithelial changes are seen consistent with dendritic keratitis. The AS-OCT image in figure 5.36 shows thinning of the epithelium in the area of the early dendrite. On the next day (Fig. 5.37),

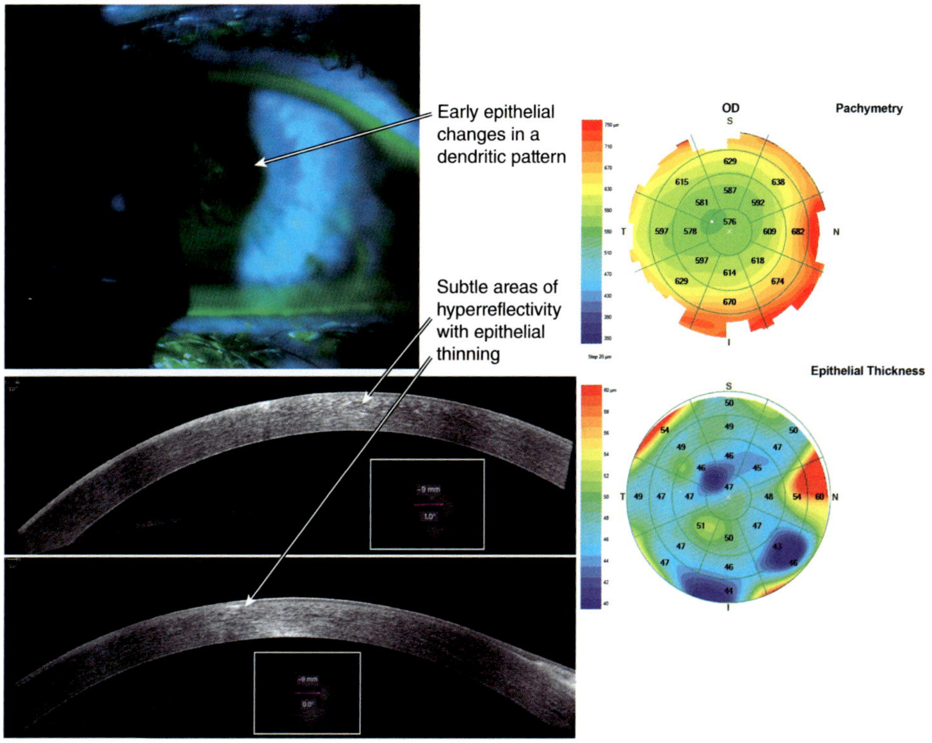

Fig. 5.36 HSV dendrite, day one.

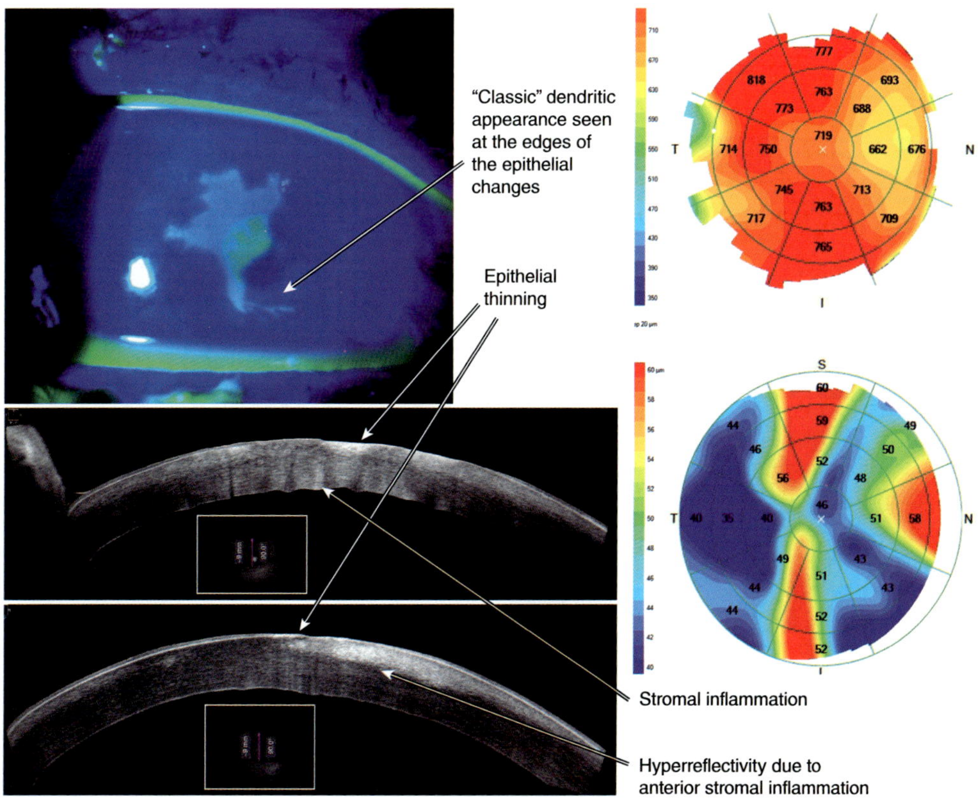

Fig. 5.37 HSV dendrite, day two.

a more classic dendrite is seen, and further thinning of the epithelium is noted with stromal edema and hyperreflectivity on AS-OCT secondary to anterior stromal inflammation.

However, the epithelial changes seen in herpes zoster, although still having a dendritic appearance, will show *thickening* rather than thinning. The thickening of the epithelium creates the classic pseudodendrite with negative staining on the most elevated area of the epithelium and pooling of fluoroscein in the areas of relative thinning. AS-OCT shows this epithelial thickening (Fig. 5.38).

XII. CORNEAL EPITHELIAL DEFECTS

Trauma to the epithelium can occur and cause a partial- or full-thickness loss of the epithelium. The loss of the epithelium in an epithelial defect can be clearly seen on AS-OCT, and the Bowman's Layer often appears hyperreflective. The epithelial defect often appears to be full thickness clinically; however, on AS-OCT, variations can be seen, with some layers of the epithelium still intact.

Fig. 5.39 shows a linear epithelial defect in a patient with prior LASIK who was poked in the eye by his son. AS-OCT also can show inflammation at the level of the flap when present

Fig. 5.40 shows image from a patient who poked herself in the eye with a hairbrush. The epithelium appears irregular at the edges; on AS-OCT, there is thickening of the epithelium, and loss of epithelium is seen on AS-OCT corresponding with the positive staining on slit-lamp exam. Although this patient had been examined in the past and no EBMD had been seen, it was later noted that she had an occult underlying EBMD. Of note, both of these images (Figs. 5.39 and 5.40) show positive staining of fluorescein with sharp borders of the epithelial defect.

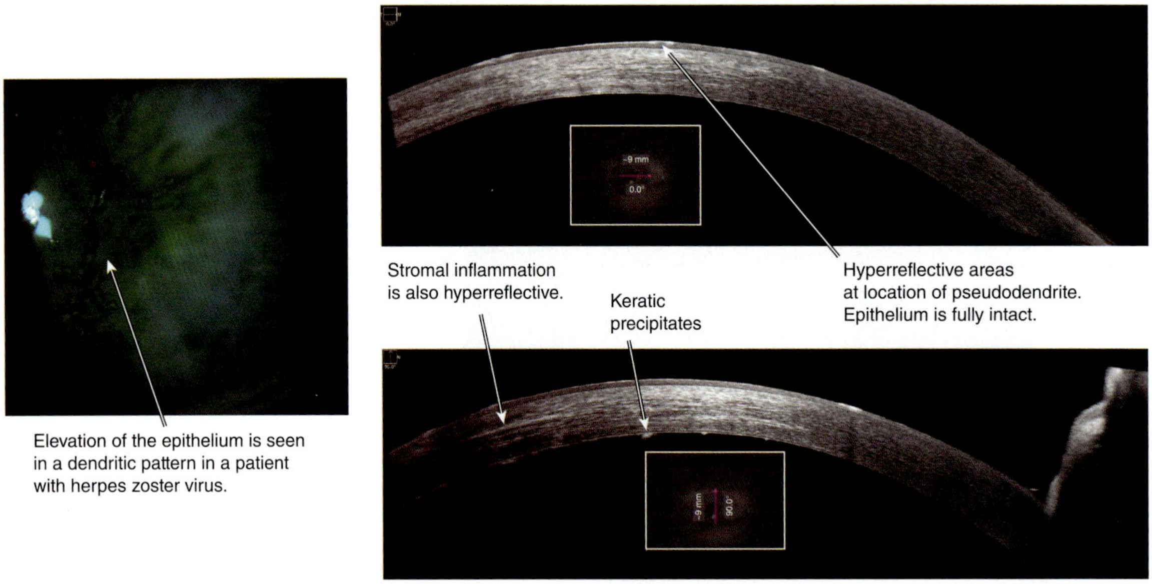

Fig. 5.38 Pseudodendrite.

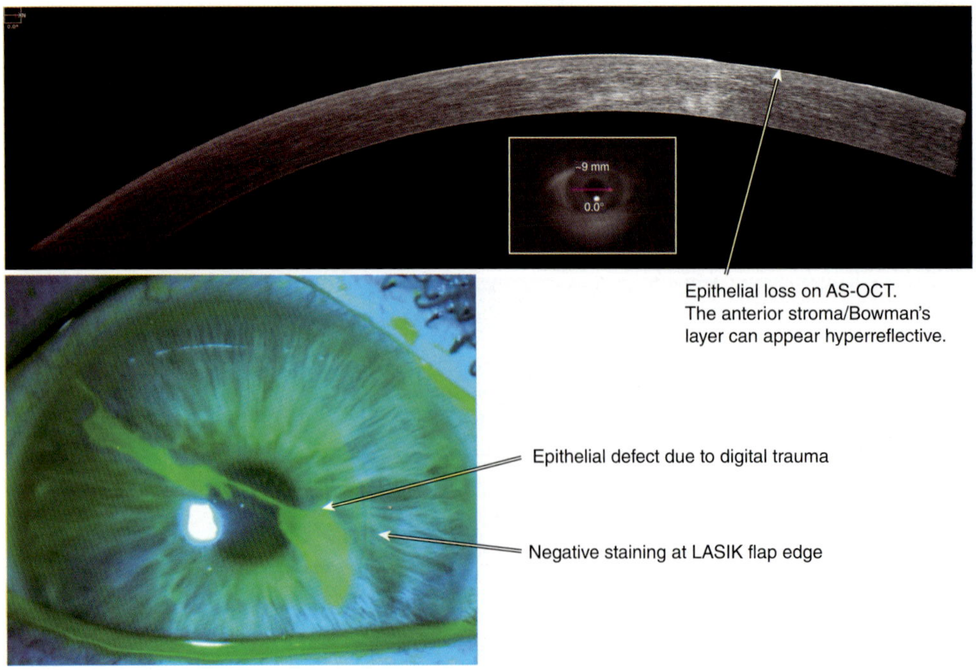

Fig. 5.39 Epithelial defect in a patient with prior LASIK.

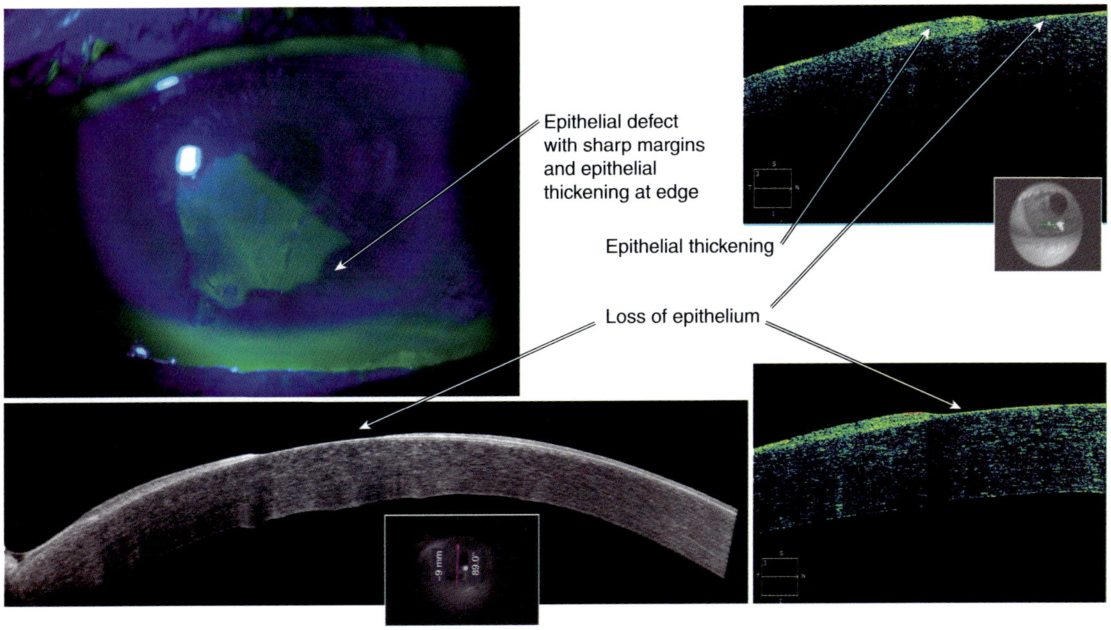

Fig. 5.40 Epithelial defect in a patient with occult EBMD.

> **CLINICAL PEARL**
>
> Healthy epithelium is hard to remove and is strongly adherent to the underlying Bowman's membrane. Clinical suspicion should be high for an underlying pathologic condition in a patient with an epithelial defect, especially recurrent ones.

In unhealthy corneas, especially with prior herpetic keratitis, the cornea can have reduced sensation and a neurotrophic "ulcer" can be seen. (The authors prefer the term *neurotrophic epithelial defect* to distinguish this clinical entity from infectious keratitis, in which the term *ulcer* is often used.) The epithelial defect is often round or oval with rounded edges. On AS-OCT, the cornea often appears unhealthy, and stromal loss from prior inflammatory episodes can be seen; keratic precipitates can be seen if there is active inflammation. The epithelium can be hypertrophied in some places and thin in others. Treatment is focused on encouraging healing of the unhealthy epithelium. Interestingly, despite the sharp margins with rounded edges seen clinically, a neurotrophic defect on AS-OCT does not always show a discrete demarcation between intact epithelium and the epithelial defect. In fact, the epithelium can be seen to be partially intact, and there is variable thickness of the epithelium in contrast to a traditional epithelial defect in which the epithelium is normally completely absent from the Bowman membrane (Fig. 5.41).

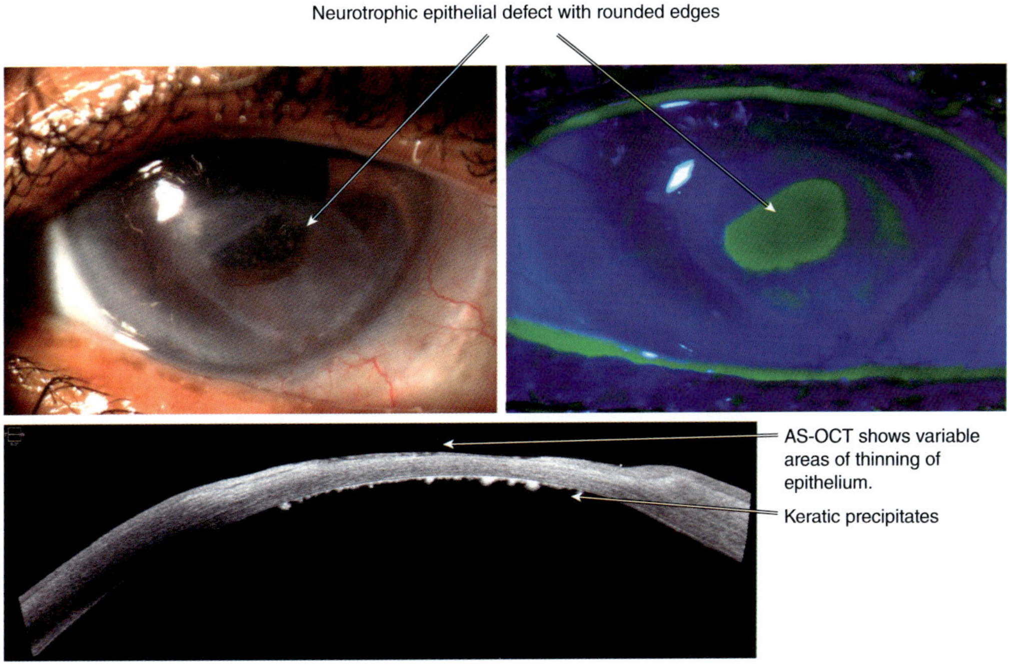

Fig. 5.41 Neurotrophic epithelial defect.

Amniotic membrane is an excellent modality to encourage resolution of slow-healing neurotrophic epithelial defects; amniotic membrane is well visualized on AS-OCT (Fig. 5.42).

XIII. CORNEAL EPITHELIAL BULLAE

Regardless of etiology, corneal edema can cause fluid to separate the epithelium from the anterior stroma (bulla). The fluid will appear hyporeflective on AS-OCT, and the epithelium can clearly be seen separated from the hyperreflective Bowman's Layer. On slit-lamp examination, negative staining can be seen, but the epithelium is clearly intact but loose. Sometimes, taking an image with the "five-line raster function" is also useful because it allows a view of five images at once and also provides a more magnified view of the corneal pathologic conditions. The color five-line raster images more closely show the fluid-filled bullae and the endothelial pathologic conditions (Fig. 5.43).

XIV. ANTERIOR STROMAL PUNCTURE

In cases of EBMD or other conditions with loose epithelium, such as corneal edema, one classic therapy has been to use a thin-gauge needle to penetrate the anterior stroma and cause scarring; this allows the epithelium to better adhere to the Bowman membrane. The scarring from anterior stromal puncture is punctate and hyperreflective on AS-OCT (Fig. 5.44).

XV. THYGESON SUPERFICIAL PUNCTATE KERATITIS

Thygeson superficial punctate keratitis (TSPK) is a commonly discussed but uncommonly seen condition in which grayish to whitish opacities are seen intraepithelially. No epithelial or stromal edema is noted, and this has been described mostly in younger people. Symptoms include tearing, extreme photophobia, a foreign body feeling, pain, and blurry

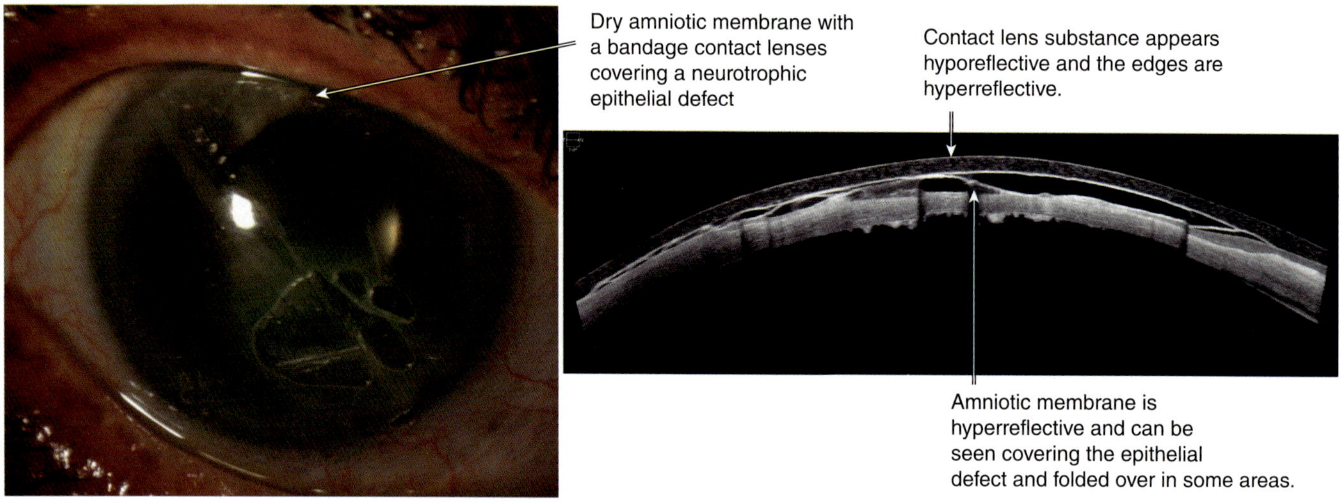

Fig. 5.42 Neurotrophic epithelial defect with amniotic membrane and bandage contact lens.

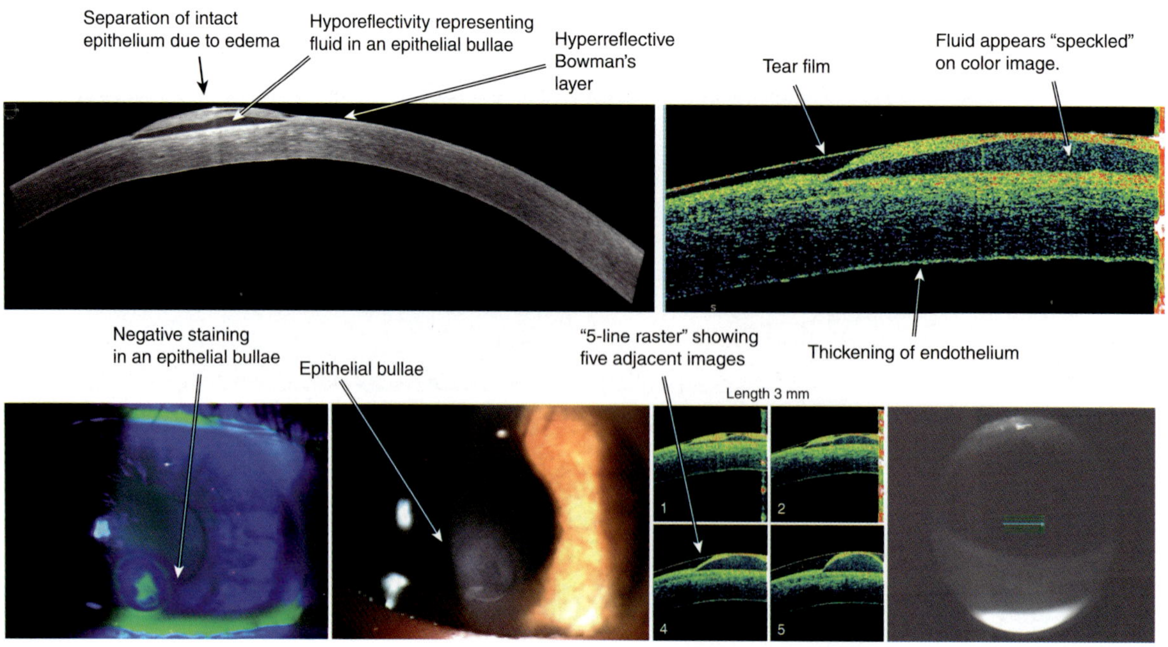

Fig. 5.43 Epithelial bullae.

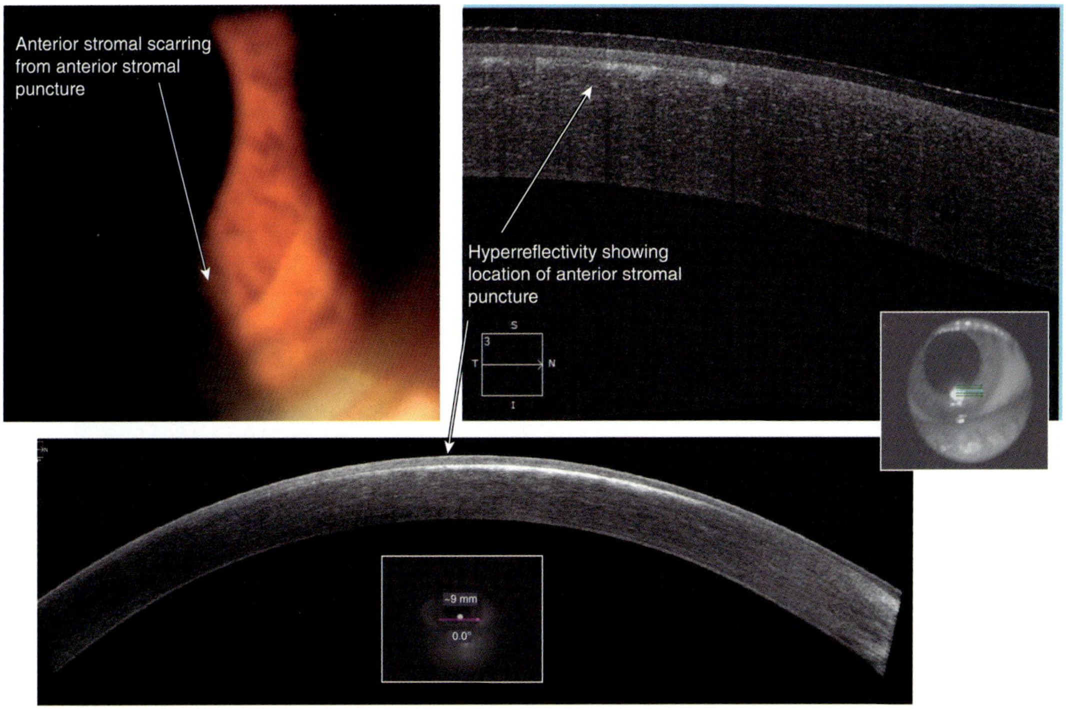

Fig. 5.44 Anterior stromal puncture.

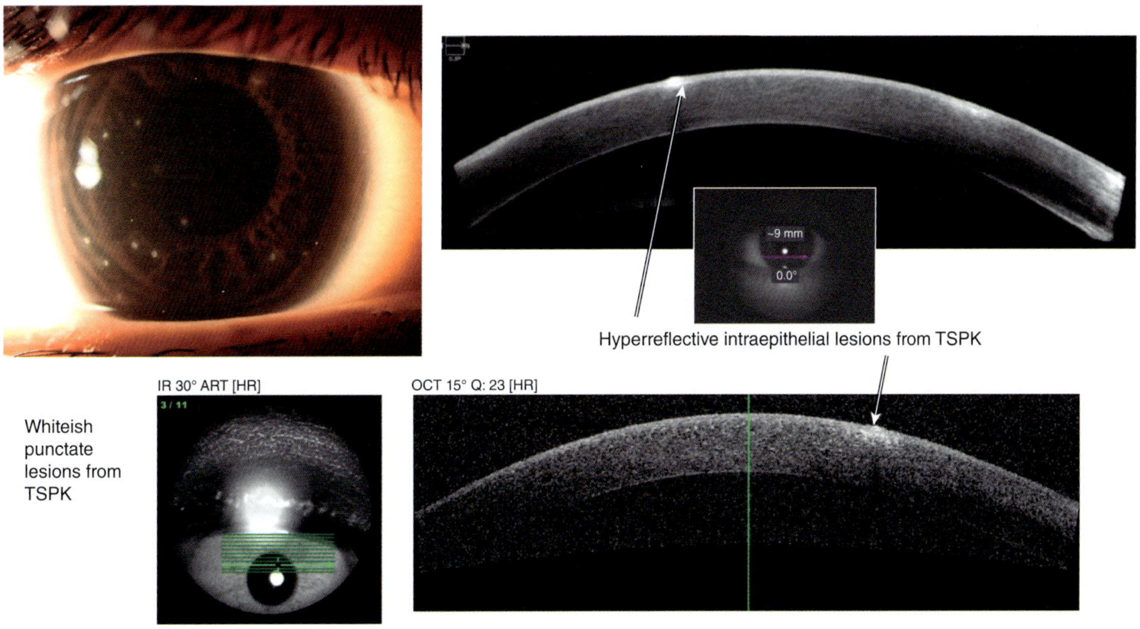

Fig. 5.45 Thygeson superficial punctate keratitis.

vision. TSPK will have negative fluorescein staining on slit-lamp examination. On AS-OCT, the hyperreflective lesions are clearly intraepithelial (Fig. 5.45).

XVI. HORNERS-TRANTAS DOTS

Horners-Trantas dots are indicative of an allergic response in the conjunctiva and are often seen in limbal-vernal keratoconjunctivitis, but they can be seen in atopic conjunctivitis as well. These elevated areas at the limbus are often "jelly-like" in appearance, are gray to whitish, will have negative fluorescein staining, and are thought to be collections of eosinophils. On AS-OCT, Horners-Trantas dots are easily seen as intraepithelial lesions with elevation of the epithelium (Fig. 5.46).

XVII. LISCH EPITHELIAL CORNEAL DYSTROPHY

Lisch epithelial corneal dystrophy (LECD) is an extremely rare dystrophy that primarily affects the corneal epithelium. Classic findings include gray-whorled or feathery-shaped lesions with a finger-like shape extending from the peripheral limbus into the central cornea. Patients usually present with gradually worsening vision without a history of epithelial erosions. The lesions are dense collections of intraepithelial microcysts that are best seen on retro-illumination with a dilated pupil. Notably, the LECD lesions do not stain with fluorescein. On AS-OCT, the epithelium demonstrates a prominent, focal hyperreflectivity of normal-thickness epithelium without the involvement of the underlying corneal layers. Inversion of colors (using a white background) on AS-OCT (an option on some devices) helps to better characterize the area of affected epithelium. Treatment options are limited and variable in the reported literature, ranging from visual rehabilitation with glasses/contact lenses, epitheliectomy with cauterization of the limbal origin of the lesion, and PTK with or without the use of mitomycin-c (Fig. 5.47).

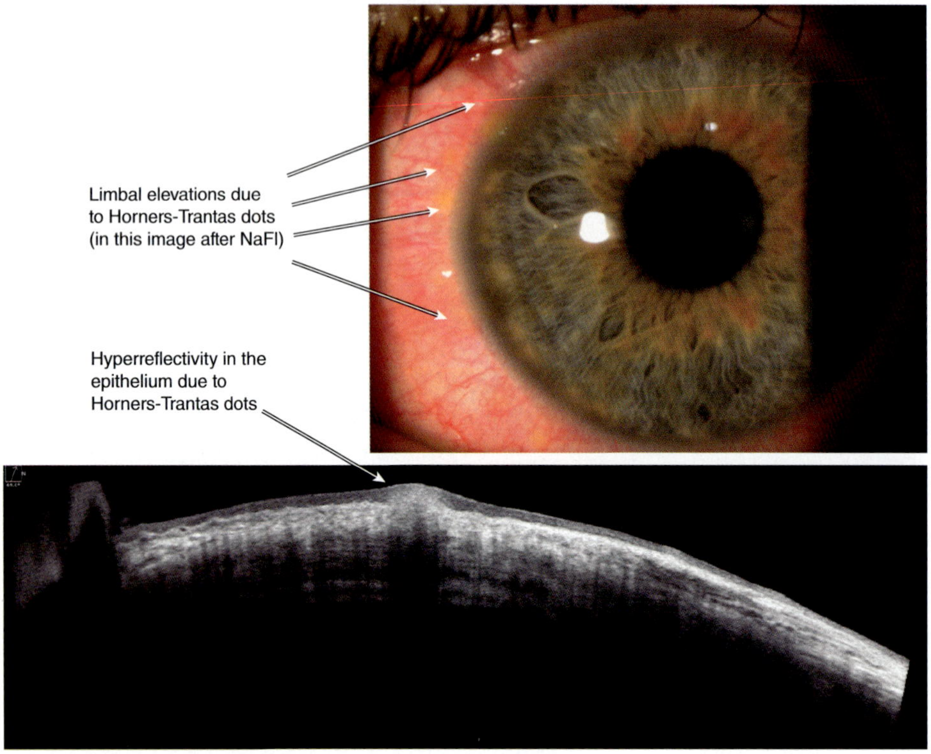

Fig. 5.46 Appearance Horners-Trantas dots on slit-lamp exam and AS-OCT.

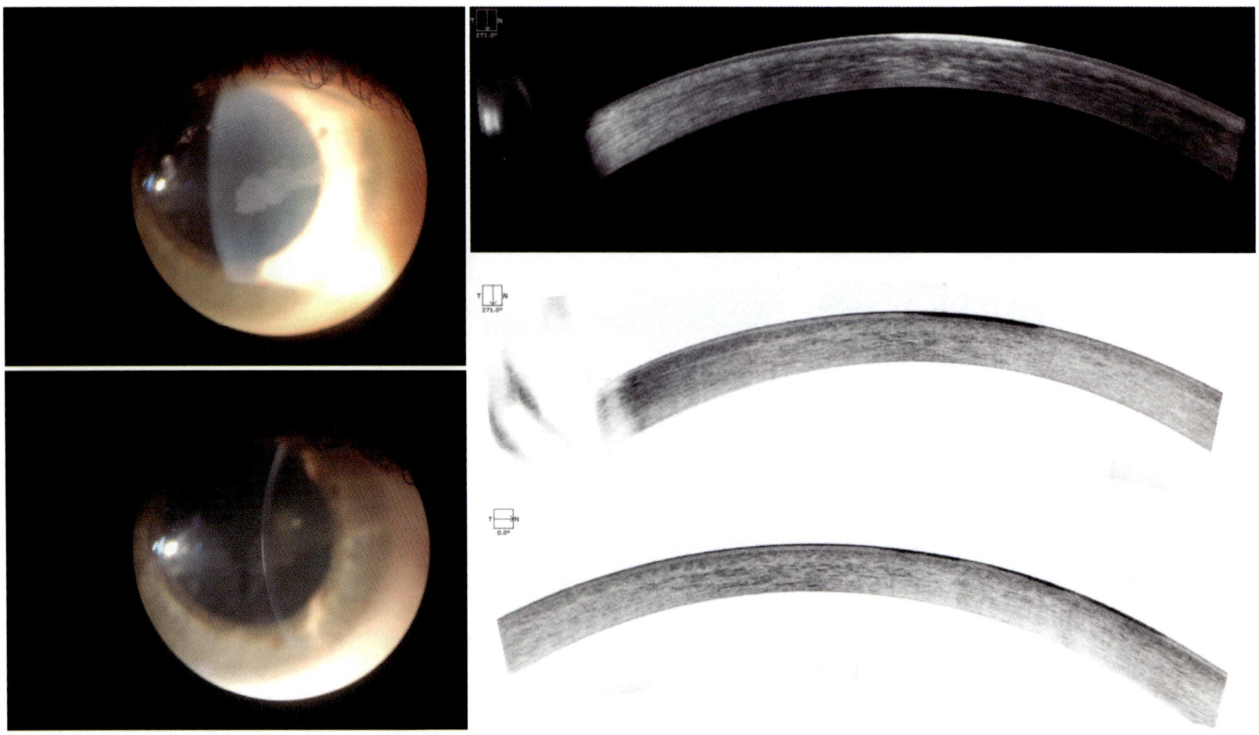

Fig. 5.47 Lisch epithelial corneal dystrophy. *(Photograph courtesy Adam Moss, MD, McCannel Eye Clinic and University of Minnesota, Minneapolis, Minnesota, United States.)* (Courtesy Dr. Adam Moss.)

BIBLIOGRAPHY

Cogan DG, Donaldson DD, Kuwabara T, Marshall D. Microcystic dystrophy of the corneal epithelium. *Trans Am Ophthalmol Soc*. 1964;63:213.

Diez-Feijóo E, Durán JA. Optical coherence tomography findings in recurrent corneal erosion syndrome. *Cornea*. 2015;34(3):290-295.

Ficker L, Seal D, Wright P. Staphylococcal infection and the limbus: study of the cell-mediated immune response. *Eye (Lond)*. 1989; 3(Pt 2):190-193.

Graue-Hernández EO, Mannis MJ, Eliasieh K, et al. Salzmann nodular degeneration. *Cornea*. 2010;29(3):283-289.

Gupta Y, Kishore A, Kumari P, et al. Peripheral ulcerative keratitis. *Surv Ophthalmol*. 2021;66(6):977-998.

Ho L, Jalbert I, Watt K, Hui A. Current understanding and therapeutic management of contact lens associated sterile corneal infiltrates and microbial keratitis. *Clin Exp Optom*. 2021;104(3):323-333.

Jhanji V, Rapuano CJ, Vajpayee RB. Corneal calcific band keratopathy. *Curr Opin Ophthalmol*. 2011;22(4):283-289.

Krachmer MA. Cornea. In: Krachmer MA, eds. *Cornea*. 2nd ed. Vol 1. Philadelphia: Elsevier Mosby; 2005:898-902.

Laibson P. Microcystic corneal dystrophy. *Trans AM Ophthalmol Soc*. 1976;74:488-531.

Lin SR, Aldave AJ, Chodosh J. Recurrent corneal erosion syndrome. *Br J Ophthalmol*. 2019;103(9):1204-1208.

Møller HU, Wittebolpost D, Weidle EG. Reis-Bücklers' dystrophy. *Cornea*. 2006;25(4):499.

Rice NS, Ashton N, Jay B, Blach RK. Reis-Bücklers' dystrophy. A clinicopathological study. *Br J Ophthalmol*. 1968;52(8):577-603.

Thygeson P. Superficial punctate keratitis. *J Am Med Assoc*. 1950; 144(18):1544-1549.

SECTION **3**

Stromal and Endothelial Disorders

6 Stromal Dystrophies, Degenerations, and Depositions

J. Christian Berry | Kamran M. Riaz

I. STROMAL DYSTROPHIES

Corneal dystrophies are inherited, noninflammatory, bilateral, fairly symmetric, and slowly progressive disorders that begin early in life and worsen with age. A complete discussion of the classification, systemic associations, genetic findings, and controversies regarding corneal dystrophies is beyond the scope of this chapter (Weiss JS, Møller HU, Aldave AJ, 2015).

Stromal dystrophies are characterized by abnormal protein deposition that primarily affects the stroma, though extension may also involve anterior and posterior corneal layers (Kanski J, Bowling B, 2016). As a result, stromal dystrophies may cause clinical symptoms similar to epithelial-Bowman dystrophies (e.g., recurrent corneal erosions seen with classic lattice corneal dystrophy [LCD]) and endothelial dystrophies (e.g., significantly decreased vision, as seen with macular dystrophy). Stromal dystrophies can cause a range of visual morbidity in patients, including blurred vision, painful erosions, and irregular astigmatism.

Clinical findings of stromal dystrophies vary significantly. Although the slit-lamp examination is usually sufficient to help identify classic findings, anterior segment optical coherence tomography (AS-OCT) can be a useful supplementary tool to help the clinician diagnose and treat this patient population. Furthermore, AS-OCT can assess patient response to therapeutic interventions and monitor disease progression and recurrence.

In general, treatment for stromal dystrophies is supportive, such as managing recurrent erosions with bandage contact lenses, using lubrication, and optimizing vision with glasses and/or contact lenses (Krachmer JH, Mannis MJ, Holland EJ, 2011; Weisenthal RW, Daly MK, de Freitas D, 2019). Surgical intervention may include phototherapeutic keratectomy (PTK) to debulk or remove lesions, especially if limited to the anterior stromal layers. PTK may need to be repeated after several years because recurrence is common. Epithelial debridement, combined with diamond burr polishing, can be effective in treating stromal dystrophies, especially epithelial and sub-Bowman's layer changes. Partial-thickness or full-thickness corneal transplantation (superficial anterior lamellar keratectomy [SALK], deep anterior lamellar keratectomy [DALK], or penetrating keratoplasty (PKP) may be necessary for advanced cases of visual decline. A complete discussion of the best therapeutic option for each stromal dystrophy is beyond the scope of this chapter.

The most commonly encountered stromal dystrophies are lattice dystrophy, granular dystrophy, macular dystrophy, and Schnyder corneal dystrophy (SCD). Congenital stromal corneal dystrophy and fleck dystrophy are extremely rare.

A. Lattice Corneal Dystrophy

Classic LCD1 is typically observed early in life. It is characterized by branching lines in the corneal stroma, which result from amyloid depositions that stain with Congo red, periodic acid–Schiff (PAS), and thioflavin T. These lines are best seen with retro-illumination or indirect illumination on slit-lamp examination. These deposits may appear as round, white, and filamentous refractile lesions (Fig. 6.1). The stroma can have a "ground-glass" appearance, but the periphery is typically spared. The corneal sensation can be reduced, and painful recurrent erosions are sometimes seen.

On AS-OCT imaging, LCD lesions can be appreciated as hyperreflective areas surrounded by areas of haze, with involvement of various depths of the stroma (Fig. 6.2). Lattice lines are accentuated as hyporeflective (dark) branching lines on red-free images (see Fig. 6.2, *left panels*) obtained with some AS-OCT devices, which may further identify subtle deposits that may be missed on the clinical examination alone. The AS-OCT images further show the depth, distribution, and morphology of the lattice deposits that occupy most of the stroma and extend

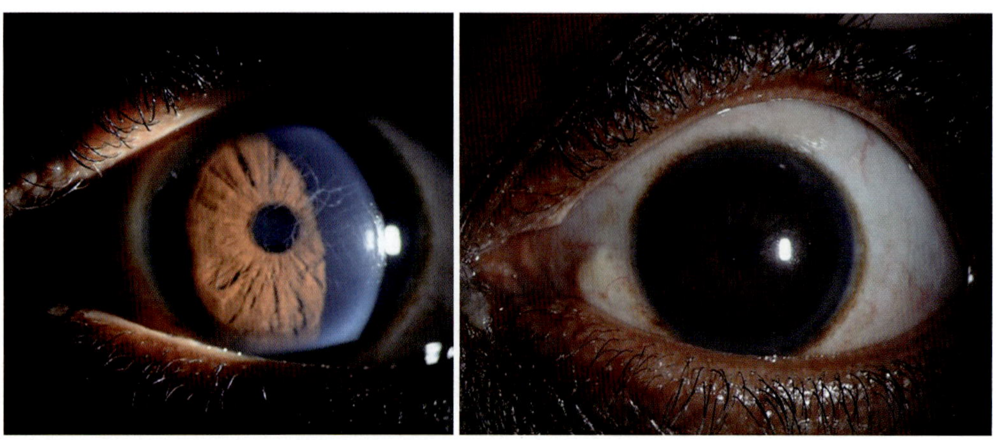

Fig. 6.1 Slit-lamp photograph of classic lattice corneal dystrophy. Indirect *(left panel)* and retro-illumination (especially after dilation) techniques may be more effective in delineating the extent of the lattice lesions compared with direct illumination techniques *(right panel)*.

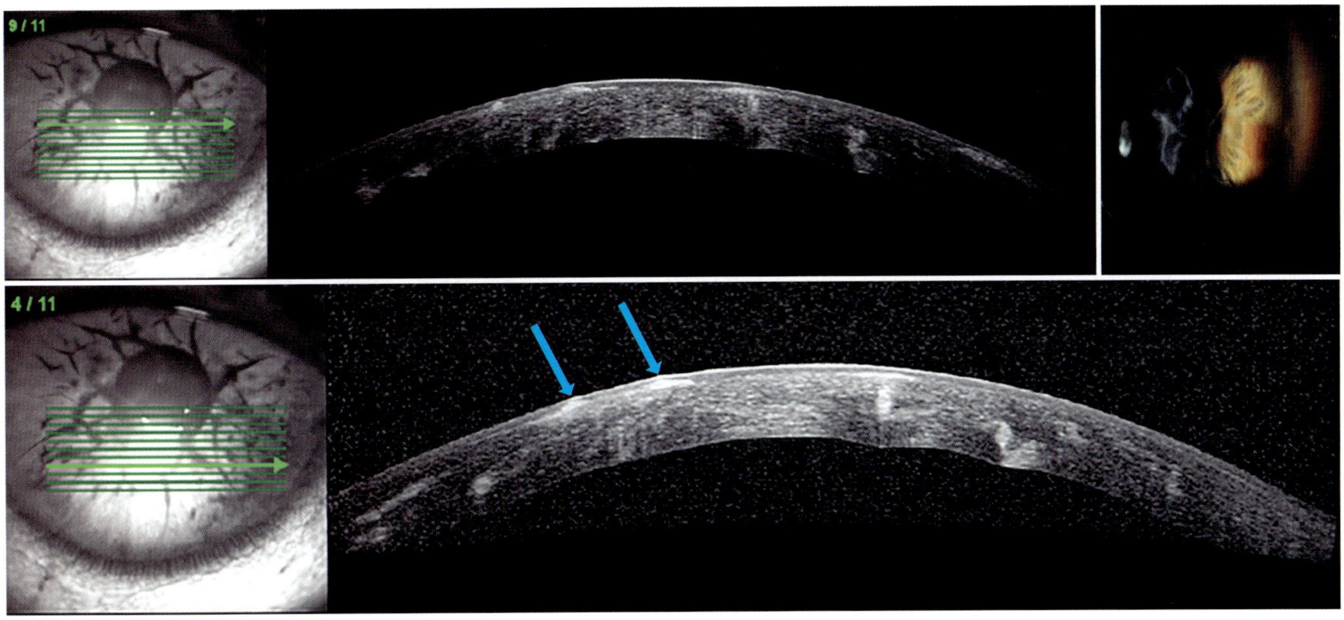

Fig. 6.2 AS-OCT can help identify the extent and depth of the lattice lesions seen on clinical examination. Lattice lesions demonstrate hyperreflectivity with the involvement of both superficial and deep stromal layers. The Bowman layer is absent or disrupted in several areas. Focal areas of epithelial hypertrophy and remodeling are observed *(arrows)*. Red-free images obtained with some AS-OCT devices can also better highlight observed pathologic findings.

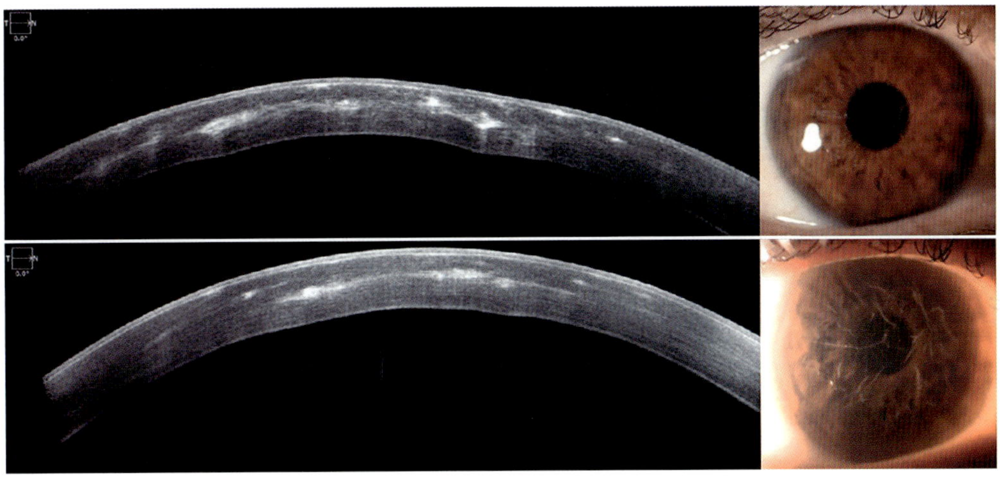

Fig. 6.3 Lattice corneal dystrophy. Slit-lamp photographs and AS-OCT images of the right eye. Visual acuity (with contact lenses) was 20/60. AS-OCT highlights the extent and depth of lattice lesions primarily located in the anterior and middle stroma.

into the subepithelial/epithelial layers. Particularly dense lattice deposits may cause secondary shadowing of the corneal layers posterior to the deposits.

Although lattice lesions are seen bilaterally, asymmetric disease is common in most patients, with one eye having more lesions and worse vision than the other. Figs. 6.3 and 6.4 show a patient with LCD in both eyes, with the left eye more affected than the right eye. AS-OCT highlights the widespread extent and depth of lattice lesions in the left eye, including involvement of the posterior stroma, that subsequently required PKP.

Although PTK can be effectively used to debulk and remove lattice lesions, mainly when they are confined to the superficial stromal layers, recurrence of lesions is very common. AS-OCT can be used to assess and monitor recurrence in patients after treatment. The patient in Fig. 6.5 has a recurrence of lattice lesions after having undergone PTK several years previously. In contrast to the previous example, the slit-lamp findings and AS-OCT show significantly fewer stromal deposits. The AS-OCT image demonstrates subepithelial haze with less prominence of lattice deposits in the anterior stroma. Deposits in the deeper stromal layers may remain.

B. Granular Corneal Dystrophy

Granular corneal dystrophy type 1 (GCD1), also known as the classic type, occurs early in life with white crumb-like opacities in the anterior central stroma, which are hyaline deposits that stain with Masson trichrome and PAS. The corneal periphery is spared. Deposits are classically described as having a “crushed bread crumb” appearance. As the disease progresses, the lesions become more confluent. Patients can report worsening visual acuity, glare, photophobia, and recurrent erosions as the disease progresses.

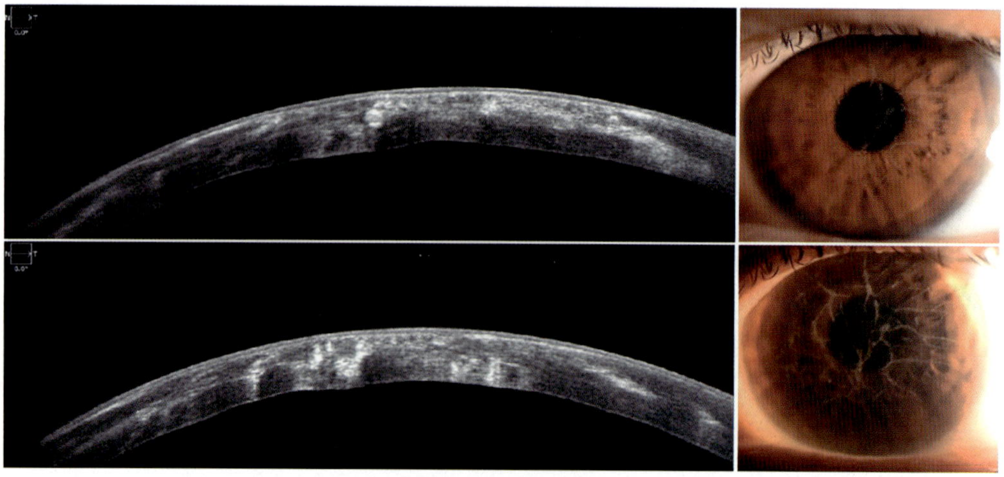

Fig. 6.4 Lattice corneal dystrophy. Slit-lamp photographs and AS-OCT images of the left eye of the patient in Fig. 6.3. AS-OCT highlights the more widespread extent and depth (including involvement of the posterior stroma) than the lesions in the right eye. The best corrected visual acuity was 20/400, and the patient underwent subsequent penetrating keratoplasty in this eye.

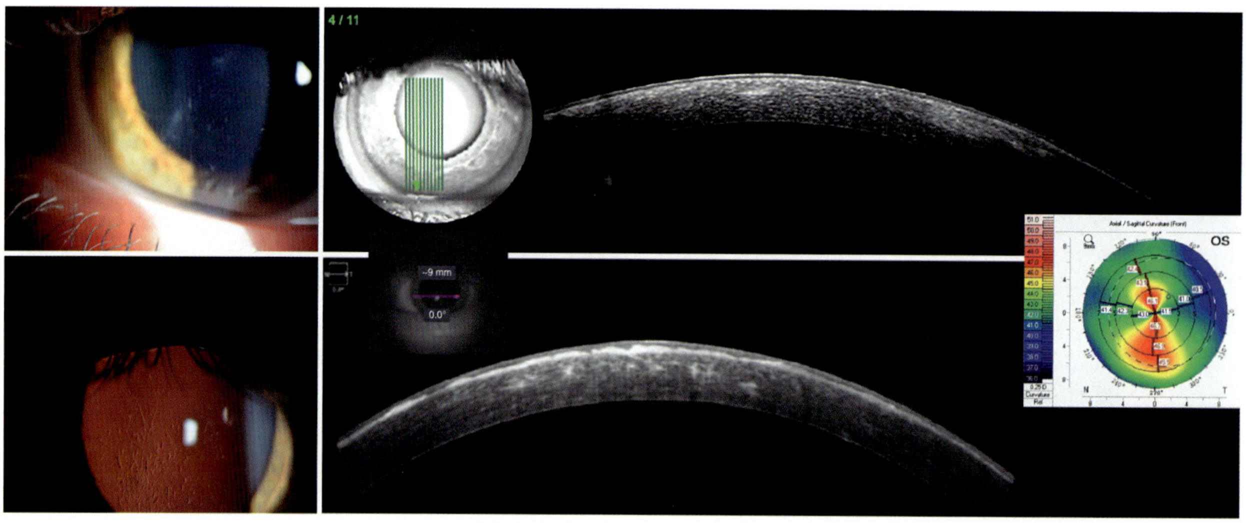

Fig. 6.5 Recurrence of lattice lesions in a patient who had undergone phototherapeutic keratectomy several years previously *(top left panel).* Note the use of retro-illumination *(bottom left panel)* to highlight better the lesions seen on direct illumination technique *(top left panel).* AS-OCT can be used to identify lesions in deeper stromal layers. In the anterior stromal layers, lesions are less prominent, but a considerable amount of subepithelial haze can be appreciated. Images from two different AS-OCT imaging devices in the same patient highlight the variation in the appearance of the lattice lesions. Topography imaging demonstrates prominent and irregular astigmatism changes.

CLINICAL PEARL

AS-OCT can be used to visualize and appreciate the "clear spaces" present in granular corneal dystrophy in cases in which slit-lamp examination may be equivocal or difficult because of haze and scarring.

On AS-OCT, multiple discrete hyperreflective deposits with intervening clear spaces are observed in the anterior stroma (Fig. 6.6). These deposits also exhibit blockage of the signal posterior to the lesions (Fig. 6.7). The posterior stroma is uninvolved.

As the lesions in GCD1 are primarily located in the superficial stromal layers, PTK may be effectively used to debulk and remove granular deposits. Fig. 6.8 shows pretreatment and posttreatment images of a GCD1 patient who underwent PTK. AS-OCT highlights the improved stromal pathologic findings and areas of nasal haze resulting from postsurgical healing.

PTK also can be used for repeat treatment in patients with recurrence of GCD1 lesions. Fig. 6.9 shows a patient who had distant (10+ years previously, in 2008) PTK with recurrence of his granular dystrophy *(top left and top right panels).* After undergoing repeat PTK (in 2019), there was a notable reduction in granular deposits *(bottom left and bottom right panels),* with an improvement in visual acuity from 20/80 to 20/30. Red-free images similarly show a decrease in granular deposits within the central cornea. Three years later (2022), the patient presented with a recurrence of GCD1 lesions and decreased visual acuity of 20/50 in both eyes. Imaging at this time (Fig. 6.10) shows the recurrence of granular deposits. The appearance of deposits with this AS-OCT device differs slightly from those seen in Figs. 6.6 to 6.9, highlighting the variability between devices. Clinicians should be mindful of these variations. Repeat AS-OCT can be used to determine suitability for additional PTK treatment or keratoplasty options.

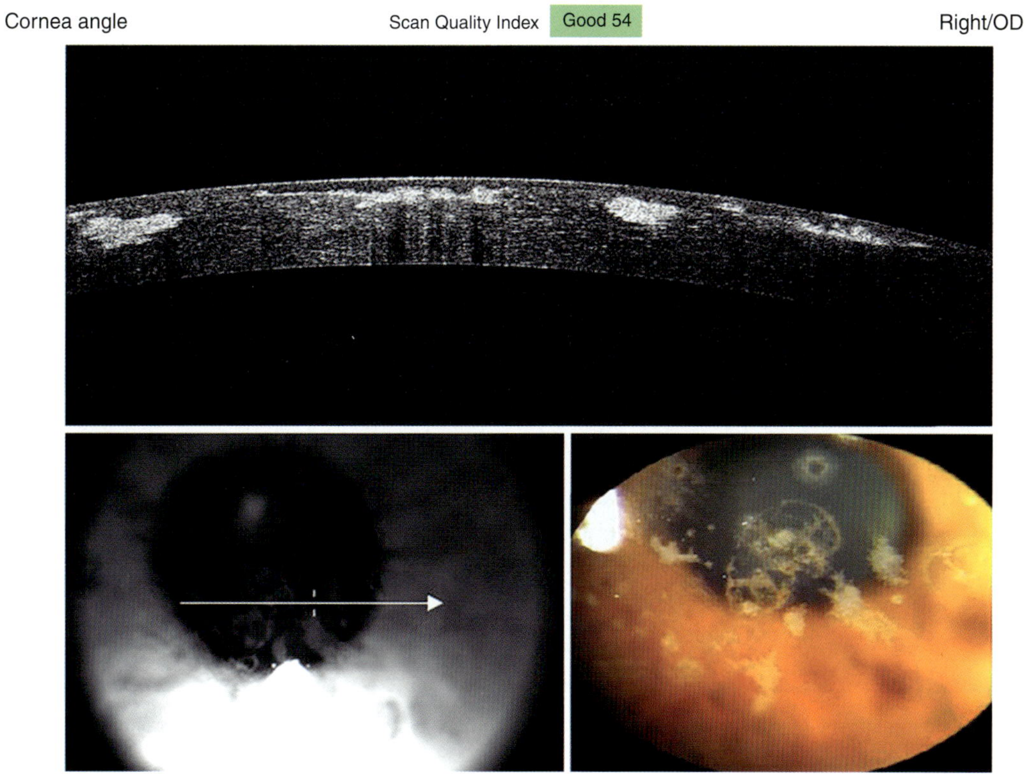

Fig. 6.6 Granular corneal dystrophy type 1 appears as bread crumb–like deposits in the anterior stroma with intervening clear spaces. AS-OCT highlights granular deposits as areas of hyperreflectivity primarily located in the epithelium, Bowman layer, and anterior stroma, with intervening clear spaces readily observed. Partial, multifocal disruption of the Bowman layer is also noted.

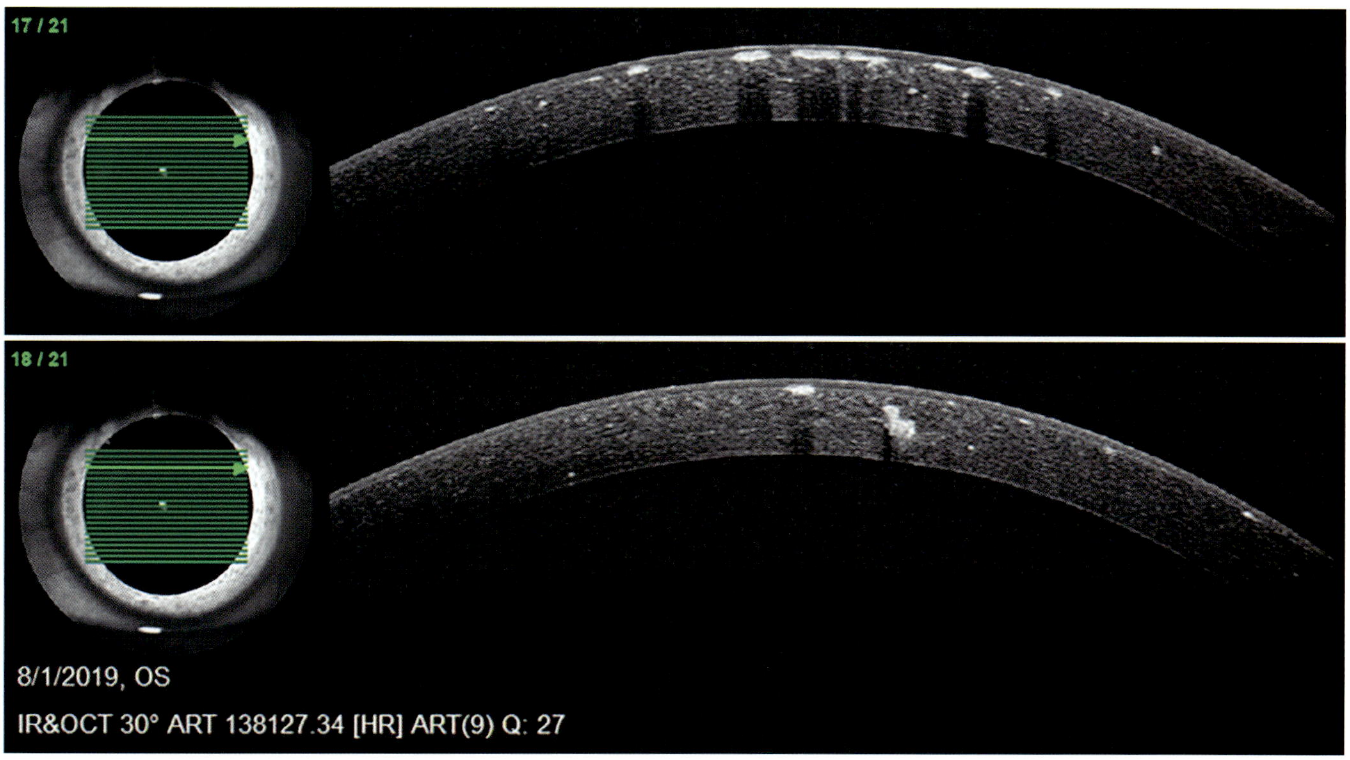

Fig. 6.7 AS-OCT demonstrates the primary clustering of granular lesions in the superficial stromal layers. Note the blockage of signal posterior to the lesions. The posterior stroma is uninvolved. (Courtesy Albert Cheung, MD, Eastern Virginia Medical School, Virginia, United States.)

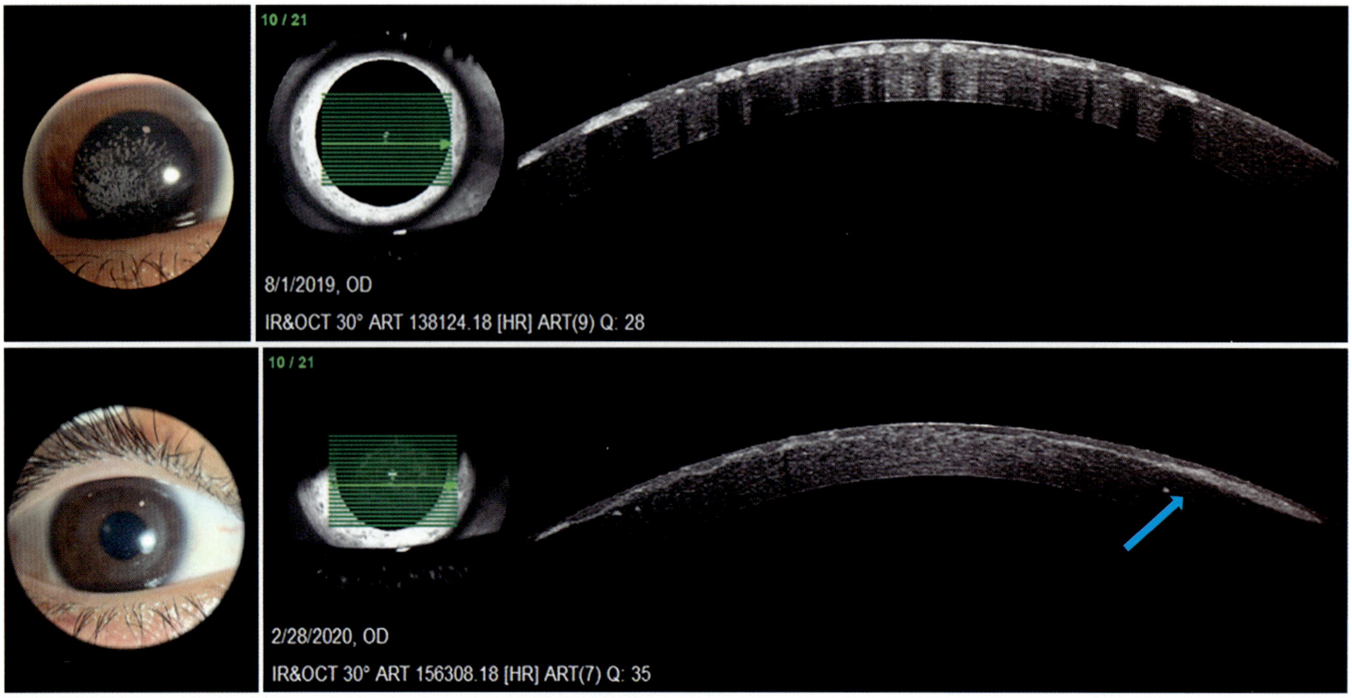

Fig. 6.8 Pretreatment and posttreatment images of a patient with granular corneal dystrophy type 1 treated with phototherapeutic keratectomy (PTK). In the *top right panel,* AS-OCT demonstrates the granular deposits as seen in Fig. 6.6; however, there are considerably fewer intervening clear spaces between the deposits, representing the advanced disease state. Nearly 7 months after PTK treatment, AS-OCT shows a dramatic improvement in the anterior stromal layer pathologic condition. The nasal haze seen on the slit-lamp photograph is viewed on the AS-OCT image *(blue arrow)* in the *bottom right panel* as an area of increased hyperreflectivity in the subepithelial space. (Courtesy Albert Cheung, MD, Eastern Virginia Medical School, Virginia, United States.)

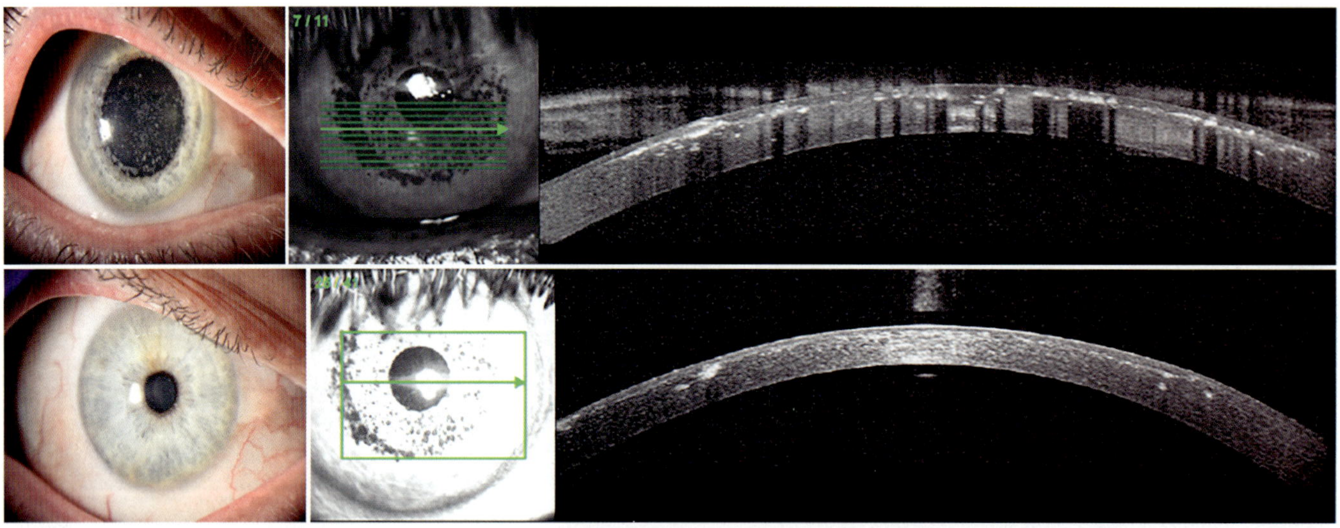

Fig. 6.9 Recurrence of granular corneal dystrophy type 1. The *top panels* show slit-lamp photographs and AS-OCT images of a patient who had undergone phototherapeutic keratectomy (PTK) for granular corneal dystrophy type 1 more than 10 years previously and now presented with recurrence and accompanying decreased vision. AS-OCT was used to measure the depth of lesions, which were noted to be primarily within the anterior stroma (approximately 100 μm). PTK was performed with an ablation depth set for 80 μm. The *bottom panels* show the post-treatment photos and AS-OCT images. Note the significantly decreased concentration of granular deposits in the posttreatment AS-OCT image *(bottom right panel).* Subepithelial haze is present as well. Deeper lesions remain. (The top left AS-OCT image has an artifactual "after-image" of the cornea, which is sometimes seen in image acquisition.)

CLINICAL PEARL

AS-OCT can be used to visualize areas of subepithelial haze that may not be as easily seen on slit-lamp examination. The appearance of granular deposits may vary depending on the AS-OCT device used for imaging.

AS-OCT is extremely helpful for the preoperative planning of granular corneal dystrophy, which often has disease limited to the superficial stromal layers. Surgical planning should focus on debulking, rather than eliminating, the granular deposits from the anterior stroma to improve vision and avoid potentially dangerous corneal thinning. In the previous patient (see Fig. 6.9), most lesions were noted to be within the anterior stroma (approximately 100-μm depth) on AS-OCT imaging. This allowed for surgical planning with an ablation depth set for 80 μm, considering the preoperative myopic refractive error and central corneal thickness.

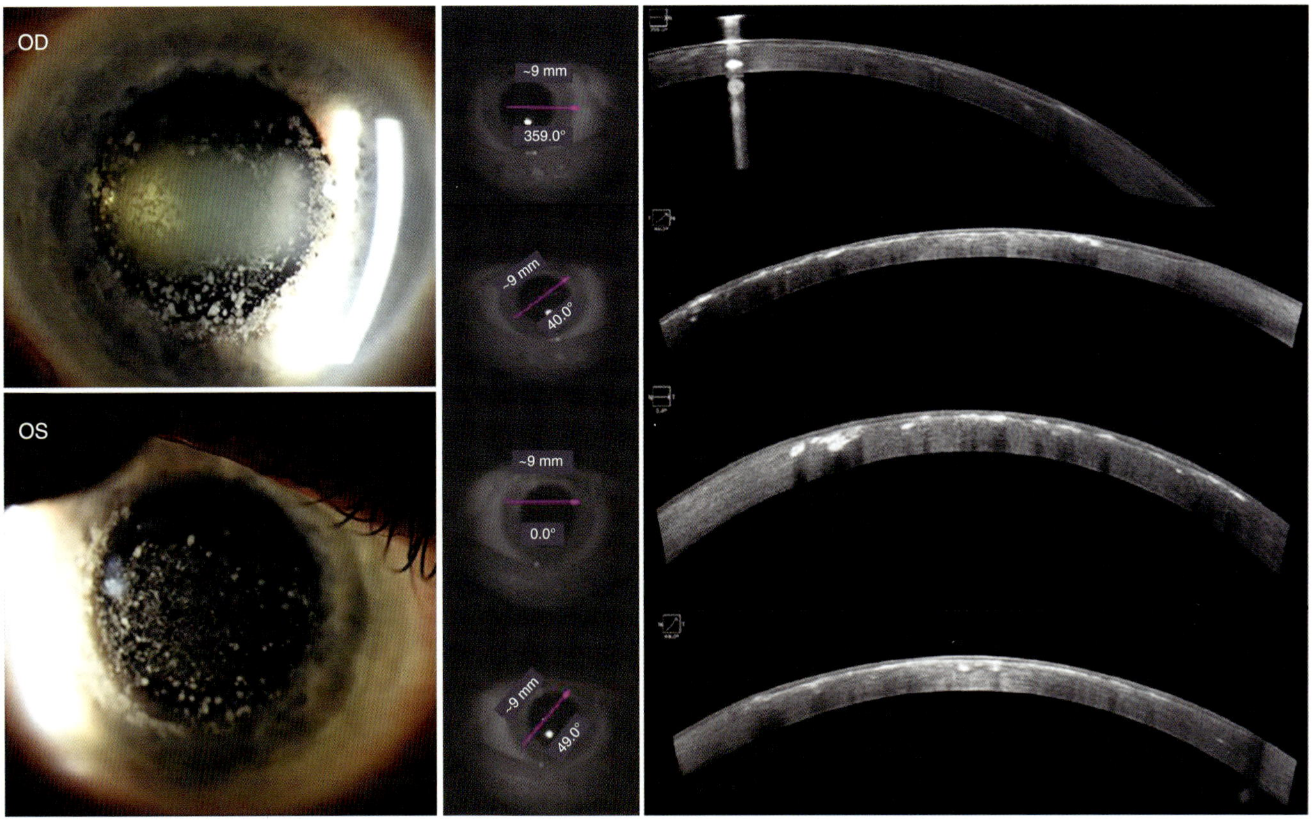

Fig. 6.10 Recurrent granular corneal dystrophy type 1 lesions after phototherapeutic keratectomy (3 years later). Slit-lamp photographs of the right and left eye show recurrence of granular deposits compared with pretreatment photographs in Fig. 6.9. AS-OCT images with a different device show the location of the granular deposits is limited to the anterior stroma, with characteristic intervening clear spaces.

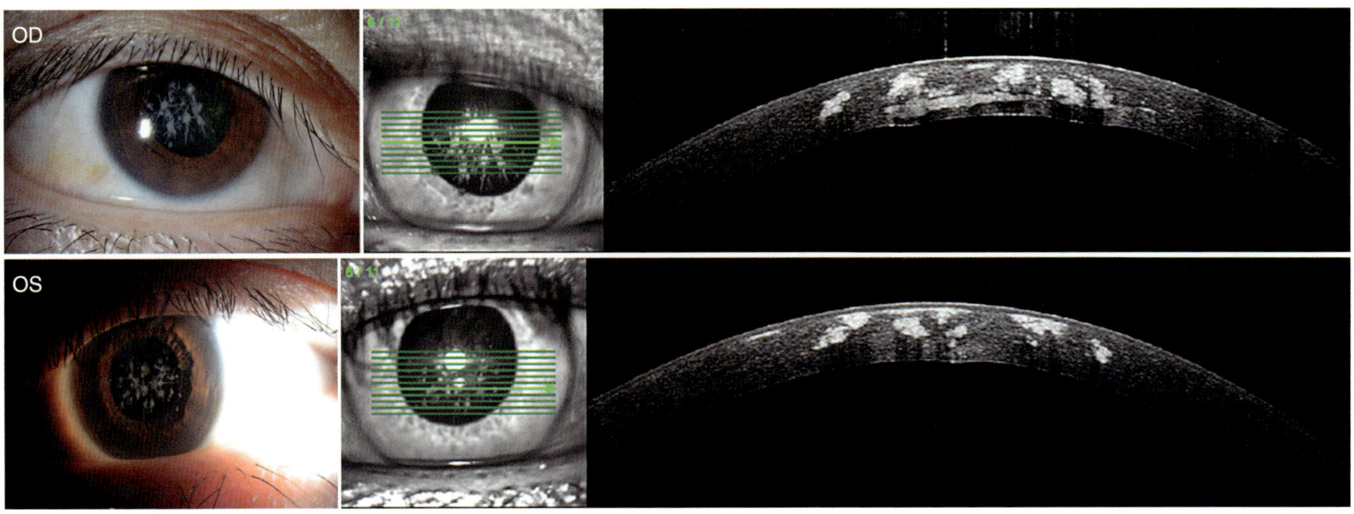

Fig. 6.11 In granular corneal dystrophy type 2, features of both lattice and granular dystrophy are seen on clinical examination. AS-OCT can highlight both pathologic conditions; granular deposits are primarily in the anterior stromal layers with intervening clear spaces, whereas lattice deposits are seen throughout the stroma, especially in the middle and posterior stroma. The Bowman layer is irregular in multiple areas with partial disruption.

Granular corneal dystrophy type 2 (GCD2), also known as granular-lattice dystrophy, exhibits features of both granular and lattice dystrophies. Pathologically, both hyaline and amyloid deposits are found. In the first two decades of life, white snowflake opacities appear in the central cornea in the anterior and middle stroma. After this, lattice lines and haze develop, often deeper than the snowflake opacities.

AS-OCT particularly showcases the features of both lattice and granular lesions (Fig. 6.11). Again, the granular deposits are hyperreflective with intervening areas of clear space. *Lattice deposits* are seen in *the middle and posterior stromal layers*, and *granular deposits* are mainly seen in the *anterior stromal layers*. Areas of dense hyperreflectivity similarly create a shadowing effect on the posterior corneal layers. Accompanying slit-lamp photographs in this figure show stellate-shaped stromal opacities.

CLINICAL PEARL

Among the stromal dystrophies, lattice and granular are most amenable to treatment with PTK because both entities have pathologic findings primarily in the anterior one-third of the cornea. If patients have significant thinning or deep opacities, PTK should be avoided. When planning PTK in these patients, preoperative ultrasound pachymetry is critical for accurately measuring corneal thickness. AS-OCT can be effectively used to assess the depth and distribution of lesions. This knowledge can allow a surgeon to plan a desired depth of treatment effectively. The goal should be to debulk the lesions in the area of the highest concentration while avoiding unnecessary tissue removal and undesirable hyperopic shift. Deeper treatments may be used in patients with preexisting myopic refractive errors but should be cautiously avoided in emmetropic and hyperopic patients. Treatment of even two-thirds to three-fourths of the depth of the lesions may be sufficient. For example, if a patient has a preoperative pachymetry of 550 μm and the bulk of the lesions are shown by AS-OCT to be limited to 80-μm depth, surgical planning can be done to remove approximately 60 to 80 μm of tissue with PTK. Whereas some surgeons prefer to remove the epithelium, others prefer to perform a transepithelial ablation. In the previous example, the surgeon can ablate approximately 60-μm and then assess the corneal surface, either at the surgical microscope or at the slit lamp. Additional treatment in 10-μm increments can be performed in a step-wise manner, stopping after each treatment to inspect the corneal surface visually. The surgical endpoint is subjective because the goal is to appreciate a clearer corneal surface with the understanding that complete removal of the lesions is either impossible or may cause significant and precarious thinning. Additionally, emoving deeper lesions may require "extra" tissue removal. In the previous example, the last 20 μm (of the original 80-μm depth of lesions) may require an additional 40 to 60 μm of treatment. For situations where a surgeon may have to remove significant layers of tissue, an additional peripheral treatment (2- to 2.5-mm spot size) can be performed on the peripheral cornea in a "donut pattern" to smooth this area and reduce the amount of induced hyperopia. Finally, mitomycin-C may be used with PTK to minimize the risk of postoperative haze and corneal scarring.

C. Macular Corneal Dystrophy

Macular corneal dystrophy is inherited in an autosomal recessive manner. The deposits are composed of glycosaminoglycans or acid mucopolysaccharides that stain with colloidal iron or Alcian blue. Mutations in the carbohydrate sulfotransferase gene *(CHST6)* cause deficient or abnormal production of keratan sulfate, which is a critical factor in maintaining corneal transparency. Uniquely, this condition involves the entire corneal stroma and periphery and can even affect the endothelium. It begins during the first decade of life as superficial white flecks that progress into gray-white, superficial, stromal opacities (macules). In contrast with granular dystrophy, there are no intervening clear areas between the opacities, and the cornea is variably cloudy (Fig. 6.12). AS-OCT imaging demonstrates hyperreflective deposits dispersed throughout the width and depth of the corneal stroma, along with loss of corneal transparency.

CLINICAL PEARL

AS-OCT can be used to assess the presence or absence of corneal transparency. In lattice and granular corneal dystrophies, the cornea remains relatively clear in areas without lesions. In macular corneal dystrophy, corneal clouding can be seen between the lesions on slit-lamp examination. On AS-OCT, this is seen as a diffuse hyperreflectivity with macular corneal dystrophy, compared with stromal hyporeflectivity seen with lattice and granular corneal dystrophies.

Clinically, vision typically declines between ages 10 and 30. Eventually, central corneal thinning also may be seen.

D. Schnyder Corneal Dystrophy

Schnyder corneal dystrophy (SCD) is a slowly progressive stromal dystrophy that can appear as early as the first year of life. However, it is typically diagnosed in the second or third decade. SCD is possibly due to a local abnormality in corneal lipid metabolism.

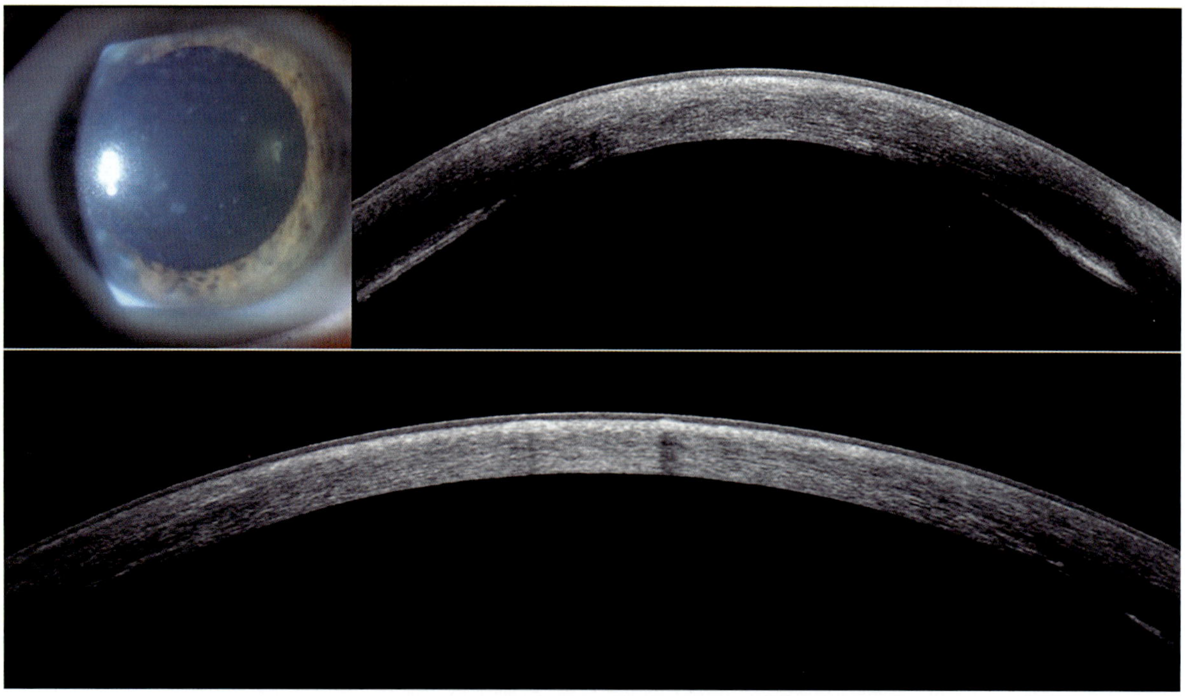

Fig. 6.12 Macular corneal dystrophy seen on clinical examination as deposits in the cornea with associated corneal clouding. Slit-lamp appearance shows multiple, round, whitish corneal opacities. Note the loss of corneal transparency seen in this dystrophy, compared with the relatively good corneal transparency seen in Figs. 6.1 to 6.11. AS-OCT can be used to assess the deposits scattered throughout the corneal stroma as focal areas of hyperreflectivity in the corneal stroma. Overall, the entire cornea stroma has increased hyperreflectivity, especially compared with the previous images of lattice and granular corneal dystrophies. (Image Credit: Christopher J. Rapuano, MD, Wills Eye Hospital, Philadelphia, PA, USA.)

On pathology, the opacities are composed of cholesterol and phospholipids that stain with oil red O or Sudan black stains.

As the disease progresses, variable clinical appearances may follow. At first, a ring or disc-like central corneal opacification is noted, occasionally with subepithelial crystals that may resemble secondary lipid keratopathy (Fig. 6.13). However, the lack of inflammatory signs (e.g., corneal neovascularization) distinguishes the two entities. In later stages of the disease, denser corneal arcus lipoides are seen. Eventually, the midperiphery of the cornea becomes opacified, affecting all layers. AS-OCT imaging demonstrates a homogeneous, hyperreflective accumulation of deposits limited mainly to the anterior stroma without discrete lesions and sparing of the peripheral cornea and deeper stroma. Another example of the clinical appearance and imaging is shown in Fig. 6.14. In the right eye, there is a denser accumulation of deposits on slit-lamp examination compared with the left

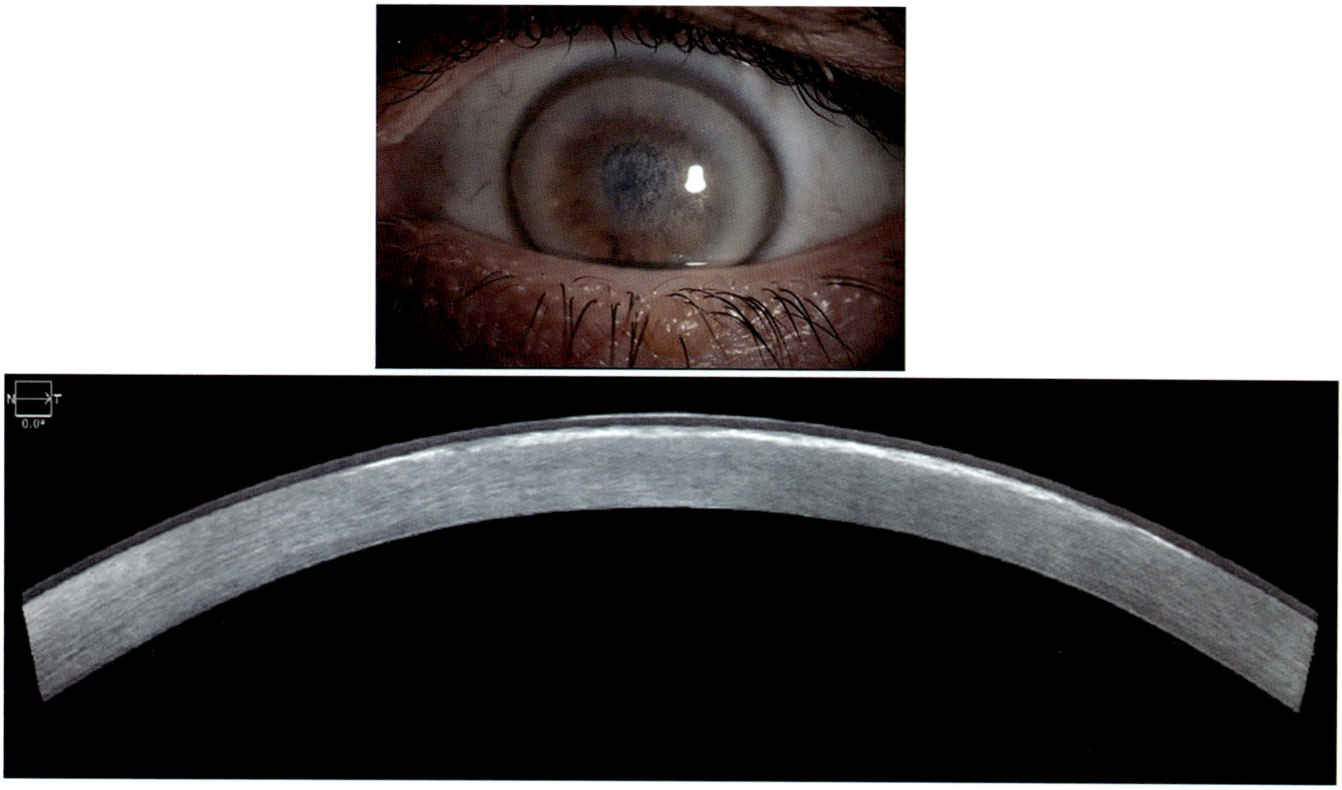

Fig. 6.13 Schnyder corneal dystrophy can be appreciated as a central, circular opacification with subepithelial crystals. AS-OCT demonstrates a homogenous accumulation of coalesced, dense, and hyperreflective deposits primarily located in the anterior stroma without involvement of the epithelium, Bowman layer, and deeper stroma. The peripheral cornea is also relatively unaffected. Note the lack of shadowing posterior to the deposits, as seen with previous dystrophies such as lattice and granular corneal dystrophies.

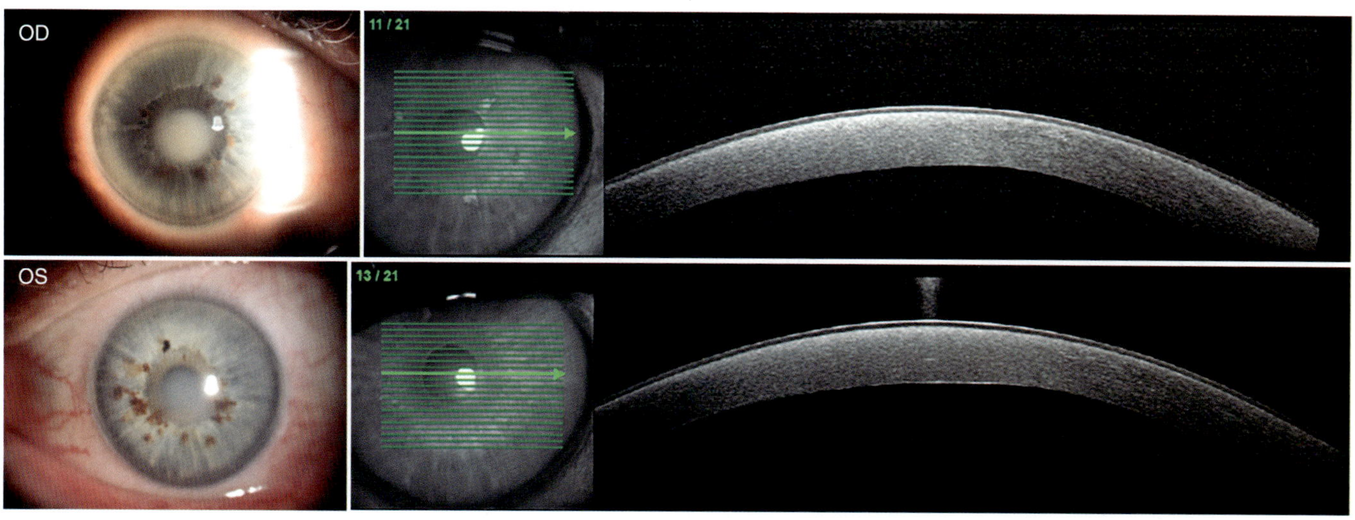

Fig. 6.14 In this patient, the right eye has a denser accumulation of cholesterol deposits seen on slit-lamp examination compared with the left eye. AS-OCT similarly shows areas of relatively increased hyperreflectivity of the lesions in the right eye compared with the left eye. A fasting lipid profile should be obtained on all Schnyder corneal dystrophy patients.

eye, which corresponds similarly to the AS-OCT image demonstrating increased hyperreflectivity of the deposits in the right compared with the left eye.

Clinically, a progressive loss of vision and corneal sensation is seen. Patients may be especially photophobic because of glare from the progressing haze. A fasting lipid profile also should be obtained on all SCD patients to screen for systemic disorders.

E. Unclassified

Assigning a singular, precise, and definitive diagnosis based solely on clinical examination may be difficult in some patients. In such cases, examination of family members and/or genetic testing may be helpful because the clinical appearance may be highly variable and demonstrate features of several dystrophies. This is unsurprising given the variable molecular pathologic processes in transforming growth factor, β-induced (TGF-β1, formerly BIGH3), a protein encoded by the *TGFBI* gene (locus 5q31). As the stromal dystrophies share a deficiency in a common gene product, the clinical presentation can be quite variable and characteristics of different "classic" dystrophies can be present in one cornea.

The following figures represent images of an 84-year-old white woman with no known family history of corneal dystrophy who was referred for evaluation of "corneal scarring" by her primary eye care provider. The vision was 20/50 in both eyes. Slit-lamp photographs (Fig. 6.15) demonstrate prominent features of lattice corneal dystrophy but also some elements of granular deposits. This combination of lattice and granular corneal findings was formerly known as Avellino dystrophy (named after a town in Italy) but has since been changed, given its global prevalence. AS-OCT shows multiple areas of hyperfluorescent deposits in the middle and posterior stroma that are not prominent in classic lattice dystrophy (Fig. 6.16). However, it is difficult to classify this based solely on these clinical features, though the clinical findings favored lattice corneal dystrophy primarily. Genetic testing was advised to the patient, but she declined to pursue this option at the time of the photographs. Because the patient also had dry, age-related macular degeneration changes, conservative management with spectacles was advised after she declined contact lens evaluation.

II. STROMAL DEGENERATIONS

Although corneal degenerations may affect multiple layers, entities such as spheroidal degeneration (Labrador keratopathy) and Salzmann nodular degeneration primarily affect the epithelial and Bowman layers. This chapter's discussion will be limited to Terrien marginal degeneration and lipid keratopathy because these primarily affect the stromal layers and leave the epithelium intact.

A. Terrien Marginal Degeneration

Terrien marginal degeneration is an idiopathic, progressive thinning of the peripheral cornea that typically affects individuals older than 40. Classically, the thinning begins in the superior or superonasal peripheral cornea and spreads circumferentially, though it may start in other locations. Bilateral disease is usually present, though asymmetric disease is commonly encountered

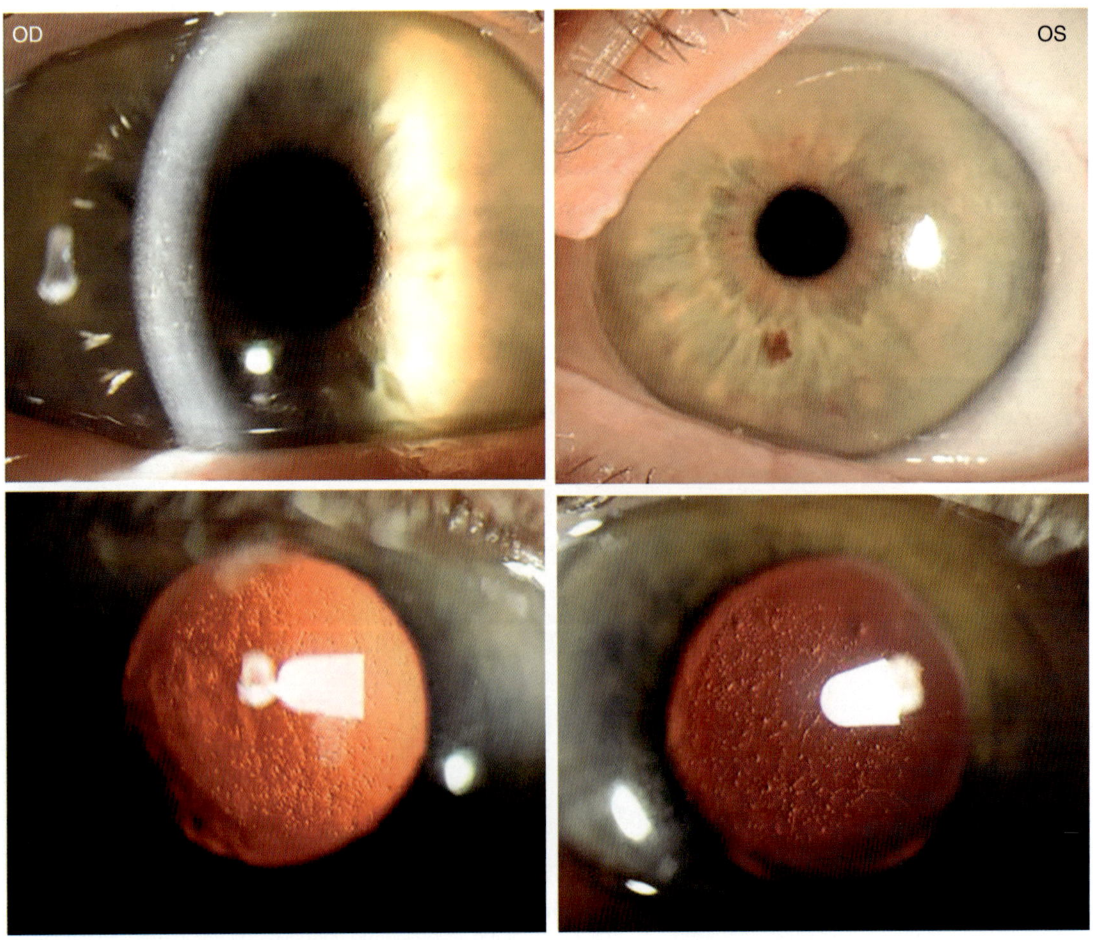

Fig. 6.15 Combined lattice and granular dystrophy changes. Slit-lamp photographs of a patient with features consistent primarily with lattice corneal dystrophy (e.g., branching lines best seen with retro-illumination) and some subtle, questionable granular deposits.

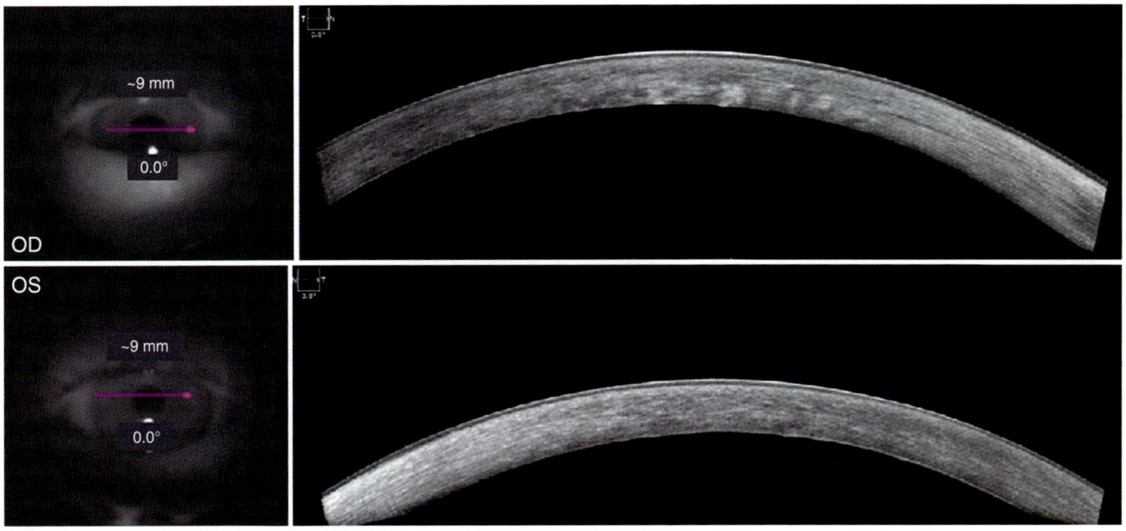

Fig. 6.16 AS-OCT shows multiple hyperfluorescent deposits in both eyes' middle and posterior stroma. AS-OCT findings are not as prominent as the classic lattice AS-OCT changes.

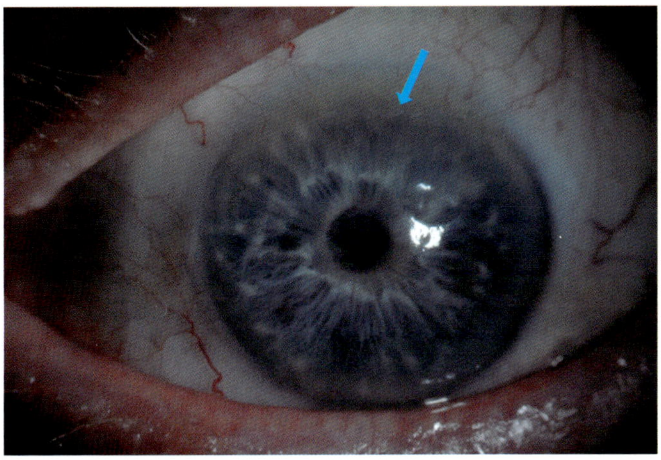

Fig. 6.17 Terrien marginal degeneration. Findings on clinical examination include a pannus of superficial vessels that overlies an area of stromal thinning with a line of lipid deposits *(arrow)* at the leading edge of the pannus. Although this condition usually occurs in the superior cornea, other locations may be encountered.

in clinical practice. As peripheral corneal thinning progresses, limbal neovascularization may secondarily appear.

Examination findings include a pannus of superficial vessels that overlies the area of stromal thinning, along with a line of lipid deposits at the leading edge of the pannus (Fig. 6.17). Progressive thinning may cause superior corneal flattening with associated steepening 90 degrees away (resulting in a secondary increase in against-the-rule keratometric astigmatism). Because the epithelium is unaffected, this condition is typically not painful for patients, (as would be expected with recurrent corneal erosions due to LCD1) but recurrent painful episodes of inflammation, similar to recurrent keratouveitis, may occur.

Conservative management may be used in the early phases, including observation and correction of refractive error with glasses and/or contact lenses. Surgical intervention may be required in the late stages because of the risk of perforation or intolerable astigmatism. Crescentic lamellar and annular lamellar keratoplasty may be necessary. For cases of perforation, corneoscleral patch grafts may be required.

Clinical findings of Terrien marginal degeneration may be further appreciated and followed on AS-OCT imaging. Fig. 6.18 shows a case of atypical Terrien marginal degeneration with inferior thinning on the slit-lamp examination. AS-OCT highlights this area of stromal thinning with secondary remodeling changes, sparing of epithelium/endothelium, and preservation of central corneal anatomy. Adjacent lipid deposition appears as a hyperreflective area. Measurement of thinning on AS-OCT also may be helpful for documentation and monitoring of disease, including surgical planning (e.g., the thickness of crescentic graft).

Fig. 6.19 shows another example of a patient with bilateral disease primarily affecting the inferior cornea in both eyes. In the right eye, mild to moderate thinning with marked epithelial hyperplasia and minimal neovascularization can be seen on slit-lamp photographs and AS-OCT. However, there is prominent vascularization in the left eye and severe thinning and overlying epithelial hyperplasia. The patient underwent a lamellar keratoplasty because of the significant thinning in the left eye; postoperative images, including AS-OCT images, are shown in Fig. 6.20.

CLINICAL PEARL

AS-OCT can be used to measure corneal thickness in cases of Terrien marginal degeneration and other peripheral thinning disorders, both in the area of maximum thinning and the adjacent healthy cornea. This can allow a surgeon to cut a crescentic lamellar graft of a desired thickness to improve graft-host apposition.

B. Lipid Keratopathy

Lipid keratopathy (LK) appears as a creamy yellow or white opacification of the stroma and is typically associated with an afferent blood vessel. LK has primary and secondary forms, with the latter being more common. Secondary LK results from prior corneal infection (usually herpes simplex virus [HSV] or varicella zoster virus [VZV]), inflammation, trauma, or other insults, which cause neovascularization of the cornea. If no clear cause can be identified, it can be described as primary LK, manifesting as a severe, prominent, arcus-like deposition.

This condition can be observed unless there is decreased vision or other visual symptoms. Topical steroids can be used to control corneal neovascularization and halt the further deposition of lipids. Other therapies such as argon laser treatment, photodynamic therapy, subconjunctival/topical bevacizumab, and intravascular embolization with mitomycin C ("MICE" treatment, as described by Dean Ouano, which is discussed more in

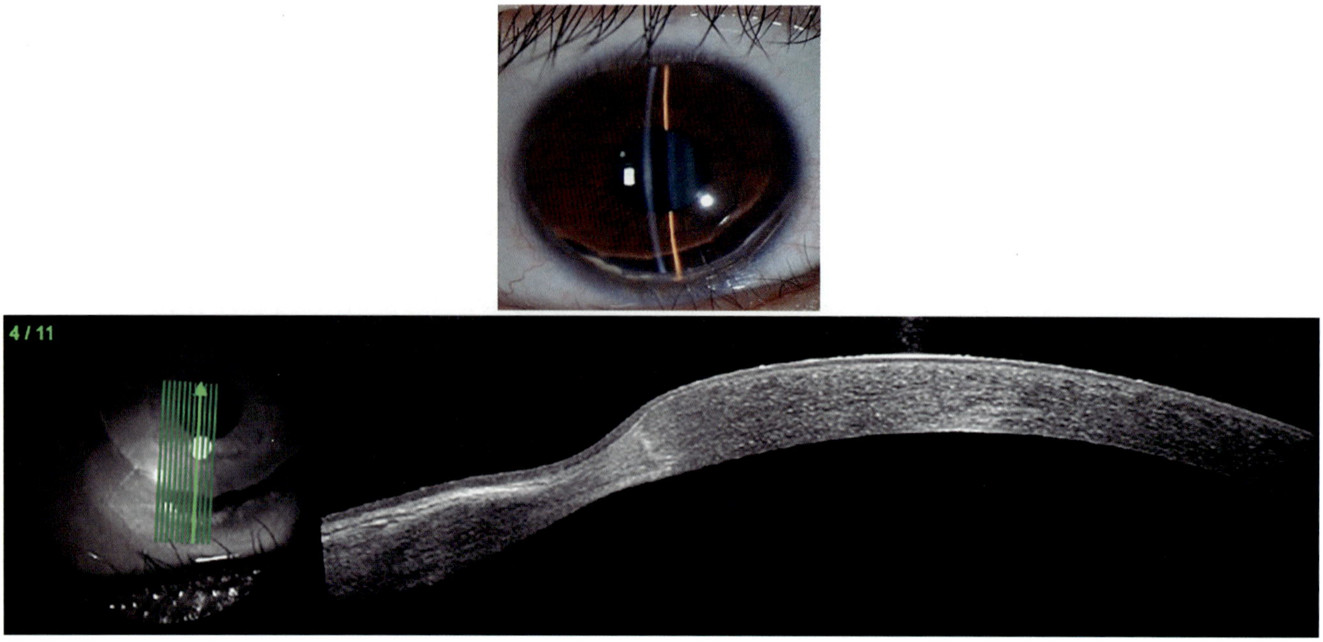

Fig. 6.18 Inferior Terrien's Marginal Degeneration. Although Terrien marginal degeneration is usually located superiorly, it may infrequently occur in the inferior cornea. AS-OCT demonstrates stromal thinning without epithelial involvement. Lipid deposition appears as areas of increased hyperreflectivity. Intact epithelium is clearly visualized on AS-OCT, helping to confirm the diagnosis.

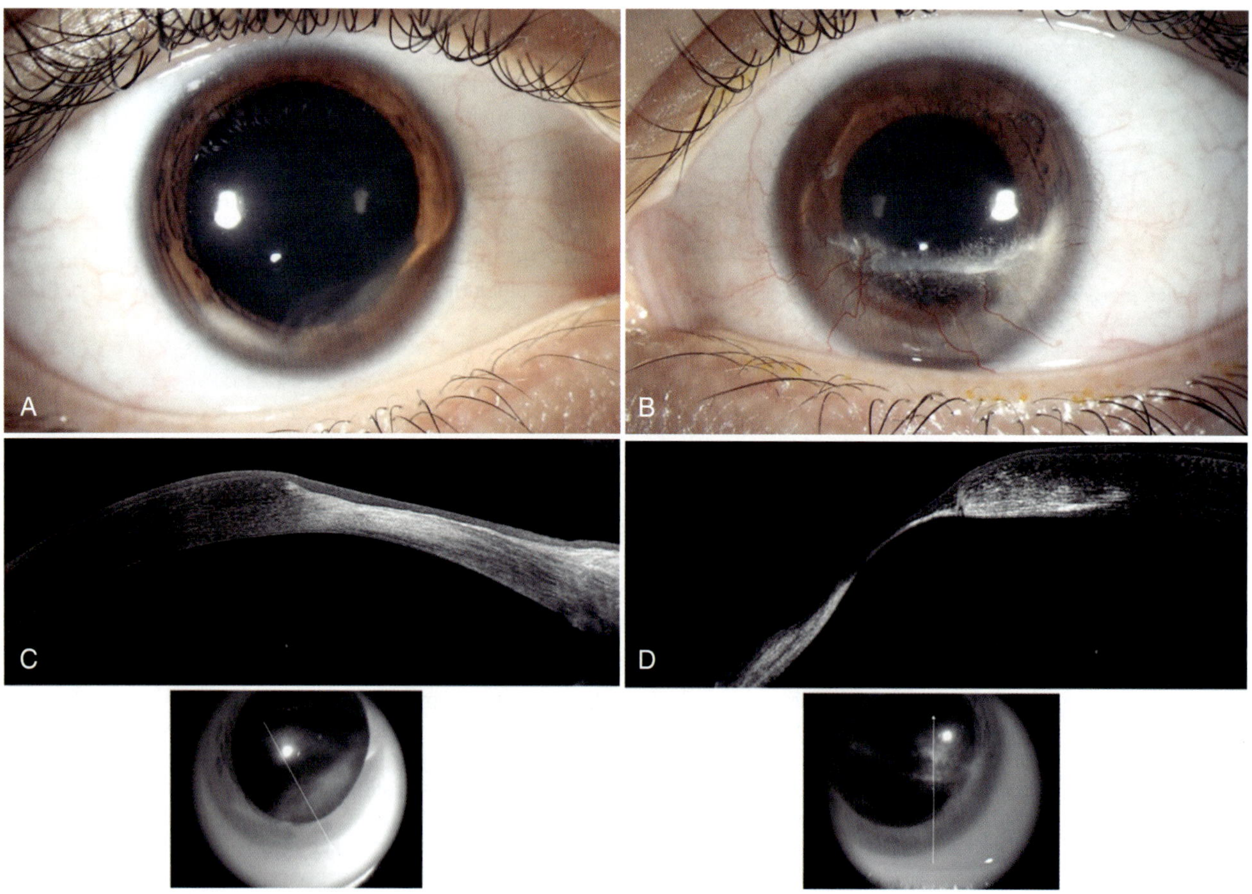

Fig. 6.19 Terrien marginal degeneration. Slit-lamp photographs of the right and left eye are shown in *panels A and B,* respectively. Clinical findings include peripheral thinning, superficial vascularization, lipid deposition at the edge of the affected area, and intact corneal epithelium without apparent inflammation. AS-OCT images of the right and left eye (*panels C and D,* respectively) show significant stromal thinning, stromal cicatrization, and intact overlying epithelium. In slit-lamp and AS-OCT images, the left eye is significantly more affected than the right eye. Note the increased epithelial thickness overlying the area of thinning. (Courtesy Guillermo Amescua, MD, Bascom Palmer Eye Institute, University of Miami, Miami, Florida, United States.)

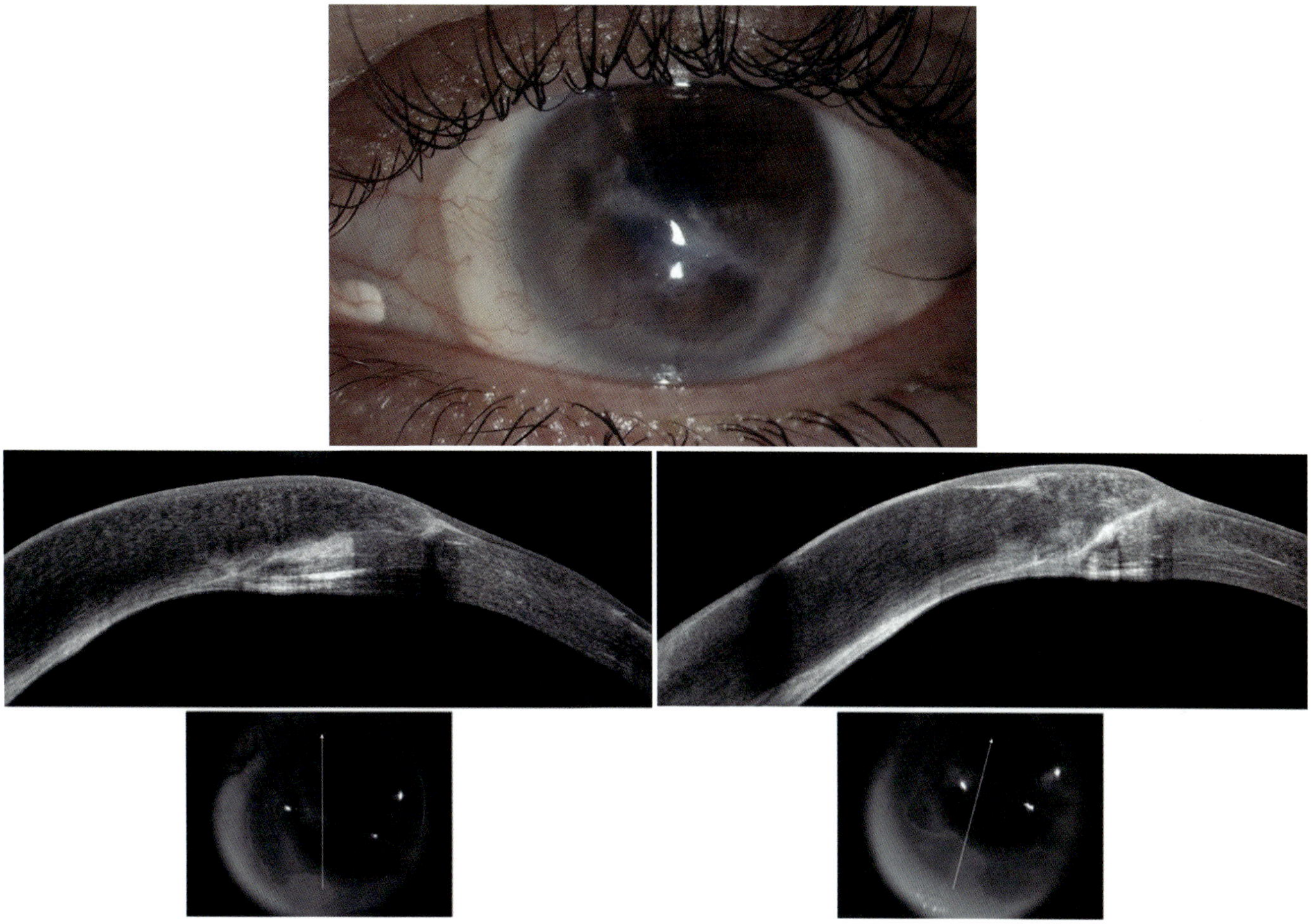

Fig. 6.20 Postlamellar keratoplasty images of the left eye shown in Fig. 6.19. Note the improvement in corneal thickness seen on AS-OCT images in this figure compared with the AS-OCT images shown in Fig. 6.19. (Courtesy Guillermo Amescua, MD, Bascom Palmer Eye Institute, University of Miami, Miami, Florida, United States.)

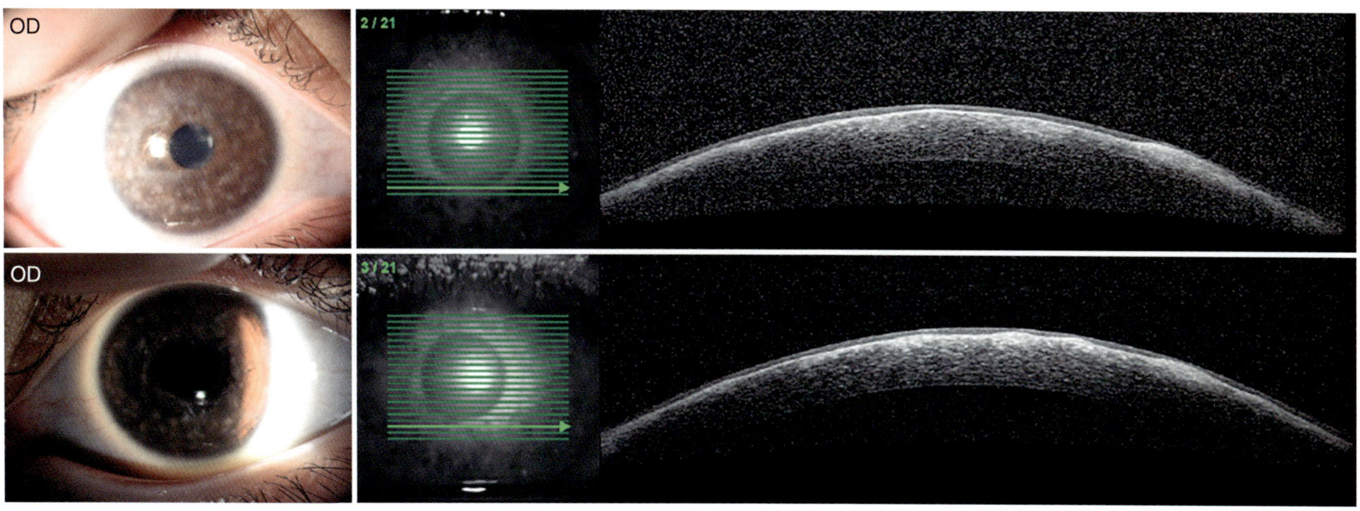

Fig. 6.21 Lipid keratopathy appears as multiple, coalescent lesions on slit-lamp examination with 360-degree involvement of the mid-peripheral cornea and relative sparing of the central cornea. AS-OCT taken over the lesions demonstrates irregularities and elevations in the anterior stroma, with an intact and smooth epithelial layer overlying. These images represent pretreatment photographs of a patient who underwent therapy with topical steroids and prophylactic systemic antiviral medications.

Chapter 20) have also been used to reduce corneal neovascularization and lipid deposits.

Fig. 6.21 illustrates the clinical appearance on slit-lamp examination as multiple deposits located in a circular pattern in the mid-peripheral cornea with relative sparing of the corneal center ("donut-like pattern"). AS-OCT demonstrates the diffuse hyperreflective nature of the lipid deposits, which can be seen mainly in the anterior stroma. Additionally, these deposits can cause irregularities and elevations in the anterior stroma interface with an intact and smooth overlying epithelium. With appropriate

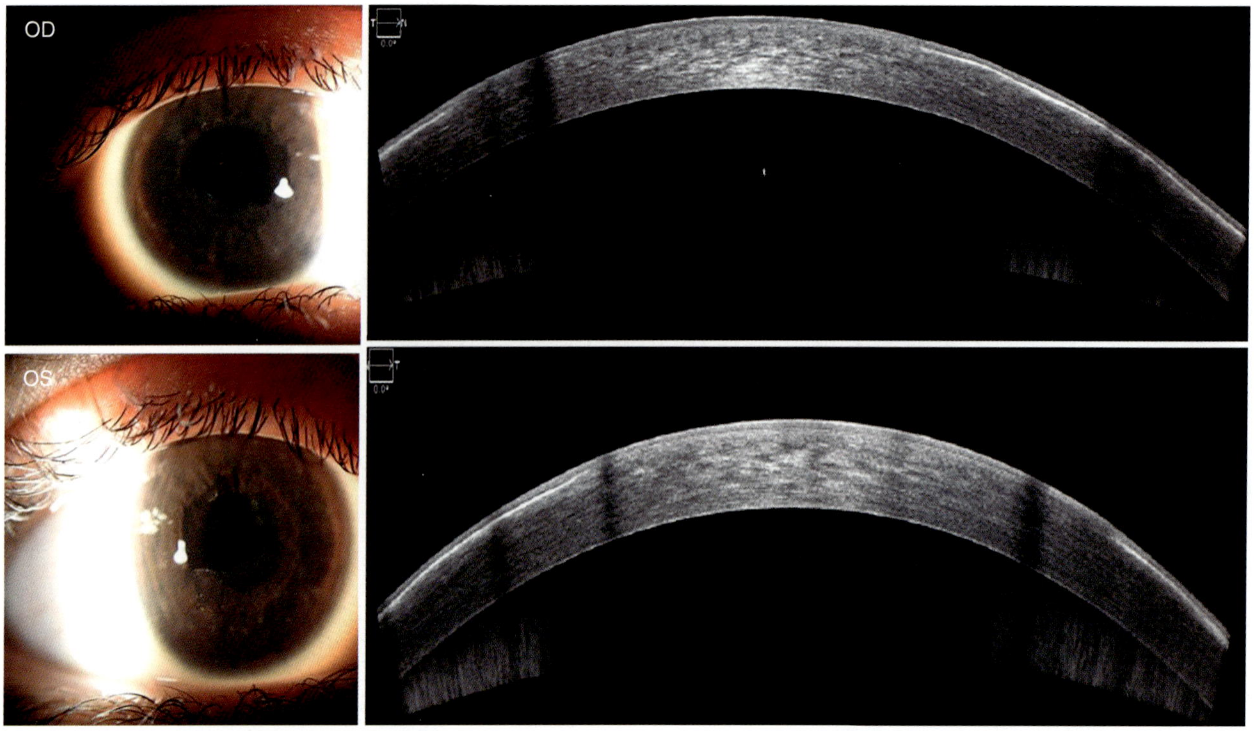

Fig. 6.22 Posttreatment slit-lamp photographs and AS-OCT images of the patient shown in Fig. 6.21. Note the significant reduction in density and number of lipid deposits on slit-lamp images. AS-OCT similarly shows improvement of the previously seen pathologic condition, although some lipid deposits remain as areas of hyperreflectivity in the corneal periphery.

medical therapy, lipid deposits can regress dramatically and visual acuity can significantly improve (Fig. 6.22).

C. Polymorphic Amyloid Degeneration

This is a relatively rare and usually visually insignificant degeneration in which amyloid deposits are seen in the middle and posterior stromal layers. They appear as white-gray, glass-like, refractile deposits of various shapes in the deep corneal stroma in both eyes, best seen on retro-illumination. Fig. 6.23 shows images from the right eye of a patient with this degeneration; AS-OCT can be used to localize the deposits primarily involving the deep stroma. Similar findings were seen in the left eye (not shown).

III. STROMAL DEPOSITIONS

Stromal depositions may occur due to various ocular and systemic inflammatory, metabolic, neoplastic, and toxic causes that lead to the accumulation of abnormal proteins (or other material) within the corneal stroma. Clinical presentation may vary widely in these cases: acute versus chronic, symptomatic versus asymptomatic, and vision-sparing versus vision-threatening. A few selected examples are presented in this section.

A. Monoclonal Gammopathy of Undetermined Significance

Although relatively uncommon, hematologic disorders such as monoclonal gammopathy of undetermined significance (MGUS), multiple myeloma (MM), and Waldenström macroglobulinemia can be associated with crystalline corneal deposits. Given an excess production of immunoglobulins, these can be deposited in corneal tissues. However, due to the protean nature of this disease process, various clinical findings may be observed, including depositions that resemble crystalline keratopathy, lipid keratopathy, and other nonspecific arrangements.

Fig. 6.24 displays the slit-lamp and AS-OCT images of a 70-year-old white woman who presented for a second opinion from her primary eye care provider to evaluate bilateral, asymmetric corneal deposits. The patient had no clinical symptoms, and visual acuity was 20/20. Slit-lamp findings were notable for multiple, discrete nodular opacities without associated neovascularization that involved multiple corneal layers with preservation of both epithelium and endothelium (see Fig. 6.24, *top left and bottom left panels*). AS-OCT aided in better characterizing the lesions' discrete nature and variable location, including preservation of epithelium/endothelium, including the varying depths of the lesions *(top right and bottom right panels).* Notably, in the right eye, the lesions were limited to the anterior stroma; in the left eye, lesions also involved the posterior stroma without affecting the middle stroma. The endothelium/pre-Descemet layer (Dua layer) complex is preserved in both eyes. An inflammatory and neoplastic laboratory workup was performed, including serum testing and urine protein electrophoresis, and there was a subsequent referral to an oncologist, who confirmed the diagnosis of MGUS. More malignant entities, such as MM, may be similarly assessed and diagnosed promptly, rendering the ophthalmologist a vital "gatekeeper" for appropriate referral and potentially life-saving treatment.

B. Cystinosis

Cystinosis is an autosomal recessive metabolic disorder in which cystine crystals are deposited in various parts of the eye, most notably in the cornea. Although these deposits are located throughout the stroma with a fine, crystalline appearance on examination, they are often densest in the periphery (Fig. 6.25).

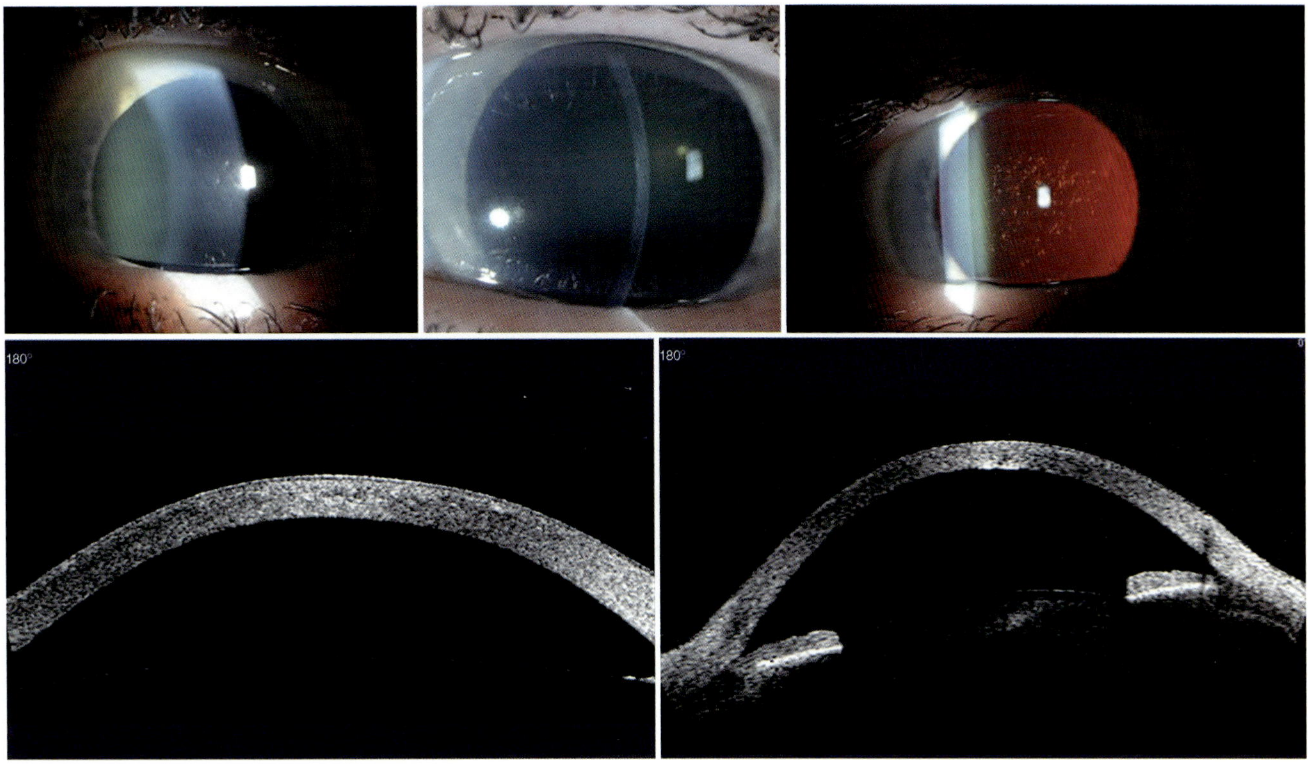

Fig. 6.23 Polymorphic amyloid degeneration. Slit-lamp photographs of the patient's right eye demonstrate white-gray deposits primarily involving the posterior stromal layers. The retro-illumination view further defines the number and location of these deposits. On AS-OCT images, the deposits are seen as focal areas of increased hyperreflectivity primarily involving the posterior stroma. Similar findings were seen in the left eye (not shown). Visual acuity was minimally affected.

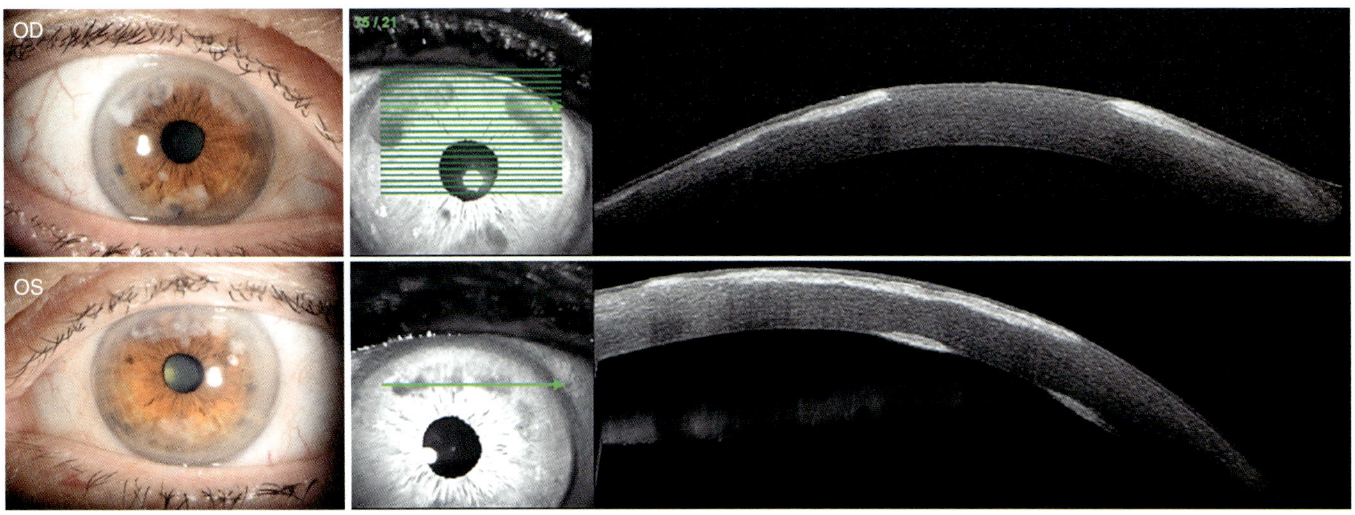

Fig. 6.24 Corneal deposits with monoclonal gammopathy of undetermined significance. Hematologic disorders, including benign entities (e.g., monoclonal gammopathy of undetermined significance [MGUS], etc.) and malignant processes (e.g., multiple myeloma, etc.), may present with nonspecific corneal deposits with involvement of multiple layers. Clinically, there is a lack of inflammation, including corneal neovascularization. Slit-lamp examination may reveal multiple, discrete, partially light-blocking opacities primarily in the mid-peripheral stroma, with a Salzmann-like appearance. AS-OCT can be used to evaluate such lesions and order appropriate laboratory testing, including serum testing and urine protein electrophoresis.

AS-OCT imaging demonstrates a diffuse, homogenous pattern of crystal deposition (hyperreflective areas) that encompasses the anterior two-thirds of the stroma. Notably, cystine deposits are not usually found in the posterior stroma. The Descemet membrane–endothelium complex is intact.

Patients often have severe photophobia and episodic pain due to recurrent corneal erosions. Topical cysteamine drops reduce intralysosomal cystine concentration and subsequent corneal crystal deposition

C. Chlorpromazine (Thorazine) Deposition

Chlorpromazine (Thorazine) is an antipsychotic drug that can cause ocular toxicity, especially with long-term use. Ocular findings may be seen in the cornea, the lens, or the retina.

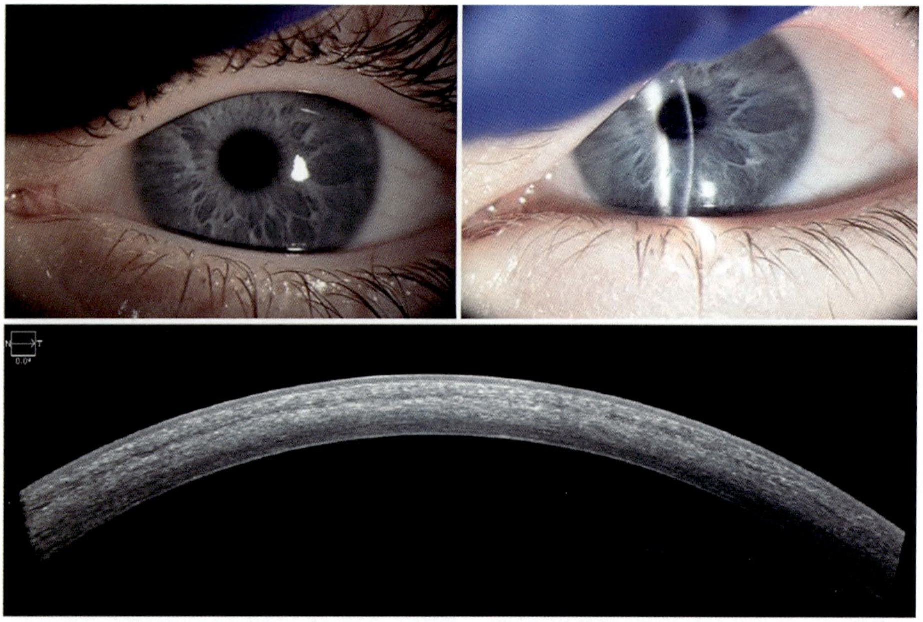

Fig. 6.25 Cystinosis findings on clinical examination classically involve the deposition of fine crystalline deposits in the anterior stroma. AS-OCT can be used to identify the location and depth of these lesions. Notably, the posterior stroma is usually uninvolved.

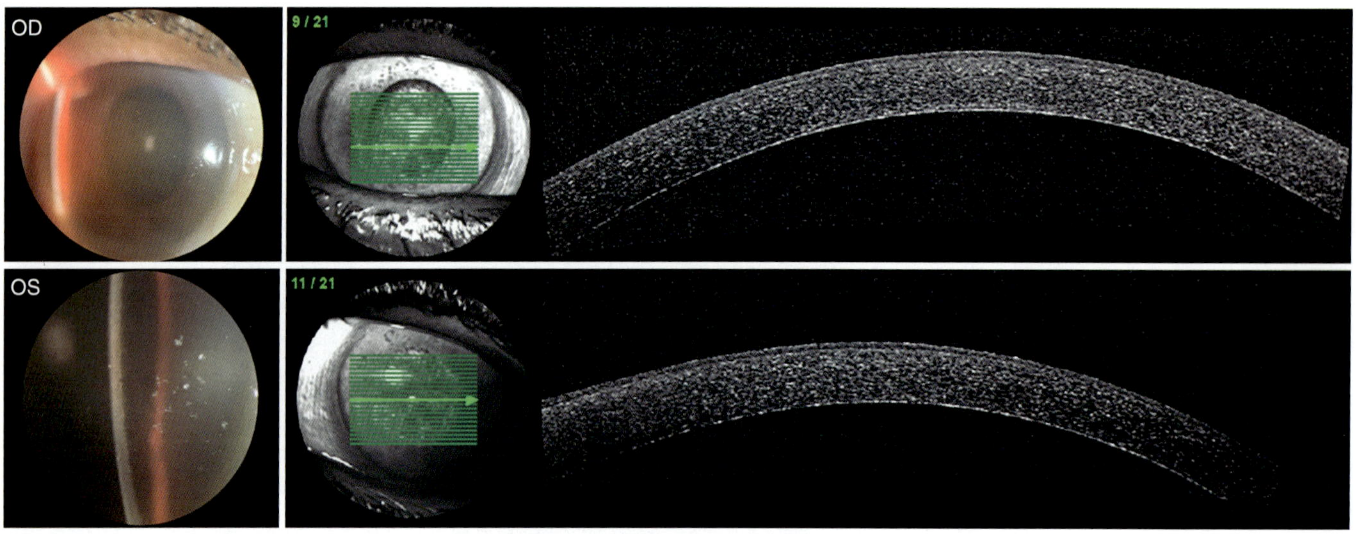

Fig. 6.26 Chlorpromazine (Thorazine) toxicity appears as fine, brownish, refractile deposits on the endothelium on slit-lamp examination. AS-OCT can be used to highlight the confluent hyperreflectivity of these deposits limited to the corneal endothelium.

In the cornea, chlorpromazine deposition is seen as diffuse, pigmented punctate deposits in the corneal endothelium, Descemet membrane, and deep stroma, typically confined within the interpalpebral cornea. A stellate pattern of pigmentary deposition may be observed on the anterior lens and lens capsule. Pigmentary changes can persist long after the cessation of therapy.

Fig. 6.26 displays clinical images of a patient who had been on chlorpromazine for 35 years. Slit-lamp photographs show fine, discrete, brownish refractile deposits in the corneal endothelium that may appear similar to guttae initially. AS-OCT imaging shows a subtle layer of hyperreflectivity of the endothelium and Descemet membrane, where these deposits are concentrated. Corneal edema is usually absent, and the corneal thickness is unchanged.

D. Intracorneal Hemorrhage

In rare cases, a patient may be at risk for intracorneal hemorrhage, especially when abnormal blood vessels have encroached into the cornea from the limbus. Clinical situations such as infection, neovascularization, and prior trauma can be the underlying cause.

Corneal surgery may contribute to intracorneal hemorrhage. The patient in Fig. 6.27 had a remote history of femtosecond laser astigmatic keratotomy (FSL-AK) in the mid-peripheral cornea. Two years later, the patient presented with a significant intracorneal hemorrhage. Slit-lamp photographs show chronologic improvement of hemorrhage with time.

In the AS-OCT images (see Fig. 6.27), the FSL-AK intrastromal incision is seen with surrounding hyporeflective (dark) areas of hemorrhage in the *lower left panel (blue arrow).* With resorption of heme, lipid deposits appear as hyperreflective areas.

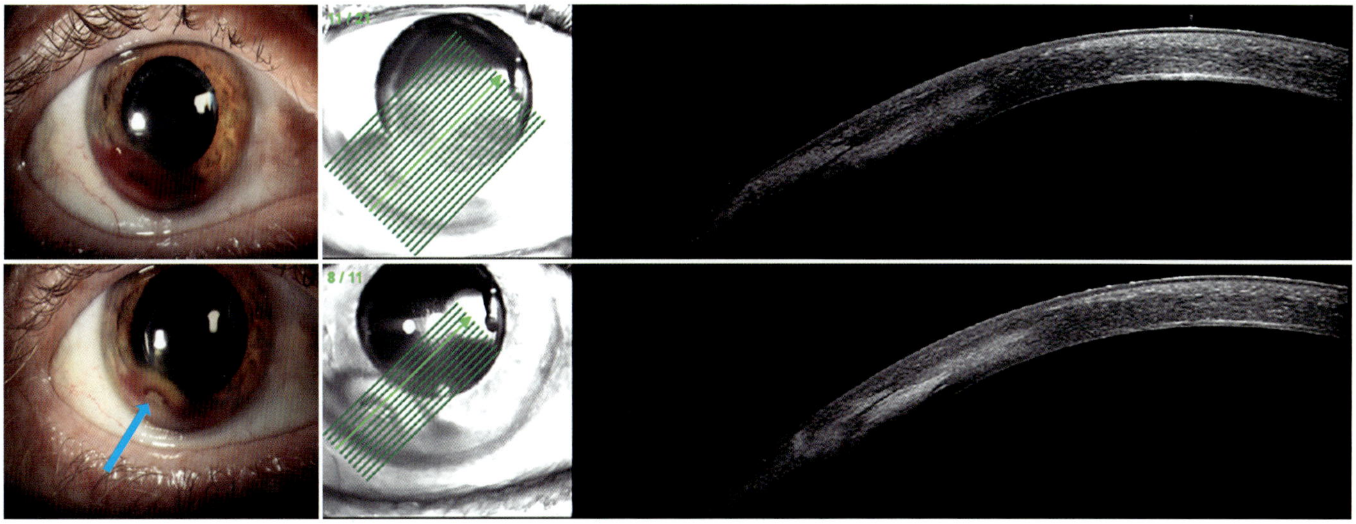

Fig. 6.27 Intracorneal hemorrhage. Hemorrhage is seen as a collection of fluid in the corneal stroma on slit-lamp examination *(top left panel)*. AS-OCT shows an area of hyporeflectivity in this area. Three months later *(bottom left panel)*, there is interval clearing of the hemorrhage *(arrow)* with associated stromal haze and scarring. AS-OCT demonstrates this scarring as increased hyperreflectivity *(bottom right panel)*.

IV. MISCELLANEOUS STROMAL PATHOLOGIC CONDITIONS

A. Stromal Edema and Bullous Keratopathy

Stromal edema may occur as a result of various corneal pathologic conditions affecting endothelial function, including primary disease (e.g., Fuchs endothelial dystrophy) and secondary conditions (HSV-associated stromal keratitis, pseudophakic bullous keratopathy, etc.). Clinical examination at the slit lamp can be sufficient to visualize stromal edema, stromal folds, and loss of corneal clarity. Corneal thickness is usually increased on pachymetry.

Fig. 6.28 shows typical slit-lamp findings *(top left panel)* associated with stromal edema. AS-OCT *(top right and bottom right panels)* can be used to assess these changes further. Corneal thickness is increased, especially in the area of the appreciable pathologic findings *(bottom left panel)*.

Although primary bullous keratopathy may occur, this condition usually happens in the context of prolonged inflammation after intraocular surgery (pseudophakic or aphakic bullous keratopathy). Clinical findings are similar to those seen in stromal edema; notably, there are increased pockets (bullae) of fluid in the epithelial space that can be appreciated on AS-OCT as areas of hyporeflectivity in the anterior cornea (Fig. 6.29)

B. Limbal Girdle of Vogt

Limbal girdle of Vogt (LGOV) is a common, benign, bilateral, age-related peripheral corneal degeneration. Crescent-shaped whitish opacities are seen mainly at the nasal and temporal limbus on clinical examination. A characteristic "clear space" between LGOV lesions and the limbus may be seen. The lesions consist of degenerated collagen with calcium particles. LGOV may represent a forme-fruste variant or precursor to calcific band keratopathy. Although they are readily detected on clinical examination, AS-OCT shows features of focal hyperreflectivity in the peripheral cornea (Fig. 6.30).

C. Stromal Thinning and Melting

Stromal thinning may occur secondary to several inflammatory, infectious, ectatic, iatrogenic, and idiopathic processes (Fig. 6.31). Ocular surface disease, especially exposure keratopathy, can significantly exacerbate disease progression. Corneal wound healing and stromal remodeling occur with appropriate treatment, including ocular surface rehabilitation and inflammation control. This may result in an abnormal corneal contour secondary to corneal scarring (Fig. 6.32).

In severe cases, stromal thinning, especially when caused by ocular and/or systemic inflammation, may cause stromal melting (Fig. 6.33). The stromal layer may be significantly attenuated with or without an intact epithelium. In very severe cases, stromal integrity may be lost altogether (Fig. 6.34). Expedited control of ocular and systemic inflammation is warranted in these cases. In cases of very severe thinning, corneal glue (e.g., cyanoacrylate glue, etc.) may be required (Fig. 6.35).

D. Stromal Scarring

Stromal scarring can occur secondary to multiple factors, such as trauma, infection, and long-standing corneal edema. Evaluating the depth and extent of stromal scars may help guide management decision-making.

For example, in cases of postinfectious stromal scarring, stromal thinning occurs with associated epithelial thickening. In Fig. 6.36, AS-OCT can be used to evaluate subepithelial scarring and associated epithelial thickening. In such cases, the scarring may be too deep for effective use of PTK because it may require undesirable removal of excessive healthy tissue. Such cases may be better managed with contact lenses or anterior lamellar keratoplasty.

AS-OCT also can be used to help guide appropriate management in corneal scarring and thinning cases secondary to chemical burns and limbal stem cell deficiency (Fig. 6.37).

CLINICAL PEARL

Secondary increase in epithelial thickness can mask stromal thinning that occurs with some types of stromal scarring. The epithelium thickens to create a more uniform anterior corneal surface. PTK may not be advisable for cases with deep scarring (subepithelial thickening) because it may be ineffective in sufficiently removing the target tissue and/or necessitate removing too much healthy tissue. SALK may be a better surgical option. Nonsurgically, visual rehabilitation with hard contact lenses or scleral contact lenses may be effective.

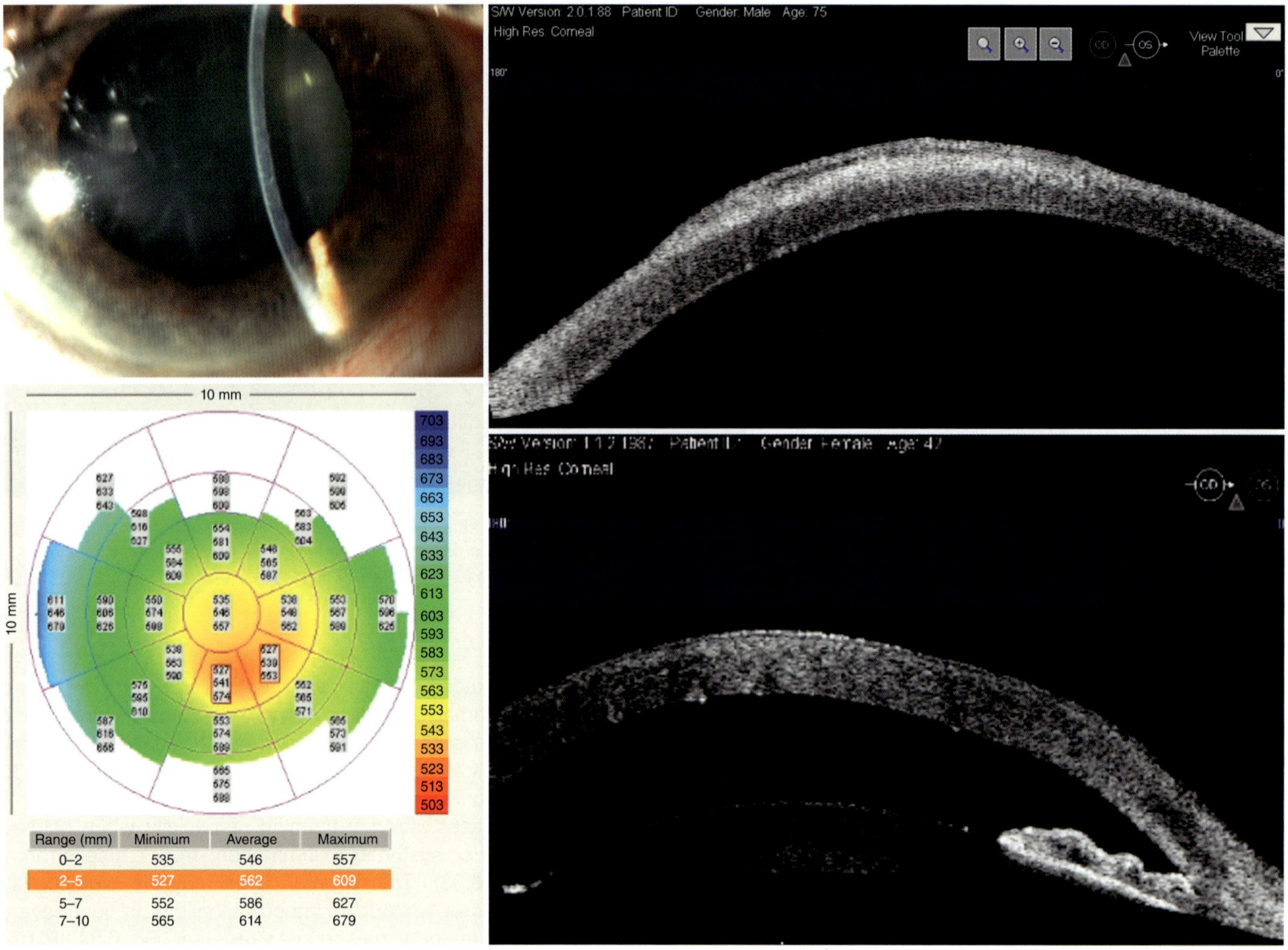

Range (mm)	Minimum	Average	Maximum
0–2	535	546	557
2–5	527	562	609
5–7	552	586	627
7–10	565	614	679

Fig. 6.28 Stromal edema detected by slit-lamp examination alone *(top panel)* with associated increased corneal thickness *(bottom left panel).* AS-OCT demonstrates stromal thickening. In the *top right panel,* a small pocket of fluid (bullous keratopathy) is also present. (Image Credit: Helena Prior Filipe, MD, MMEd. West Lisbon Hospitals Center (CHLO). Hospital Egas Moniz. Portugal; Egas Moniz Center for Interdisciplinary Research (CiiEM). Portugal.)

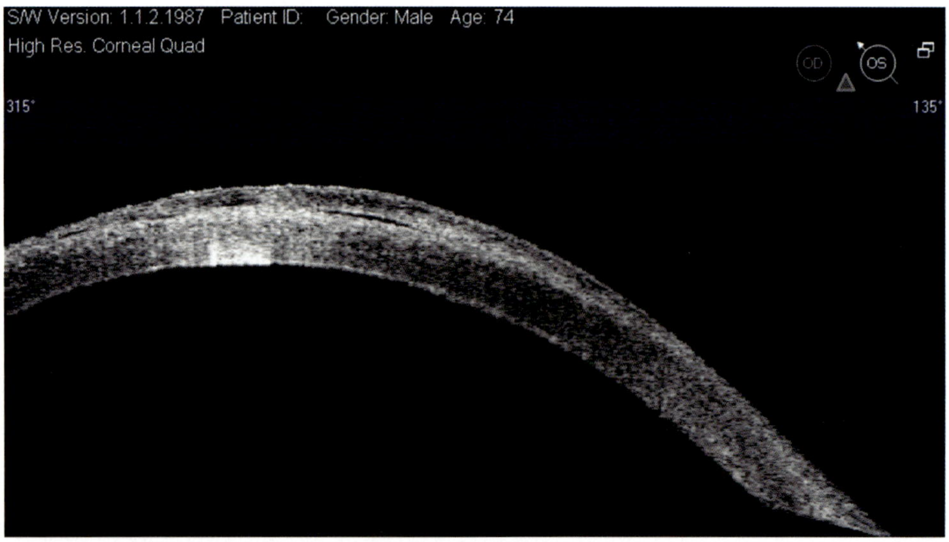

Fig. 6.29 Bullous keratopathy, usually seen in the presence of stromal edema. AS-OCT demonstrates focal areas of fluid as hyporeflective areas in the anterior stroma. (Image Credit: Helena Prior Filipe, MD, MMEd.West Lisbon Hospitals Center (CHLO). Hospital Egas Moniz. Portugal; Egas Moniz Center for Interdisciplinary Research (CiiEM). Portugal.)

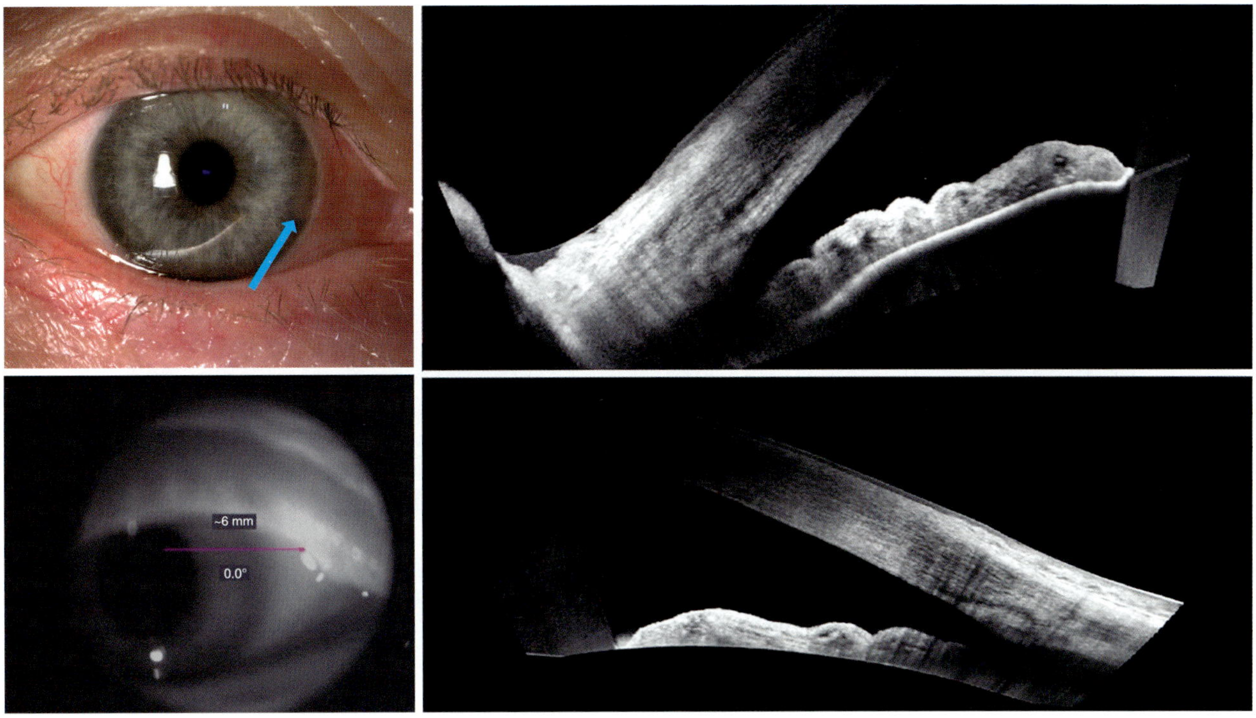

Fig. 6.30 Limbal girdle of Vogt (LGOV). LGOV is an age-related degeneration typically seen at the nasal and temporal limbus *(top left panel, arrow).* AS-OCT demonstrates a focal area of increased hyperreflectivity in the peripheral cornea, usually at the nasal and temporal limbus.

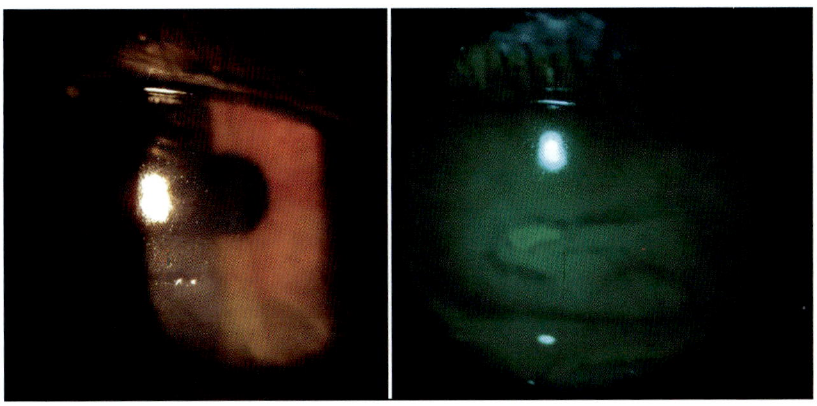

Fig. 6.31 Stromal thinning. Stromal thinning may occur as a result of a variety of factors. Fluorescein staining can highlight the area of epithelial defect.

Stromal scarring may also occur in cases of long-standing corneal edema, such as in patients with decompensation of Fuchs endothelial dystrophy. In cases with extensive stromal scarring, endothelial keratoplasty (Descemet stripping [automated] endothelial keratoplasty [DSAEK/DMEK]) may be challenging or insufficient to improve vision because the anterior stromal scarring remains, and a full-thickness graft may be considered instead (Fig. 6.38). In cases with subepithelial scarring with relatively clear stroma, DSAEK or DMEK may be effectively performed. AS-OCT can help assess the presence and extent of stromal scarring. In Fig. 6.32, note the extensive stromal scarring (increased stromal hyperreflectivity) in the *top panel* compared with the subepithelial scarring with relatively clear stroma (normal stromal reflectivity) in the *bottom panel.*

Extensive stromal scarring may also occur after multiple corneal refractive surgeries. Fig. 6.39 shows images of a patient who underwent radial keratotomy with astigmatic keratotomy and then underwent laser-assisted in situ keratomileusis (LASIK) many years later. Significant areas of scarring causing irregular astigmatism can be seen on clinical examination and topography, respectively. AS-OCT can be used in such cases to assess the depth and extent of scarring and determine the best course of visual rehabilitation. In this patient, cataract surgery followed by scleral contact lens fitting was sufficient to improve the vision to 20/40 and avoid corneal transplant surgery.

E. Descemetocele

A descemetocele occurs when an intact Descemet membrane herniates through an area of an overlying stromal defect. Clinical examination reveals a central clear zone within surrounding areas of thinning. This rare but severe outcome can occur with progressive stromal tissue loss secondary to infectious keratitis, neurotrophic corneal disease, severe corneal inflammation, and sometimes rarely in severe dry eye disease with exposure

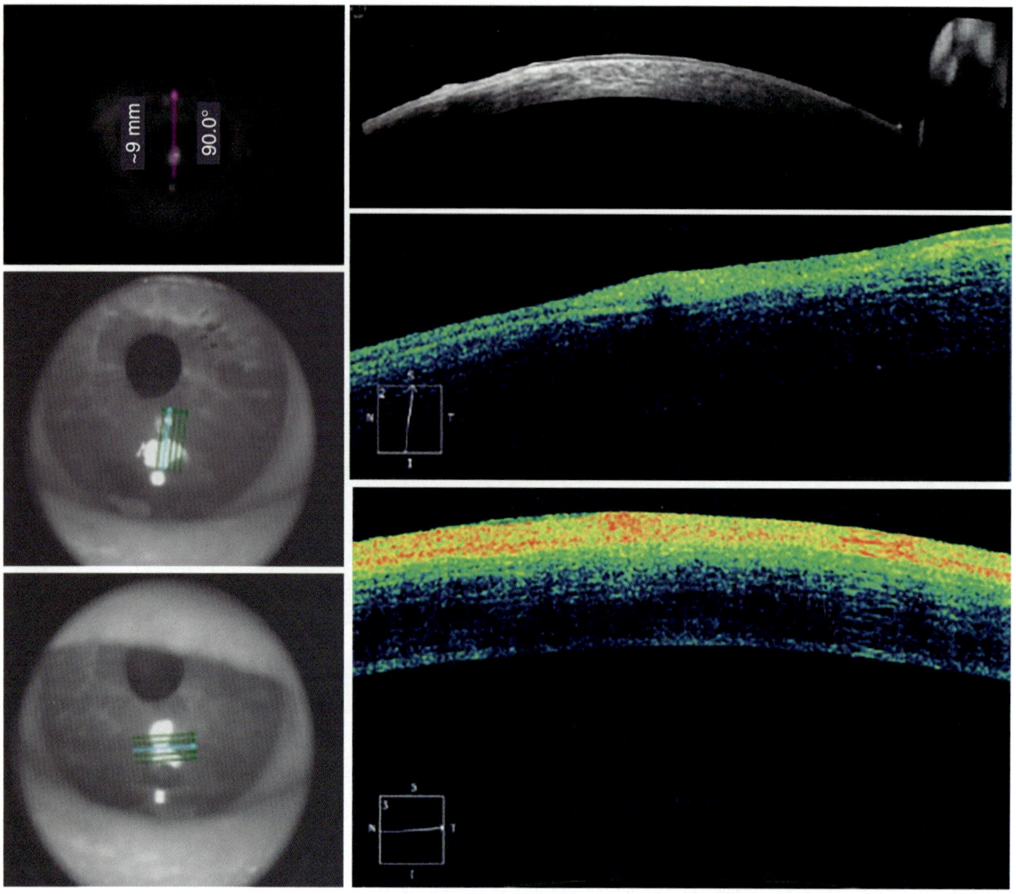

Fig. 6.32 Posttreatment images of the patient in Fig. 6.31. After successful treatment of the patient in the previous figure, AS-OCT images with two different devices demonstrate scarring changes associated with corneal wound healing. In the *top right panel,* AS-OCT highlights the irregular, protruding contour of the inferior corneal surface. In the *middle and bottom right panels,* AS-OCT shows the elevated contour and corneal scarring, respectively.

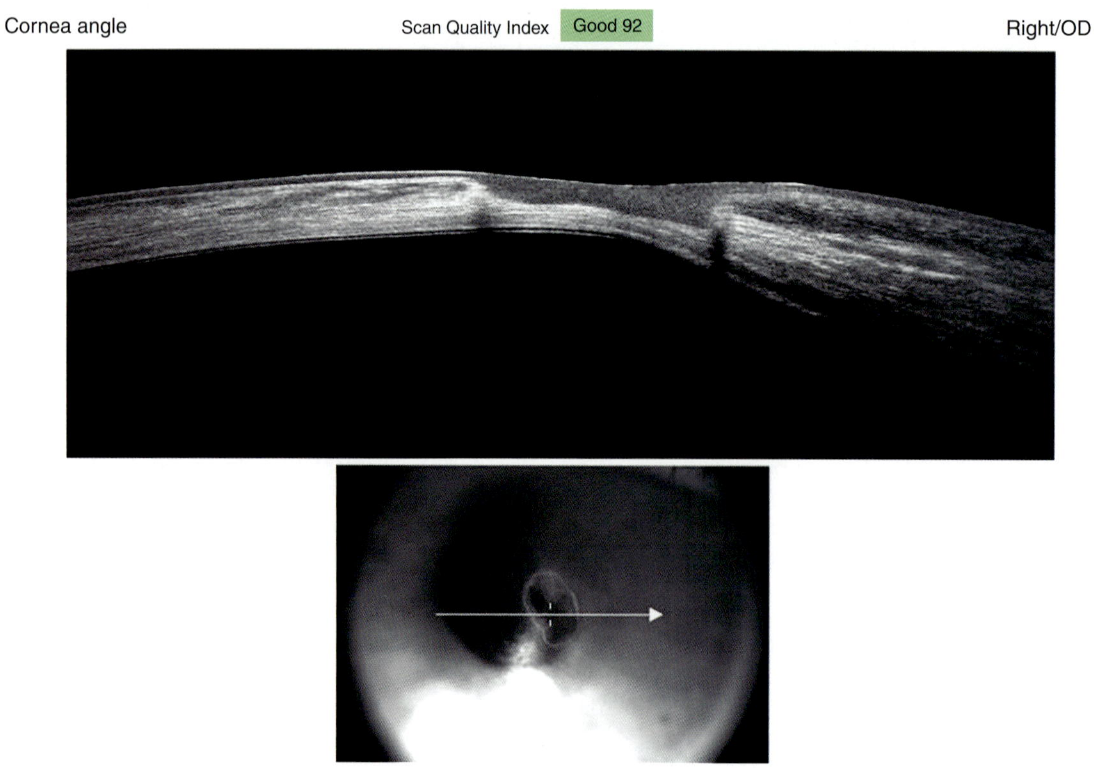

Fig. 6.33 AS-OCT of stromal melting. Images demonstrate significant thinning of the stroma with intact epithelium overlying.

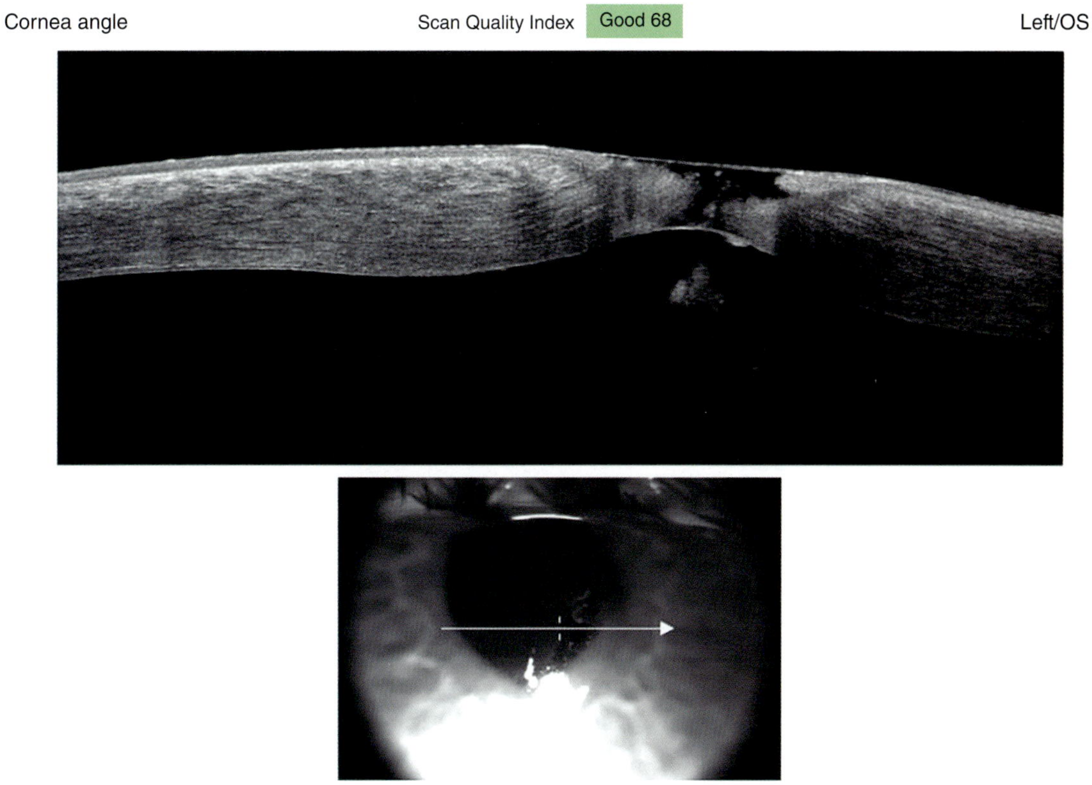

Fig. 6.34 AS-OCT of very severe stromal melting, demonstrating disruption of stromal integrity. The epithelium and endothelium are still intact. This finding warrants urgent corneal glue placement because the risk of corneal perforation is very high. Prompt reduction and control of associated ocular and systemic inflammation are paramount in these situations.

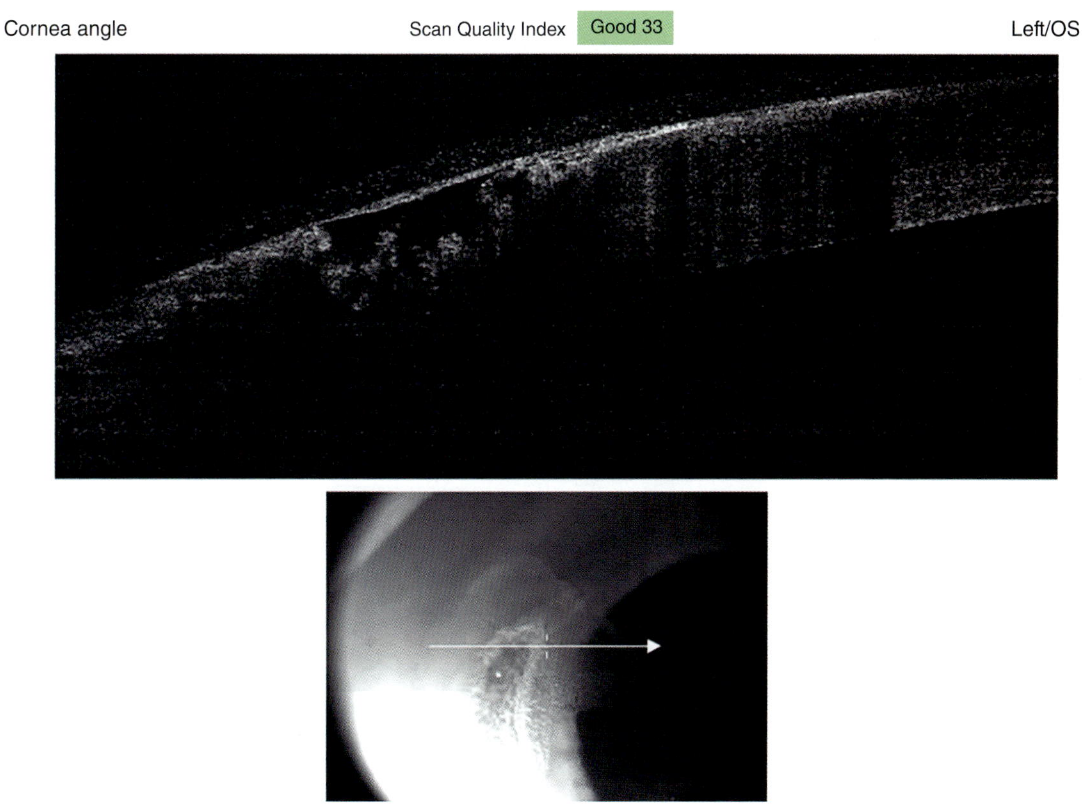

Fig. 6.35 Application of corneal glue in stromal melting. Corneal glue may be required in significant cases of stromal melting to prevent corneal perforation. The glue can be seen on AS-OCT as an additional "layer" over the intact corneal epithelium.

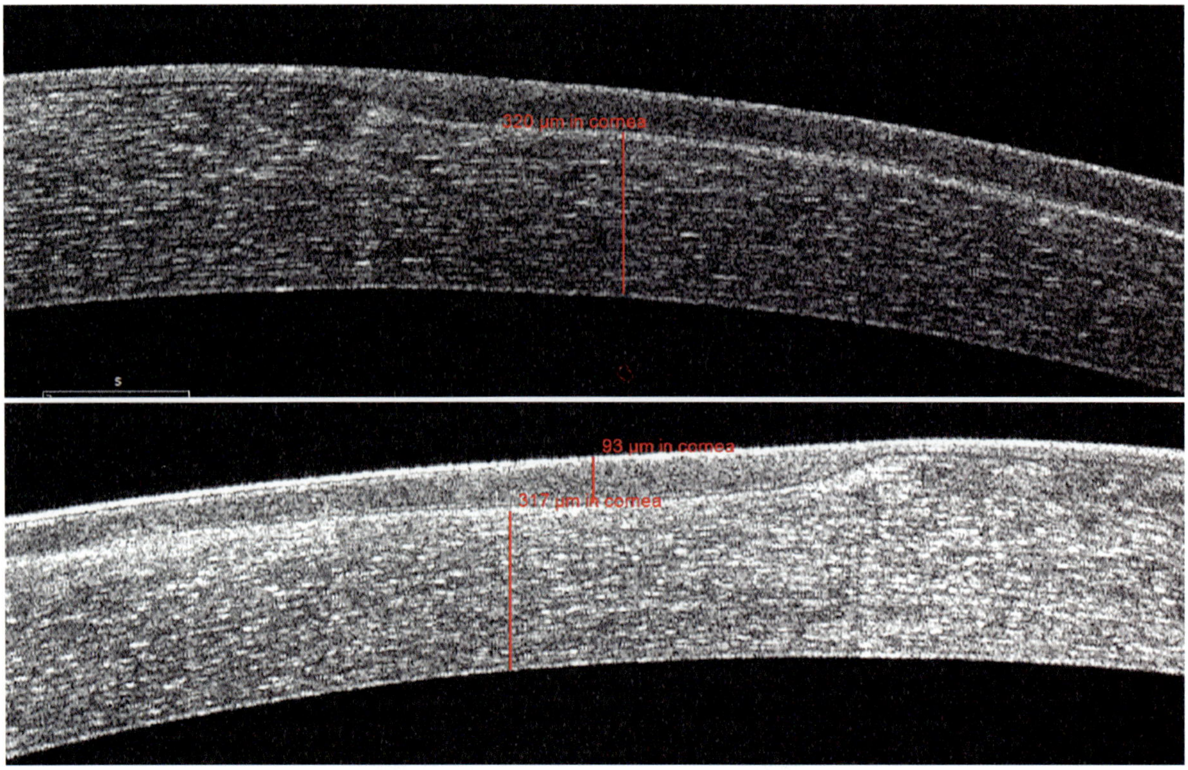

Fig. 6.36 Stromal scarring with thinning. In cases of stromal scarring with thinning, secondary epithelial thickening occurs to create a more uniform anterior corneal surface. AS-OCT can be used to measure the depth and extent of the subepithelial scarring. In this case, the scarring is quite deep and may not be amenable to phototherapeutic keratectomy. (Courtesy of Nikhil Gokhale, Gokhale Eye Hospial, Mumbai, India.)

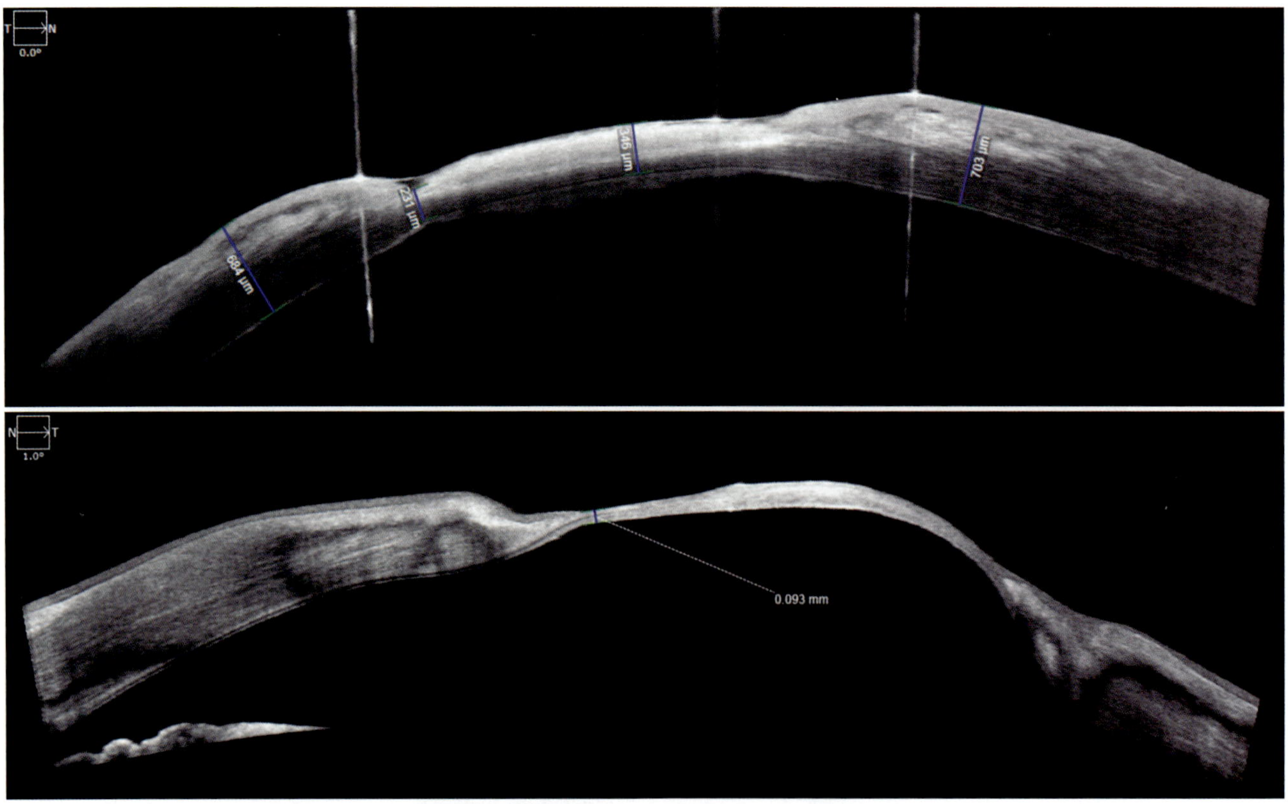

Fig. 6.37 Corneal scarring and thinning. AS-OCT can be used to evaluate corneal thickness and ocular surface anatomy in cases of corneal scarring and thinning secondary to infectious keratitis, chemical burns, and/or limbal stem cell deficiency. These images show two different areas of severe stromal thinning after contact lens associated–*Pseudomonas* keratitis.

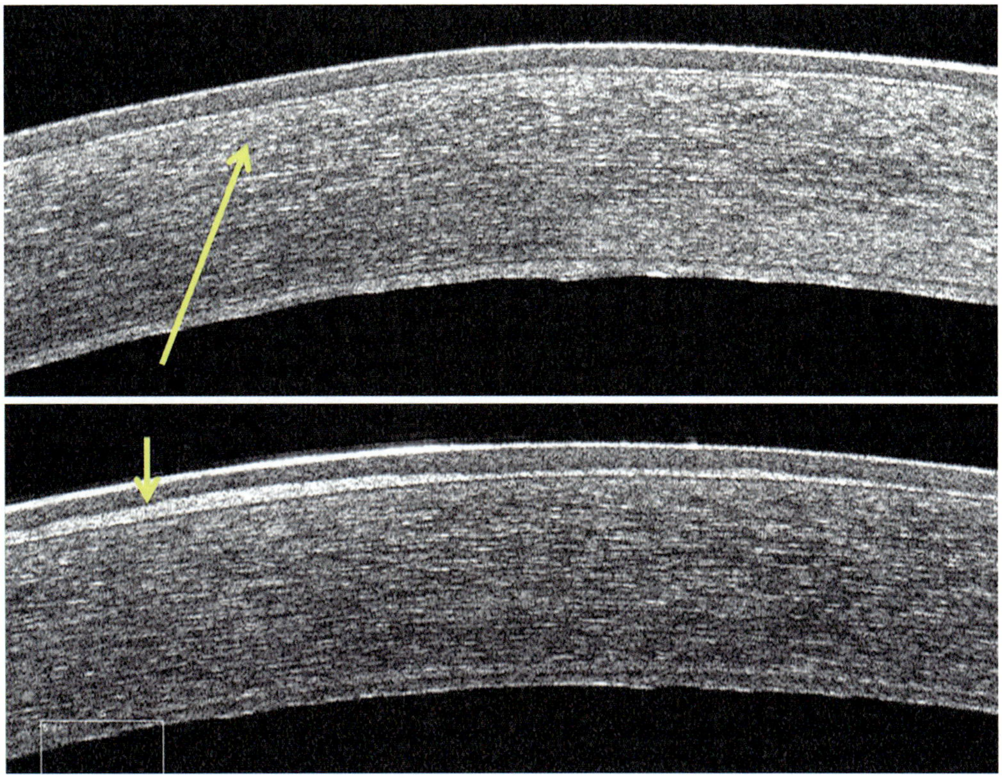

Fig. 6.38 Subepithelial and stromal scarring. Long-standing corneal edema in patients with decompensated Fuchs endothelial dystrophy may result in secondary subepithelial and stromal scarring. In the *top panel,* AS-OCT demonstrates significant stromal scarring (increased hyperreflectivity, yellow arrow) in the anterior stroma. Endothelial keratoplasty (EK) may be insufficient to improve the vision in this patient; even with a successful EK, the surgeon may have to address the stromal scarring with contact lens rehabilitation. In the *bottom panel,* there is prominent but limited subepithelial scarring (small yellow arrow) with relatively clear stroma (normal intensity of stromal reflectivity). In this case, EK may be effectively performed, although phototherapeutic keratectomy and/or contact lens rehabilitation may be required postoperatively. (Courtesy of Nikhil Gokhale, Gokhale Eye Hospital, Mumbai, India.)

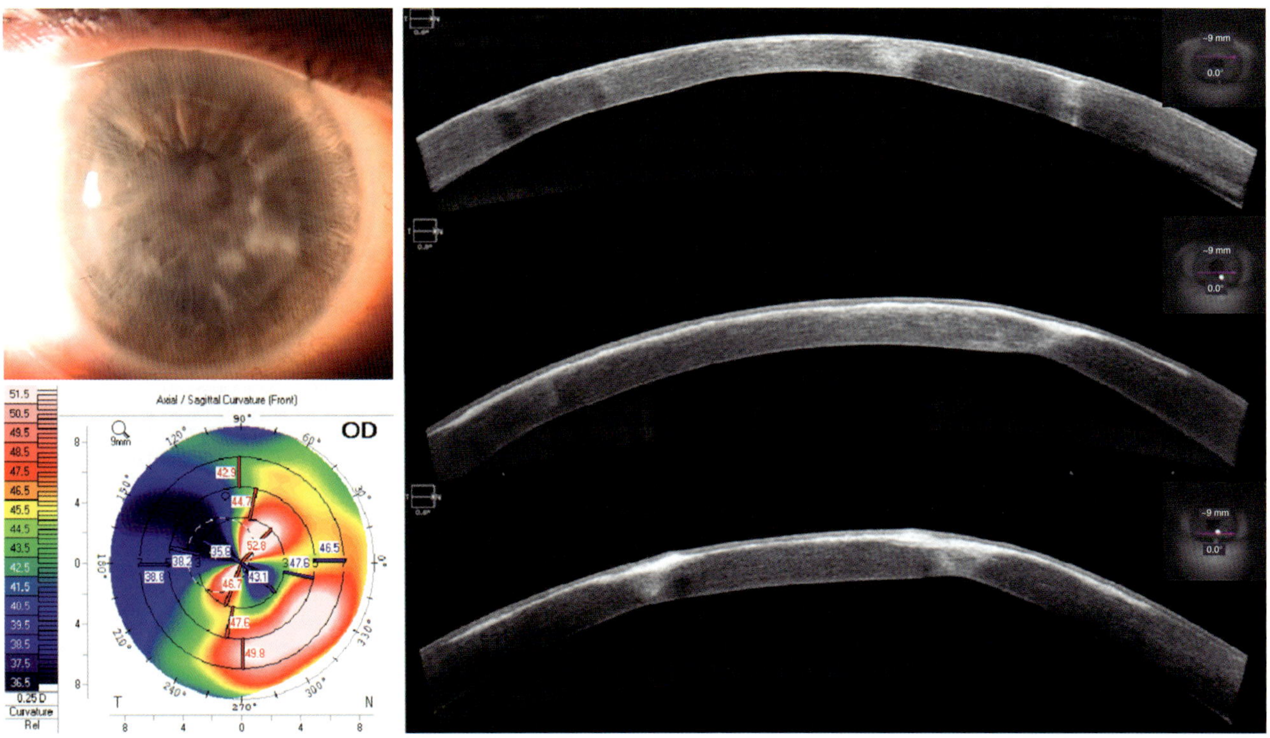

Fig. 6.39 Corneal scarring secondary to radial keratotomy, astigmatic keratotomy, and LASIK procedure. Slit-lamp photograph *(top left panel)* shows extensive stromal scarring with partial light-blocking effect throughout the central cornea. Topography *(bottom left panel)* shows significant irregular astigmatism. AS-OCT images demonstrate the extent and depth of scarring; this information can be used for clinical versus surgical decision-making.

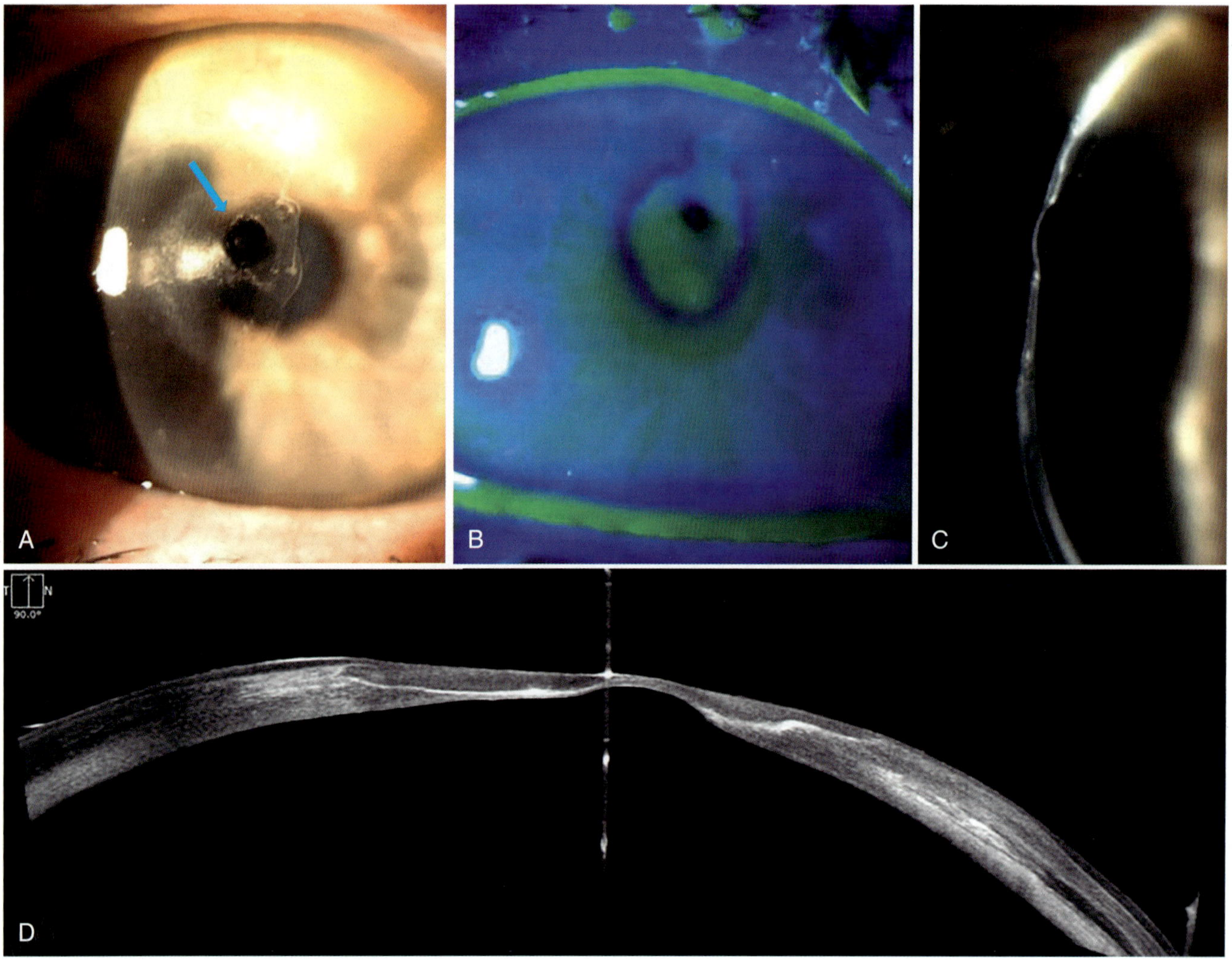

Fig. 6.40 Descemetocele secondary to recurrent herpes simplex virus keratitis. Slit-lamp photograph with broad-beam illumination *(panel A)* shows a relatively clear central area *(blue arrow)* corresponding to the anterior herniation of the Descemet membrane, within a surrounding area of thinning and haze. After fluorescein staining, cobalt-blue illumination *(panel B)* shows an area of negative staining corresponding to the descemetocele. Secondary staining of the surrounding thinning is also present. With the thin-slit technique *(panel C)*, a cross-sectional view at the slit-lamp further highlights the anterior protrusion of the Descemet membrane with a thin but intact overlying stromal layer. AS-OCT *(panel D)* through the descemetocele better captures these changes in cross-section. In addition to the anterior herniation of the Descemet membrane, other salient features of AS-OCT include prominent stromal hyperreflectivity corresponding to stromal scarring and epithelial remodeling.

keratopathy. Corneal inflammation secondary to immune-mediated systemic disease is also a well-known cause. An untreated descemetocele may eventually cause corneal perforation, warranting prompt surgical intervention in the office setting (corneal glue) or operating room (patch graft or penetrating keratoplasty).

Fig. 6.40 shows slit-lamp and AS-OCT findings in a patient who developed a descemetocele secondary to recurrent, progressive HSV keratitis. AS-OCT further highlights features seen on the thin-slit technique on slit-lamp examination, including Descemet membrane herniation, stromal thinning, and stromal scarring.

BIBLIOGRAPHY

Krachmer JH, Mannis MJ, Holland EJ. *Cornea: Fundamentals, Diagnosis and Management*. 3rd ed. Mosby Elsevier; 2011.

Kanski J, Bowling B. Cornea. In: *Kanski's Clinical Ophthalmology: A Systematic Approach*. 8th ed. Saunders; 2016:167-238.

Weiss JS, Møller HU, Aldave AJ, et al. IC3D classification of corneal dystrophies–edition 2. *Cornea*. 2015;34(3):117-159.

Weisenthal RW, Daly MK, de Freitas D, et al. *External Disease and Cornea – Basic and Clinical Science Course: 2019-2020*. Vol 8. American Academy of Ophthalmology; 2019.

7 Corneal Ectasias

Kamran M. Riaz

I. INTRODUCTION

The term *corneal ectasias* refers to several disease processes characterized by progressive, noninflammatory thinning changes in the central or peripheral cornea. Broadly, ectasia refers to a "dilation or expansion of a tubular organ". Clinically, thinning caused by corneal ectasias leads to protrusion or bulging of the affected region(s) of the cornea. While the disease process is usually bilateral, a high degree of asymmetry in detectable pathology usually exists, especially in early and subclinical disease states. Furthermore, progression in early disease states may occur extremely slowly, so clinically significant changes may not be readily detected on routine slit-lamp examination.

Corneal imaging remains the gold standard for diagnosing corneal ectasias. Corneal *topography* allows for a quantitative and qualitative evaluation of the anterior corneal surface and readily displays information using color-coded maps to aid clinical decision-making. Corneal *tomography* additionally measures corneal thickness and gives information about the posterior cornea. Information gained from both of these imaging techniques allows clinicians to diagnose ectatic disease, assess disease progression, and determine appropriate nonsurgical/surgical interventions. Additionally, both are used to critically screen candidates who present for laser refractive surgery, especially to determine which candidates have an increased risk for iatrogenic post-refractive corneal ectasia.

Both topography and tomography are not without limitations. For example, irregular ocular surface (e.g., ocular surface disease, poor tear film, corneal scars) may lead to poor image acquisition. Image acquisition time varies from device to device and may be a limiting factor in certain patients who may not be able to cooperate for imaging. Finally, neither of these imaging techniques provides information and visualization of the various corneal layers.

Anterior segment optical coherence tomography (AS-OCT) technology complements and supplements information gleaned from topography and tomography. By providing clinicians with a cross-sectional and (reconstructed) three-dimensional view of the cornea, additional information, especially for subclinical disease, is obtained. Given that these processes preferentially affect various corneal layers depending on the stage of disease, AS-OCT can be advantageously used with topography and tomography to yield a strategic "trifecta" in diagnosing and managing these challenging diseases.

This chapter will primarily focus on corneal ectasias with central and paracentral corneal involvement. Terrien marginal degeneration, which mainly involves thinning of the peripheral corneal stroma, is discussed in Chapter 6.

II. KERATOCONUS

In clinical practice, keratoconus (KCN) is the most frequently encountered corneal ectasia. KCN is a bilateral, progressive, noninflammatory disease that classically causes stromal thinning leading to an irregular conical shape in the inferior cornea. Various genetic, environmental, ethnic, and hormonal factors have been implicated. While bilateral disease exists in most KCN patients, significant asymmetry in corneal changes is frequently seen.

Several systemic conditions (e.g., systemic atopic disease, Down syndrome, Marfan syndrome, sleep apnea) and ocular conditions (e.g., floppy eyelid syndrome, vernal keratoconjunctivitis, atopic eye disease) have been noted to have an increased incidence of cornea ectasia. Of note, there is a nearly universal tendency for KCN patients to demonstrate eye rubbing; in many cases, the asymmetric disease may be attributed to patients' preferential rubbing of the more affected eye.

In the early stages of KCN, patients may report progressively worsening vision with complaints of blurry vision; increasing eye strain; headaches; and glare/halos/starbursts, especially at night. In these stages, glasses and/or contact lenses may progressively fail to improve best corrected visual acuity. As KCN progresses, vision loss results from increasing myopia, irregular astigmatism, and corneal scarring.

While several clinical signs (e.g., Munson sign, Rizutti sign, Fleischer ring, Vogt striae, and oil droplet red reflex) have been described, these clinical signs often do not present in the early stages of KCN. Thus, similar to other corneal ectasias, corneal imaging is an invaluable tool for detecting subclinical and early KCN. Topography and tomography can demonstrate a variety of findings, including but not limited to irregular astigmatism, inferior corneal steepening, inferior corneal thinning, and anterior/posterior surface changes. Several KCN classification systems and criteria using topography and tomography data have been advocated in the literature, but these are beyond the scope of this chapter.

Recently, an international coalition described KCN as a disease process characterized by posterior elevation and abnormal corneal thickness distribution. As such, AS-OCT is uniquely suited to aid clinicians in early diagnosis.

A. Appearance of Keratoconus Changes on Imaging

Various AS-OCT findings can be seen depending on the stage of KCN disease. It should be noted that there is a significant overlap between imaging findings and disease severity.

I. AS-OCT CHANGES ASSOCIATED WITH MILD-MODERATE KERATOCONUS

In early (mild) KCN, AS-OCT can be used to visualize epithelial *thinning over the apex* of the conical changes, typically in the inferotemporal quadrants (Figs. 7.1 and 7.2). This may be due to underlying stromal remodeling in the area of the steepening and protrusion as the cornea attempts to "reshape" the early stages of anterior surface irregularities. In the area of the cone apex, subtle epithelial thinning can be seen as compared to the adjacent *normal* or *slightly thickened* epithelium (Figs. 7.3 and 7.4). These changes can mask stromal thinning such that pachymetry

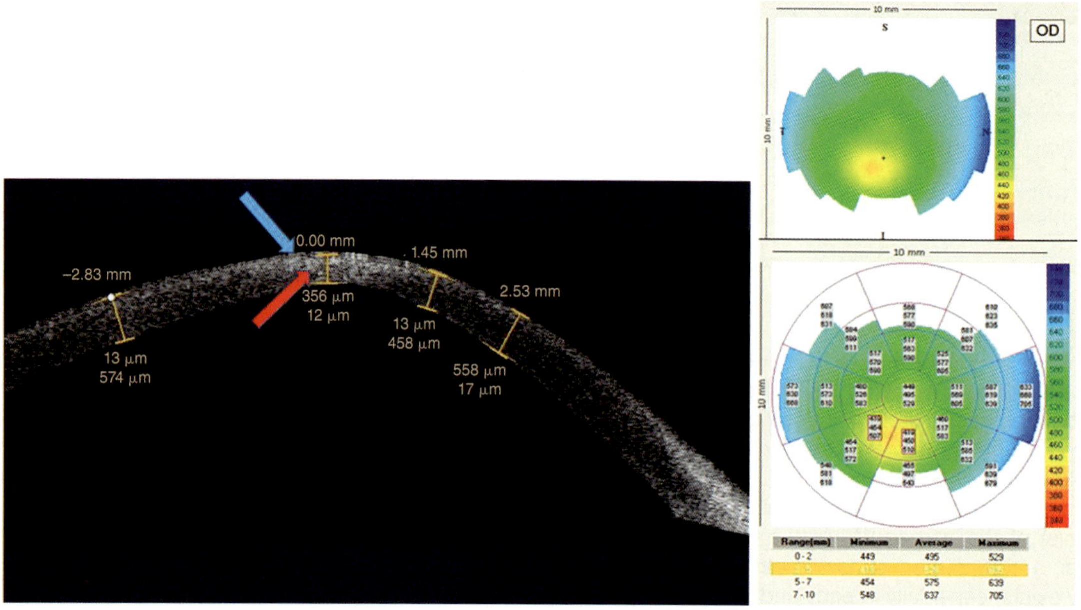

Fig. 7.1 AS-OCT imaging in patients with mild keratoconus. AS-OCT often demonstrates stromal thinning *(red arrow)* corresponding to early apical cone changes seen on topography *(top right panel)*. Epithelial thickness mapping additionally shows epithelial thinning over the area of the protrusion as the cornea remodels itself to create a smoother anterior surface. AS-OCT demonstrates subtle thinning *(blue arrow)* of the epithelial thickness over the area of the apical cone. (Courtesy Helena Filipe, MD, Lisbon, Portugal.)

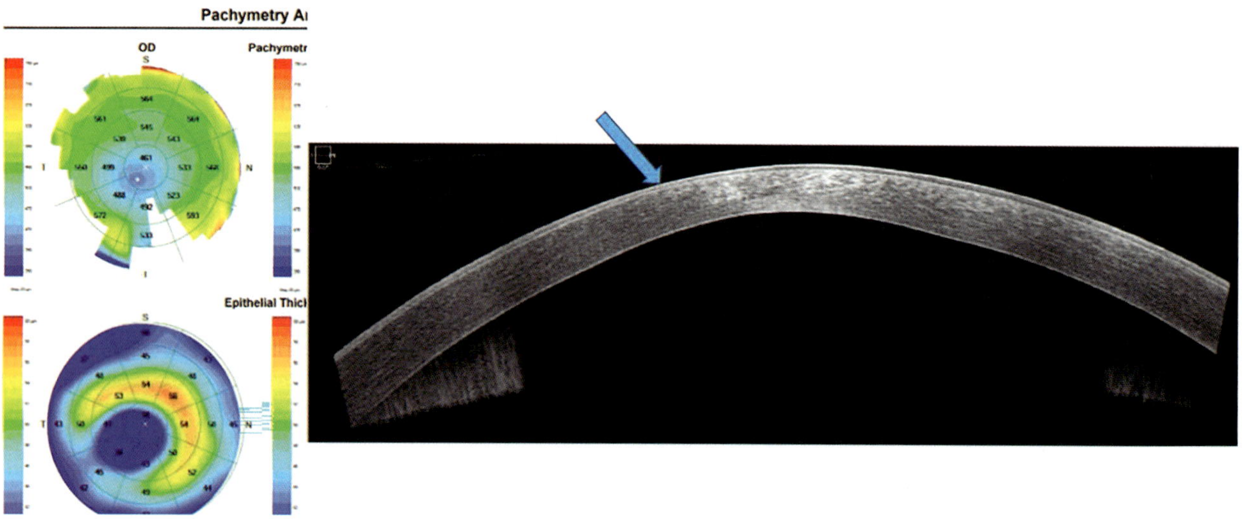

Fig. 7.2 AS-OCT imaging in patients with mild keratoconus. AS-OCT often demonstrates epithelial thinning *(blue arrow)* over the area of the apical cone. Epithelial thickness mapping additionally shows epithelial thinning over the area of the protrusion as the cornea remodels itself to create a smoother anterior surface.

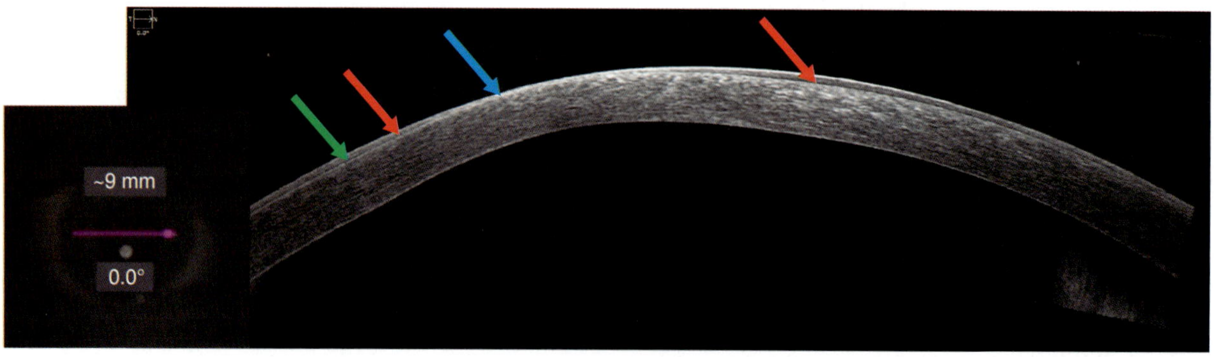

Fig. 7.3 Epithelial thinning *(blue arrow)* can be appreciated over the apex of the cone. The adjacent epithelium *(red arrows)* maintains normal thickness. The Bowman layer is not clearly visualized under the area of the cone but can be appreciated as a hyperreflective line *(green arrow)* underlying areas of normal epithelium and overlying areas of stroma without thinning

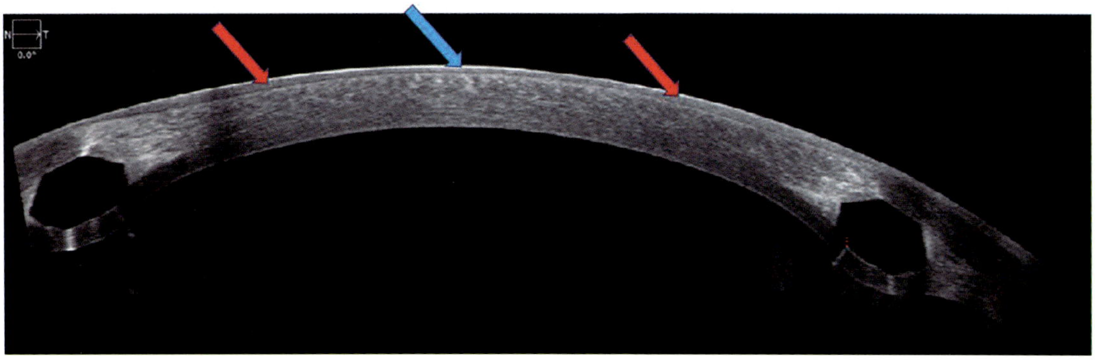

Fig. 7.4 Subtle epithelial thinning in keratoconus (KCN). In mild to moderate stages of KCN, subtle epithelial thinning *(blue arrow)* may be appreciated directly under the apex of the cone. Adjacent to this, the epithelium may be normal or even slightly thickened *(red arrows).* This patient has also undergone an intrastromal ring segment placement (to be discussed later in the chapter). Note the continuity and clear demarcation of the Bowman layer compared with the previous image.

readings are relatively normal. However, the AS-OCT images can be used to visualize the aforementioned epithelial and stromal changes, which may provide information for accurate diagnosis of mild KCN, especially in cases where topography/tomography shows questionable changes in patients presenting for refractive surgery.

CLINICAL PEARL

AS-OCT can be used to visualize epithelial thinning over the apex of the cone with associated normal or slightly thickened epithelium in the surrounding areas.

These changes can also be seen in corneal epithelial thickness mapping (ETM), which can further highlight inferotemporal epithelial *thinning* and superonasal epithelial *thickening*. This epithelial thickness profile across the central 8 mm follows a "donut-pattern" characterized by a thin central region ("the hole") surrounded by a ring of thickened tissue ("the donut"). As such, clinicians may use AS-OCT and ETM to supplement topography/tomography to aid in accurate diagnosis.

Additional changes in mild to moderate KCN include subepithelial scarring underlying the area of apical protrusion and thinning (Figs. 7.5 and 7.6). AS-OCT helps highlight the location and depth of these subsurface scarring changes. This scarring may be seen in conjunction with stromal thinning (Figs. 7.7 and 7.8). In moderate KCN, both scarring and thinning may be appreciated in the stroma, with secondary epithelial thickening (Fig. 7.9). This hypertrophic remodeling likely occurs to establish a smoother anterior corneal surface.

Subepithelial scarring should be distinguished from the raised subepithelial nodular scars that often develop in KCN patients at or near the apex of the cone. Such fibrotic scars may lead to contact lens intolerance and recurrent erosions. These nodular scars are located in the subepithelial space; a vital feature of these scars is the presence of an intact Bowman layer, which distinguishes these from other forms of reticular scarring. ETM will usually demonstrate epithelial *thinning* in the area of the scar with associated *thickening* in a concentric area around the scar (Figs. 7.10 and 7.11). AS-OCT reflects this pattern of epithelial thinning-thickening, and it highlights the presence of an intact epithelium and Bowman layer. These patients may benefit from scleral contact lenses that allow for vaulting of the lens over the lesion. Surgical intervention (manual nodule removal or phototherapeutic keratectomy) may be required in some cases.

II. AS-OCT CHANGES ASSOCIATED WITH SEVERE KERATOCONUS

In moderate to severe KCN, subepithelial scarring (secondary epithelial thickening) occurs due to ruptures in the Bowman

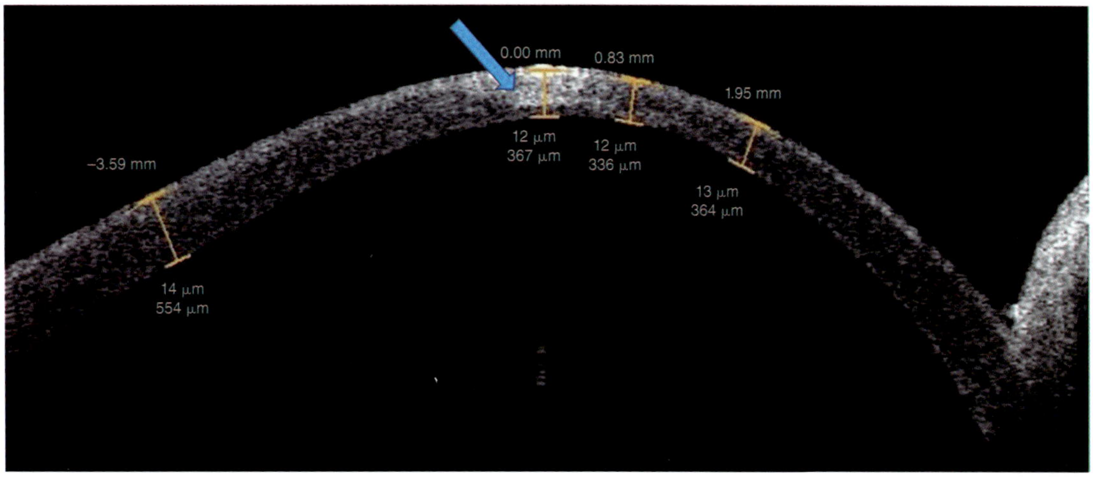

Fig. 7.5 Subepithelial scarring in mild keratoconus (KCN). AS-OCT highlights the area of subepithelial scarring in mild KCN disease as a hyperreflective region *(blue arrow)* underlying the area of the apical cone and thinning. (Courtesy Helena Filipe, MD, Lisbon, Portugal.)

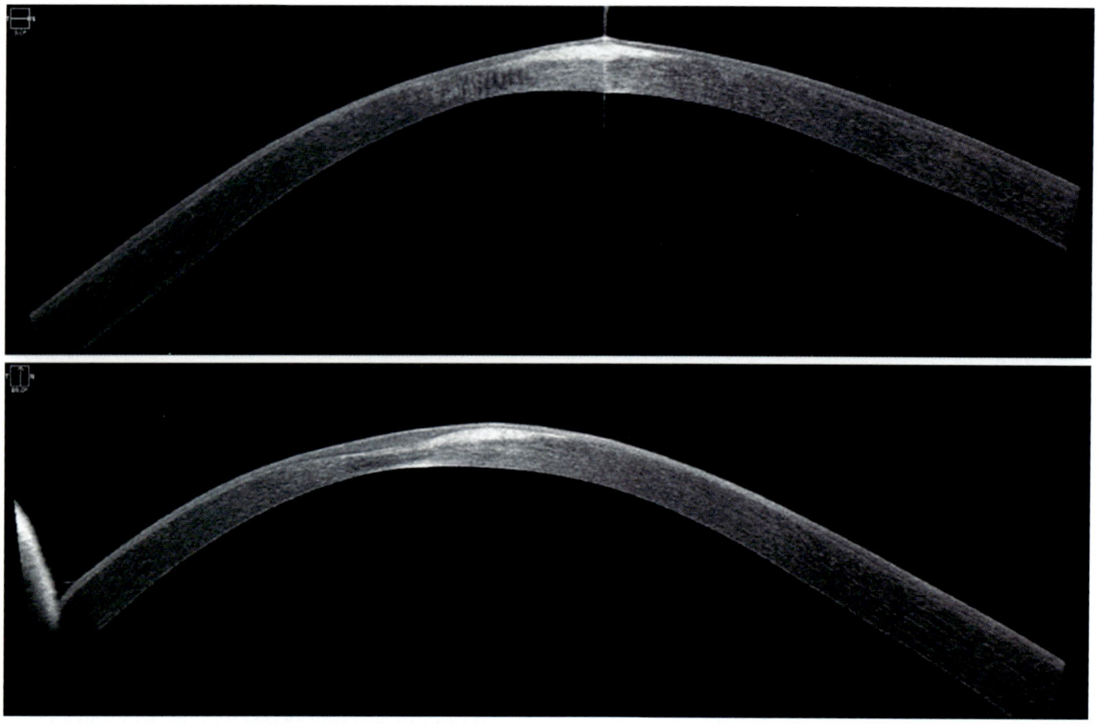

Fig. 7.6 Subepithelial scarring in moderate keratoconus. Scarring appears as an area of increased hyperreflectivity with thinning of the overlying epithelium in the *top panel* (horizontal slice). In the *bottom panel* (vertical slice), there is similar hyperreflectivity of the subepithelial scarring. Notice the thickened epithelium immediately inferior to the scar, thus allowing for a relatively smooth anterior corneal surface.

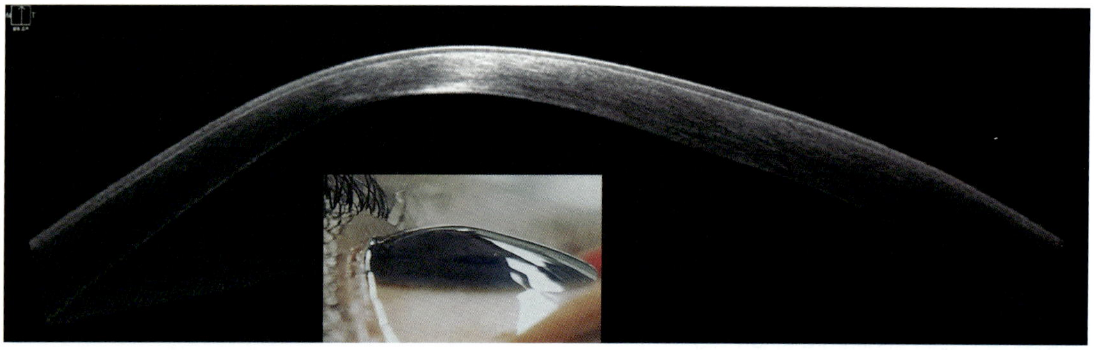

Fig. 7.7 In moderate keratoconus, subepithelial scarring (hyperreflective area) associated with stromal thinning. Note the relative central thinning compared with the thickness and translucency of the peripheral cornea. AS-OCT findings correlate with changes seen on clinical examination.

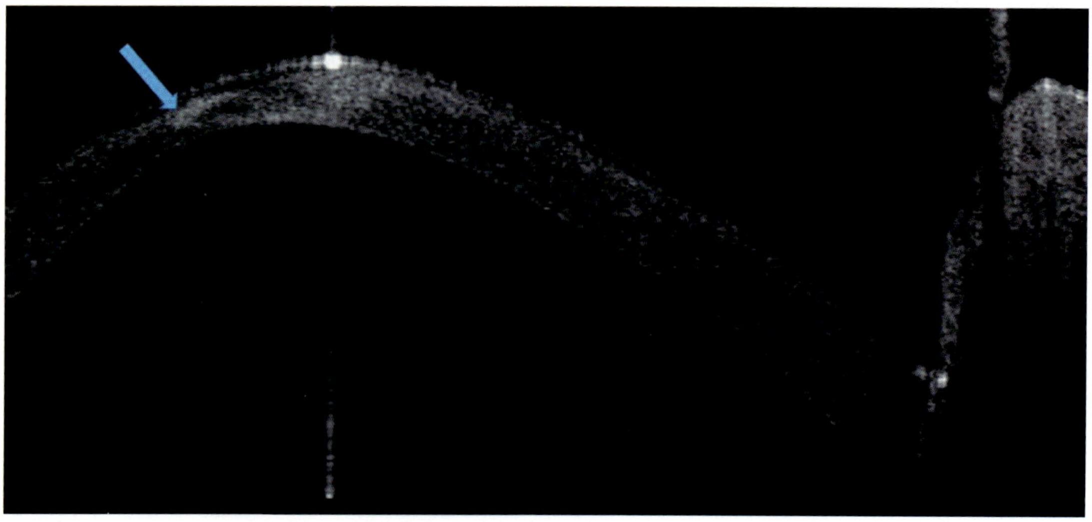

Fig. 7.8 In moderate keratoconus disease states, further apical thinning, protrusion, and subepithelial changes (hyperreflectivity; *blue arrow*) can be seen. (Courtesy Helena Filipe, MD, Lisbon, Portugal.)

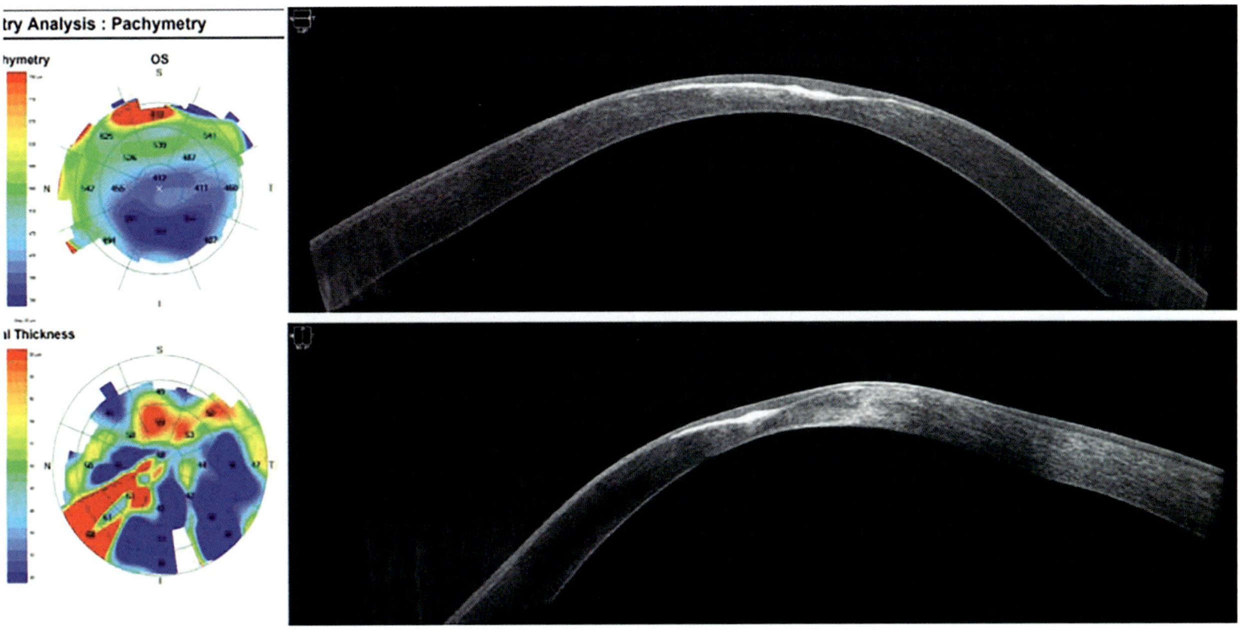

Pachymetry OS

Range (mm)	Min. (μm)	Avg. (μm)	Max. (μm)	S-I (μm)	SN-IT (μm)
0.0–2.0	384	412	483	-	-
2.0–5.0	303	438	571	192	172
5.0–7.0	0	554	1636	-	218

Minimum thickness (μm)	0	Y Min (μm)	3300
Pachy min-median (μm)	–132	Central corneal thickness (μm)	406

Epithelial thickness OS

Range (mm)	Min. (μm)	Avg. (μm)	Max. (μm)	S-I (μm)	SN-IT (μm)
0.0–2.0	37	48	66	-	-
2.0–5.0	32	50	90	17	8
5.0–7.0	27	45	102	16	6
7.0–9.0	27	47	103	-	-

Minimum thickness (μm)	27	Y Min (mm)	–3.5
Min-median (μm)	–17	Central thickness (μm)	55

Fig. 7.9 In moderate keratoconus, both stromal thinning and stromal scarring are present. The scarring appears to have a prominent area of hyperreflectivity within the corneal stroma. Horizontal slice and vertical slice views of the same eye are shown in the *top right and bottom right panels,* respectively. Pachymetry and epithelial thickness mapping can be used to quantify the qualitative changes seen on AS-OCT and topography.

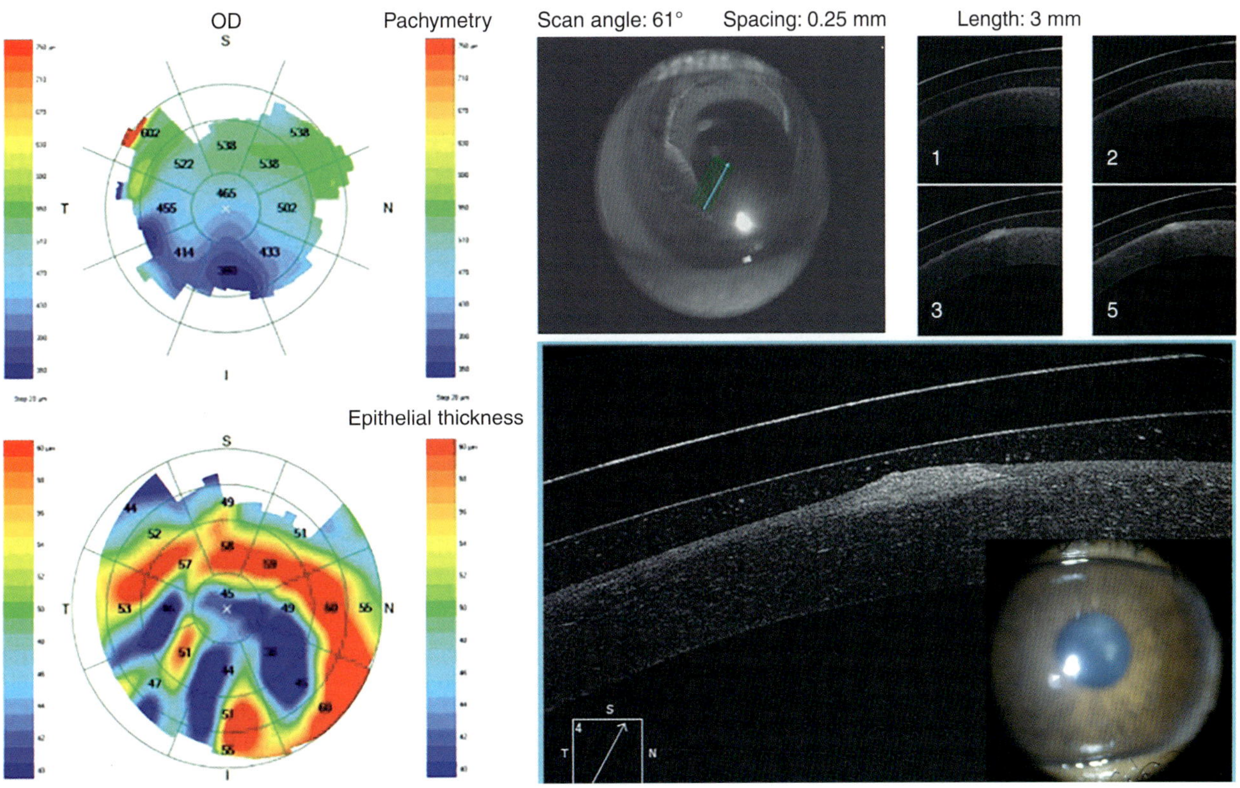

Fig. 7.10 Raised subepithelial nodular scars in keratoconus (KCN). Scars may develop over the apex of the cone in some patients with KCN. Epithelial thickness mapping *(lower left panel)* often demonstrates epithelial *thinning (blue zones)* directly underneath the scar with a concentric region of epithelial *thickening (red zones)* around the scar. AS-OCT *(right panel)* highlights the extent, location, and depth of the scar. These scars may preclude using soft toric and rigid gas-permeable contact lenses. A scleral contact lens (as shown in the AS-OCT) allows for vaulting of the lens over the scar to improve visual acuity.

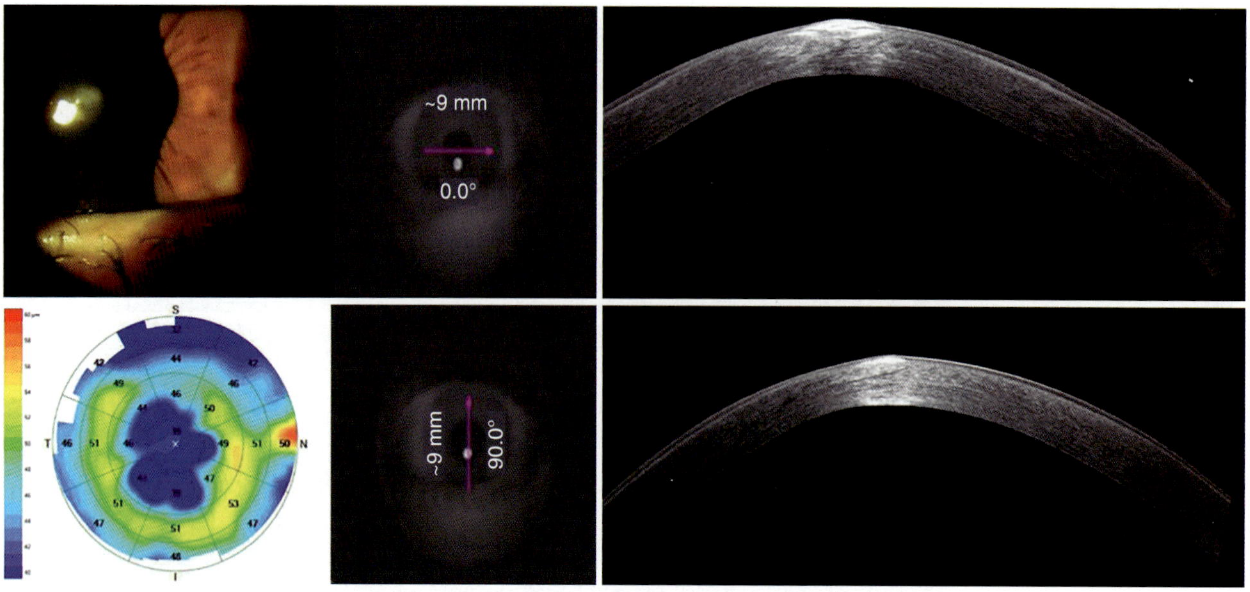

Fig. 7.11 Subepithelial nodular scars seen on slit-lamp examination. Scars *(top left panel)* will cause surface protrusion and localized epithelial *thinning* with adjacent concentric epithelial *thickening.* AS-OCT of horizontal and vertical views (*top right and bottom right panels,* respectively) highlight the location, depth, and extent of the scar (hyperreflective area underlying the apex of the cone). Note the slight protrusion of the epithelial surface in the *top panel.* The corneal thickness is relatively uniform in this patient.

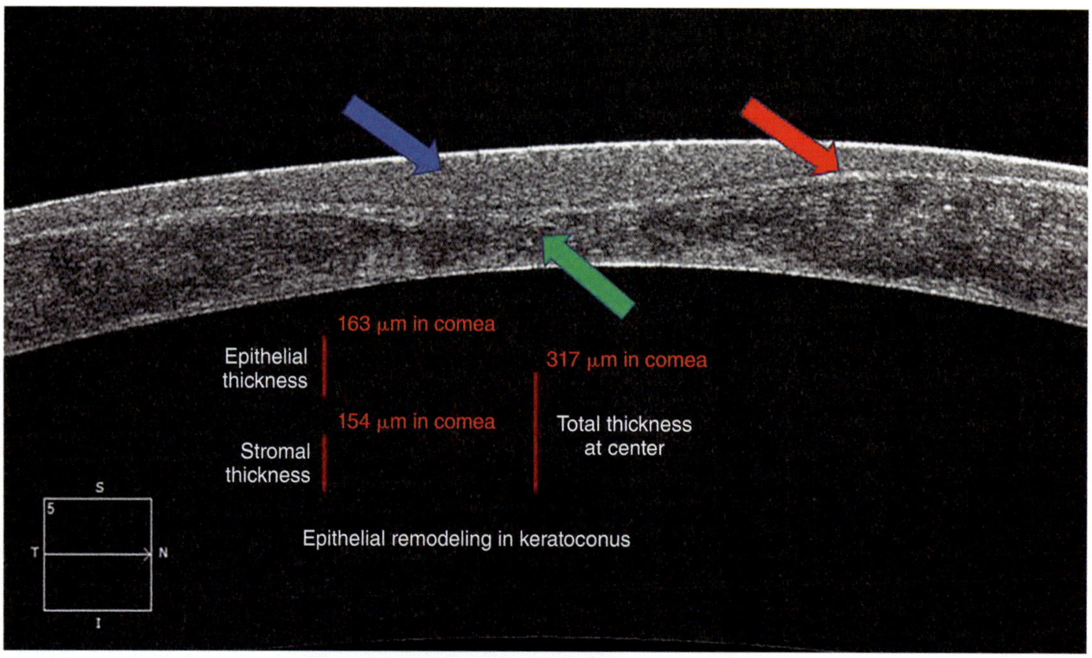

Fig. 7.12 In moderate to severe keratoconus, several notable pathologic features are seen on AS-OCT. This image shows epithelial thickening *(blue arrow),* stromal thinning *(green arrow),* and a hyperreflective Bowman layer *(red arrow).* (Courtesy Nikhil Gokhale, MD, Gokhale Eye Hospital, Mumbai, India.)

layer and progressive stromal thinning. AS-OCT helps to visualize the stromal thinning and epithelial remodeling (Figs. 7.12 and 7.13) in these cases. The Bowman layer demonstrates increased hyperreflectivity as well.

III. CORNEAL HYDROPS

In severe cases, acute corneal hydrops may occur secondary to the rupture of the relatively robust Descemet membrane (DM), causing ingress of aqueous humor into the cornea with profound stromal edema and epithelial bullae. While hydrops may be seen in other corneal ectasias, it is classically and more commonly seen in KCN.

Diagnosis of corneal hydrops can primarily be made by slit-lamp examination. AS-OCT can be used to assess the extent of corneal edema and to monitor the healing process. Resolution of hydrops occurs in about three months in the vast majority of patients without active intervention as the detached DM eventually reattaches to the posterior stroma; this process is accompanied by endothelial migration from the reattached DM to reestablish endothelial layer integrity. Based on the degree of hydrops,

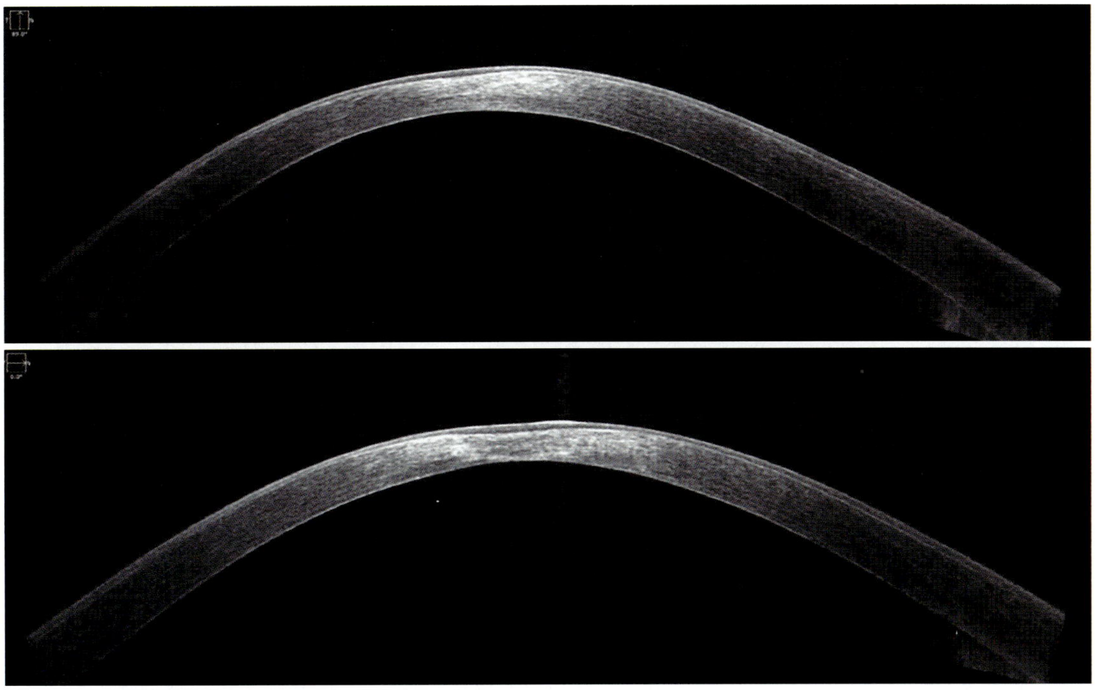

Fig. 7.13 Progressive stromal thinning in moderate to severe keratoconus. Stromal thinning is appreciated as an area of hyperreflectivity underlying the apex of the cone. Note the epithelial thickening overlying this region that allows for a smooth contour of the anterior corneal surface.

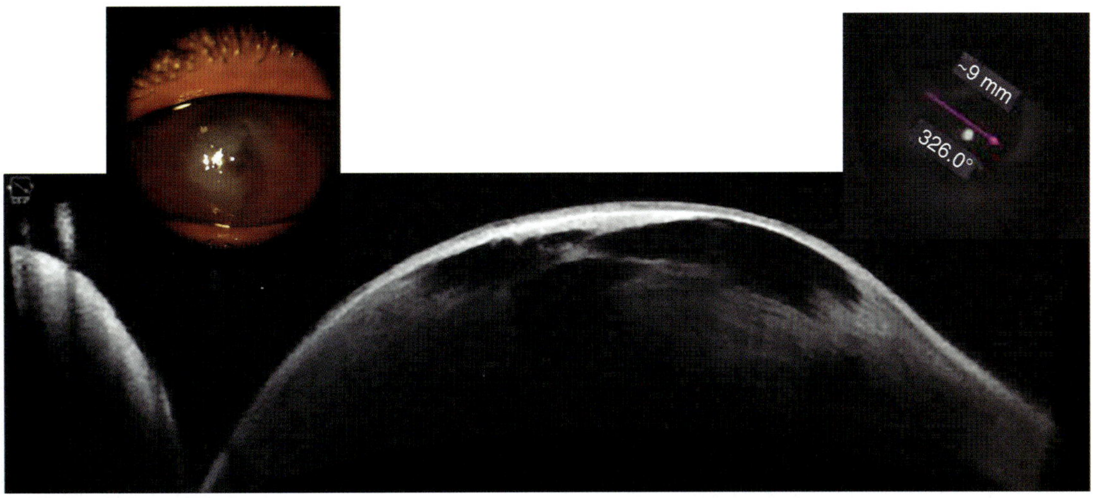

Fig. 7.14 Corneal hydrops. Slit-lamp examination *(left panel)* highlights prominent corneal edema with overlying bullae and associated microcystic edema. AS-OCT *(right panel)* highlights the cystic intrastromal accumulation of fluid in multiple areas, which appears as translucent pockets of edema within the distended stroma. Note the obscuration of the underlying corneal layers secondary to the shadowing effect of the edema.

corneal scarring results in variable levels of visual compromise. Severe cases may benefit from active intervention such as intracameral gas or even endothelial keratoplasty to resolve hydrops. Corneal scarring that is not improved with nonsurgical therapies, such as contact lenses, may ultimately require corneal transplantation (deep anterior lamellar keratoplasty [DALK] or penetrating keratoplasty [PKP]).

Examination at the time of acute hydrops reveals significant corneal edema with overlying bullae and associated microcystic edema (Figs. 7.14 and 7.15). AS-OCT highlights the fluid-filled spaces as translucent areas of edema within the swollen, distended stroma. A break in DM also may be visualized on the AS-OCT images (Fig. 7.16).

Historically, medical therapy, such as hypertonic saline, aqueous suppressants, bandage contact lenses (with antibiotics), and cycloplegic drops, are used to resolve corneal edema and for patient comfort. The use of topical steroids is debated intensely among many authorities. AS-OCT can be especially helpful for assessing the progress of corneal hydrops resolution during serial examinations (Fig. 7.17 to 7.19). Intracameral gas may be used in select cases to increase time to resolution, and AS-OCT can be used after gas injection to monitor resolution. In some patients, hydrops may not resolve even after three to six months of intensive medical therapy; these patients may ultimately require DALK or PKP (Fig. 7.20).

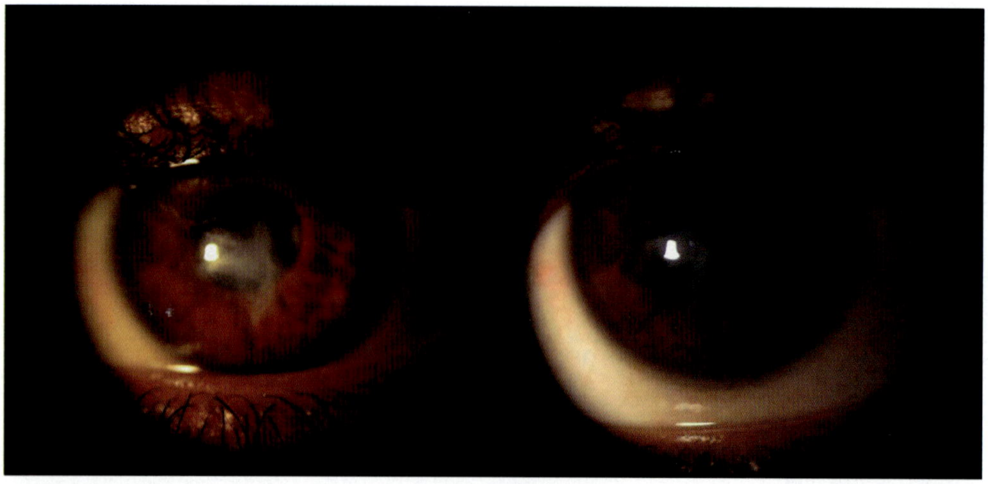

Fig. 7.15 Scarring in corneal hydrops. Corneal hydrops resolves in most cases, though a variable degree of corneal scarring may occur. The *left panel* shows the clinical progression of the patient shown in Fig. 7.14 three months after the initial hydrops incident. The right panel shows the appearance of the corneal scar nine months after the initial incident. Note the interval thinning and shrinkage of the initial pathologic findings over this time frame.

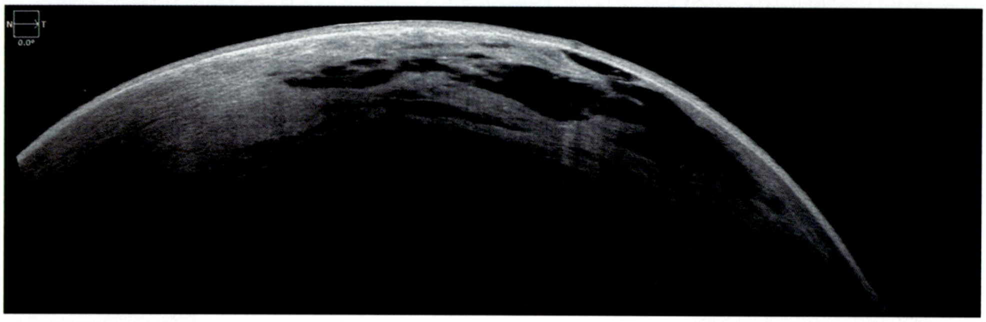

Fig. 7.16 Corneal hydrops. Multiple fluid-filled spaces are seen along with separation of the stromal layers among the areas of edema. The underlying Descemet membrane layer shows a subtle break. With eventual closure of this break and reestablishment of the endothelial layer, the stromal edema usually resolves, although corneal scarring of varying degrees may result. (Courtesy Nikhil Gokhale, MD, Gokhale Eye Hospital, Mumbai, India.)

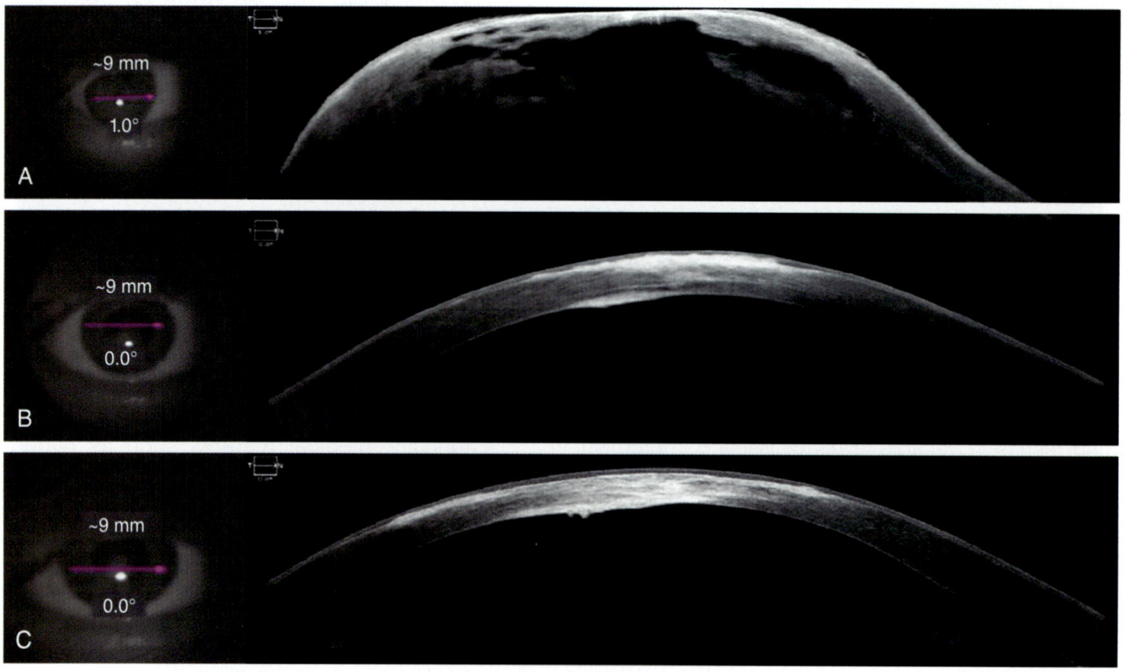

Fig. 7.17 Serial AS-OCT imaging can be used to monitor progression of hydrops resolution. At the time of the initial presentation *(panel A),* note the large area of translucent intrastromal cystic fluid spaces. After initiation of medical therapy with hypertonic saline, aqueous suppressants, and cycloplegic drops, significant improvement of hydrops was noted at the one-month visit *(panel B).* At the three-month visit, the edema had completely resolved, but a large area of stromal scarring (seen as a hyperreflective area) *(panel C)* resulted. Visual acuity improved from counting fingers at the initial presentation to 20/200 at the three-month visit. *Panels B and C* correspond to the slit-lamp photographs in Fig. 7.15 (*left panel and right panel,* respectively).

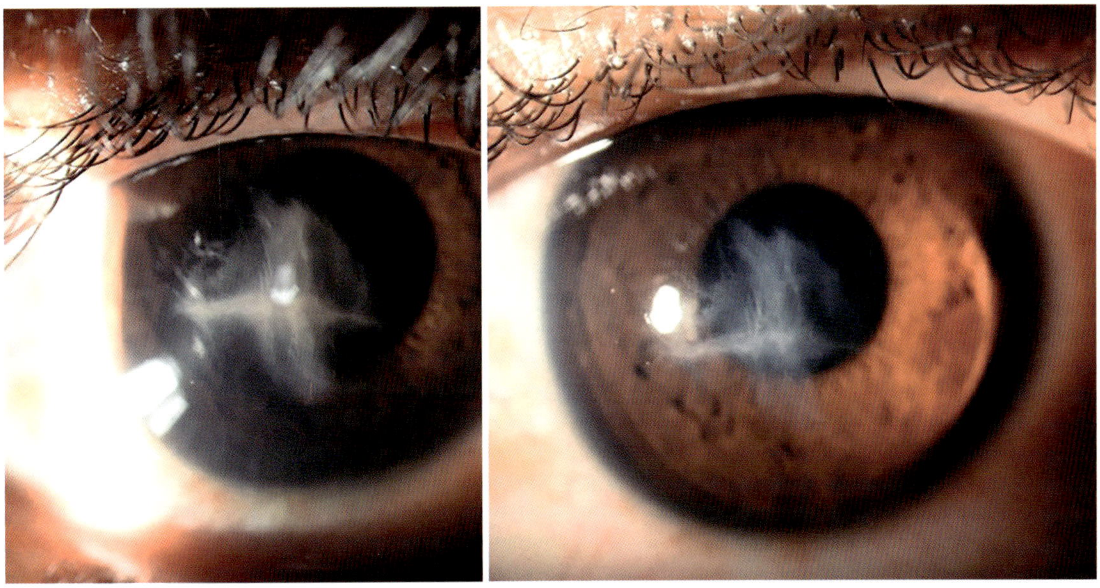

Fig. 7.18 Slit-lamp photograph taken one month *(left panel)* after the initial corneal hydrops of the patient presented in Fig. 7.14. By three months *(right panel),* full resolution of the corneal edema has occurred, with resultant stromal scarring involving a significant portion of the visual axis.

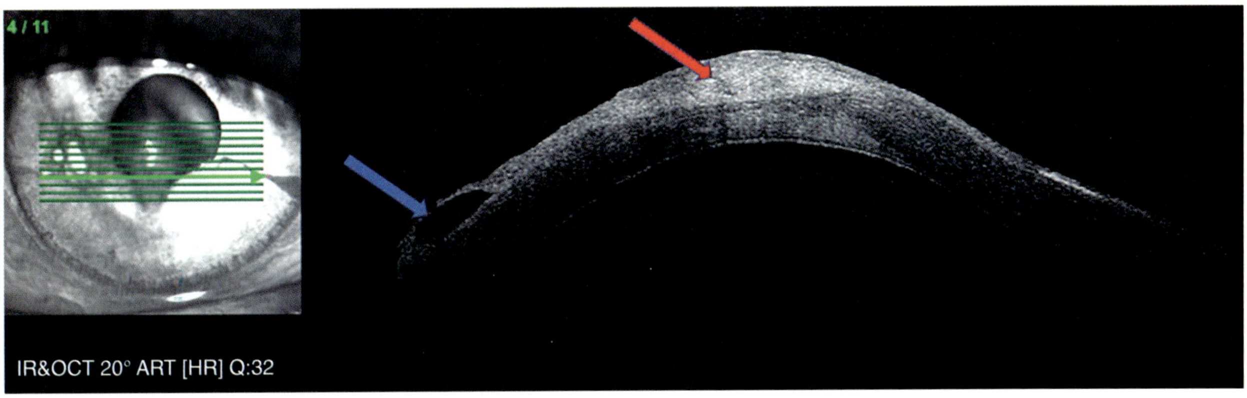

Fig. 7.19 Resolving hydrops. AS-OCT in a patient with resolving hydrops shows areas of persistent fluid *(blue arrow)* along with corneal scarring in areas of resolved stromal edema *(red arrow).*

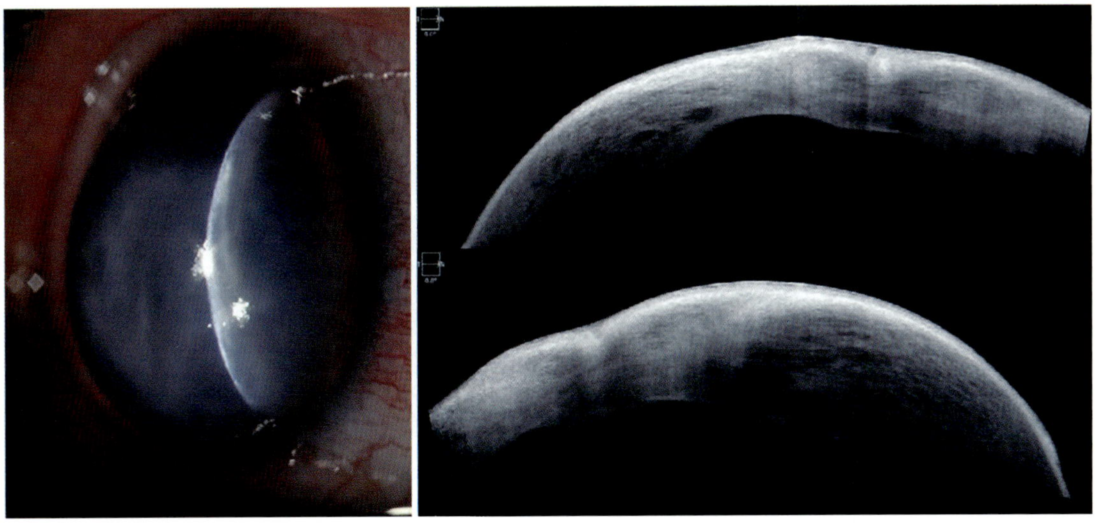

Fig. 7.20 AS-OCT demonstrates persistent pockets of stromal edema despite large areas of corneal scarring. If corneal hydrops fails to improve despite medical therapy, corneal transplant surgery may be required. Visual acuity was still hand motions in this patient. After penetrating keratoplasty, the best corrected visual acuity (with scleral contact lens) improved to 20/30 nine months later.

> **CLINICAL PEARL**
>
> AS-OCT can be used to serially monitor KCN patients who develop hydrops to assess the resolution of intrastromal fluid, especially in cases in which intracameral gas is used.

B. Use of AS-OCT in Keratoconus Interventions

Glasses and contact lenses may be sufficient for patients with forme fruste and mild KCN. However, because many KCN patients have significant amounts of irregular astigmatism, rigid gas-permeable contact lenses have historically been used to improve vision. Scleral contact lenses (ScCLs) have recently gained popularity, as they combine comfort and improved vision. ScCL fitting heavily relies on AS-OCT imaging; contact lens practitioners will use AS-OCT to assess the fitting and vaulting of ScCLs. The nuances of using AS-OCT for contact lens fitting are discussed in Chapter 18.

I. CORNEAL COLLAGEN CROSS LINKING

While used by clinicians around the world for more than a decade, the US Food and Drug Administration's approval of corneal collagen cross linking (CXL) in 2016 has changed the management of mild-moderate KCN disease in the United States. Broadly speaking, CXL involves topical application of riboflavin drops followed by exposure to ultraviolet A (UVA) irradiation; however, various treatment protocols, including "epithelium-on" and "epithelium-off," are employed by corneal specialists. CXL prevents disease progression by forming chemical bonds ("cross links") among stromal collagen fibrils. Numerous studies have demonstrated the repeatable safety and efficacy of CXL for halting disease progression and reducing the risk of KCN progression.

> **CLINICAL PEARL**
>
> The line of demarcation within the corneal stroma is a useful sign detectable on AS-OCT after CXL to determine whether the CXL had the intended effect. This line is seen within the first few weeks after CXL and disappears after 6 months.

While clinicians continue to rely on topography/tomography to determine which patients would benefit from CXL, AS-OCT can be a remarkably useful imaging tool to assess and confirm the effects of the procedure. The most recognized change on AS-OCT is the "line of demarcation" within the corneal stroma, distinguishing the treated anterior and untreated posterior stroma. While its appearance and location are variable, this landmark appears as a prominently hyperreflective line within the stroma (Fig. 7.21 and 7.22). Clinicians may use this line to determine whether the CXL had the desired effect by measuring its depth from the corneal surface (Fig. 7.23). The line of demarcation may fade considerably after three to six months and may be replaced by subtle, irregular, and faint hyperreflective fragmented lines within the mid-posterior stroma (Fig. 7.24).

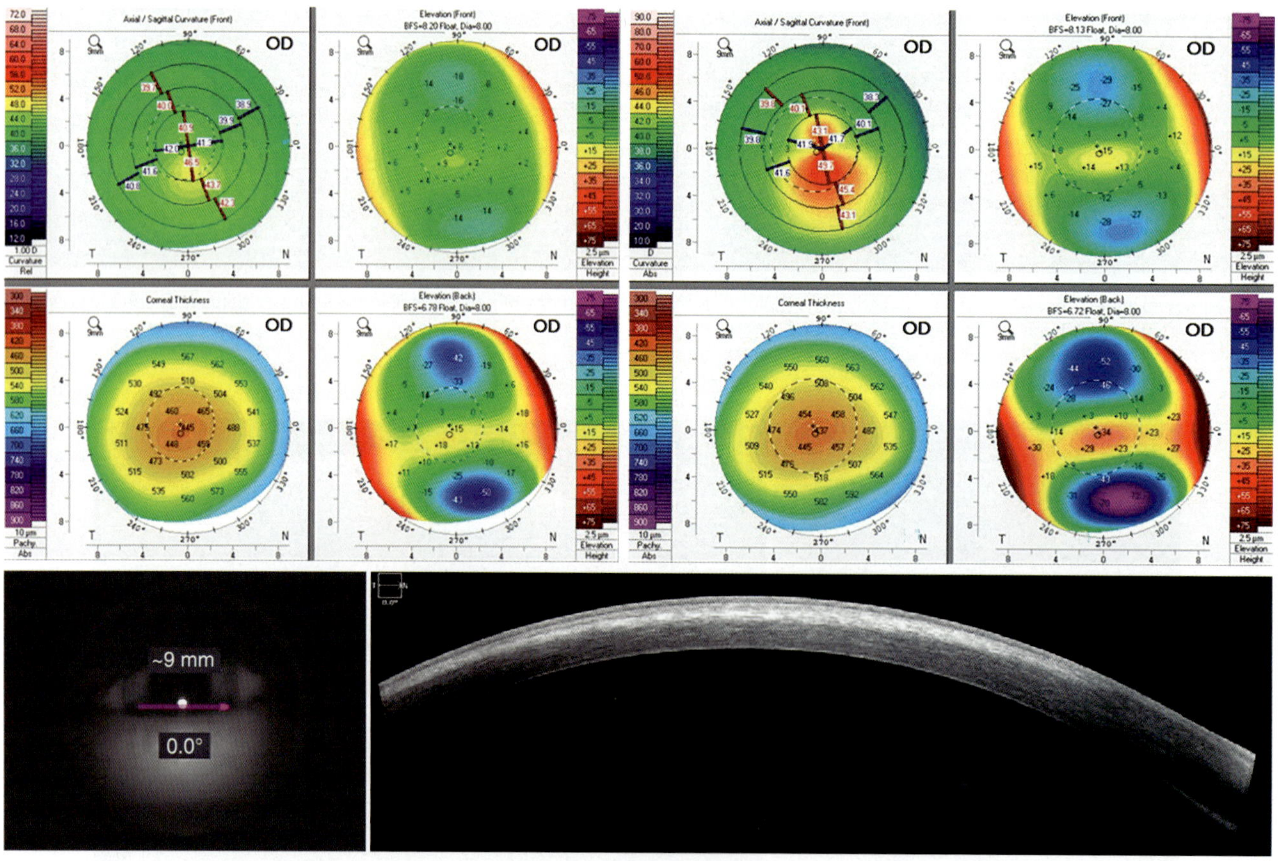

Fig. 7.21 Progression of keratoconus and before/after cross linking (CXL) treatment. In the *top left panel,* a patient presented with early signs of forme fruste keratoconus, evidenced by inferior steepening and subtle anterior/posterior elevation. One year later *(top right panel),* the disease process had significantly progressed, thus meeting the criteria for CXL. The patient underwent CXL, and one month later *(bottom panels),* AS-OCT was performed to visualize the line of demarcation, which may be used to assess and confirm the intended CXL effects. This line is appreciated as an extremely bright (hyperreflective) line in the corneal stroma. It is postulated that this represents the border between the anterior treated and posterior untreated stroma. This line may fade after three to six months and may be replaced by faint, irregular hyperreflective lines in the posterior stroma.

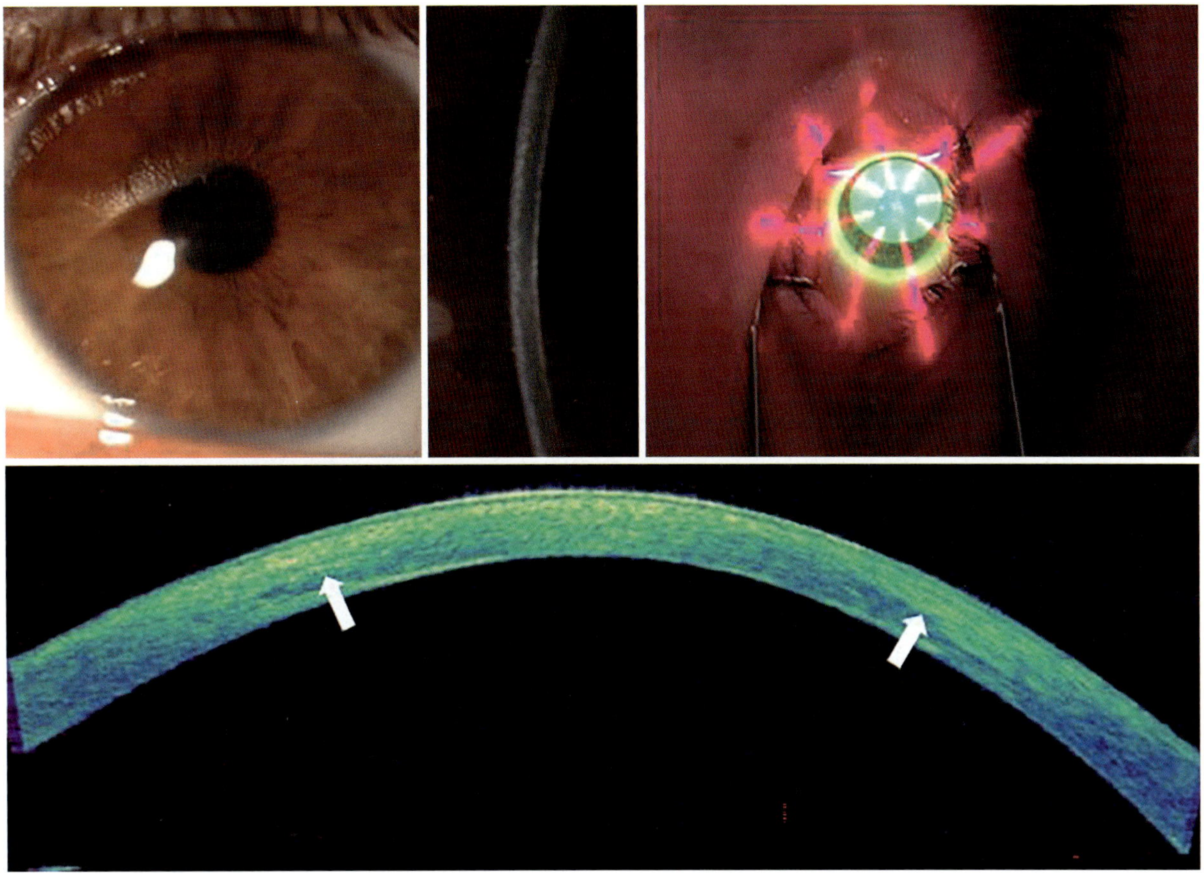

Fig. 7.22 The line of demarcation appears as a prominently hyperreflective line within the stroma. The treatment has affected approximately half of the stromal thickness in this patient.

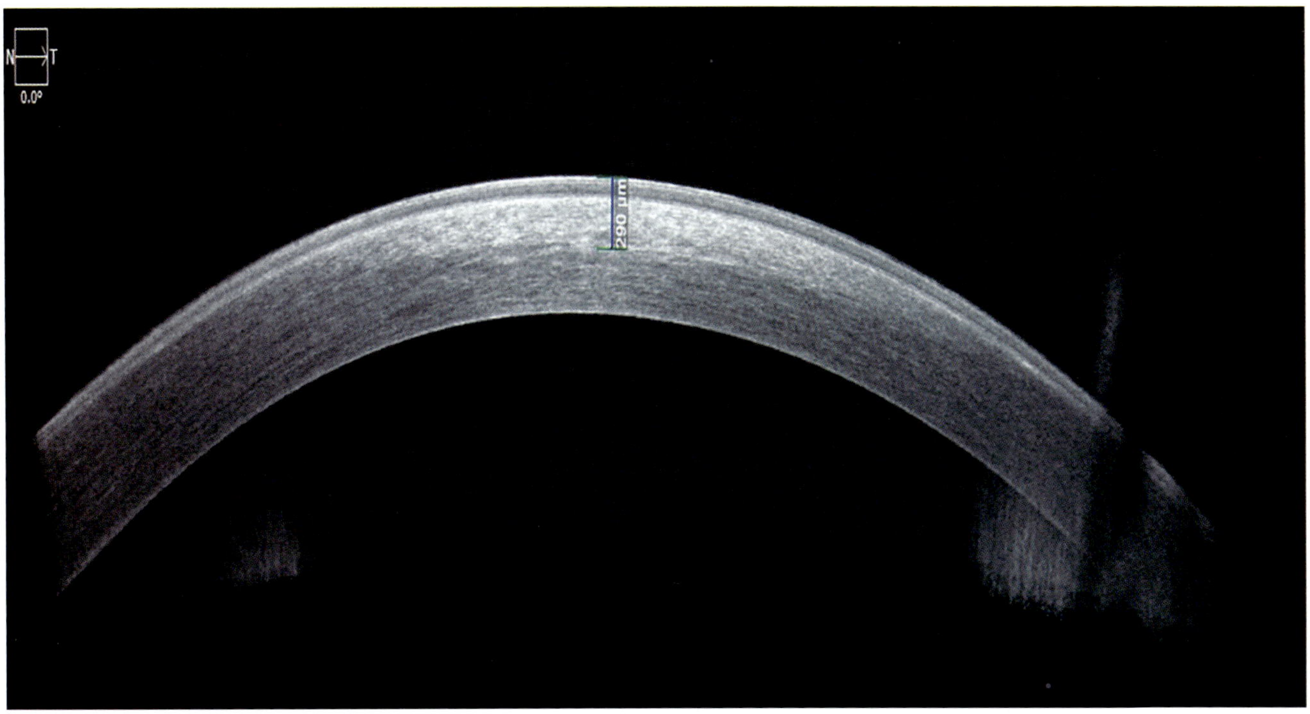

Fig. 7.23 The line of demarcation appears as a hyperreflective line within the stroma. The depth of this line can be used to measure the treatment area. (Courtesy Nikhil Gokhale, MD, Gokhale Eye Hospital, Mumbai, India.)

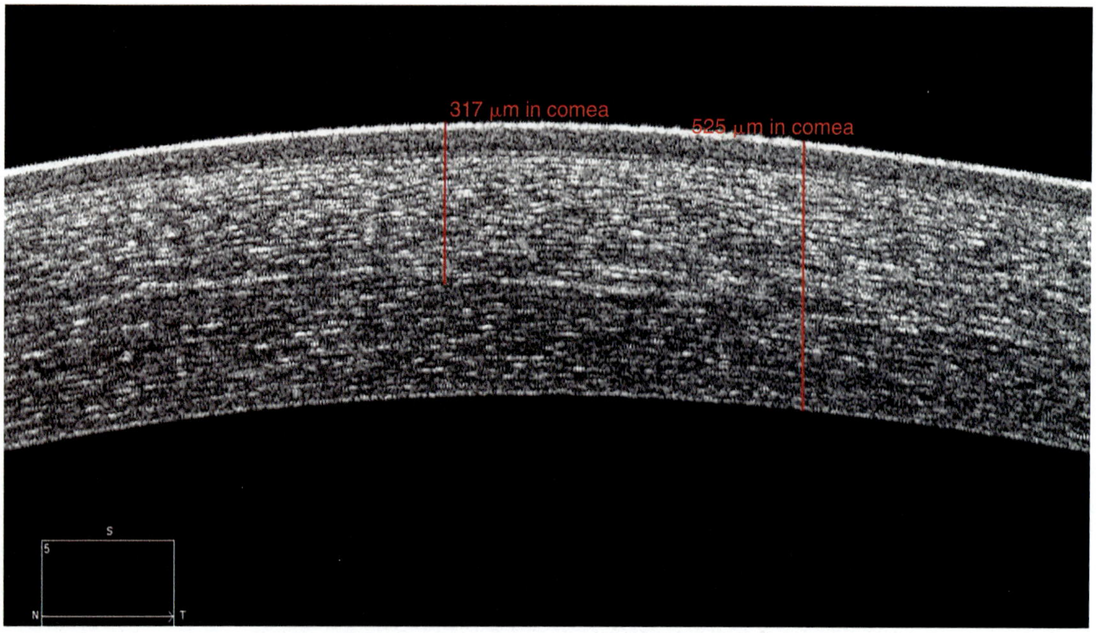

Fig. 7.24 Progression of line of demarcation postoperatively. By three to six months, the line of demarcation may fade considerably and may be replaced by subtle, irregular, and faint hyperreflective fragmented lines within the mid-posterior stroma. This depth can be measured using the ruler function on most AS-OCT devices. (Courtesy Nikhil Gokhale, MD, Gokhale Eye Hospital, Mumbai, India.)

II. INTRASTROMAL CORNEAL RING SEGMENTS

Intrastromal corneal ring segments (ICRSs) are polymethyl methacrylate (PMMA) semicircular implants placed in the posterior stroma to flatten and reduce corneal curvature. Initially designed for the treatment of myopia, ICRSs have found a role in the management of KCN by inducing flattening of the steep area(s) of the cornea and reducing corneal distortions, which in turn improve both uncorrected and best corrected visual acuity in KCN patients. ICRSs are best used in patients with moderate-severe KCN who can no longer tolerate contact lenses; flattening the cornea in such patients aims to improve vision and facilitate continued wearing of contact lenses. Multiple studies have demonstrated the efficacy of visual improvement in ICRS patients.

One limitation of ICRS procedures is that they do not halt the KCN disease process. Therefore many patients may initially improve with ICRS but may worsen over time as the KCN process has not been controlled. Thus ICRSs are not endorsed by some practitioners because of the unknown long-term effects. However, in the era of CXL, many corneal specialists are placing Intacs (CorneaGen, Seattle, Washington, United States) followed by simultaneous or sequential CXL in an effort to combine corneal flattening and halting of disease progression.

Four main types of ICRS devices are available: Intacs, Ferrara Rings (Ferrara Ophthalmics, Belo Horizonte, Brazil), Kerarings (Mediphakos Inc., Belo Horizonte, Brazil), and the MyoRing (DIOPTEX GmBh, Linz, Austria).

In the United States, Intacs is the only approved ICRS device available to corneal surgeons. These consist of 150-degree arc segments with 8.1-mm external and 6.8-mm internal diameter. Intrastromal corneal tunnels for Intacs placement can be created mechanically or with a femtosecond laser; the latter is the preferred method by many surgeons because the former is associated with additional risks, including but not limited to persistent epithelial defects and segment extrusion. Intacs may be placed as asymmetric (210/450) or symmetric (450/450) segments. Whereas tomography is used for surgical planning, AS-OCT can be used to confirm the proper placement of the ring segments in the posterior stroma (Fig. 7.25). Because these segments displace posterior stromal fibers, AS-OCT imaging may also demonstrate a slight protrusion of the corneal endothelium toward the anterior chamber (Fig. 7.26). Fig. 7.25 demonstrates asymmetric Intacs segments (210/450), and Fig. 7.26 demonstrates symmetric (450/450) segments.

> **CLINICAL PEARL**
>
> AS-OCT can be used after ICRS placement to assess that the rings are placed at the appropriate depth. Shallow placement of ICRS may increase the risk for epithelial erosions and segment extrusion.

ICRSs, including Intacs, are not without potential postoperative limitations and complications. Some patients may report intractable glare, halos, and starbursts in mesopic light conditions. Fig. 7.27 shows the AS-OCT images of a patient with an initial good response to the ring segments with appropriate placement depth. Postoperatively, the patient experienced debilitating nighttime glare, and the Intacs were removed approximately three months later. The *bottom panel* AS-OCT shows the post-Intacs removal changes. The areas of stromal hyperreflectivity represent scarring from the collapsed stromal tunnels after Intacs removal.

Trauma can dislodge or shift ICRS segments. Fig. 7.28 display images of the left eye from a patient with initially good Intacs placement who subsequently experienced blunt force trauma two months later that caused dislodging and shifting of the segments, necessitating surgical removal. Slit-lamp photographs demonstrate shifting of the segments such that the temporal segment is underneath the nasal segment longitudinally. AS-OCT shows the temporal ring segment having slipped underneath the nasal segment

Ferrara rings have smaller external and internal diameters (5.4 and 4.4 mm, respectively) than Intacs. As they are placed in a

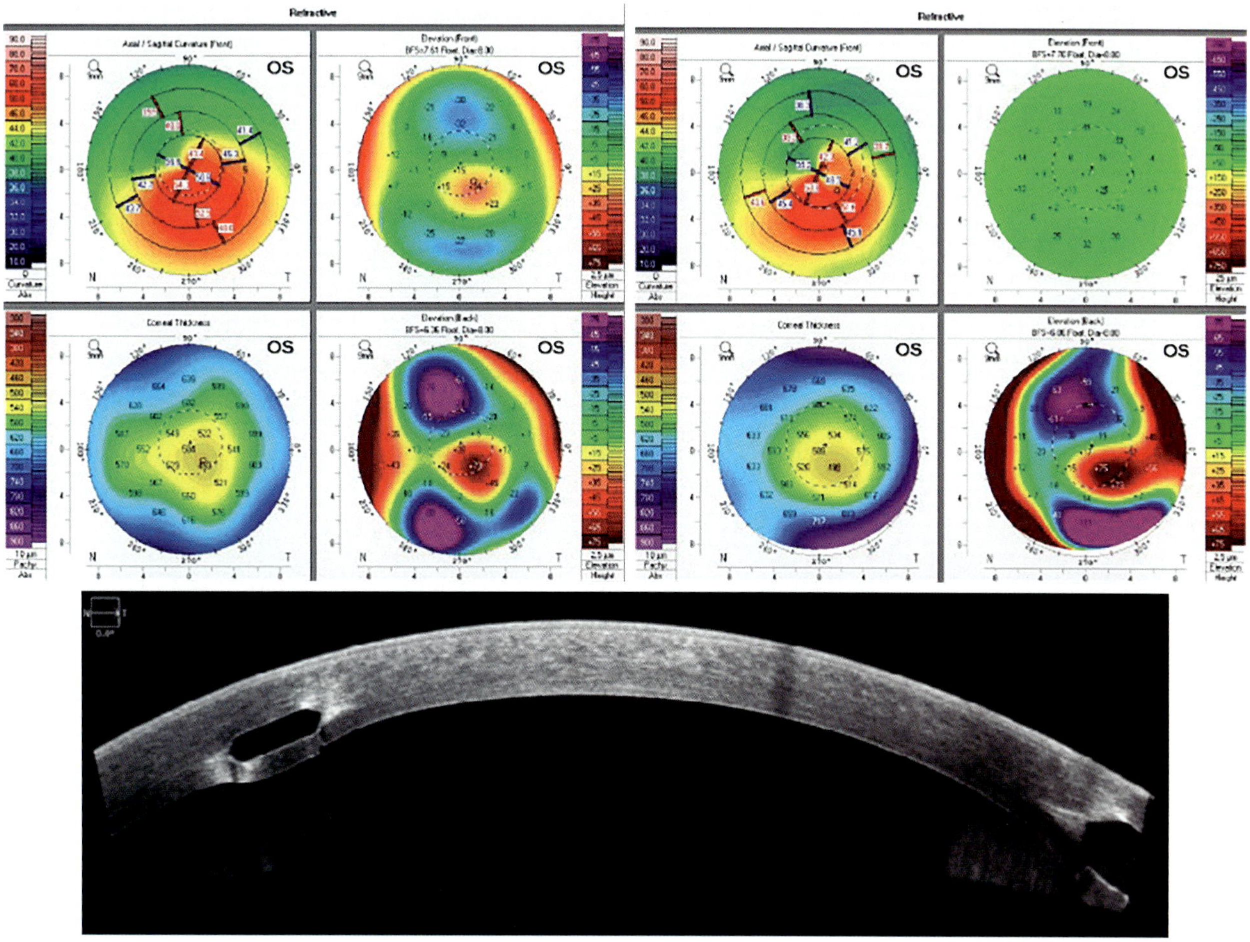

Fig. 7.25 Placement of asymmetric 210/450 Intacs segments for a patient with moderate keratoconus. Preoperative topography/tomography maps are shown in the *top left panel.* The manifest refraction before the surgery was –2.50 + 4.00 × 154, yielding 20/50 vision. The postoperative topography and tomography maps are displayed in the *top right panel.* Note the reduction of steepening on the axial map and flattening of the front surface elevation. The manifest refraction one month after Intacs placement was –1.00 + 2.25 × 160, yielding 20/25 vision. AS-OCT can be used to visualize the asymmetric segments in the deep stroma, which have a hexagonal appearance on a cross-sectional view. In the *bottom panel,* the thinner (210-micron) segment is seen on the *left,* and a portion of the thicker (450-micron) segment is seen on the *right.* As these ring segments displace stromal fibers, secondary distention of the corneal endothelium toward the anterior chamber also may be noted. This patient underwent cross linking approximately three months after the Intacs procedure.

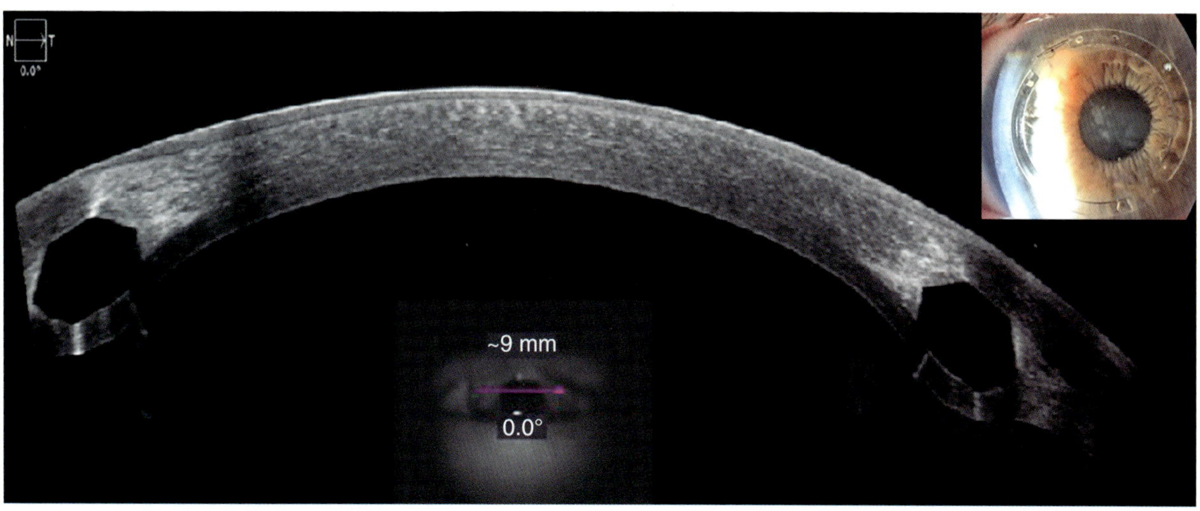

Fig. 7.26 For advanced cases, bilateral 450-micron segments may be placed to cause additional flattening. AS-OCT confirms the appropriate placement of these segments in the posterior stroma with similar changes as described in Fig. 7.25. In this patient, the manifest refraction before Intacs placement was –2.75 + 4.25 × 43 yielding 20/60 best corrected visual acuity. Six weeks after Intacs placement, repeat manifest refraction was –1.75 + 1.75 × 180, yielding 20/30 best corrected visual acuity.

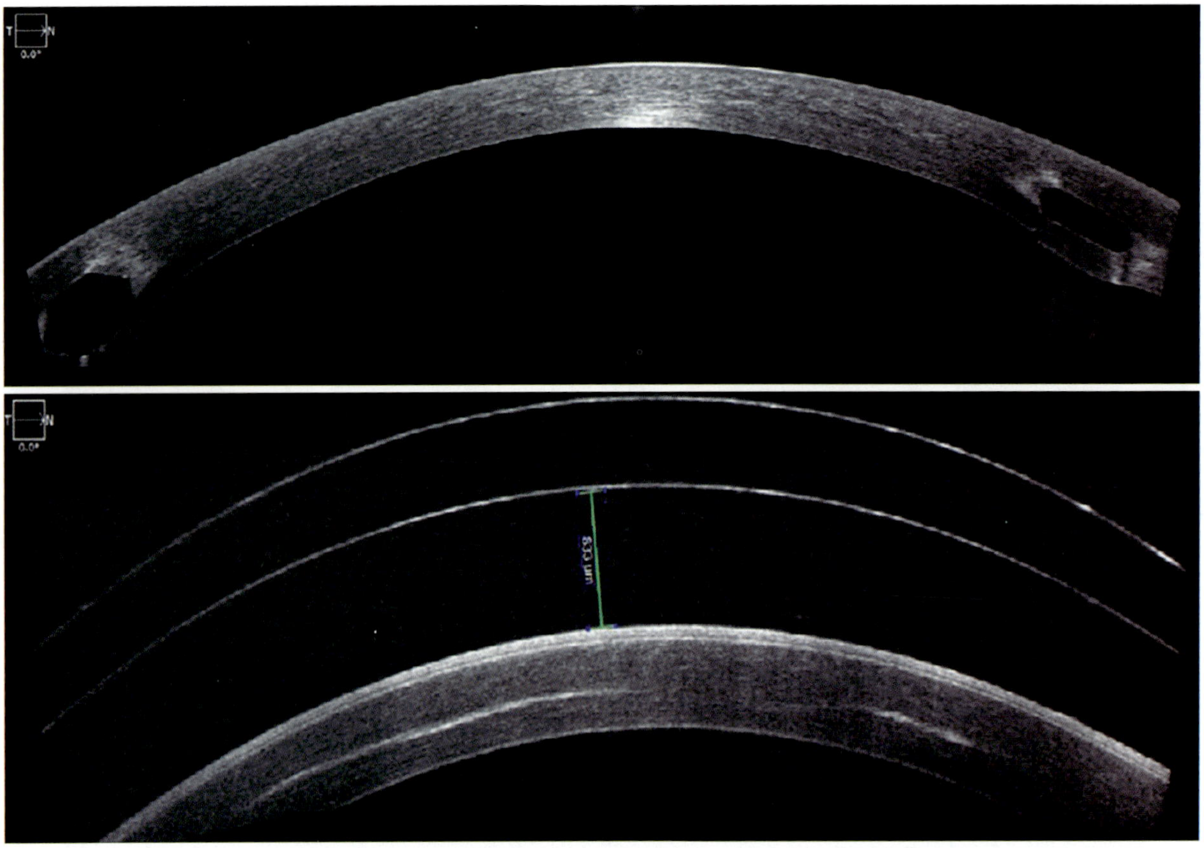

Fig. 7.27 AS-OCT images *(top panel)* after routine Intacs placement. Although the patient had a good objective response to the ring segments (e.g., reduction of corneal steepening, improved visual acuity), he reported debilitating glare, halos, and starbursts at nighttime that prevented safe driving. The patient thus underwent the removal of Intacs. Three months later, he underwent cross linking and was eventually fitted with a scleral contact lens. The *bottom panel* shows the post-Intacs removal (4 months after removal) images. Note the areas of hyperreflectivity indicating the stromal scarring in the areas of the collapsed corneal tunnels. A scleral contact lens with a good vault is also present at the time of image acquisition.

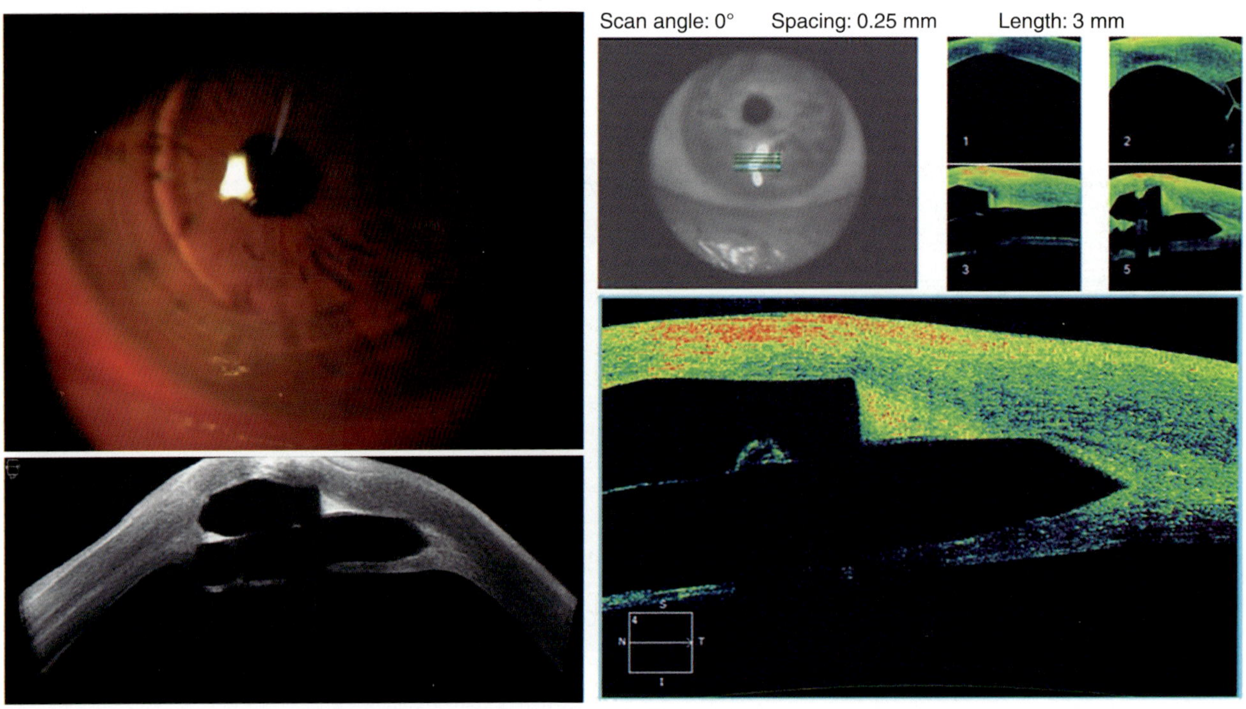

Fig. 7.28 Slippage of the temporal ring segment. Slit-lamp image *(top left panel)* shows slippage of the temporal ring segment. AS-OCT imaging demonstrates the location of the temporal segment underneath the nasal segment.

manner similar to Intacs, AS-OCT can be used to confirm placement at the desired depth. These segments can be appreciated on AS-OCT as having a triangular shape on cross-section imaging (Fig. 7.29). These can also be combined with phakic intraocular lenses (pIOLs) to further correct refractive error (Fig. 7.30).

III. CORNEAL TRANSPLANT SURGERY: POSTOPERATIVE MANAGEMENT

The use of intraoperative AS-OCT in corneal transplant surgery for corneal ectasia, especially lamellar keratoplasty (e.g., superficial anterior lamellar keratoplasty [SALK] and DALK) is discussed in Chapters 13 and 14. In certain circumstances, AS-OCT can be used to further diagnose and evaluate patients after DALK and PKP.

In Fig. 7.31, a patient with severe KCN was scheduled for DALK surgery. A successful type I big bubble was performed, but during the removal of the anterior stromal tissue, there was inadvertent perforation of the endothelium, and the case was converted to PKP. The full-thickness donor tissue was sutured uneventfully. In the postoperative examination, a "double anterior chamber" was noted. AS-OCT confirmed the presence of a significant amount of incompletely removed host DM-endothelium complex. The patient underwent removal of this complex successfully.

III. POST-LASIK ECTASIA

Post-LASIK ectasia may unfortunately be seen as a devastating complication after LASIK. These patients may present with increasing refractive error, especially irregular astigmatism, and progressive loss of best corrected visual acuity after laser-assisted in situ keratomileusis (LASIK) surgery, in both the short-term and late-term postoperative period.

Diagnosis of post-LASIK ectasia is similarly made by combining clinical exam findings and imaging changes seen on topography and tomography. AS-OCT may help aid the diagnosis of this condition, like the previous discussion on the diagnosis of KCN. Imaging changes in this condition are similar to the previously discussed images.

In rare cases, disease progression may continue to such an extent that a corneal hydrops event occurs. Figs. 7.32 to 7.36 show the course of a post-LASIK ectasia patient who experienced corneal hydrops. This patient developed loss of uncorrected distance vision two years after her LASIK, and her decrease in vision from her ectasia was so profound that she developed an exotropia. She presented 9 years after her LASIK with severe pain from hydrops. The initial slit-lamp findings (Fig. 7.32) are confirmed on AS-OCT imaging, which shows common findings of profound epithelial edema, intrastromal fluid, and DM detachment; note the additional edema between the flap and stromal bed (Fig. 7.33). The ectasia was so severe, that at the area of maximal thinning, only "wisps" of residual corneal stroma is seen on AS-OCT, Serial AS-OCT imaging (Figs. 7.34 and 7.35) can be used to monitor the resolution of the hydrops event with appropriate medical therapy. While the hydrops resolved significantly over a period of six weeks, the stromal loss

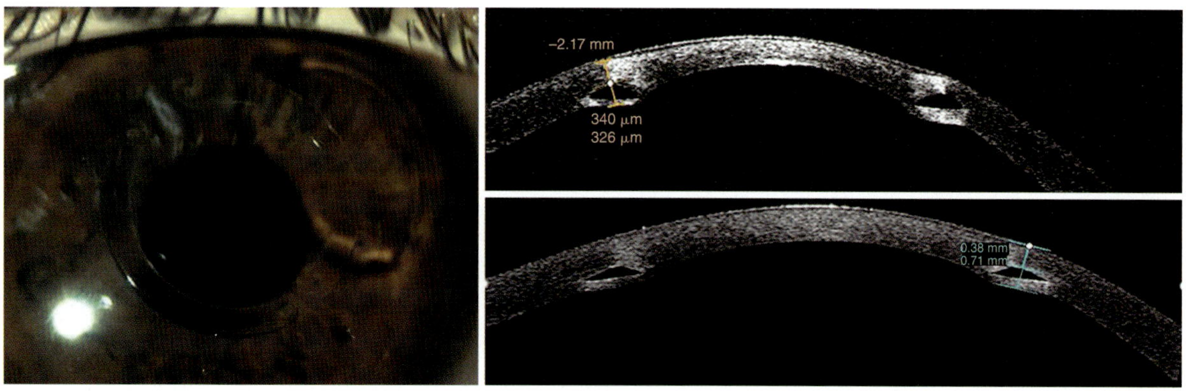

Fig. 7.29 Ferrara rings can be seen in the slit-lamp image of the cornea *(top left).* Note the smaller diameter of the segments and the closer location to the visual axis compared with the Intacs segments. AS-OCT can be similarly used to confirm the proper placement of these ring segments. Ferrara ring segments demonstrate a triangular shape on cross-section imaging. (Courtesy Helena Filipe, MD, Lisbon, Portugal.)

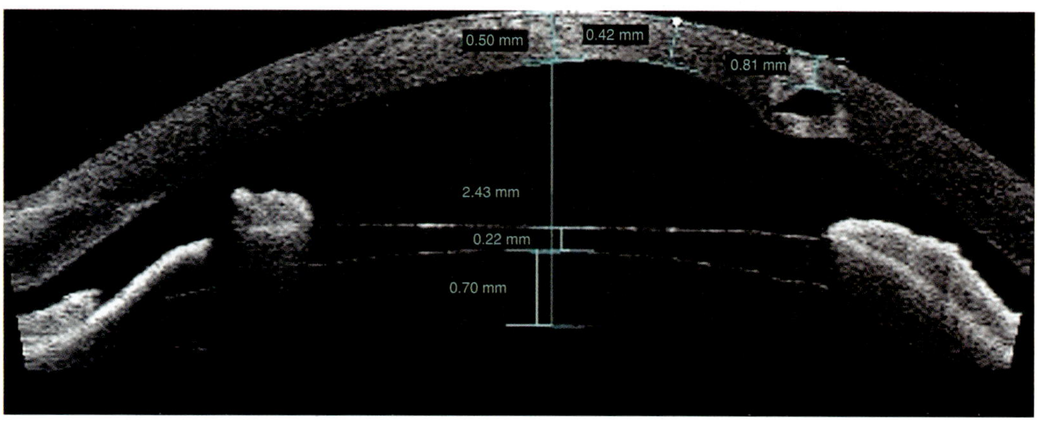

Fig. 7.30 Appearance of Ferrara ring on AS-OCT. A single Ferrara ring has been placed in this patient and has been additionally combined with a phakic intraoperative lens to treat the refractive error. (Courtesy Helena Filipe, MD, Lisbon, Portugal.)

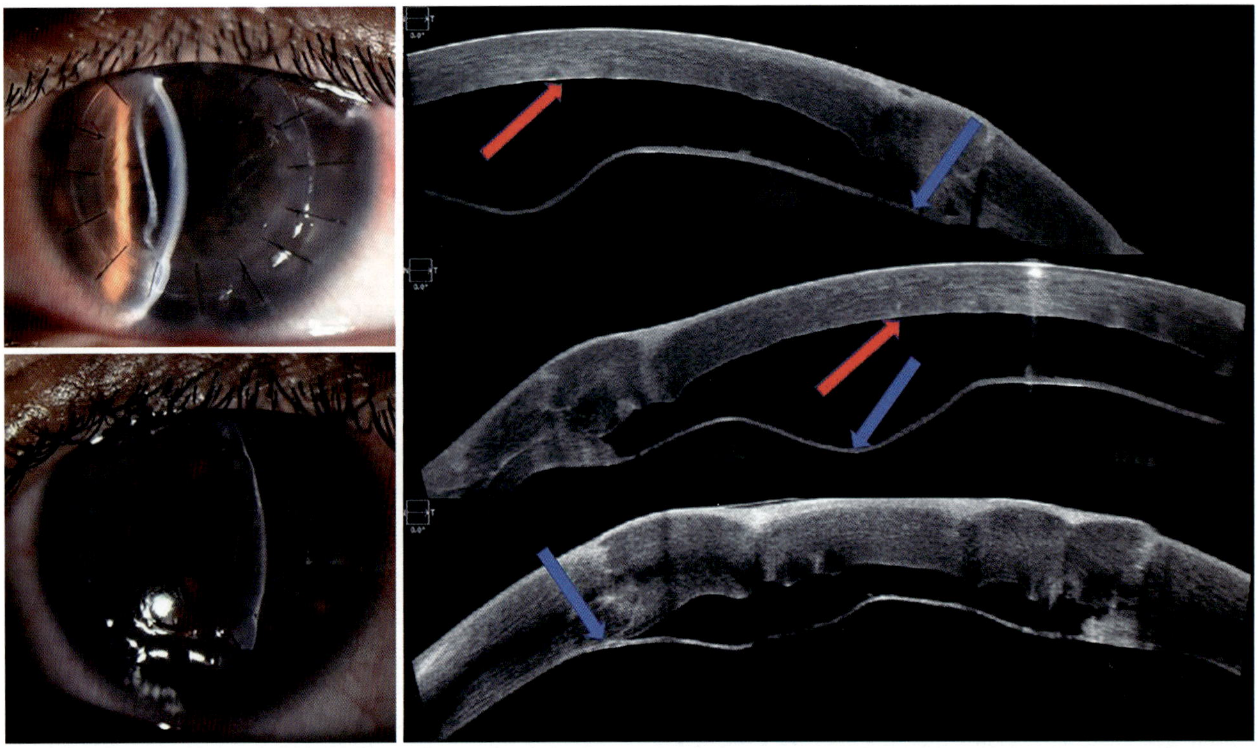

Fig. 7.31 Postoperative slit-lamp photographs and AS-OCT images of a keratoconus patient who underwent deep anterior lamellar keratoplasty with conversion to penetrating keratoplasty. Initially, a successful type I big bubble was created, but during removal of the anterior stromal cap, there was iatrogenic perforation of the host Descemet membrane (DM)–endothelium complex. A full-thickness donor graft was successfully sutured. Postoperatively, there was a "double anterior chamber" appearance on slit-lamp examination *(top left and bottom left panels).* AS-OCT confirmed the presence of a significant amount of host DM-endothelium complex *(blue arrow)* attached to the peripheral host cornea and separate from the donor endothelium *(red arrow).*

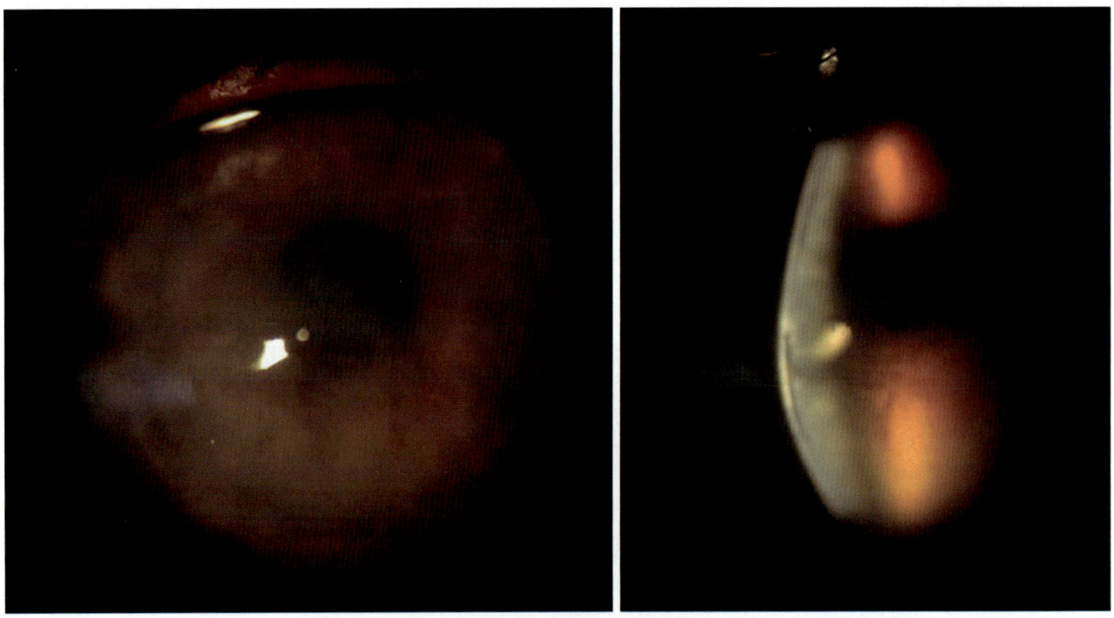

Fig. 7.32 Slit-lamp images from a patient with post-LASIK ectasia who developed corneal hydrops.

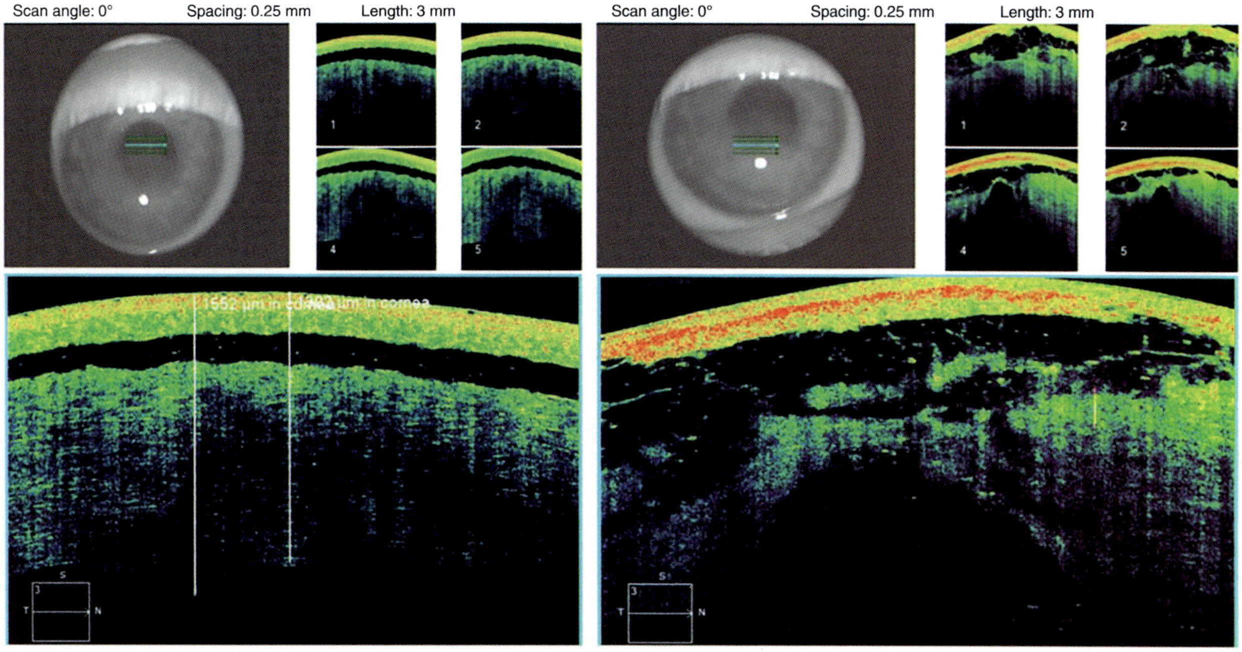

Fig. 7.33 AS-OCT taken at the time of the initial hydrops event shows similar intrastromal cystic fluid spaces (translucent spaces). Note the additional edema between the area of the LASIK flap and the underlying stroma.

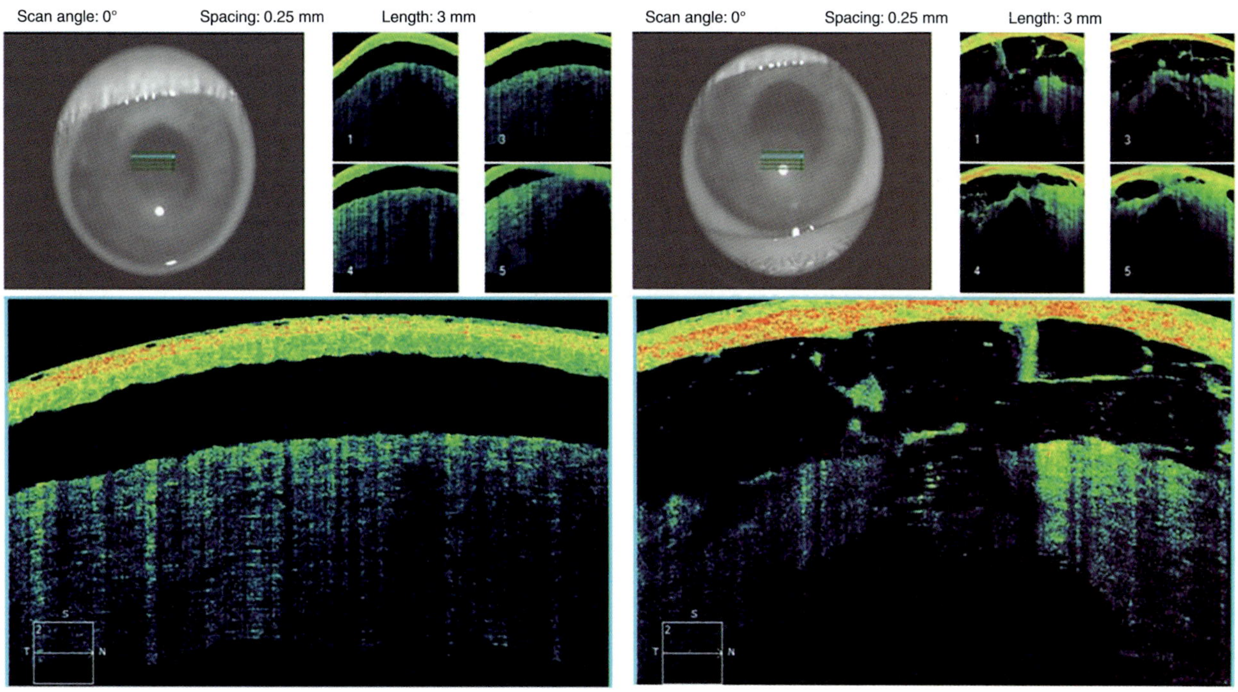

Fig. 7.34 Appearance of post-LASIK ectasia corneal hydrops one week after the initial event. Note the persistent edema between the LASIK flap and the underlying stroma. The post-LASIK ectasia in this case was so severe that at area of maximal thinning there was minimal remaining stromal tissue.

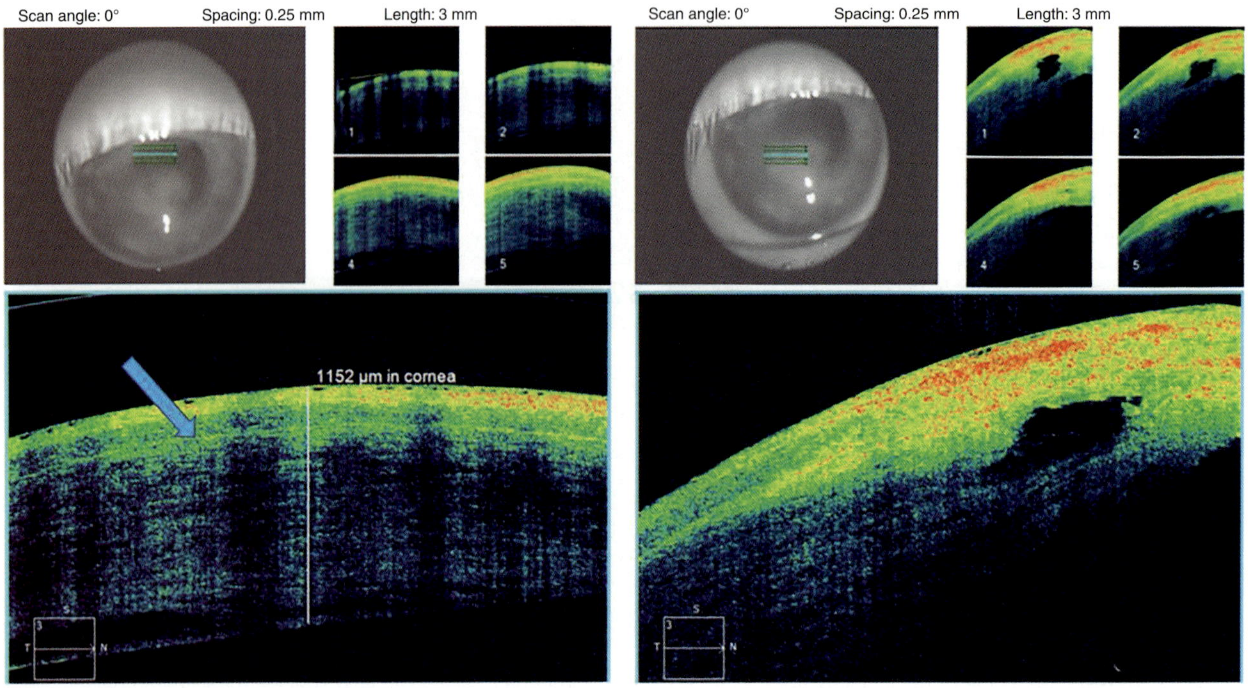

Fig. 7.35 Significant improvement hydrops at 6 weeks. Note the reapposition of the flap *(left panel)* to the underlying stromal bed. A thin line of hyperreflectivity can be seen, delineating the flap border *(blue arrow)*. Stromal edema is still resolving in some areas of the cornea *(right panel)*.

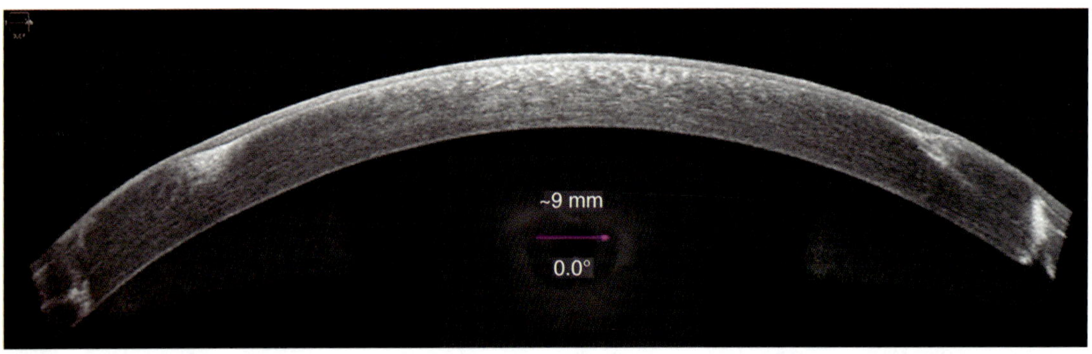

Fig. 7.36 Two years after corneal hydrops. Restoration of expected corneal anatomy has occurred, including reapposition of corneal layers and delineation of the LASIK flap. Note the areas of hyperreflectivity in the anterior stroma indicating persistent scarring.

and ectasia was so profound that she required a full-thickness keratoplasty with a return of excellent vision (Fig. 7.36).

Keratoconus in Conjunction with Other Corneal Dystrophies

In rare cases, KCN may occur with other corneal dystrophies in the same patient (see Chapters 5 and 6 for more discussion regarding epithelial–Bowman layer and stromal dystrophies, respectively). Among these concurrences, epithelial basement membrane dystrophy (EBMD) and Fuchs endothelial corneal dystrophy (FECD) have been reported as the most common types. Most comorbidity cases tend to be bilateral, with a higher percentage of cases occurring in female patients. It is unclear which disease occurs first, though KCN has a predilection for younger patients, while EBMD and FED usually occur later in life.

In Figs. 7.37 to 7.42, slit-lamp photographs, topographies, and AS-OCT of a patient with concurrent KCN and FECD are presented. The patient had moderate KCN in the right eye and forme fruste and mild KCN in the left eye. Consistent with FECD, guttae (2+ to 3+) were noted in both eyes, with associated corneal edema and increased corneal thickness on ultrasonic pachymetry (646 and 639 μm).

IV. PELLUCID MARGINAL DEGENERATION

Pellucid marginal degeneration (PMD) is a noninflammatory thinning disorder with a predilection for the *inferior* peripheral cornea. The hallmark finding in PMD is an area of corneal protrusion above the point of maximal thinning, as compared with KCN, wherein the area of corneal protrusion is within the area of maximal thinning. Clinically, patients have a high degree of against-the-rule astigmatism. The hallmark finding on topography/tomography is a unique pattern of inferior corneal steepening described as a "crab claw" or "kissing doves" shape. (However, it is important to note that KCN can also have a "crab claw" appearance, and this corneal presentation is not pathognomonic. PMD is a slit-lamp or AS-OCT diagnosis and not a topographic diagnosis.) Also, corneal hydrops may rarely occur.

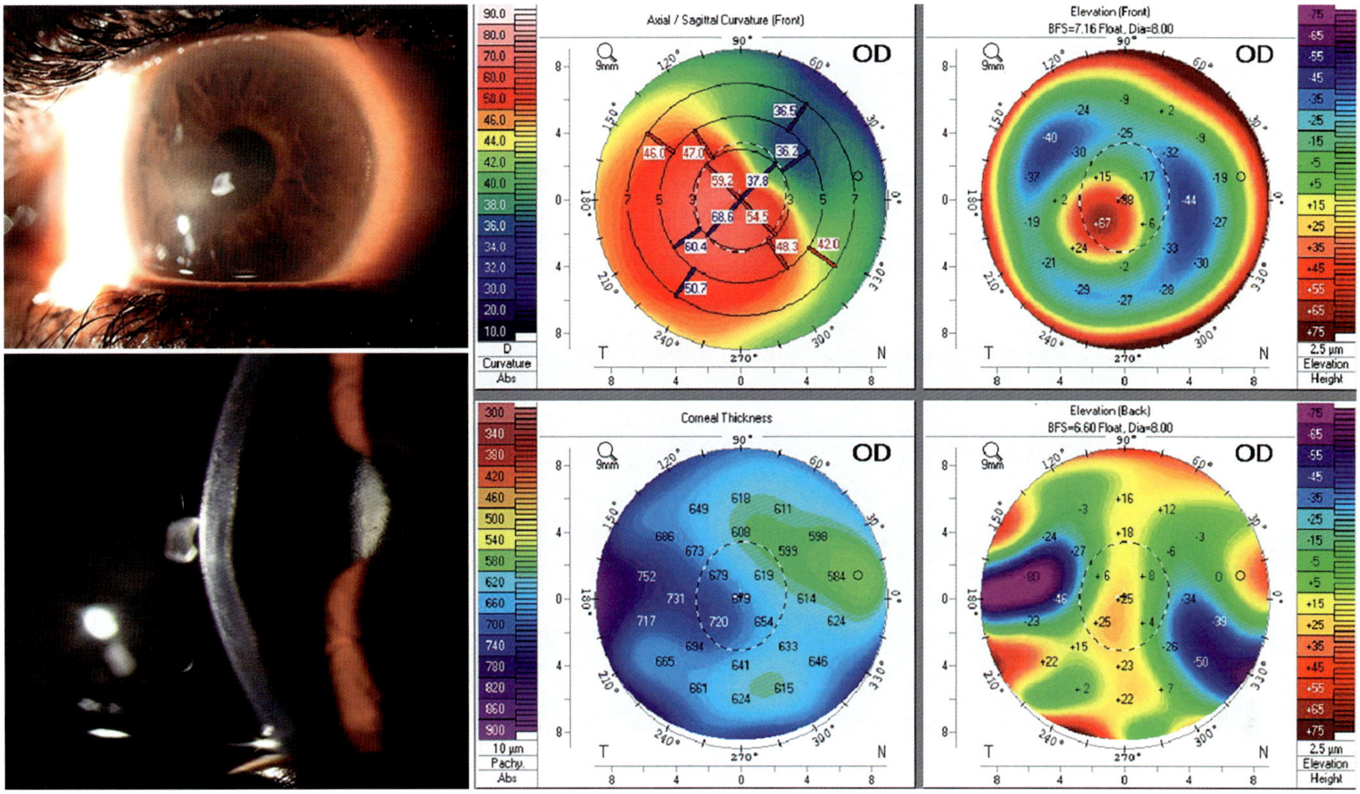

Fig. 7.37 Slit-lamp photos and tomography images from the right eye of a patient with concurrent moderate keratoconus and Fuchs endothelial corneal dystrophy. The left eye is not shown but has similar features.

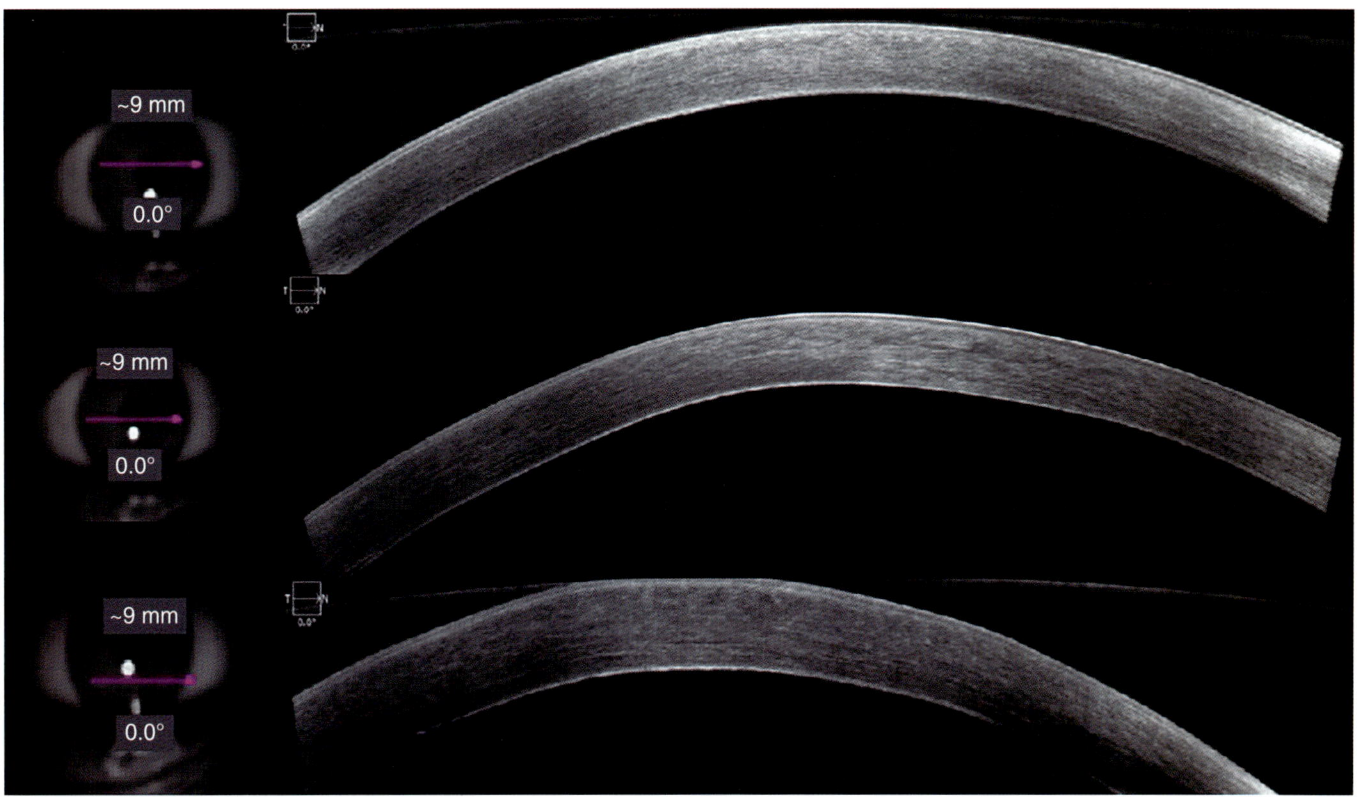

Fig. 7.38 AS-OCT images (spectral-domain, Zeiss Cirrus) from the right eye of a patient with concurrent moderate keratoconus (KCN) and Fuchs endothelial corneal dystrophy (FECD) shown in Fig 7.37. Previously mentioned features of KCN are noted in the epithelium, Bowman layer, and anterior stroma. Endothelial changes consistent with FECD are seen as increased hyperreflectivity in the thickened Descemet membrane with subtle, focal nodular changes in the endothelium (endothelial guttae).

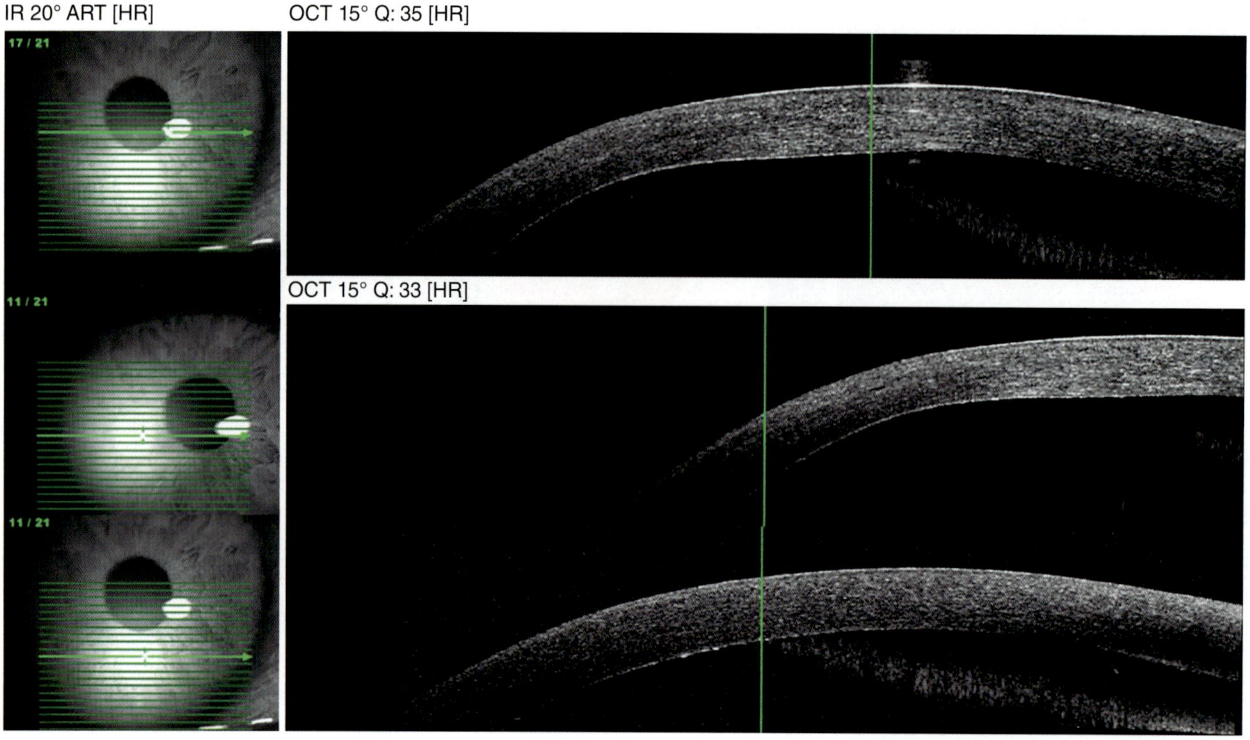

Fig. 7.39 AS-OCT images (spectral-domain, Heidelberg Spectralis) from the left eye of the same patient in Fig. 7.37 with concurrent moderate keratoconus (KCN) and Fuchs endothelial corneal dystrophy (FECD). Previously mentioned features of KCN are noted in the epithelium, Bowman layer, and anterior stroma. Endothelial changes consistent with FECD are seen as increased hyperreflectivity in the thickened Descemet membrane with subtle, focal nodular changes in the endothelium (endothelial guttae).

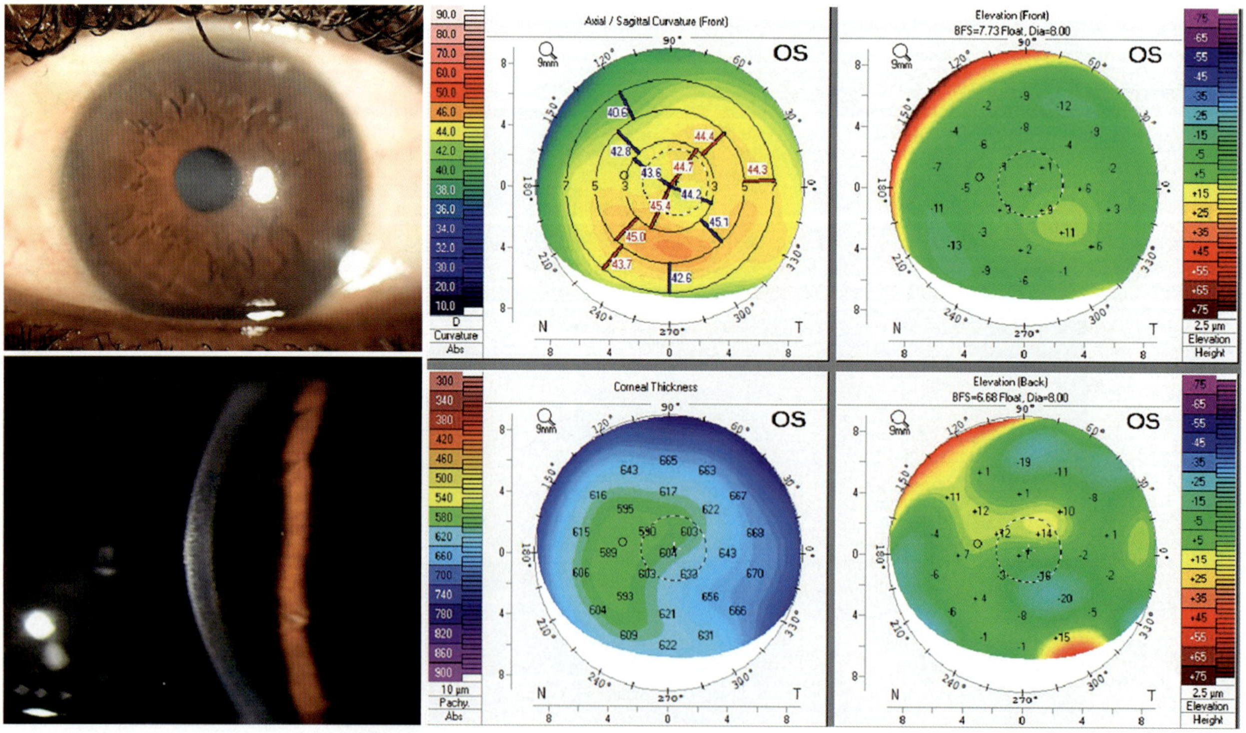

Fig. 7.40 Slit-lamp photographs and tomography images from the left eye of a patient with concurrent forme fruste keratoconus and mild-moderate Fuchs endothelial corneal dystrophy.

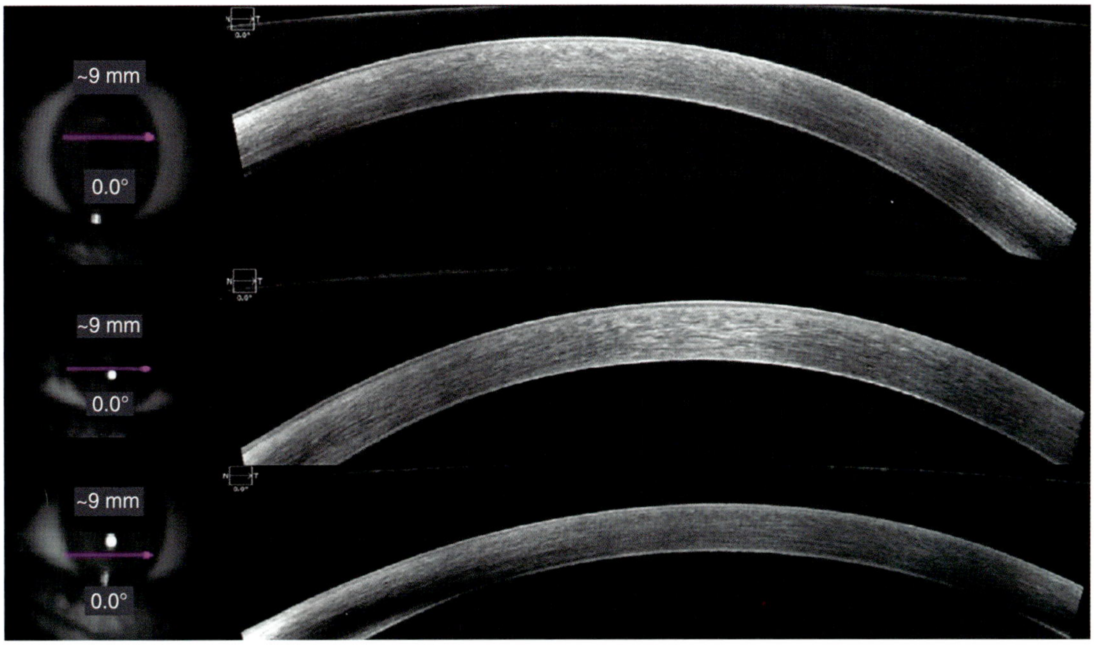

Fig. 7.41 AS-OCT images (spectral-domain, Zeiss Cirrus) from the right eye of a patient with concurrent forme fruste keratoconus (KCN) and mild Fuchs endothelial corneal dystrophy (FECD). Previously mentioned features of KCN are noted in the epithelium, Bowman layer, and anterior stroma, although to a significantly lesser degree compared with Fig. 7.38. Endothelial changes consistent with FECD are seen as increased hyperreflectivity in the thickened Descemet membrane with subtle, focal nodular changes in the endothelium (endothelial guttae).

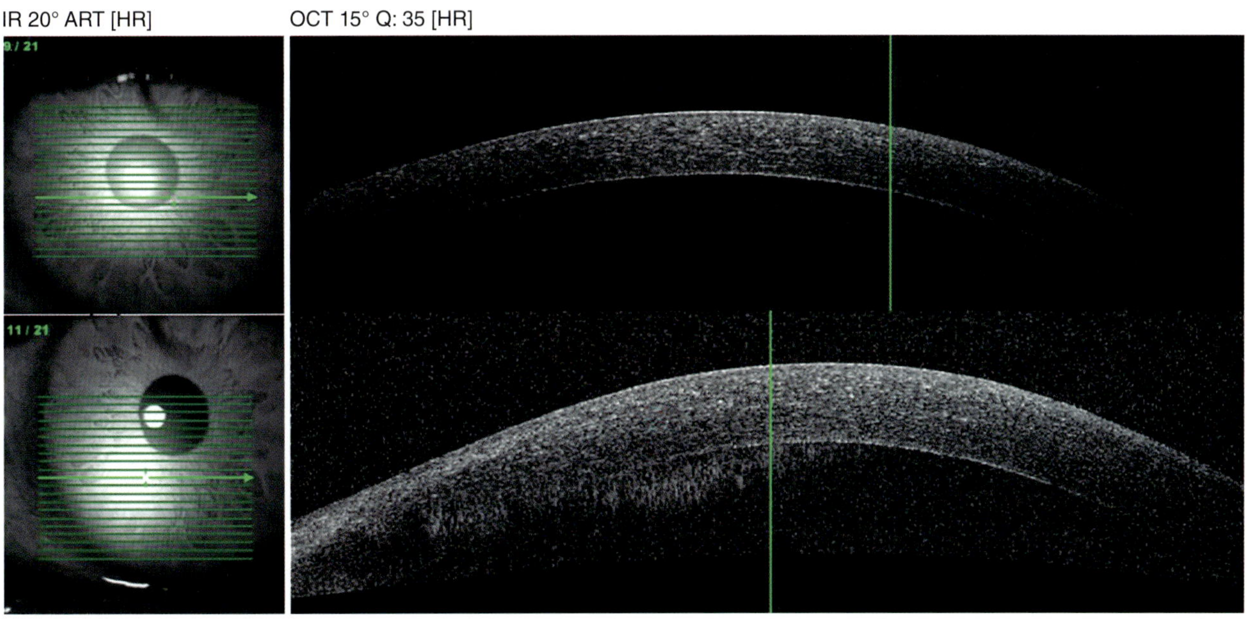

Fig. 7.42 AS-OCT images (spectral-domain, Heidelberg Spectralis) from the left eye of the same patient in Figs. 7.40 to 7.41 with concurrent forme fruste keratoconus (KCN) and mild Fuchs endothelial corneal dystrophy (FECD). Previously mentioned features of KCN are noted in the epithelium, Bowman layer, and anterior stroma, though to a significantly lesser degree compared with Fig. 7.39. Endothelial changes consistent with FECD are seen as increased hyperreflectivity in the thickened Descemet membrane with subtle, focal nodular changes in the endothelium (endothelial guttae).

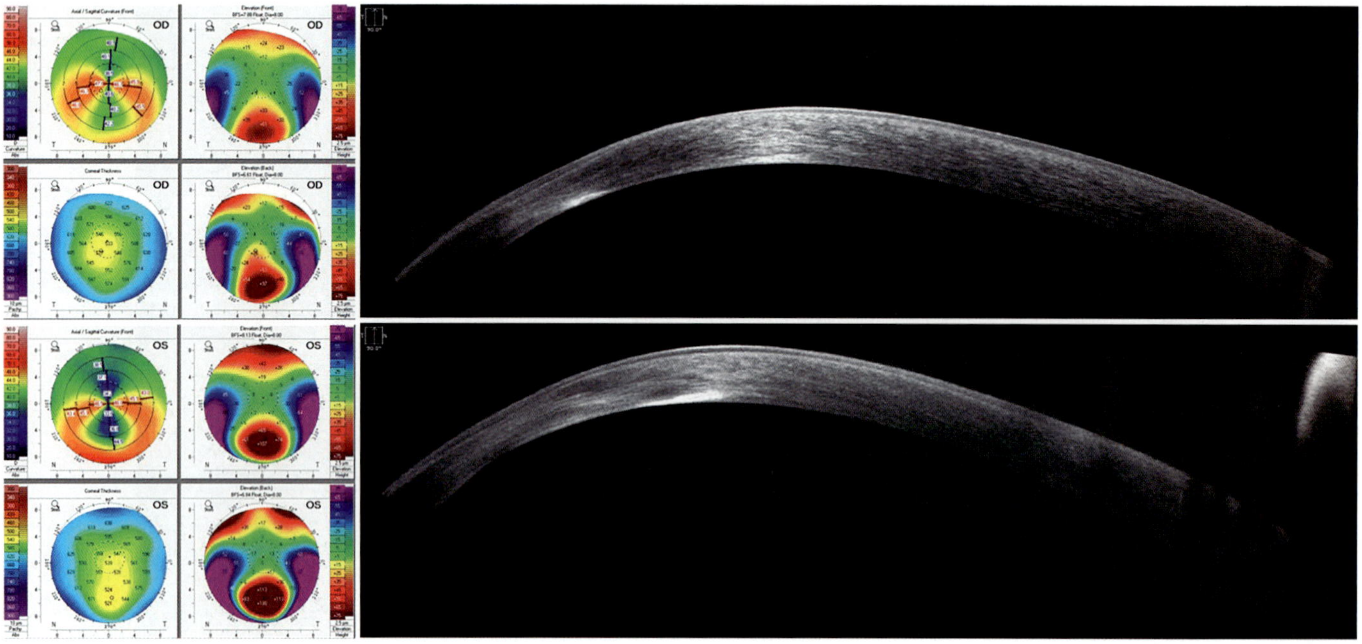

Fig. 7.43 Pellucid marginal degeneration (PMD) is characterized by peripheral thinning of the inferior cornea. The area of maximal thinning is *inferior* to the area of maximal protrusion. The classic shape on corneal topography, indicating significant against-the-rule astigmatism and inferior steepening, can be described as a "crab claw" or "kissing doves" shape. AS-OCT can be helpful to delineate the location of maximal thinning that lies just inferior to the area of maximal corneal protrusion.

While corneal topography is often sufficient to diagnose PMD, AS-OCT can highlight, in cross-sectional view, the area of maximal corneal thinning being *slightly inferior* to the area of maximal protrusion (Fig. 7.43). This can be useful in cases in which features of KCN and PMD may overlap, especially with equivocal topography changes, thus making AS-OCT visualization of the locations of thinning and protrusion extremely helpful. AS-OCT may similarly be used for disease monitoring and to aid surgical decision-making. As these patients may require crescentic lamellar grafts for transplantation, AS-OCT can be used to measure the area of thinning and select an appropriate graft thickness and size.

CLINICAL PEARL

AS-OCT can be used to visualize the unique ectasia changes seen in pellucid marginal degeneration in which the area of maximal thinning is located *inferior* to the area of maximal protrusion. While topography can be suggestive of keratoconus or pellucid marginal degeneration, there is significant overlap in the topographic appearance of these two ectacic conditions. As PMD is defined as thinning inferior to the area of the steepest part of the cornea, and the corneal morphology can be clearly viewed, AS-OCT is the more definitive imaging modality to differentiate KCN from PMD.

V. KERATOGLOBUS

Keratoglobus (KGB) is a rare, bilateral ectasia that is characterized by diffuse corneal protrusion and limbus-to-limbus thinning. As the name suggests, peripheral thinning causes the cornea to assume a more globular (spherical) shape rather than its normal aspherical shape. Interestingly, because of this spherical shape, KGB patients often have *regular* astigmatism compared to the typically encountered irregular astigmatism seen with other corneal ectasias.

Because of its rarity, the diagnosis of KGB can be difficult to make on slit-lamp examination and topography alone. AS-OCT (Fig. 7.44) can be used to visualize the peripheral cornea and assess the extent, location, and severity of the diffuse thinning at the limbus in a circumferential fashion.

VI. POSTERIOR KERATOCONUS

Posterior keratoconus (PKC) is a rare, nonprogressive ectasia defined by an increased curvature of the *posterior* corneal surface. Both localized and diffuse forms have been described in the literature. Clinically, slit-lamp examination of PKC patients may reveal a focal stromal opacity with underlying stromal thinning and posterior corneal indentation. The endothelial layer is intact and unaffected (Fig. 7.45). AS-OCT can be used to visualize the posterior corneal anatomy, including confirmation of intact endothelial layer and assessment of the depth and width of the posterior stromal changes.

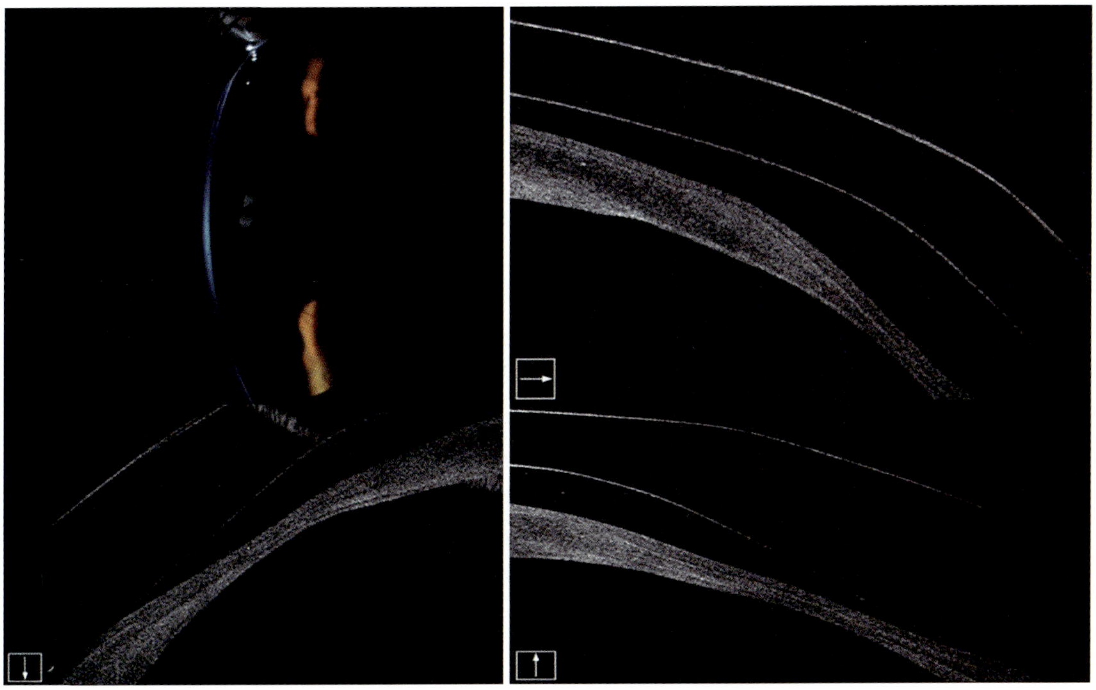

Fig. 7.44 Keratoglobus findings on clinical examination include significant peripheral limbus-to-limbus corneal thinning in a circumferential pattern. Thin slit-beam view may be used as an "optical" OCT to generate a cross-sectional image at the slit-lamp to examine the peripheral limbus. AS-OCT can be additionally used to visualize the location and severity of peripheral thinning. (Courtesy Tyler Oostra, Ohio State University, Ohio, United States and Thomas Mauger, West Virginia University, West Virginia, United States.)

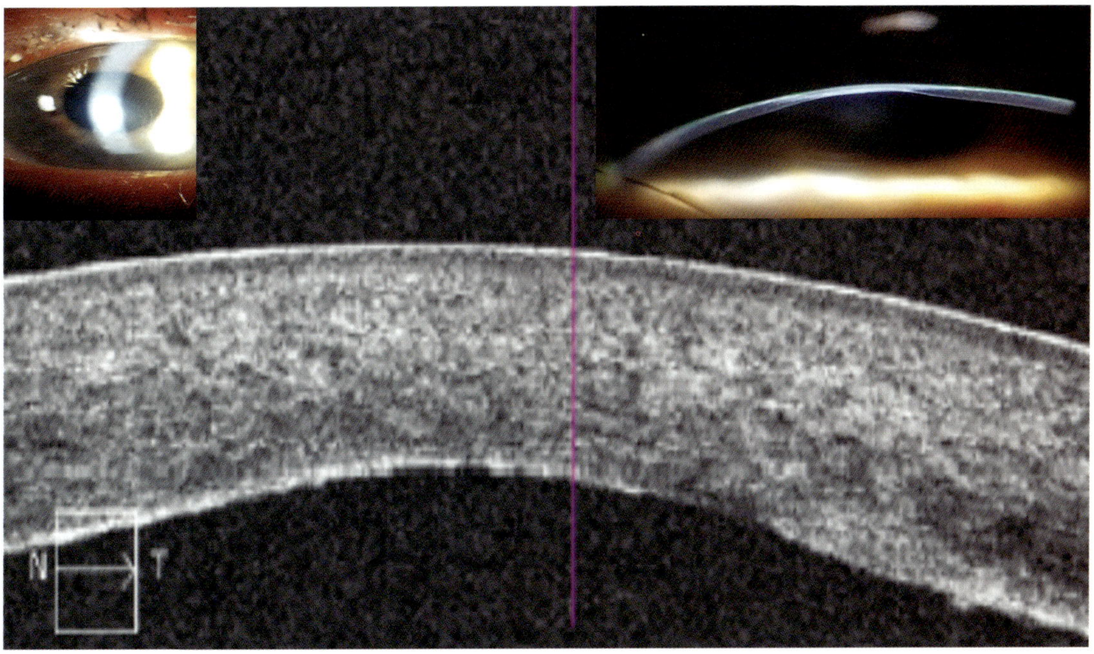

Fig. 7.45 Posterior keratoconus can be seen on clinical examination with broad beam as a focal stromal opacity. Thin-slit beam view can be used to highlight the area of posterior stromal changes and confirm the presence of an intact endothelium. AS-OCT can be used to not only confirm the diagnosis but also to delineate the extent of posterior corneal changes. Note the intact endothelial cell layer in the AS-OCT image. (AS-OCT image courtesy Asim Farooq, MD, Chicago, Illinois, United States; slit-lamp photographs from author's personal images.)

BIBLIOGRAPHY

Gomes JA, Tan D, Rapuano CJ, et al. Global consensus on keratoconus and ectatic diseases. *Cornea*. 2015;34:359-369.

Merriam-Webster. Ectasia. Available at: https://www.merriam-webster.com/medical/ectasia. Accessed March 20, 2021.

Reinstein DZ, Archer TJ, Gobbe M. Corneal epithelial thickness profile in the diagnosis of keratoconus. *J Refract Surg*. 2009;25: 604-610.

8 Pathology of the Endothelium

Allen Omid Eghrari | Michael Joseph Fliotsos

I. FUCHS ENDOTHELIAL CORNEAL DYSTROPHY

Fuchs endothelial corneal dystrophy (FECD) is an inherited condition that appears most often in middle age and results in endothelial dysfunction and loss of the pumping mechanism of the endothelium, leading to progressive corneal edema. A hallmark finding in FECD is the thickening of the Descemet membrane (DM), with a classic "beaten metal" appearance on slit-lamp examination and the formation of guttata, or excrescences of DM. Guttata are protrusions in the corneal endothelium and can be seen clinically and on anterior segment optical coherence tomography (AS-OCT) (Fig. 8.1).

CLINICAL PEARL

In the setting of endothelial failure or perceived endothelial damage, AS-OCT allows for the detection and characterization of patterns of corneal edema.

In early endothelial dystrophy, changes in the appearance of the DM and the endothelium can be seen, including guttae. The pattern of edema may vary between the center and periphery, with amantadine-associated corneal edema often affecting the center and sparing the periphery, whereas pseudophakic bullous keratopathy (PBK) tends to be diffuse and may result in epithelial bullae.

AS-OCT can assist with the identification of DM detachment (DMD) when edema makes visualization with slit-lamp biomicroscopy challenging.

Patients with FECD will report symptoms of decreasing vision, especially with blurriness in the morning, which improves as the day progresses, and increasing glare and halos. For many affected individuals, edema progresses gradually over years to decades, starting initially with the posterior cornea and extending anteriorly to include the epithelium (Figs. 8.2 to 8.5).

The thickening of Descemet's membrane leads to excresences (guttata), which are readily observed at the slit-lamp, and are visible on AS-OCT (Fig. 8.6).

In this image of a DM detachment that occurred after intraocular surgery, the anatomic layers of the DM—the anterior banded layer and the posterior nonbanded layer—can be seen clearly on AS-OCT imaging (Fig. 8.7).

II. PSEUDOPHAKIC BULLOUS KERATOPATHY

Pseudophakic bullous keratopathy (PBK) results from endothelial failure after intraocular surgery. Although PBK can certainly occur in the setting of a normal, healthy endothelium when the endothelium receives iatrogenic trauma during surgery, the risk for PBK is much higher when there is preexisting Fuchs dystrophy, which can be seen on AS-OCT. Compromise of the endothelium occurs as a result of excessive exposure to phacoemulsification energy, direct trauma to the endothelium from intraocular instruments, or toxicity from intracameral medication. Due to endothelial cell death or dysfunction, the ability of the endothelium to pump fluid from the cornea corneal stroma into the aqueous humor is decreased, leading to corneal edema. In severe disease, edema extends to the epithelium, resulting in microcystic changes or gross bullae.

Diffuse corneal edema can be seen with DM folds in Fig. 8.8. AS-OCT will show the extent and location of the corneal swelling and the characteristic changes in the endothelium and DM, as is often seen in Fuchs dystrophy.

Fig. 8.9 is the AS-OCT image of the slit-lamp photograph in Fig. 8.8. Corneal edema is seen as the stroma is thickened, and the Descemet folds appear as wavy protrusions of the posterior cornea.

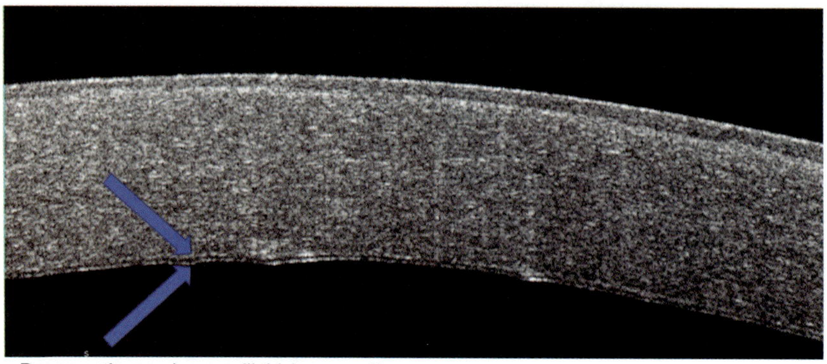

Fig. 8.1 Normal age-related changes of the Descemet membrane. With increasing age, the Descemet membrane will thicken; this is a normal physiologic change. (Courtesy Nikhil Gokhale, MD, Gokhale Eye Clinic, Mumbai, India.)

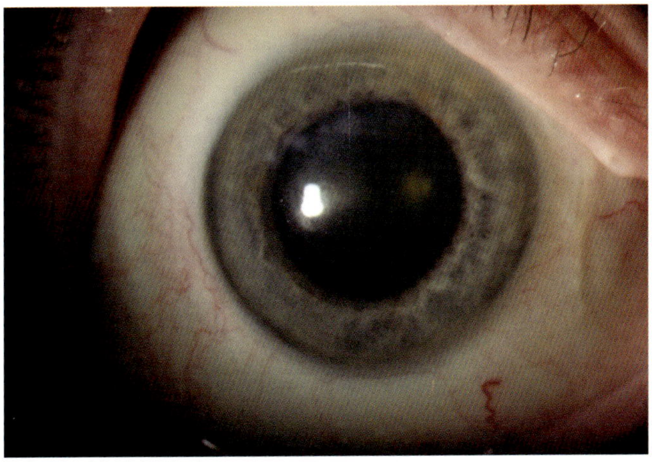

Fig. 8.2 In this slit-lamp photograph, mild corneal edema is seen in early Fuchs corneal endothelial dystrophy.

However, the clinical appearance of PBK can be quite variable, from mild to severe corneal edema. In Fig. 8.10, the corneal edema is milder, but there is significant edema causing separation of the epithelium and the clinical appearance of an epithelial bulla.

Although the previous images showed corneal edema after cataract surgery, which is why this condition is referred to as *pseudophakic,* corneal edema can occur after any intraocular surgery, particularly glaucoma surgery. In Fig. 8.11, corneal opacification and mild corneal edema can be observed in an 11-year-old female patient with history of retinopathy of prematurity who was referred for nonclearing edema/opacification after goniotomy.

III. POSTERIOR POLYMORPHOUS MEMBRANE/CORNEAL DYSTROPHY

Posterior polymorphous membrane dystrophy (PPMD, also known as posterior polymorphous corneal dystrophy or

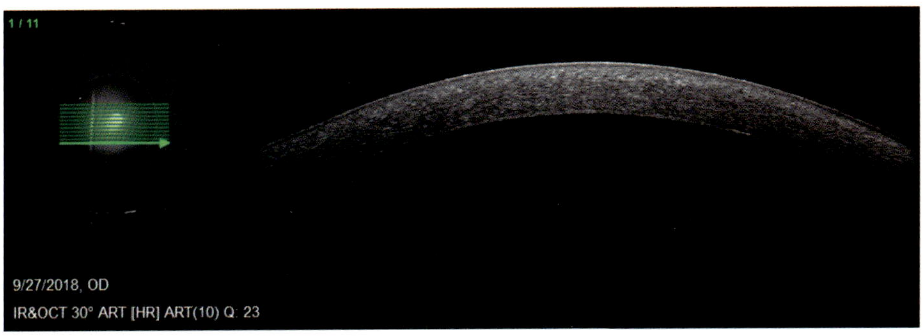

Fig. 8.3 AS-OCT can highlight areas of early corneal edema in Fuchs endothelial corneal dystrophy. Some thickening of the endothelium is seen, but no guttata are visible on AS-OCT. Guttata can be a later finding.

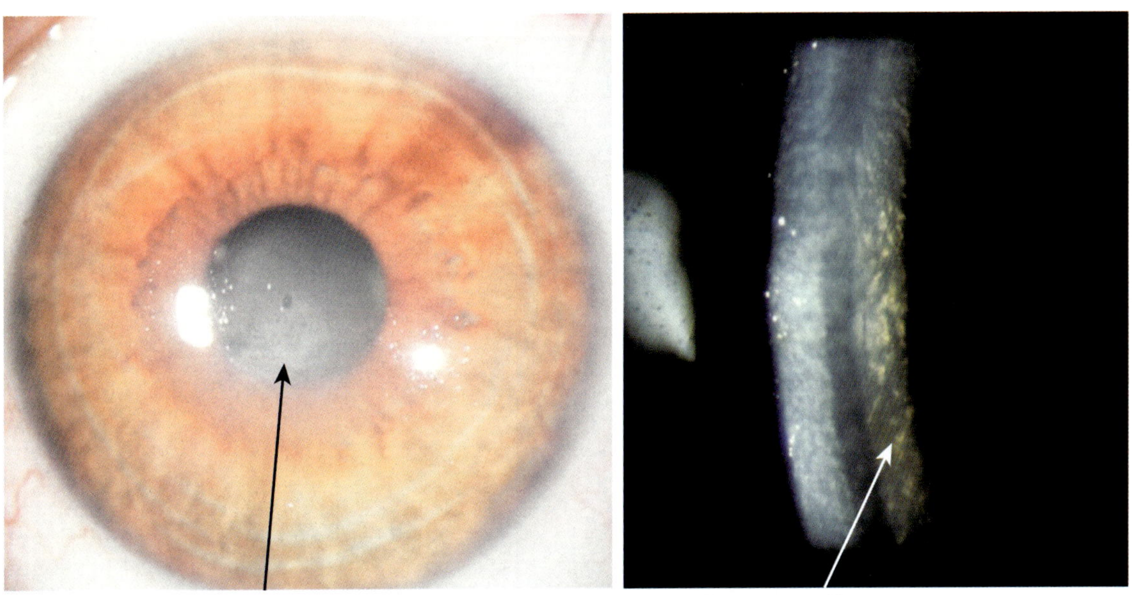

Fig. 8.4 Moderate-severe Fuchs endothelial corneal dystrophy. Slit-lamp exam demonstrates central corneal edema, microcystic edema, and the classic "beaten metal" appearance of the endothelium. (Courtesy Nikhil Gokhale, MD, Gokhale Eye Clinic, Mumbai, India.)

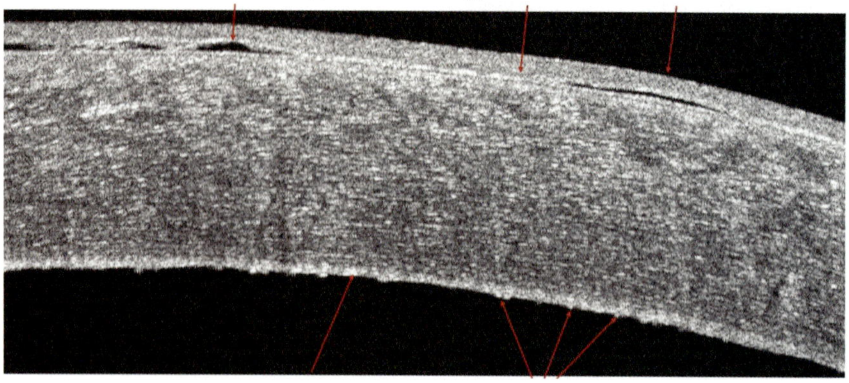

Fig. 8.5 Guttata are visible in more advanced Fuchs endothelial corneal dystrophy on AS-OCT. Several additional morphological changes are observed in the anterior corneal layers. (Nikhil Gokhale, MD, Gokhale Eye Clinic, Mumbai, India.)

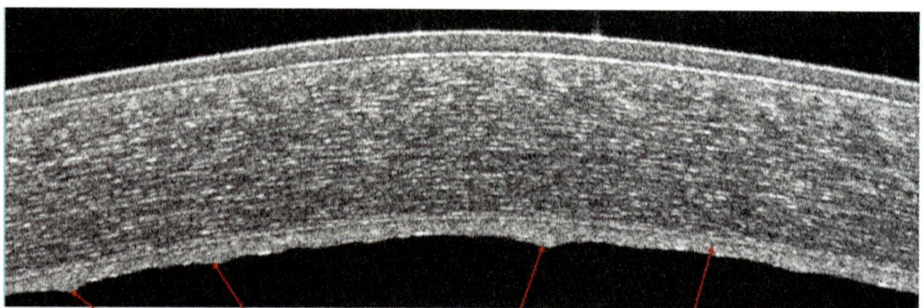

Fig. 8.6 AS-OCT demonstrates Descemet's membrane thickening and guttata (excrescence's of Descemet's membrane). (Courtesy Nikhil Gokhale, MD, Gokhale Eye Clinic, Mumbai, India)

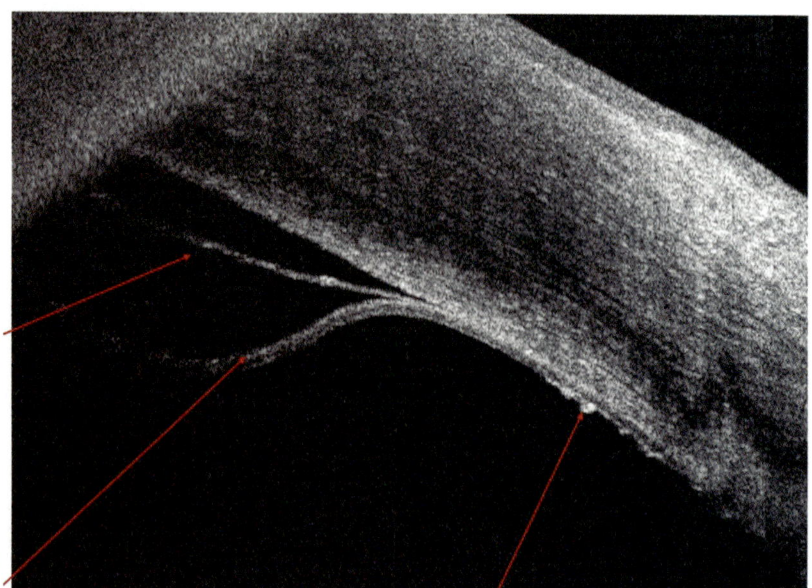

Fig. 8.7 AS-OCT demonstrates splitting of the Descemet's membrane into the anterior banded layer and posterior non-banded layer. Thickened endothelium with guttata are also observed. (Courtesy Nikhil Gokhale, MD, Gokhale Eye Clinic, Mumbai, India.)

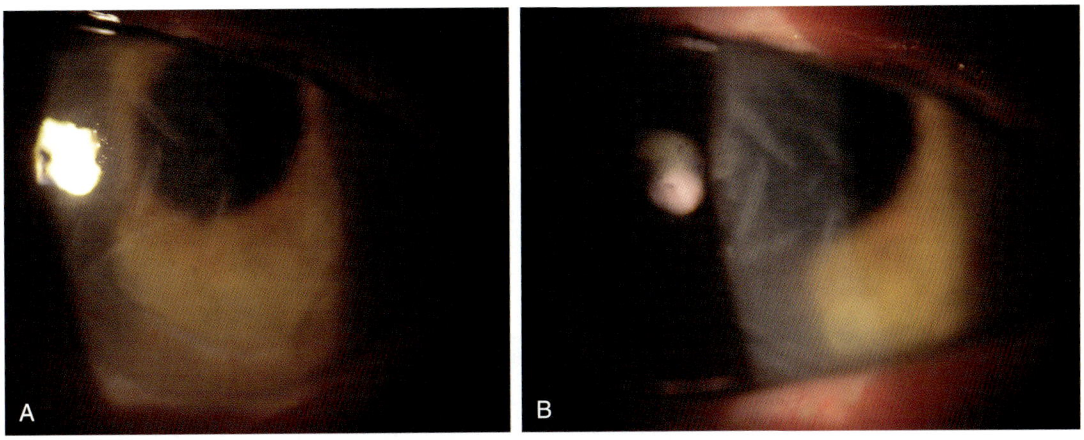

Fig. 8.8 **Pseudophakic bullous keratopathy with Descemet membrane folds.**

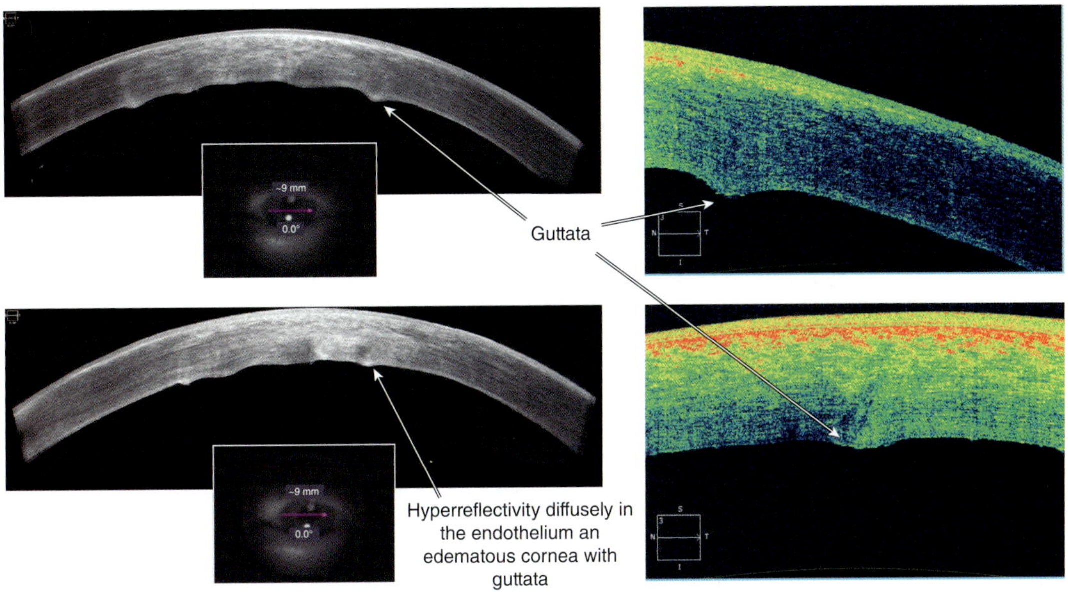

Fig. 8.9 **AS-OCT of pseudophakic bullous keratopathy with Descemet membrane folds.**

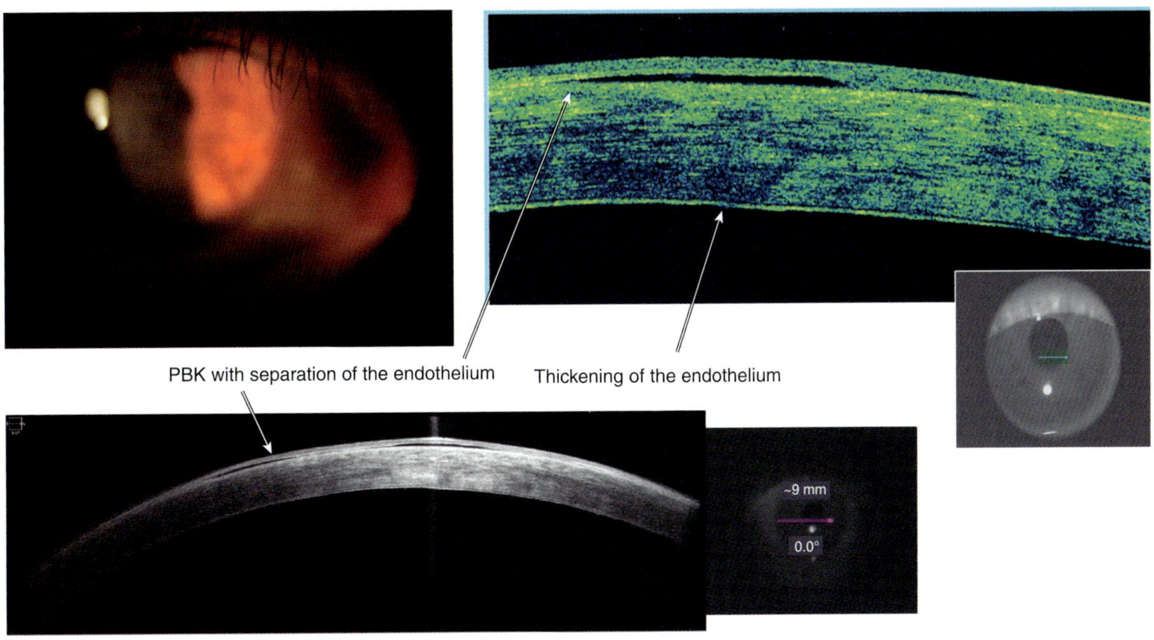

Fig. 8.10 **Pseudophakic bullous keratopathy with separation of the epithelium from the underlying corneal layers.** Thickening of Descemet's membrane is also observed..

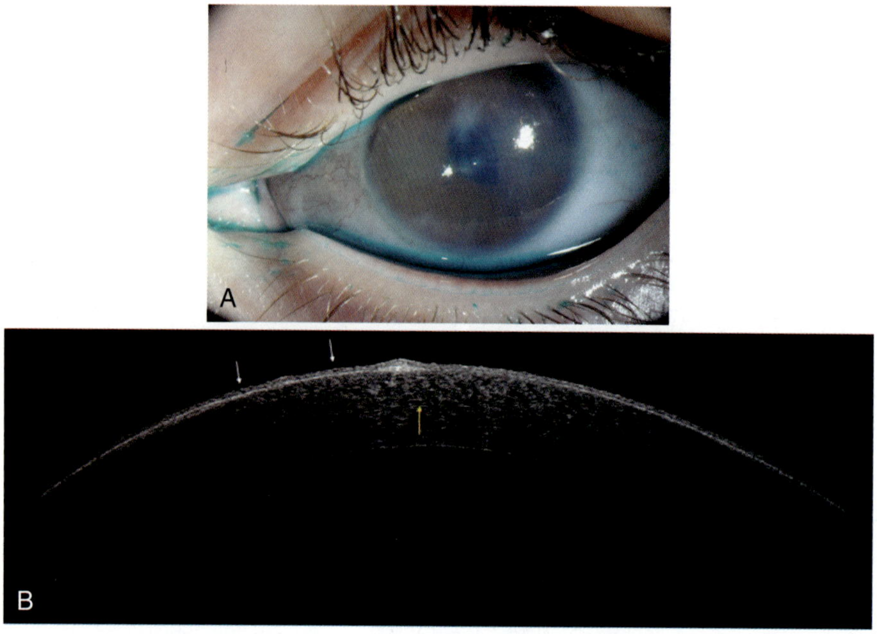

Fig. 8.11 **A. Slit-lamp photograph of bullous keratopathy. B. AS-OCT image of bullous keratopathy.** Microcystic edema is visible as black spaces in the epithelium *(white arrows)*. Stromal edema appears as black spaces in between corneal lamellae, which have been separated *(yellow arrow)*.

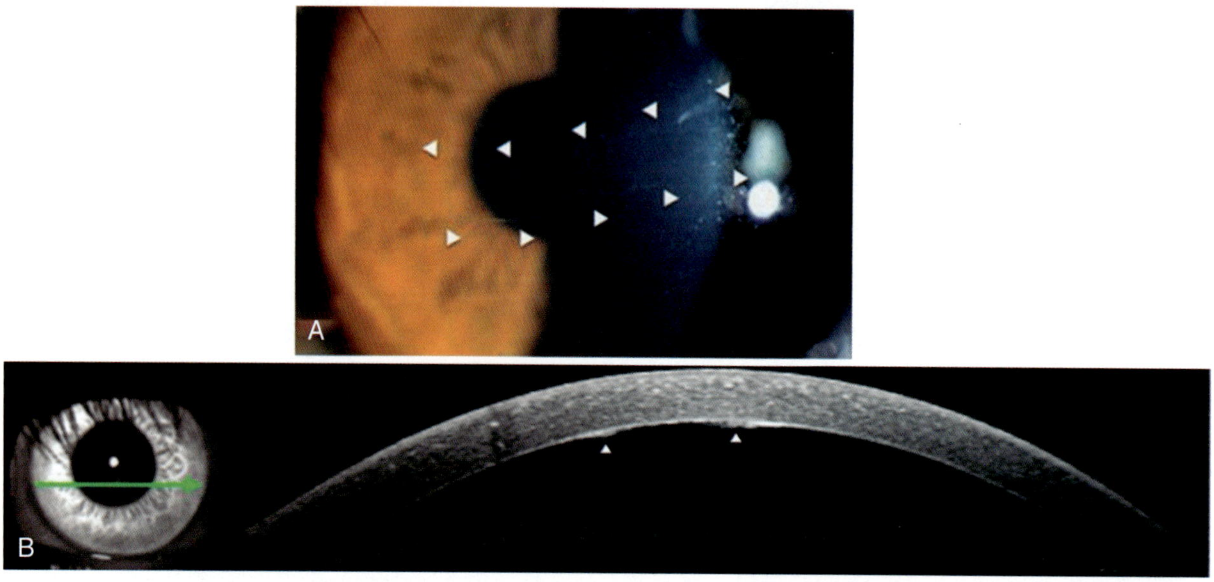

Fig. 8.12 **A. Slit-lamp photograph of a 25-year-old man with posterior polymorphous membrane dystrophy.** A horizontal bandlike lesion on the endothelium can be observed *(white arrowheads)*. B In the corresponding AS-OCT image, the epithelial-like changes on corneal endothelium are noted. *(white arrowheads)*. (Reproduced with permission from Joon Young Hyon, Department of Ophthalmology, Seoul National University College of Medicine from their publication: Jeon HS and Hyon JY. Unilateral posterior polymorphous corneal dystrophy presented as anisometropic astigmatism: 3 case reports. Case Rep Ophthalmol 2017;8:250-258. https://doi.10.1159/000472704.)

Schlichting dystrophy) is a disorder of the corneal endothelium and DM that is inherited in an autosomal dominant fashion. Normally, the slit-lamp findings are subtle, and often there is no clinical significance. PPMD occurs when the endothelium develops epithelial characteristics, and the maps, dots, and lines seen in epithelial basement membrane dystrophy (EBMD) are visualized in the endothelium. However, in some rare cases of PPMD, the epithelial-like changes on the endothelium can grow into the anatomic angle and cause corneal edema, angle closure, and increased risk for increased eye pressure and glaucoma (Fig. 8.12).

The AS-OCT images in Fig. 8.12 show epithelial-like changes in the endothelium. Note that the endothelium appears similar to that in AS-OCT images of the epithelium in EBMD (see Chapter 5).

In Fig. 8.13, subtle maps and lines reminiscent of EBMD are seen in the endothelium, and a round cluster of irregular cellular material is noted on the endothelium.

In Fig. 8.14, a crescentic-like appearance of the endothelium is seen, also consistent with PPMD. Like EBMD, PPMD is protean and can have a variable presentation, even in the same patient. The thickening and reduplication of the epithelial changes in the endothelium are seen in the AS-OCT images with variable thickening, hyper-reflectivity, and "double-layer" appearance.

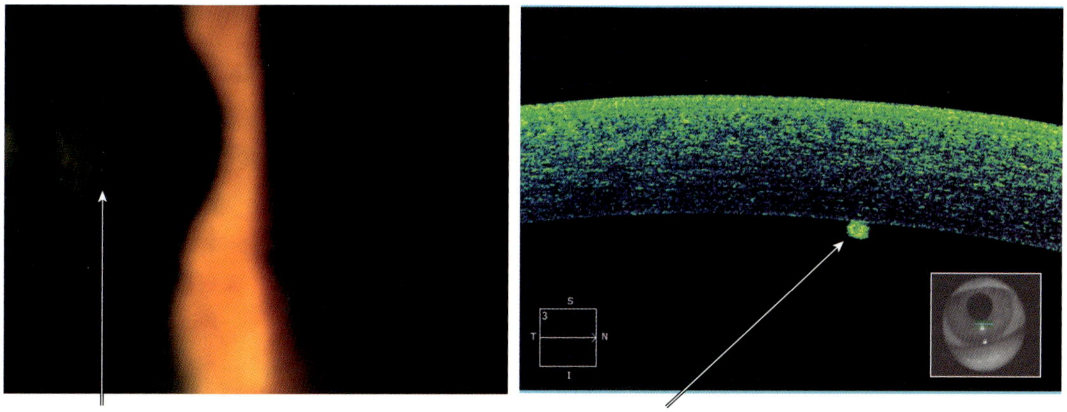

Fig. 8.13 Slit-lamp photograph (left panel) demonstrates epithelial-like changes in the endothelium in a patient with PPMD. AS-OCT (right panel) shows epithelial-like changes (focal areas of hyper-reflectivity) of the endothelium.

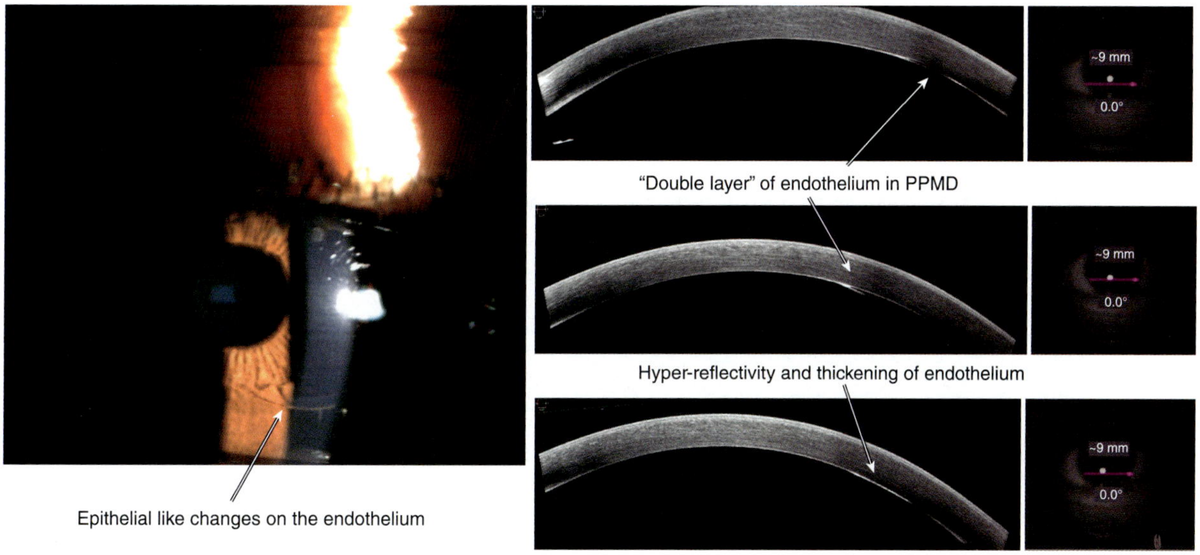

Fig. 8.14 Slit-lamp photograph demonstrates crescentic, epithelial-like changes in the posterior corneal layers. AS-OCT findings can be variable, ranging from endothelial thickening, hyper-reflectivity, and "double-layer" appearance.

IV. DESCEMET'S MEMBRANE DETACHMENT AFTER CATARACT SURGERY

Descemet's membrane detachment (DMD) is a complication of intraocular surgery. It is most often reported after cataract surgery but can occur after any intraocular surgery requiring a transcorneal incision, such as trabeculectomy, penetrating keratoplasty, pars plana vitrectomy, and iridectomy. DMD is caused by a variety of potential mechanisms, such as anterior and shelved incisions, dull blades, traumatic intraocular lens implantation, or inadvertent trauma with the irrigation/aspiration device when the DM is mistaken for an anterior capsular remnant.

Examination under the slit-lamp with direct illumination usually discloses a scrolled or unscrolled DMD, with varying degrees of accompanying corneal edema. AS-OCT will reveal a thin DMD in the anterior chamber (Figs. 8.15 and 8.16). Variable areas of scrolling and attachment are noted with fluid (black spaces) visible between the posterior stroma and DM.

V. AMANTADINE-ASSOCIATED CORNEAL EDEMA

Corneal edema in the setting of amantadine is characteristically bilateral and begins as central folds of DM, moving to diffuse stromal edema over time. It can occur at any time during chronic therapy with amantadine and improves with cessation of the medication or if required, corneal transplantation. The frequency of its occurrence among patients taking this medication is unknown (Fig. 8.17).

VI. NETARSUDIL-ASSOCIATED CORNEAL EDEMA

Netarsudil is a topical glaucoma medication that reduces intraocular pressure by targeting the trabecular pathway of aqueous humor outflow. As both a rho kinase inhibitor and a norepinephrine transport inhibitor, it is associated with conjunctival hyperemia and a cobblestone pattern of microcystic

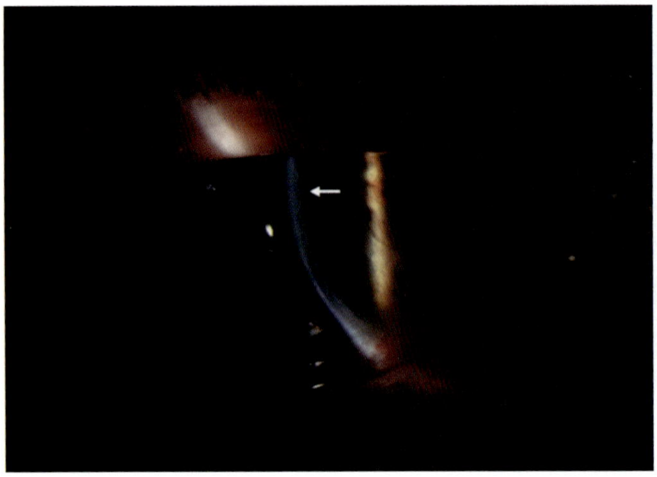

Fig. 8.15 Descemet's membrane detachment in a patient with Fuchs corneal endothelial dystrophy five days after cataract surgery. The detachment *(white arrow)* appears as a fine, white, curved line posterior to the anterior corneal layers. The patient was initially managed with an air bubble before presenting for further management.

corneal edema that both resolve with cessation of the medication. In the figure below, the patient underwent Descemet's membrane endothelial keratoplasty and was subsequently treated with netarsudil for non-clearing corneal edema postoperatively. Although the corneal edema resolved, several bullae are seen on AS-OCT (Fig. 8.18).

VII. *COL8A2*-ASSOCIATED CORNEAL DYSTROPHY

Mutations in *COL8A2* are associated with a corneal dystrophy similar in appearance to classic FECD but appearing early in life. In the L450W mutation, aberrant collagen deposition results in markedly thickened DM with guttae that are buried within its layers. Therefore, although DM has a guttate-like appearance at the slit-lamp, pathologic evaluation reveals that the guttae are buried inside DM and do not protrude posteriorly. Bullae may appear focally (Fig. 8.19).

In the AS-OCT image (Fig. 8.19) of this patient, the thickness of the DM is comparable to the epithelium, which is approximately 50 microns in thickness. In contrast, the normal DM is approximately 15 to 20 microns in thickness, and does not have excrescences (guttae) as seen in the previous images of FECD (Fig. 8.20).

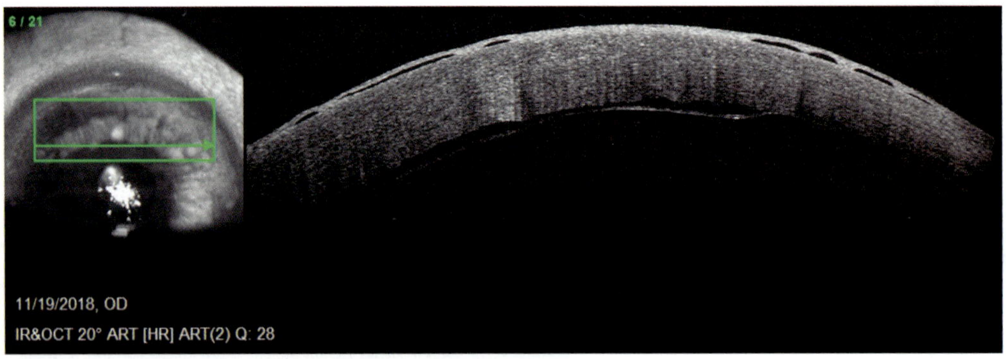

Fig. 8.16 AS-OCT image of the patient in Fig. 8.15 with Descemet membrane detachment in the superior cornea. Several notable features are observed. First, the Descemet's membrane naturally scrolls or curves toward the posterior stroma with delineation between the areas of attachment and non-attachment. Second, central stromal folds are appreciated in the posterior cornea. Third, epithelial bullae are also observed.

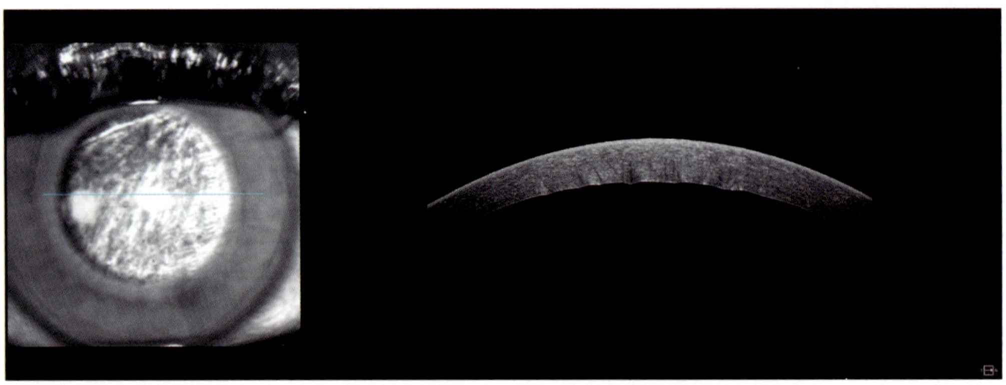

Fig. 8.17 AS-OCT image of bilateral corneal edema in a 46-year-old woman who had taken amantadine for several years. The cornea exhibits central folds of the Descemet membrane (DM). This gives a wavy appearance to both the posterior stroma and central DM. In contrast, the peripheral cornea remains relatively intact and clear.

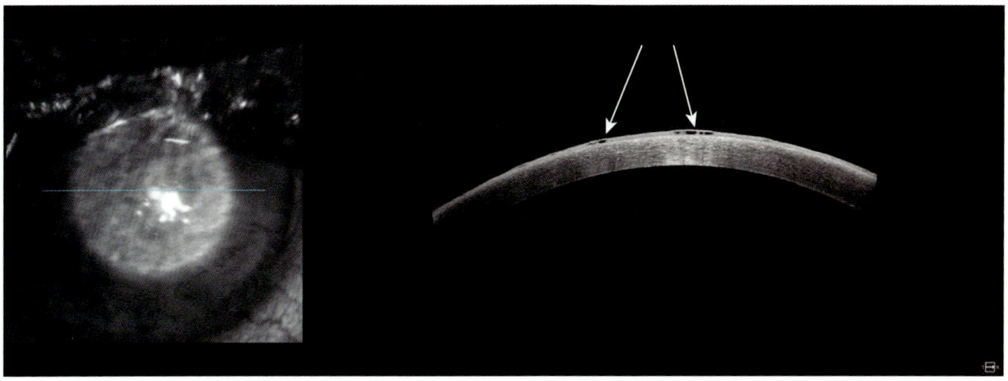

Fig. 8.18 AS-OCT image of an eye 3 months after Descemet's membrane endothelial keratoplasty (DMEK). The DMEK graft is attached, and the corneal edema, which was previously more than 100 microns, has now decreased to less than 600 microns. Notably, though the edema from the endothelial failure has resolved, the use of netarsudil resulted in the apperance of microscopic bullae, which appear as black spaces in the epithelium (red arrows).

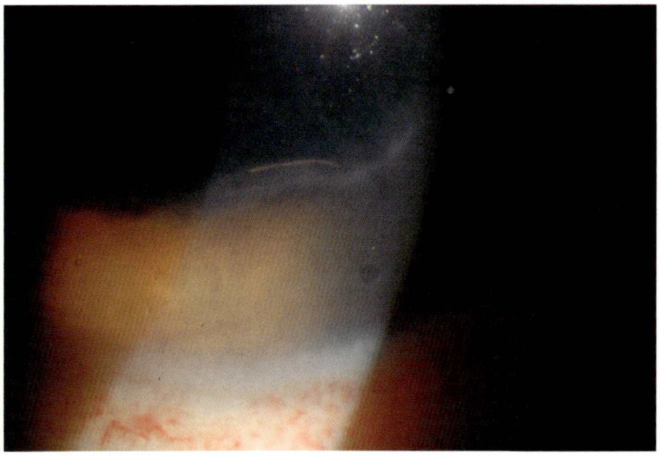

Fig. 8.19 Slit-lamp photograph of a 42-year-old man with the L450W mutation in *COL8A2*. Peripheral bullae are appreciated despite his young age.

In a 46-year-old man with the L450W mutation in *COL8A2,* the marked thickness of the DM is apparent before undergoing DMEK (Figs. 8.21 and 8.22).

After DMEK, the central donor DM is noted to be thinner than the peripheral DM, where the original host tissue remains. AS-OCT is particularly adept at visualization of this layer to determine its thickness.

VIII. IRIDOCORNEAL ENDOTHELIAL SYNDROME

Iridocorneal endothelial (ICE) syndrome is a disorder that involves irregularities of the corneal endothelium. ICE syndrome will have a common pathologic process, has a heterogeneous presentation, and is divided into three distinct variants: Chandler syndrome, essential/progressive iris atrophy, and iris nevus (also known as Cogan-Reese syndrome). Although there are unique clinical characteristics that can be used to distinguish between each subtype, all three can cause significant visual

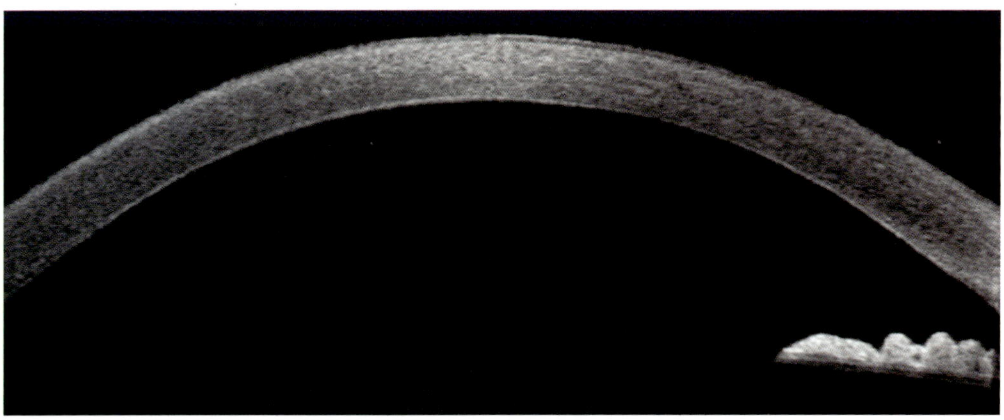

Fig. 8.20 AS-OCT image of the patient shown in Fig 8.19. AS-OCT demonstrates that although the DM is markedly thickened (with similar thickness as the epithelium), no excrescences (guttae) are observed.

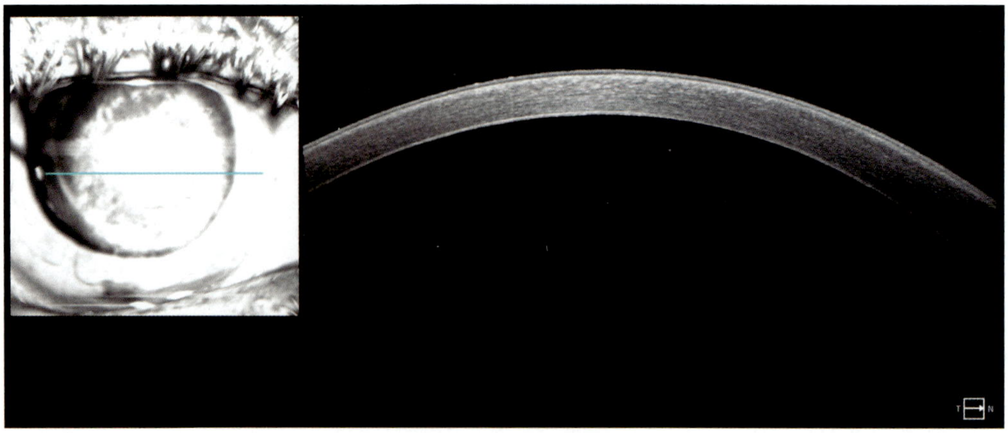

Fig. 8.21 ***COL8A2*-associated corneal dystrophy.** In this 40-year-old, patient the Descemet membrane is noted to be extremely thickened, with a thickness similar to the epithelium

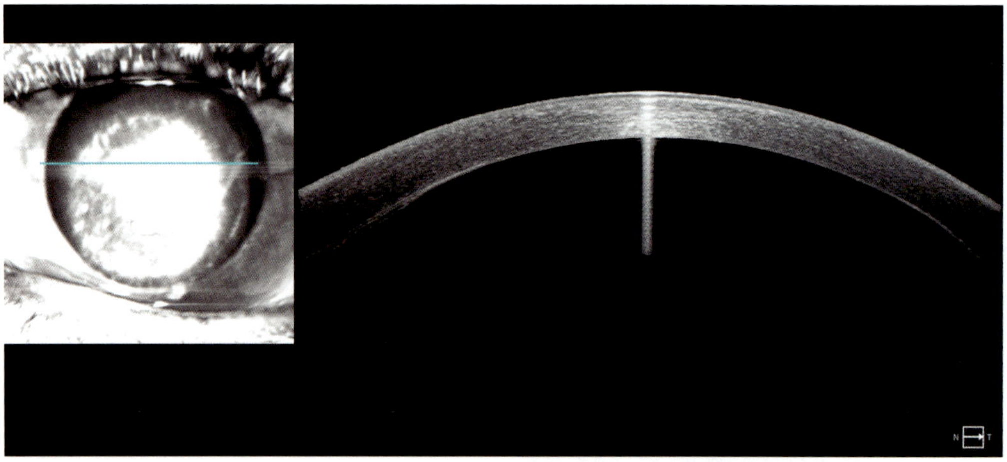

Fig. 8.22 AS-OCT image after DMEK in the patient in Fig. 8.21. The Descemet membrane (DM) is now of normal thickness centrally, in contrast to the peripheral rim of the host DM, which remains relatively thicker and similar to the overlying epithelium.

impairment from optic neuropathy secondary to glaucoma and corneal edema.

At the slit-lamp, the corneal endothelium typically has a beaten bronze or hammered silver appearance that often bears similarities to guttae in FECD, as mentioned previously. It is hypothesized that the normal endothelium is replaced with an epithelial-type layer with desmosomes, tonofilaments, and microvilli when analyzed in histopathologic studies. Migration of this altered endothelium posteriorly toward the trabecular meshwork (and sometimes onto the iris itself) and subsequent contracture results in high peripheral anterior synechiae (PAS), characteristic iris changes, and the possibility of secondary angle-closure glaucoma. A challenge in the assessment of ICE syndrome is the fact that the high PAS formation can occur without overt synechiae as the migrating endothelium closes the angle without contraction. Fig 8.23 shows the slit-lamp photograph of a 56 year old female patient with ICE syndrome. Examination demonstrated a pupil peaked at 2:00 and 10:00 with fibrous-like iris changes approximately 1 to 2 mm across with iridocorneal touch (Fig. 8.23).

Fig. 8.24 shows an AS-OCT image of the angle from the patient shown in Fig 8.23. Anterior synechiae are readily seen.

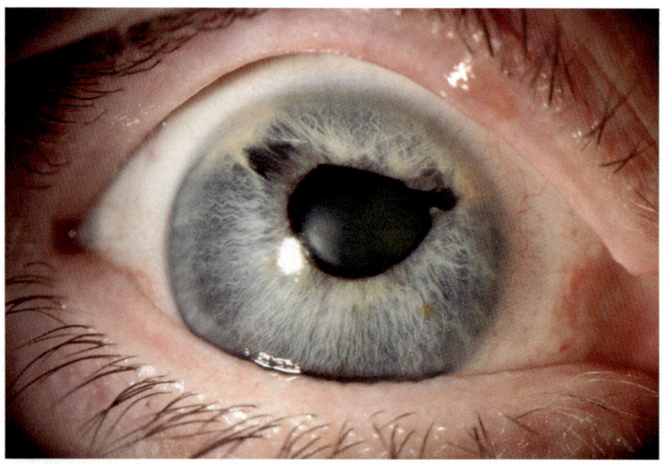

Fig. 8.23 Slit-lamp photograph of a 56 year old female patient with iridocorneal endothelial (ICE) syndrome. Correctopia, focal areas of iris atrophy, and iris holes are observed. In the corneal periphery, PAS can be seen, though these are better visualized on gonioscopy.

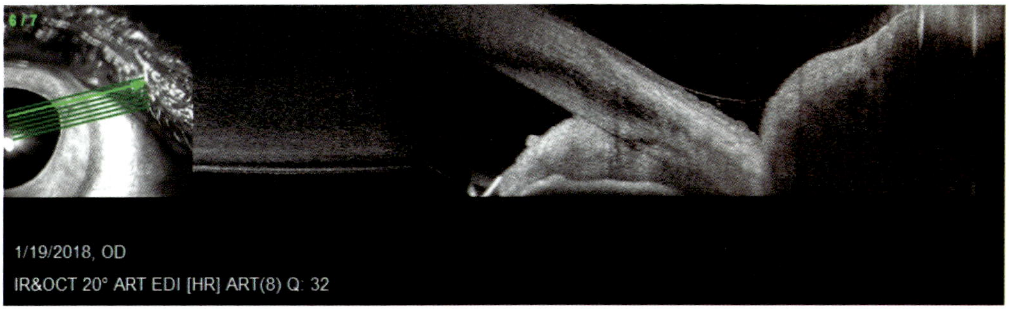

Fig. 8.24 Iridocorneal endothelial (ICE) syndrome. AS-OCT image of the anatomic angle in a patient with ICE syndrome demonstrates prominent anterior synechiae.

IX. ENDOTHELIAL DEBRIS

Pseudoexfoliation syndrome (PXF) is a systemic condition with ocular manifestations that results in the release and deposition of white, flaky material from the lens and zonules. These deposits can appear throughout the anterior segment, and although they are often appreciated on the surface of the lens capsule, they can also settle on the corneal endothelium and trabecular meshwork.

In the series of AS-OCT images in Fig. 8.25, several opacities appear on the corneal endothelium, notably of varying morphology: punctate, oval, and rectangular. This is consistent with the flaky PXF material, which may appear in the OCT image at different angles.

Keratic precipitates (KPs) are inflammatory debris that settle on the corneal endothelium in the setting of intraocular inflammation. These may appear in various forms, from small, stellate KPs to large, mutton-fat KPs.

Fig. 8.26 is a slit-lamp image of a 27-year-old man with anterior uveitis. Inflammatory material is appreciated on the posterior cornea. The KPs visualized here are deposited in a pattern called an Arlt's triangle, which is distribution pattern of mutton-fat KPs depositing and forming an inverted triangle (wedge-shape) region on the inferior corneal endothelium.

In Fig. 8.27, AS-OCT demonstrates the round, focal morphology of such deposits of these KPs using two different AS-OCT devices. This contrasts with the more variable and linear appearance of PXF material in the preceding figures. Note that the endothelium is intact with normal morphology and thickness in these images.

Fig. 8.28 shows a hypopyon with mutton-fat KPs. The layered hypopyon can be seen on the AS-OCT images as well, as can a patchy deposition of white blood cells and inflammatory material on the endothelium and clusters of white blood cells, which appear clinically as KPs. A membrane of inflammatory material also can be seen bridging the pupil. Of note, a shadow can be seen in the image of the hypopyon; this is a common artifact of the defocus of the AS-OCT.

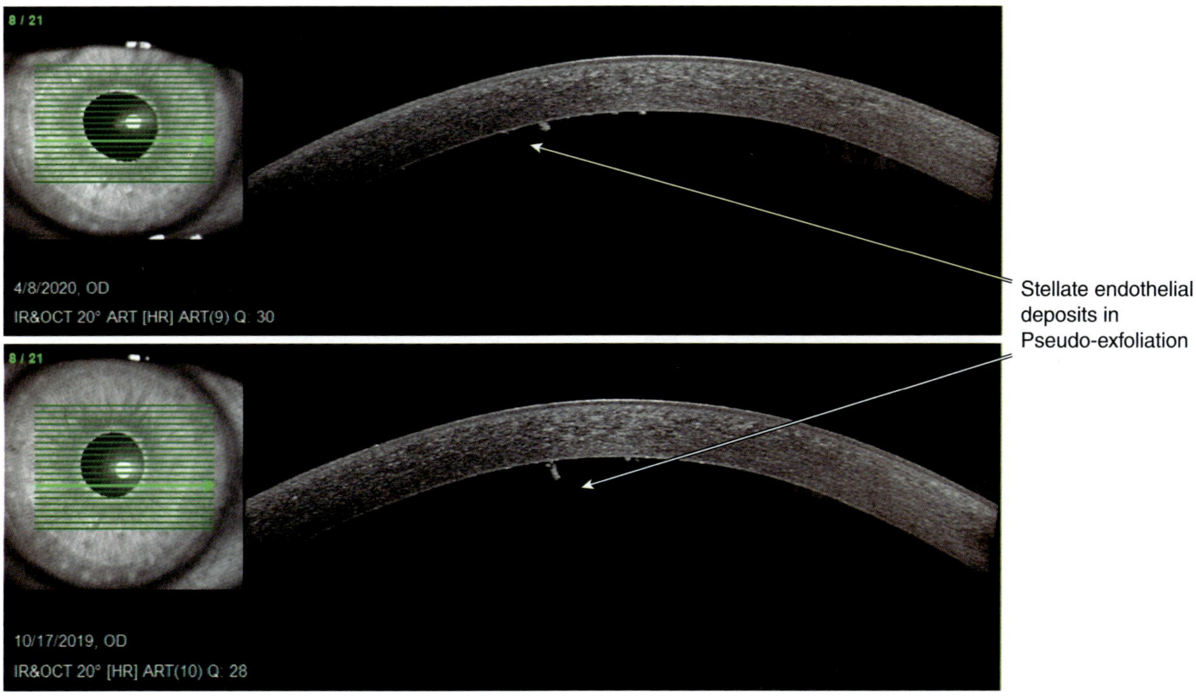

Fig. 8.25 Pseudoexfoliation deposits on the endothelium. (Courtesy Albert Cheung.)

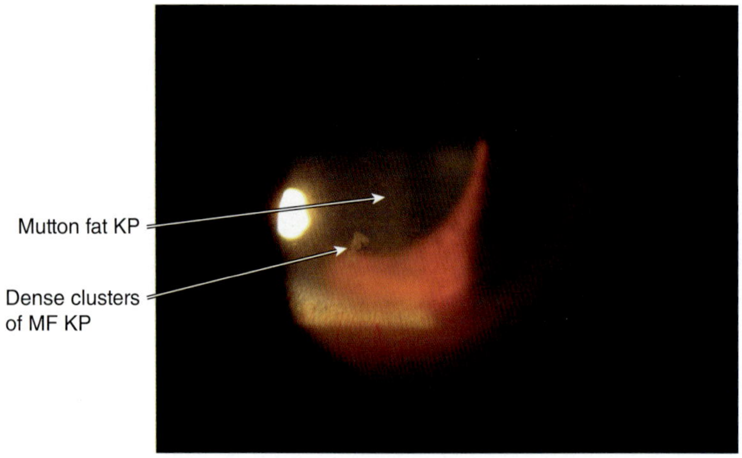

Fig. 8.26 **Mutton-fat keratic precipitates *(KPs)* in the Arlt triangle.**

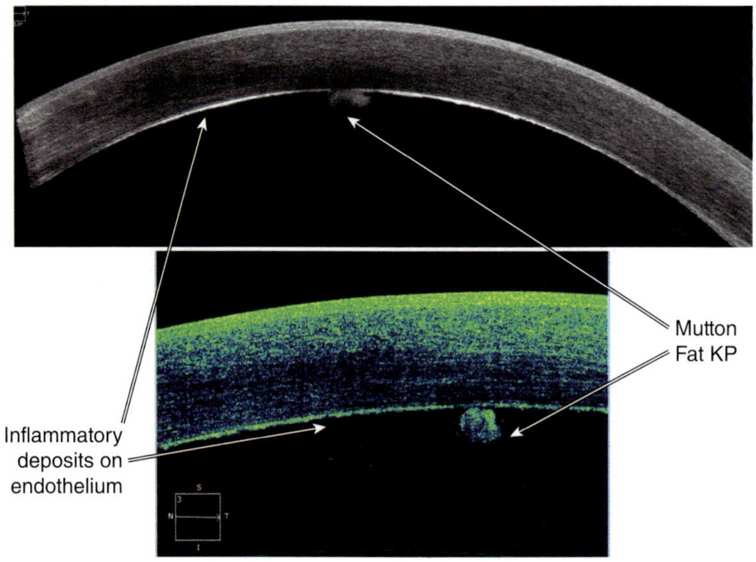

Fig. 8.27 **Mutton-fat keratic precipitates.**

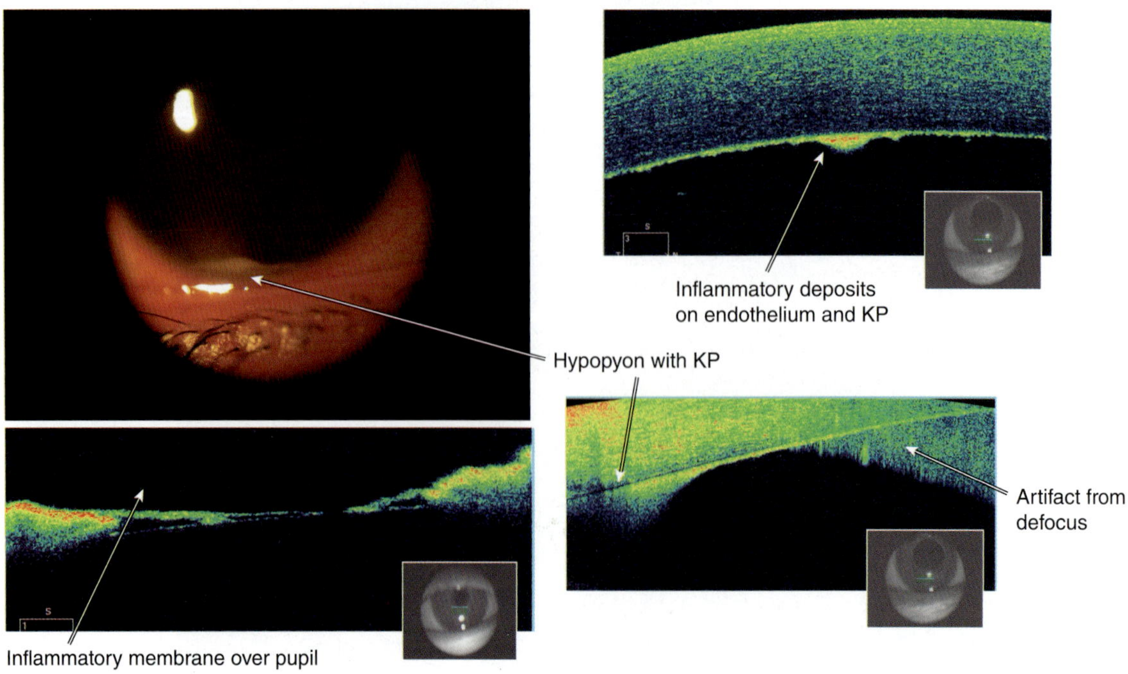

Fig. 8.28 **Appearance of hypopyon and mutton-fat keratic precipitate (KP) on slit-lamp and AS-OCT images.**

BIBLIOGRAPHY

Eghrari AO, Riazuddin SA, Gottsch JD. Distinct clinical phenotype of corneal dystrophy predicts the p.(Leu450Trp) substitution in COL8A2. *Cornea*. 2016;35(5):587-591.

Glaucoma. *Basic and Clinical Science Course (BCSC)*. San Francisco: American Academy of Ophthalmology; 2010-2011:142-144.

Hessen MM, Vahedi S, Khoo CT, et al. Clinical and genetic investigation of amantadine-associated corneal edema. *Clin Ophthalmol*. 2018;12:1367-1371.

Levy SG, Kirkness CM, Moss J, Ficker L, McCartney AC. The histopathology of the iridocorneal-endothelial syndrome. *Cornea*. 1996;15(1):46-54.

Marcon AS, Rapuano CJ, Jones MR, Laibson PR, Cohen EJ. Descemet's membrane detachment after cataract surgery: management and outcome. *Ophthalmology*. 2002;109(12): 2325-2330.

SECTION 4

Iris, Angle and Lens Abnormalities

9 Abnormalities of the Iris

Zelia M. Correa | Helena Prior Filipe

I. INTRODUCTION

There are a broad spectrum of iris lesions that ranges from cystic to solid to benign to malignant. Although a detailed slit-lamp and gonioscopy evaluation can be beneficial in diagnosing these lesions, anterior segment optical coherence tomography (AS-OCT) can be a very useful way to obtain their structural features. AS-OCT also offers clinicians a more comfortable and convenient imaging modality compared with ultrasound biomicroscopy (UBM). Surprisingly, there are only a limited number of publications in the literature comparing UBM with AS-OCT in evaluating iris and iridociliary body lesions. OCT technology is evolving quickly and is often more widely available than UBM in general ophthalmology practices; thus its use in evaluating iris lesions is expected to increase.

Standard AS-OCT features allow optical imaging with an image resolution of 18 microns and penetration depth of three to four mm, which is adequate for evaluating solid and cystic iris lesions. With the introduction of spectral-domain OCT, the axial resolution of newer AS-OCT devices can reach as deep as five to seven mm. Despite the apparent advantages offered by AS-OCT in terms of resolution, one major disadvantage is the heavy shadowing caused by the iris pigment epithelium. Although the *anterior* surface of iris lesions is depicted in great detail, high-resolution visualization of structures, including internal architecture of the structure of interest, is usually obscured.

Although not a comprehensive schema, one potentially useful system to classify iris lesions is as follows:

- Age of presentation (congenital vs. acquired)
- Cause (primary vs. secondary, including inflammatory and traumatic)
- Neoplasm risk and type (nonneoplastic, benign, and malignant)
- Internal features (cystic and solid)

In this chapter, we will present commonly encountered iris abnormalities for which AS-OCT can provide the clinician with additional information that can aid diagnosis, treatment, management, and monitoring of these conditions.

II. SOLID IRIS LESIONS

AS-OCT has been shown to be superior to UBM for imaging small lesions located in the anterior iris. UBM may be better for imaging larger iris lesions with posterior or ciliary body extension. Thus clinicians may use both imaging modalities depending on the location and extension of the lesion of interest. There are multiple primary and metastatic iris neoplasms that AS-OCT can evaluate, but because of their higher frequency, this chapter will focus on iris nevi and iris melanoma.

III. IRIS MELANOCYTIC LESIONS

AS-OCT of iris melanocytic lesions facilitates imaging because of its noncontact nature, which can be used to monitor tumor growth as a clinical surrogate of malignancy (Fig. 9.1).

The reflective features of different tissues seen on AS-OCT correlate with the degree of pigmentation and scattering, enabling a more intuitive interpretation than with UBM. AS-OCT demonstrates that melanotic lesions have a higher reflectivity, whereas amelanotic lesions have a reflectivity similar to or lower than that of normal iris stroma (Fig. 9.2). Because of the dense pigmentation with these lesions, there is noticeable obscuration of the iris stroma details on imaging. Ectropion iridis, frequently associated with iris tumors and iris neovascularization, appears as a highly reflective anterior surface at the pupillary margin (Fig. 9.3).

A study comparing multiple imaging technologies for iris tumors reported that iris nevi display high reflectivity and shadowing of the pigment epithelium, whereas iris melanomas had variable reflective areas distributed throughout the whole thickness of the mass. The authors advocated that these reflectivity patterns may be of diagnostic value, compared with UBM, which demonstrates medium to low reflectivity for both nevi and melanomas, independent of degree of pigmentation.

The most significant limitation of AS-OCT is with densely melanotic lesions. In these cases, the melanin pigment tends to obscure deeper imaging by creating an optical shadow similar to what is seen with the iris pigment epithelium, especially in lesions thicker than 2.5 mm. Another limitation of AS-OCT is poor visualization of the ciliary body, which is better visualized by UBM (Fig. 9.4). Finally, AS-OCT also has an important application in treated tumors to monitor regression and recurrence (Fig. 9.5).

IV. CYSTIC IRIS LESIONS

Iris cysts can be divided into primary and secondary types. Primary cysts include stromal cysts and pigment epithelial (iris pigment epithelium [IPE]) cysts. Stromal cysts can be congenital or acquired. This type of cyst has a characteristic smooth appearance with lucent features on or within the iris stroma, occasionally manifesting with a fluid-debris level. Stromal cysts can enlarge and have been reported to rupture, leading to secondary iritis, photophobia, pain, and glaucoma. Timely diagnosis is especially important in newborn infants because they can manifest within the first few weeks of life and cause photophobia, amblyopia, and buphthalmos. These cysts tend to have a more aggressive course when diagnosed in children younger than 10 years of age, requiring multiple surgeries and determining a poor visual outcome. If not visually significant during vision-development years, these same cysts, when detected during teenage and adult years, may be more benign, requiring intervention in 25% of cases.

IPE cysts are probably more common than previously realized with the increasing use of advanced anterior segment imaging modalities such as AS-OCT and UBM. These cysts are usually asymptomatic and arise on the posterior surface of the iris. According to their location and prevalence, IPE cysts can be categorized into peripheral (73%), midzonal (21%), marginal (3%), and dislodged and free-floating (approximately 3%).

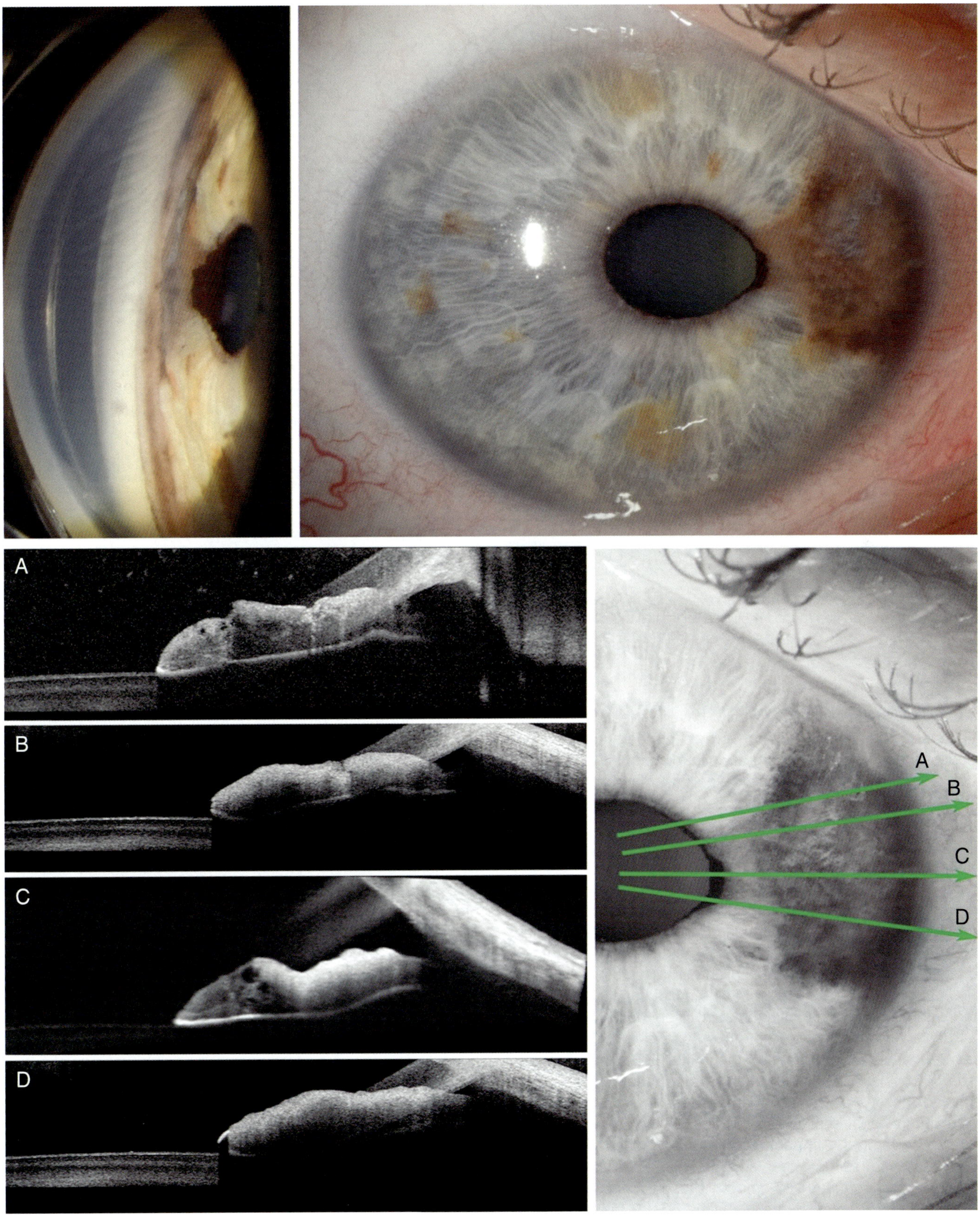

Fig. 9.1 Iris melanocytic lesion (being monitored for growth six months after fine-needle aspiration biopsy [FNAB]). Composite image showing gonioscopy and slit-lamp photograph of an iris melanocytic lesion in a patient. The slit-lamp photograph demonstrates a lesion with an irregular surface and variable pigmentation within it. Additionally, there are at least three discrete round spots on the superior aspect of the tumor consistent with previous FNAB. AS-OCT images show areas of hyporeflectivity *(panels A and B)* consistent with stromal disruption from FNAB. In *panel C,* there are prominent areas of irregular reflectivity with noticeable intralesional cystic structure. In *panel D,* there is homogeneous internal reflectivity of the choroidal lesion with a small hyperreflective shadow at the pupillary margin consistent with ectropion iridis

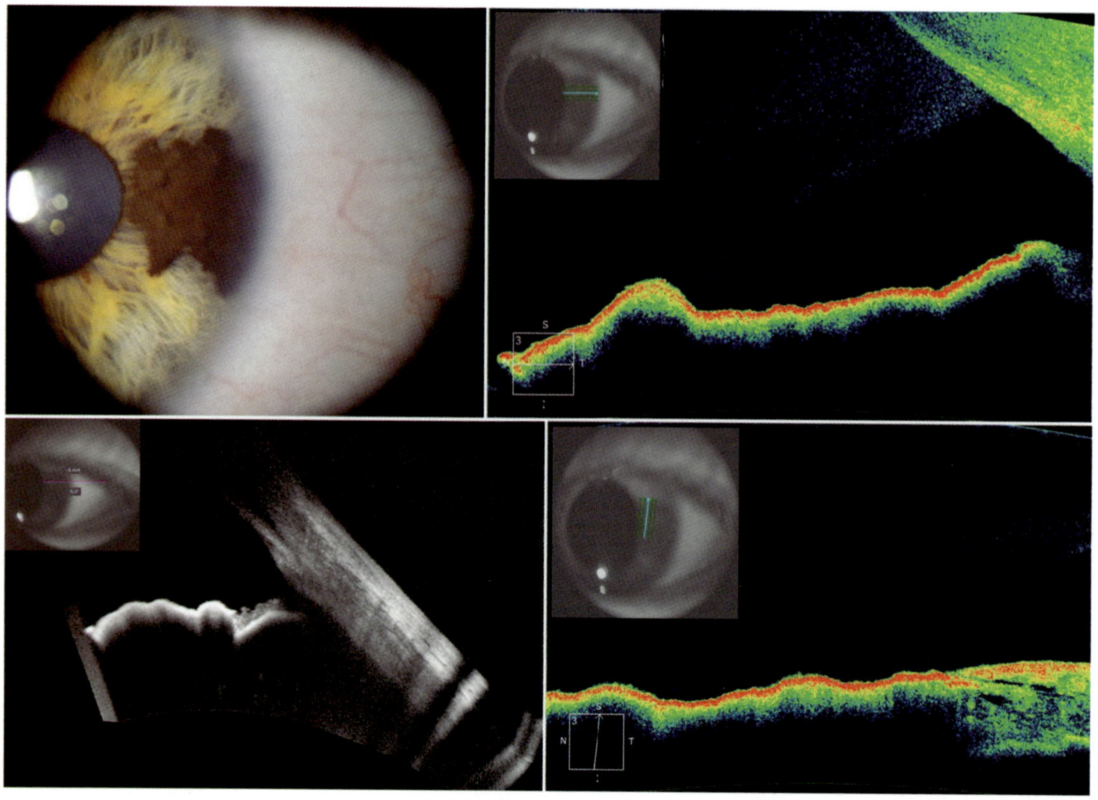

Fig. 9.2 Iris nevus. Composite image showing a slit-lamp photograph of dark-brown iris nevus with well-defined margins evaluated by AS-OCT. Note the significant obscuration of the iris stroma related to the dense pigmentation.

Pupillary margin cysts usually have a teardrop shape. Midzonal cysts have a fusiform brown appearance and may become more visible after pupillary dilation (Fig. 9.6). Peripheral cysts appear as an iris stromal bulge and may be associated with plateau iris configuration (Fig. 9.7). The characteristic retroiridic presentation should prompt careful evaluation and imaging. A free-floating cyst is a round mass moving by gravitational forces in the aqueous or vitreous (Fig. 9.8).

Surgical intervention for drainage or resection is rarely necessary for these cysts. Because of their dark brown color and similar configuration, many iris cysts used to be misdiagnosed as ciliary body melanoma when high-resolution anterior segment imaging such as AS-OCT and UBM were not available. It is important to stress that some iris cysts have been associated with iris nevus, iris melanoma, or ciliary body melanoma.

Pupillary margin cysts, also known as *iris flocculi* (Fig. 9.9), are rare, often asymptomatic, congenital IPE cysts that may undergo cycles of collapse and reformation, resulting in wrinkled masses. Even when large, these lesions typically do not result in visual impairment. Iris flocculi are usually sporadic but can be familial. Although benign, iris flocculi rarely can be associated with aortic aneurysms and dissections as a result of the shared mutation of smooth muscle gene alpha-actin 2 *(ACTA2)* and/or myosin heavy chain (*MYH11*) that affect both iris and aorta. The presence of iris flocculi should prompt the clinician to evaluate the patient for life-threatening conditions such as aortic aneurysms. AS-OCT of iris flocculi typically reveals smooth, dark, irregular cystic lesions at the pupillary margin of various sizes.

Free-floating cysts may occur in the anterior chamber or the vitreous. Anterior chamber cysts can be idiopathic or induced by trauma or surgery. Anterior chamber cysts usually consist of IPE; some may have pigment granules within them, as seen in Fig. 9.8. These cysts can detach from the iris surface, float freely, and sometimes reattach to the iris at another location. Although usually asymptomatic, patients may complain of transient floaters.

Secondary iris cysts may manifest as a result of anterior segment trauma (e.g., epithelial downgrowth) or intraocular surgery, especially in eyes with severe inflammation. They can have drug-induced, tumor-induced, or parasitic causes, or they can be due to conditions associated with systemic disorders. Among these, implantation cysts are the most common type (Fig. 9.10). They originate by an invasion of conjunctival or corneal epithelial cells after surgical trauma or a penetrating wound. Many of these cysts are associated with anterior peripheral synechiae involving the anterior chamber angle or posterior pupillary synechiae involving the lens (Fig. 9.11).

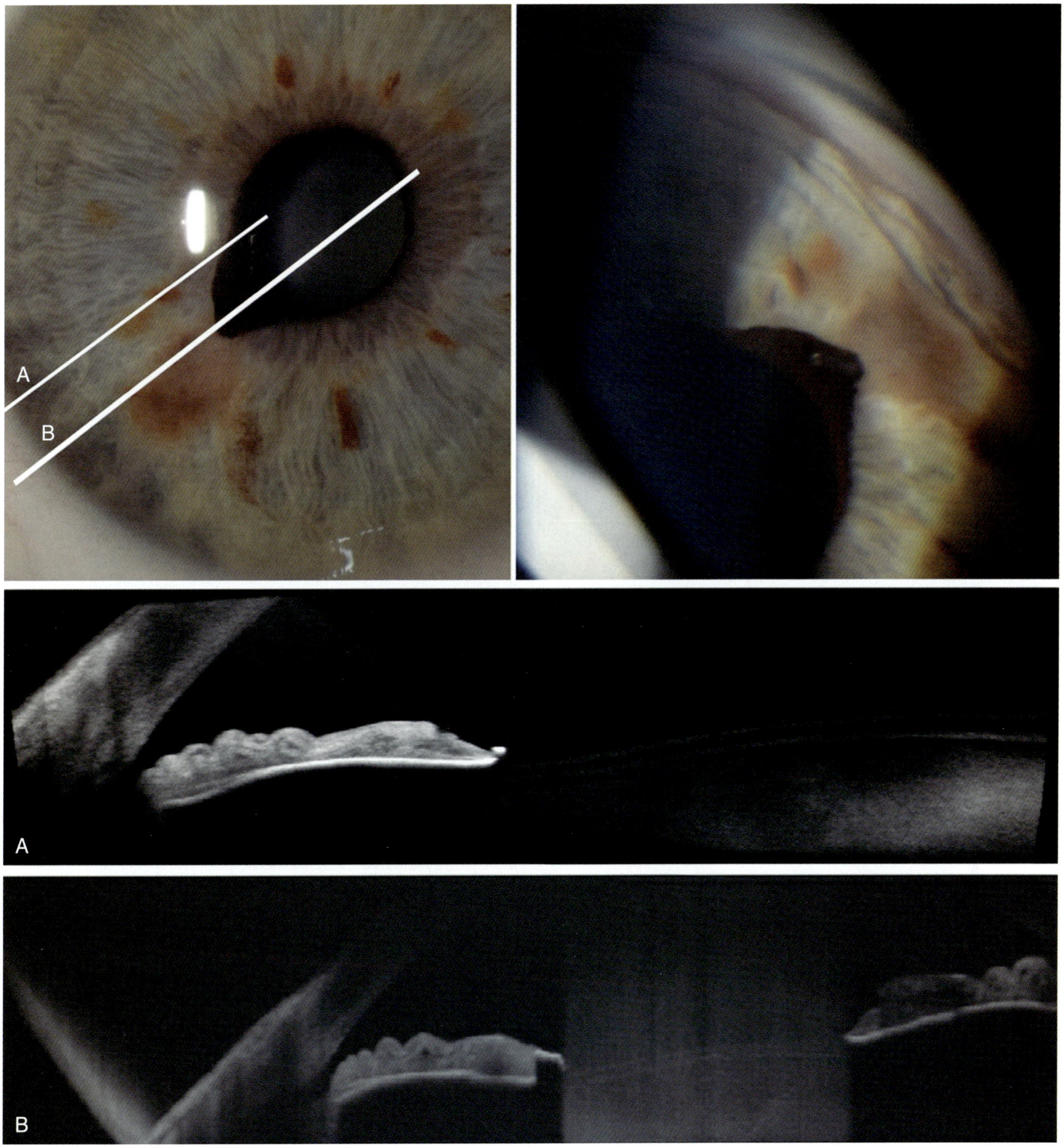

Fig. 9.3 Iris nevus associated with iris ectropion. Composite image shows a small iris nevus centered between seven and eight o'clock with distinct iris ectropion. AS-OCT shows two distinct cross-sectional images. *Panel A* shows small/flat iris freckles and iris ectropion at the pupillary margin that presents as a hyper-reflective band over the iris stroma. *Panel B* shows increased iris thickness related to iris nevus and a thin hyperreflective line at the pupillary margin consistent with iris ectropion.

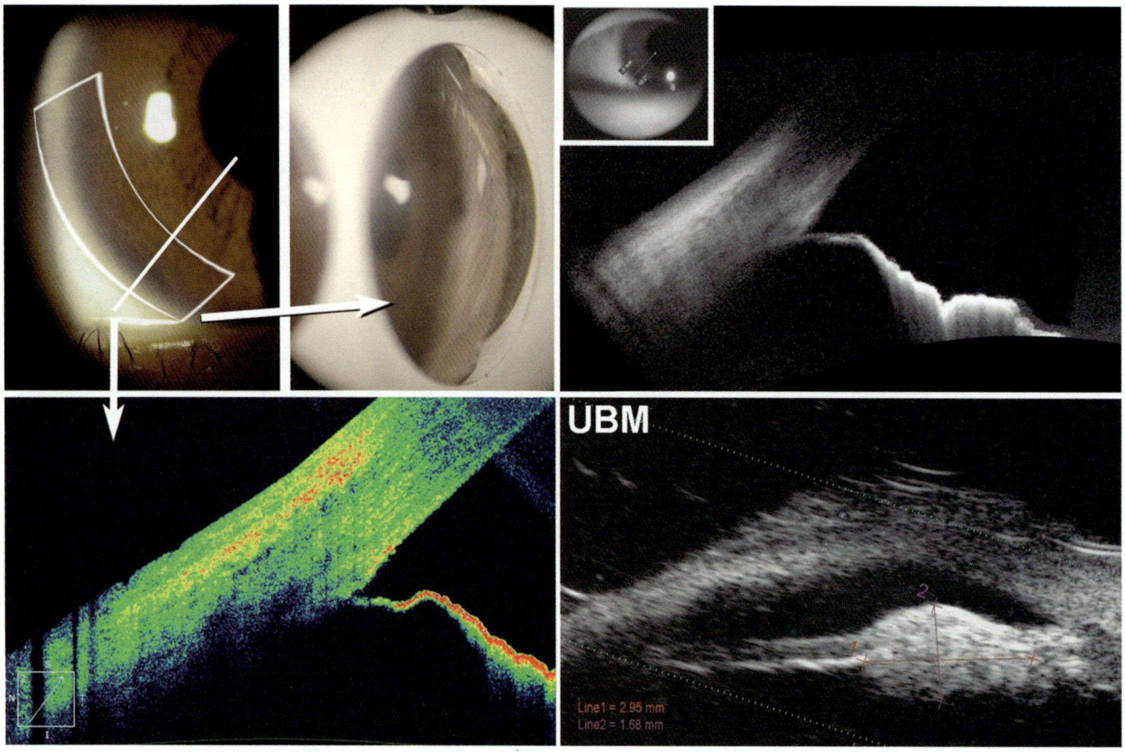

Fig. 9.4 Iris melanoma with ciliary body involvement. Composite image of iridociliary melanoma involving the root of the iris as seen on gonioscopy. AS-OCT technologies do not offer enough penetrance through hypermelanotic tissue for an accurate evaluation of this tumor but show a hyper-reflective surface with dark underlying lesion. Ultrasound biomicroscopy image in the *bottom right panel* allows evaluation and measurement of the entire tumor.

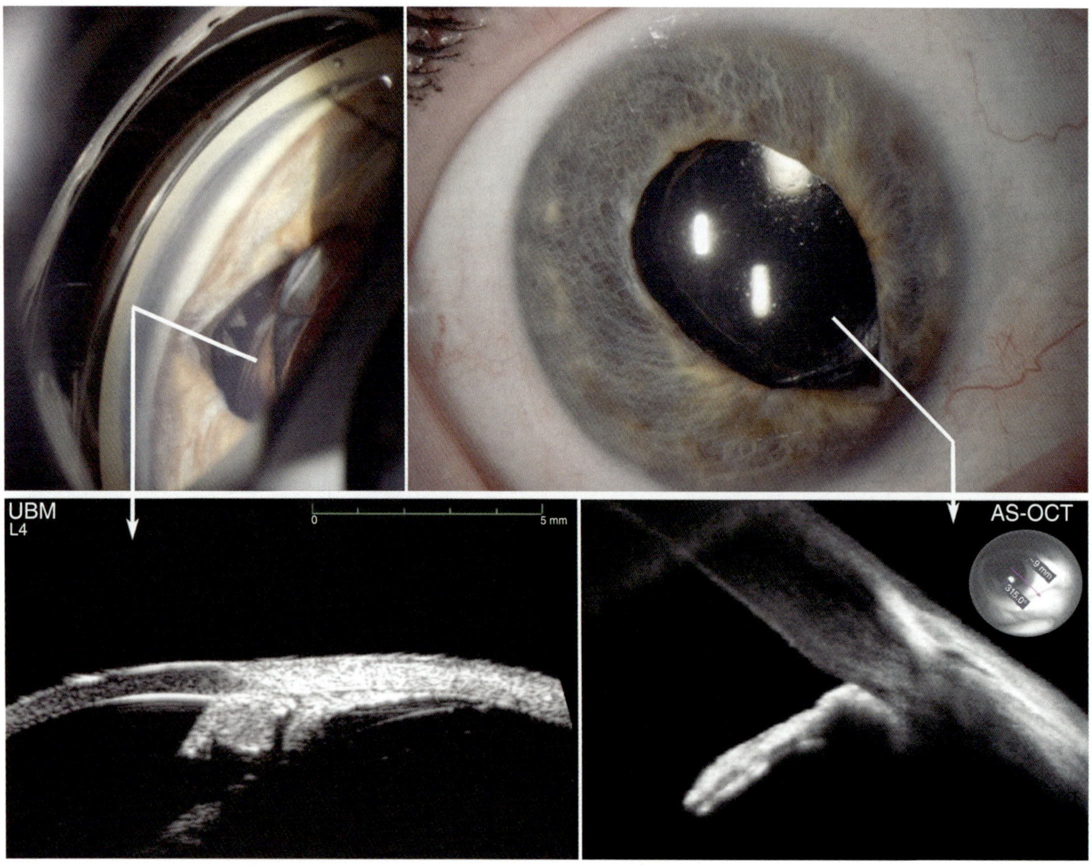

Fig. 9.5 Iris melanoma regressed after iodine-125 plaque. Composite image of an iris melanoma managed by plaque brachytherapy three years previously. The tumor regressed, causing a peaked pupil at the four-o'clock meridian. Arrows indicate the area imaged and orientation. Ultrasound biomicroscopy shows the regressed tumor, including its retro-iridic component. AS-OCT shows focal synechiae and hyperreflective tumor surface, but the intense melanotic nature of the tumor precludes a view of the ciliary body.

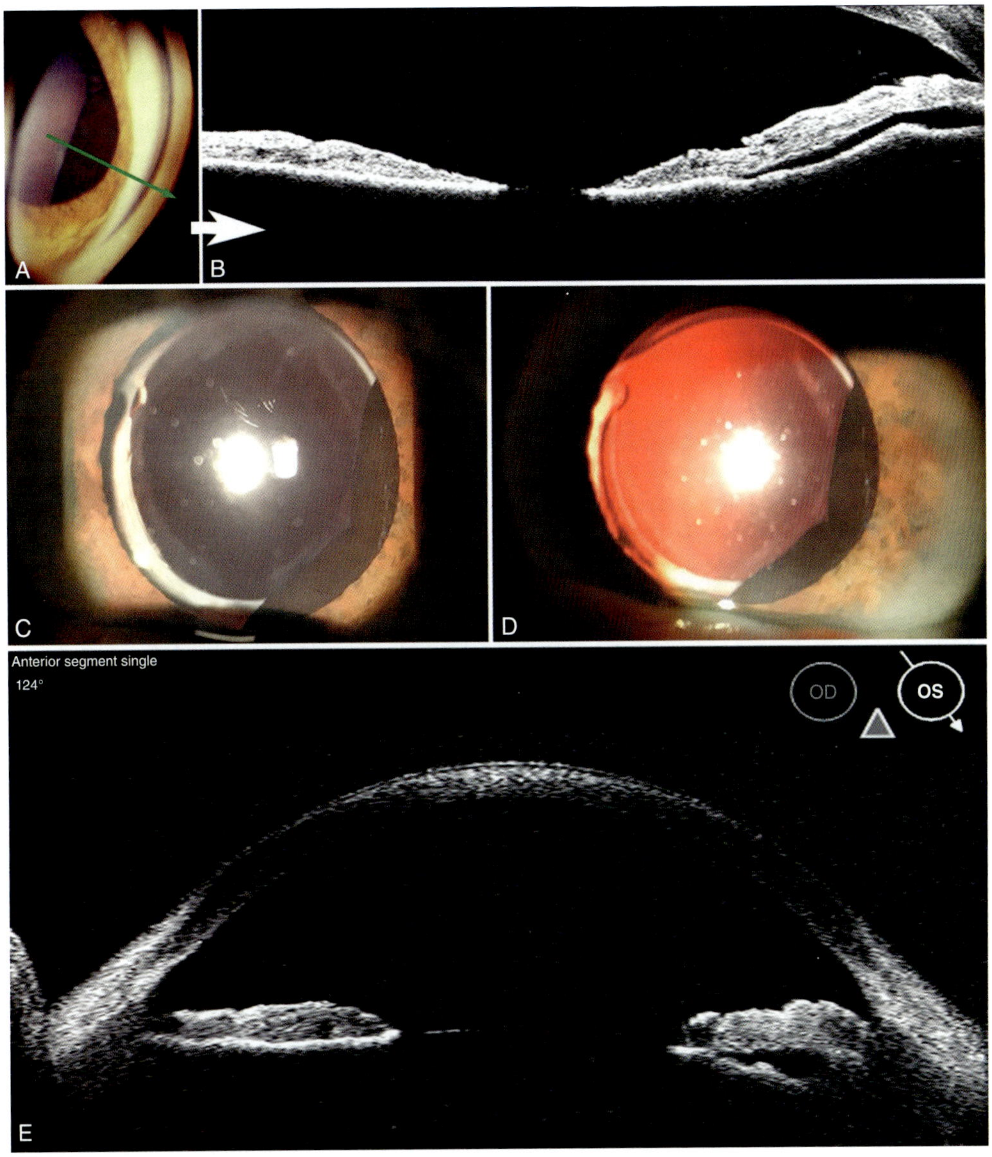

Fig. 9.6 Iris pigment epithelium (IPE) cyst—midzonal. Composite image of a cyst that creates localized anterior protrusion of the iris seen on gonioscopy *(panel A)*. Arrow indicates area imaged by AS-OCT. AS-OCT with the pupil undilated shows the cyst under the iris leaflet *(panel B)*. Dilated pupil reveals a retro-iridic smooth lesion that is dark brown and projects into the pupil *(panels C and D)*. AS-OCT shows shortening of the iris leaflet and the protrusion of the IPE midzonal cyst *(panel E)*.

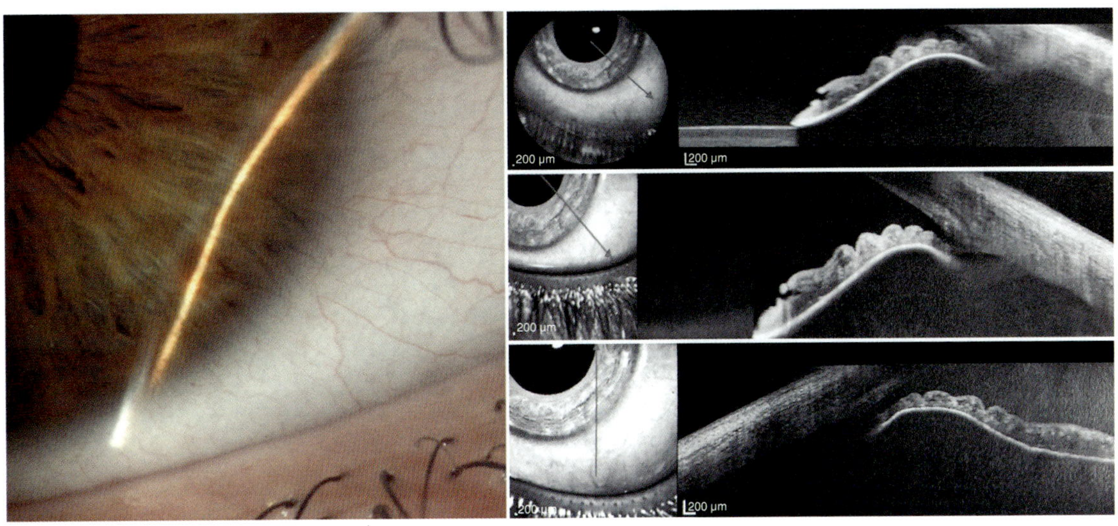

Fig. 9.7 Iris pigment epithelium cyst—peripheral. Composite image showing slight bulge of the peripheral iris and the matching AS-OCT images through the peripheral iris pigment epithelium cyst.

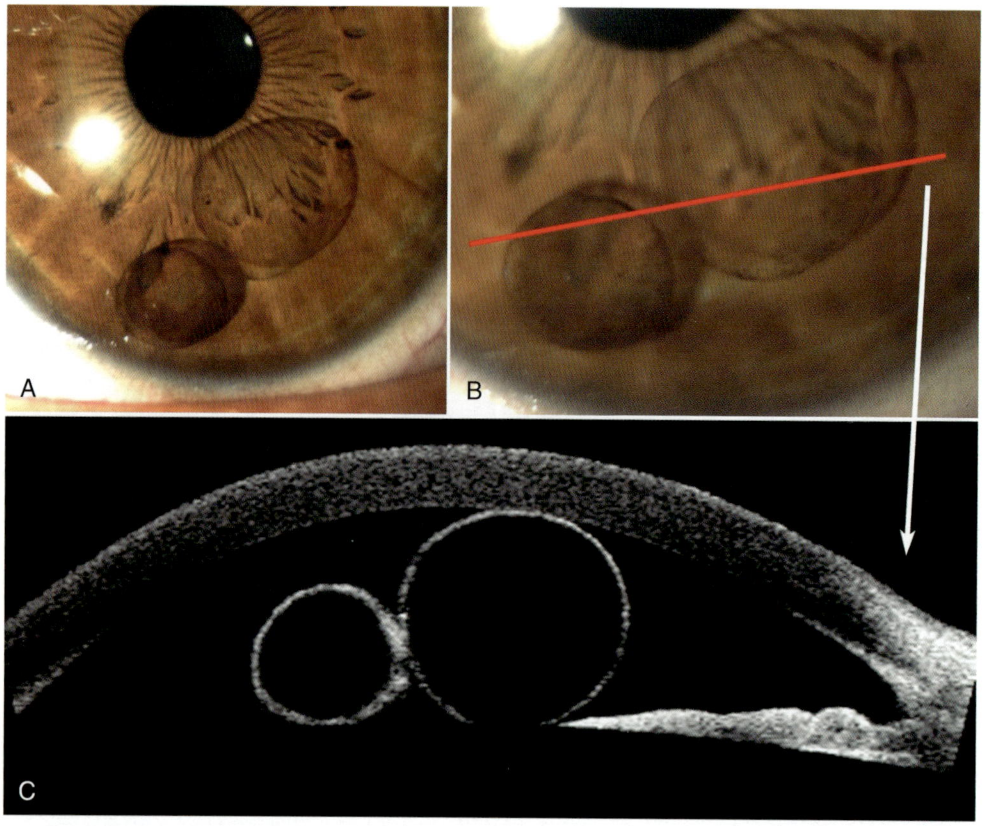

Fig. 9.8 Iris pigment epithelium cyst—free-floating. Composite images show the clinical appearance of free-floating iris cysts *(Panel A)* with melanin pigment granules in the cyst cavity. Red line in the slit-lamp photograph *(Panel B)* indicates the location imaged on AS-OCT *(Panel C)* confirming the absence of any attachment of these cysts to the iris.

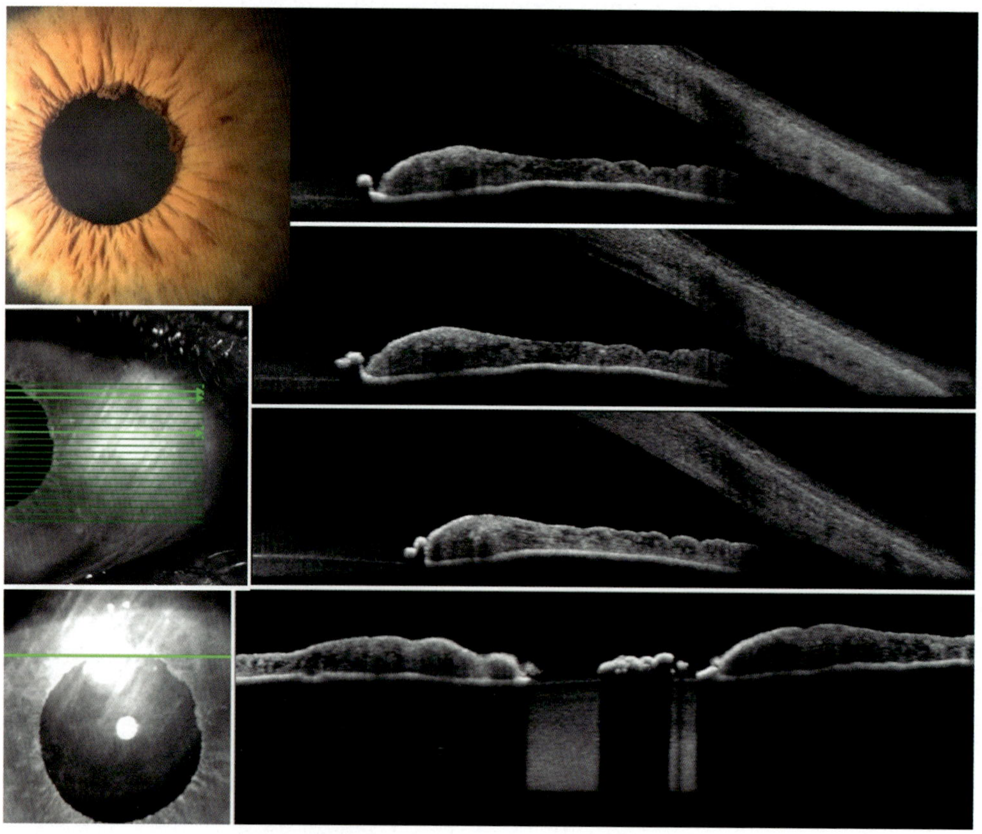

Fig. 9.9 Iris pigment epithelium (IPE) cyst—pupillary margin (iris flocculi). Composite image shows the clinical appearance of iris flocculi at the superior and temporal pupillary margin. AS-OCT images show multiple small/irregular IPE cysts. Note that the iris pigment epithelium casts a hyperreflective shadow that obscures the lens.

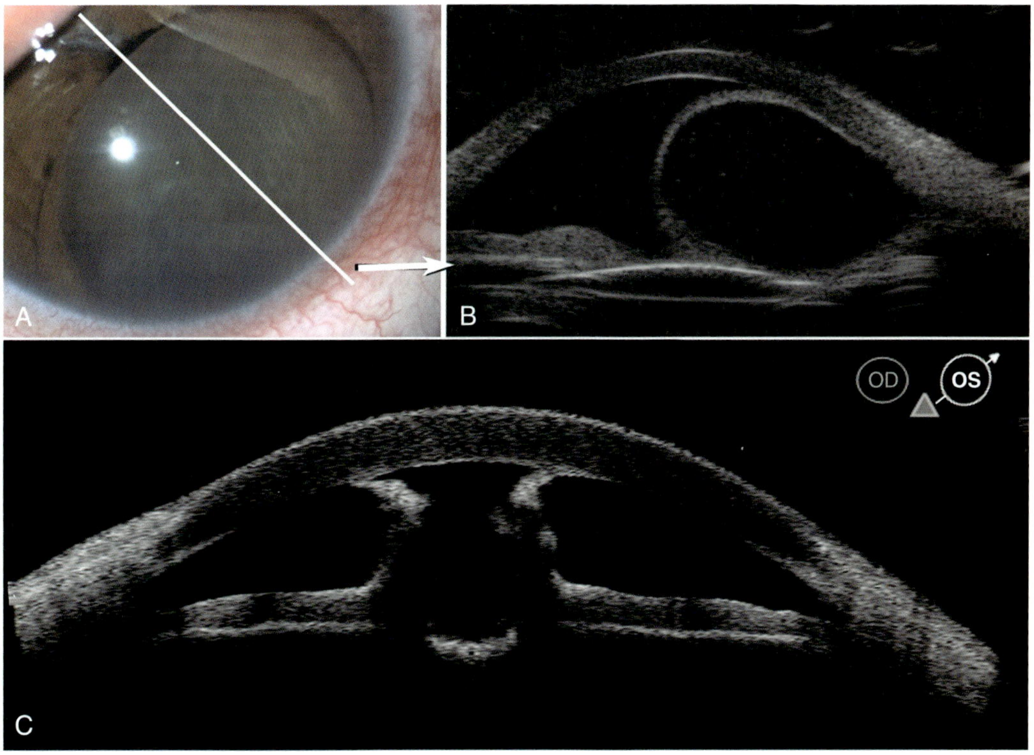

Fig. 9.10 Epithelial downgrowth. Composite image in *panel A* shows the clinical appearance of an epithelial downgrowth after ocular trauma. Ultrasound biomicroscopy shows the epithelial cyst attached to the surface of the iris and corneal endothelium *(panel B)*. The AS-OCT scan in *panel C* shows the thicker and hyperreflective cyst walls.

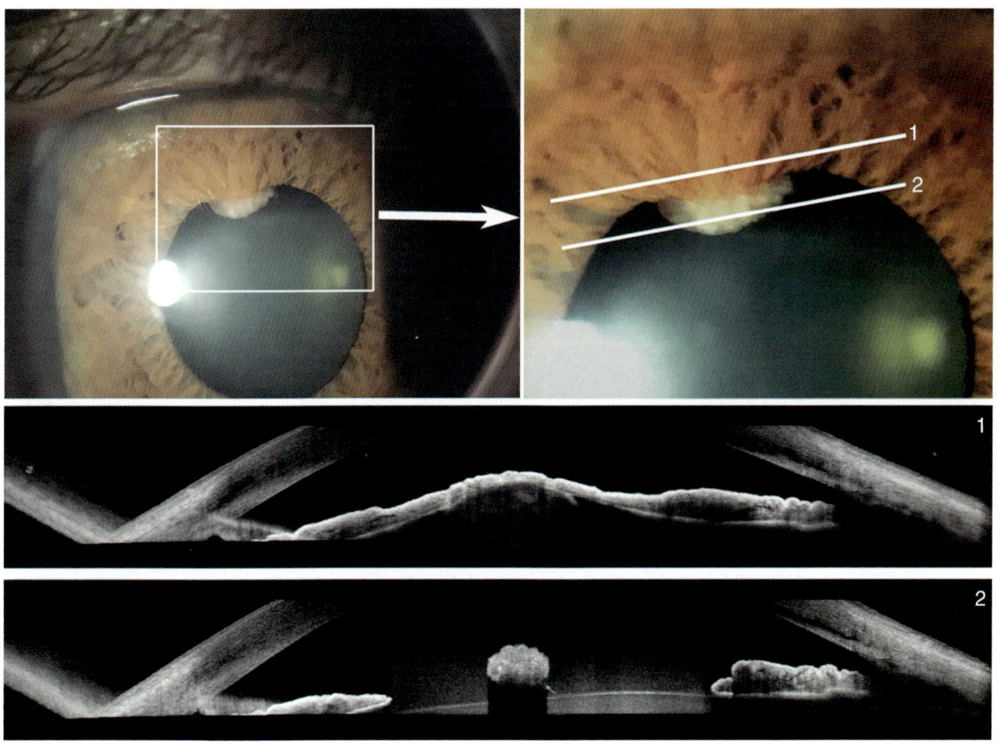

Fig. 9.11 Secondary iris cyst—with posterior pupillary synechiae. Composite images show the clinical appearance of a whitish cyst at the pupillary margin superiorly associated with posterior synechiae. The area inside the square is magnified on the right and slices 1 and 2 are representative of the AS-OCT images seen bellow. The cyst color and features could be consistent with an inflammatory cause, stromal cells, or lens epithelium.

V. CONGENITAL IRIS ABNORMALITIES

A. Iridocorneal Endothelial Syndrome

Among various nonneoplastic lesions simulating iris tumors reported in the literature, iridocorneal endothelial syndrome (ICE) is the most common diagnosis. Features observed in eyes with ICE syndrome that distinguish them from other melanocytic (and solid) iris tumors are cornea guttata, multidirectional corectopia, polycoria, broad peripheral anterior synechiae, IPE defects, and lack of elevated/solid mass. ICE syndrome is a group of three conditions: Cogan-Reese syndrome, Chandler syndrome, and essential iris atrophy. The latter is a rare, progressive disorder characterized by a corectopia, polycoria, and distorted areas of thinning and degeneration on the iris. This disorder most frequently affects only one eye (unilateral) and develops slowly over time (Fig. 9.12).

B. Aniridia

Aniridia is a rare congenital disorder related to a mutation of the *PAX6* gene that occurs during ocular development. This disorder is inherited most commonly in an autosomal dominant fashion with variable expressivity. Children with aniridia have a higher risk for childhood glaucoma because of the anterior rotation of the undeveloped iris. Interestingly, reports have shown that the formation of peripheral anterior synechiae and progressive angle closure is more related to history of ocular surgery. AS-OCT of eyes with aniridia typically shows evidence of a rudimentary iris associated with open- and closed-angle findings, as shown in Fig. 9.13.

C. Arteriovenous Malformations

Iris arteriovenous malformations (AVMs) are rare, benign, congenital vascular lesions unrelated to systemic disease or other ocular conditions. AVM is not a true neoplasm but rather anomalous lesion of abnormal vascular channels at the site of the communication. The physiopathology of these lesions relates to a local failure of mesenchymal maturation leading to an artery connecting with a vein directly bypassing the defective capillary network. The diagnosis of iris AVM is usually clinical, with careful slit-lamp examination, gonioscopy, and targeted imaging, as seen in Fig. 9.14. Although these are benign lesions, their differential diagnosis includes other causes of abnormal iris vessels such as hemangiomas, iris neovascularization, dilated normal vessels secondary to iritis or other chronic intraocular inflammation, and neoplasms. Additionally, these lesions may be associated with scleral sentinel vessels; therefore it is important to rule out concomitant malignancy.

D. Secondary Iris Abnormalities

Iris atrophy and transillumination defects often occur after major anterior segment surgery with iris manipulation or as a result of

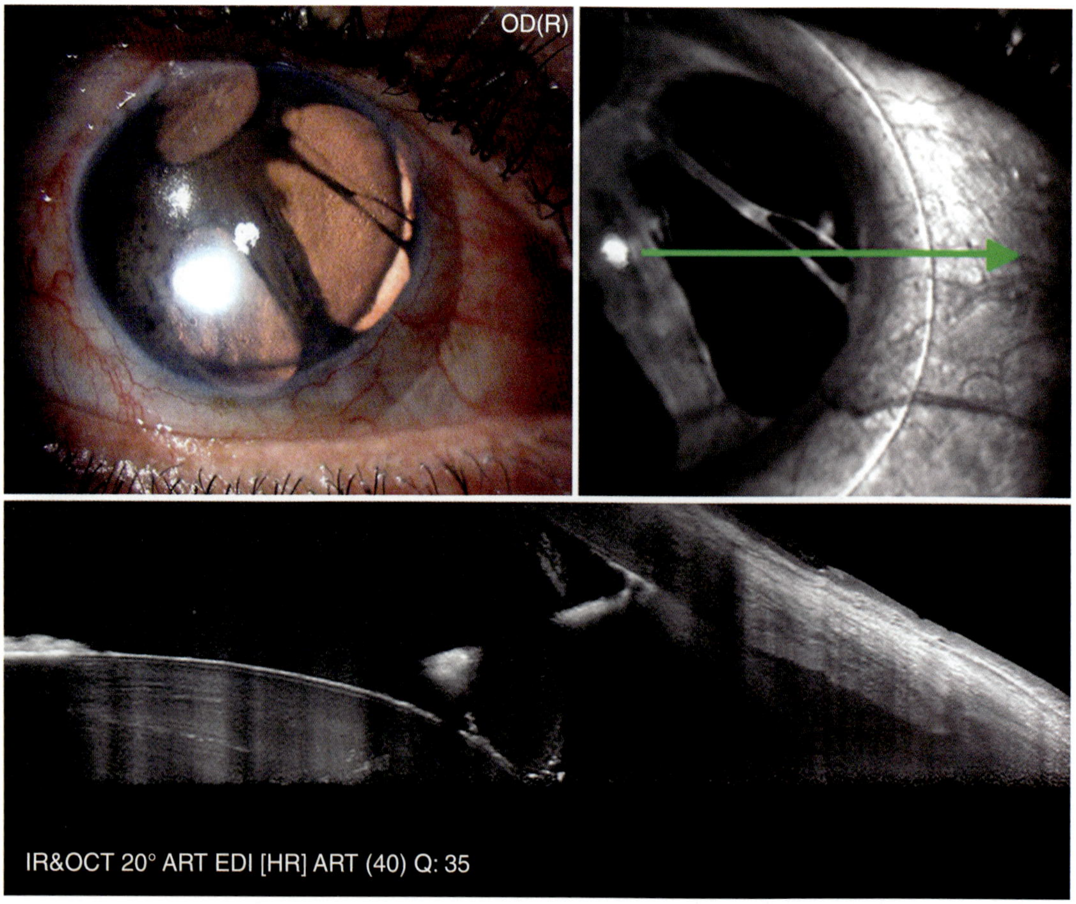

Fig. 9.12 Essential iris atrophy. Composite images show an eye with essential iris atrophy, which is a subtype of the iridocorneal endothelial syndrome. As the clinical photograph shows, this condition is characterized by the formation of multiple iris holes/defects that develop over time. AS-OCT shows the absence of iris tissue matching the dark areas in the iris. (Courtesy Claudia Gonçalves, MD, and Bruno Pereira, OD. Lisbon, Portugal)

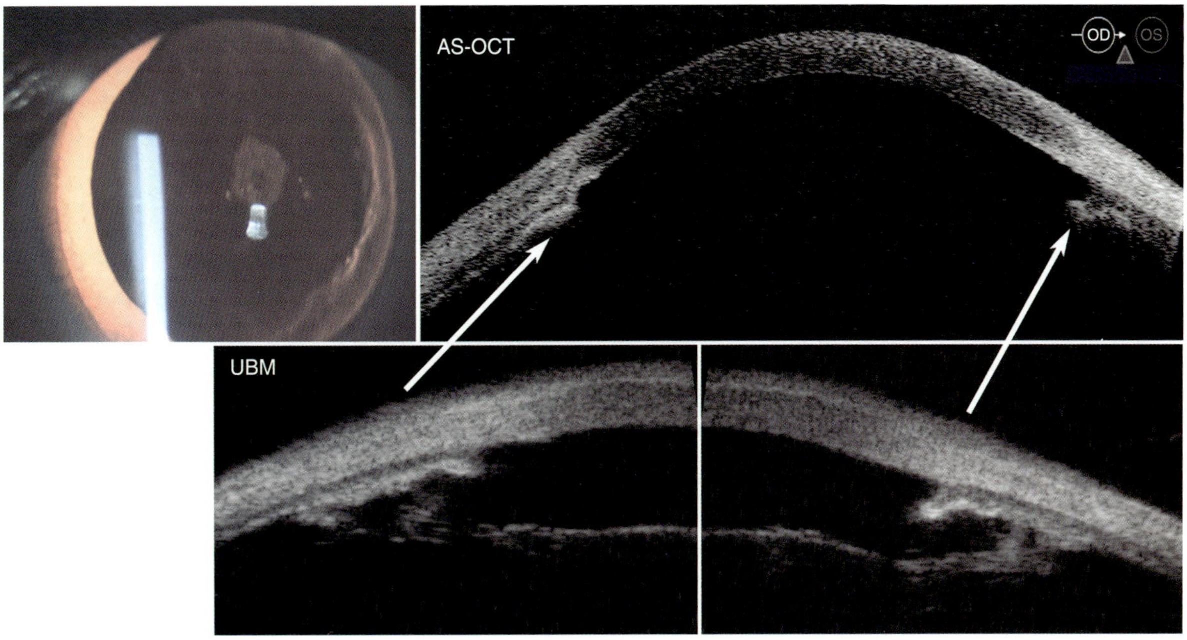

Fig. 9.13 Aniridia. Composite image shows the outline of the lens through a rudimentary iris and posterior subcapsular cataract. The arrows indicate rudimentary iris stumpt. Ultrasound biomicroscopy and AS-OCT depict similar features, but the AS-OCT has a broad 180-degree view of the anterior segment.

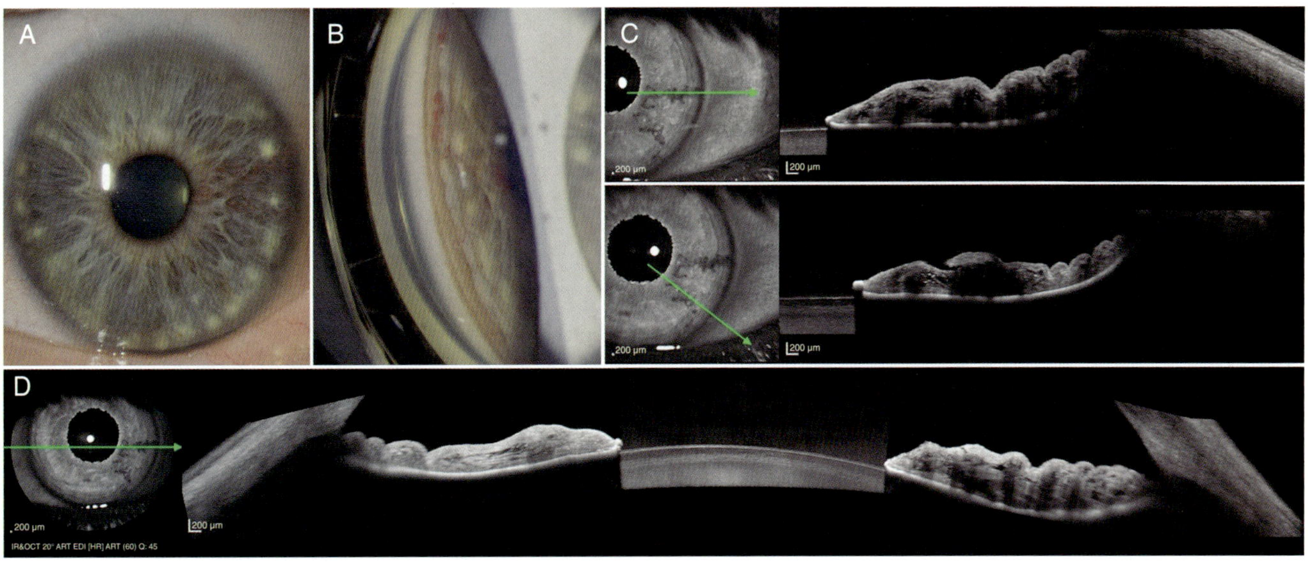

Fig. 9.14 Iris arteriovenous malformation (AVM). Composite images in *panel A* show clinical appearance of AVM as a tortuous radial blood vessel and tangle of vascular channels at the site of the communication. Gonioscopy provides a view of the tortuous vessels in the anterior chamber angle *(panel B)*. The AS-OCT in *panel C* shows thickening of the iris stroma related to the presence of numerous tangles vessels. (Courtesy Rita Anjos, MD, and Pedro Reis, OD. Lisbon, Portugal)

radiation or laser treatment. AS-OCT can document the loss of IPE and transillumination defect, ruling out iris heterochromia (Fig. 9.15).

Iris bombe is a condition in which 360 degrees of posterior pupillary synechiae affect the movement of aqueous from the posterior to the anterior chamber. The resulting impaired flow of aqueous increases the posterior pressure, bowing the iris forward and resulting in secondary angle closure. Iris bombe is caused by severe inflammation that drives the formation of iris synechiae with and without iris neovascularization. AS-OCT usually shows a thin, anteriorly bowed iris attached to the lens at the pupil causing angle closure, as shown in Fig. 9.16. Similarly, UBM shows iris bowing and complete angle closure but lacks definition compared with AS-OCT. As a clinical tool, AS-OCT mapping of the anterior chamber assists the planning of peripheral iridotomy using yttrium-aluminum-garnet (YAG) or argon laser while minimizing damage to other structures.

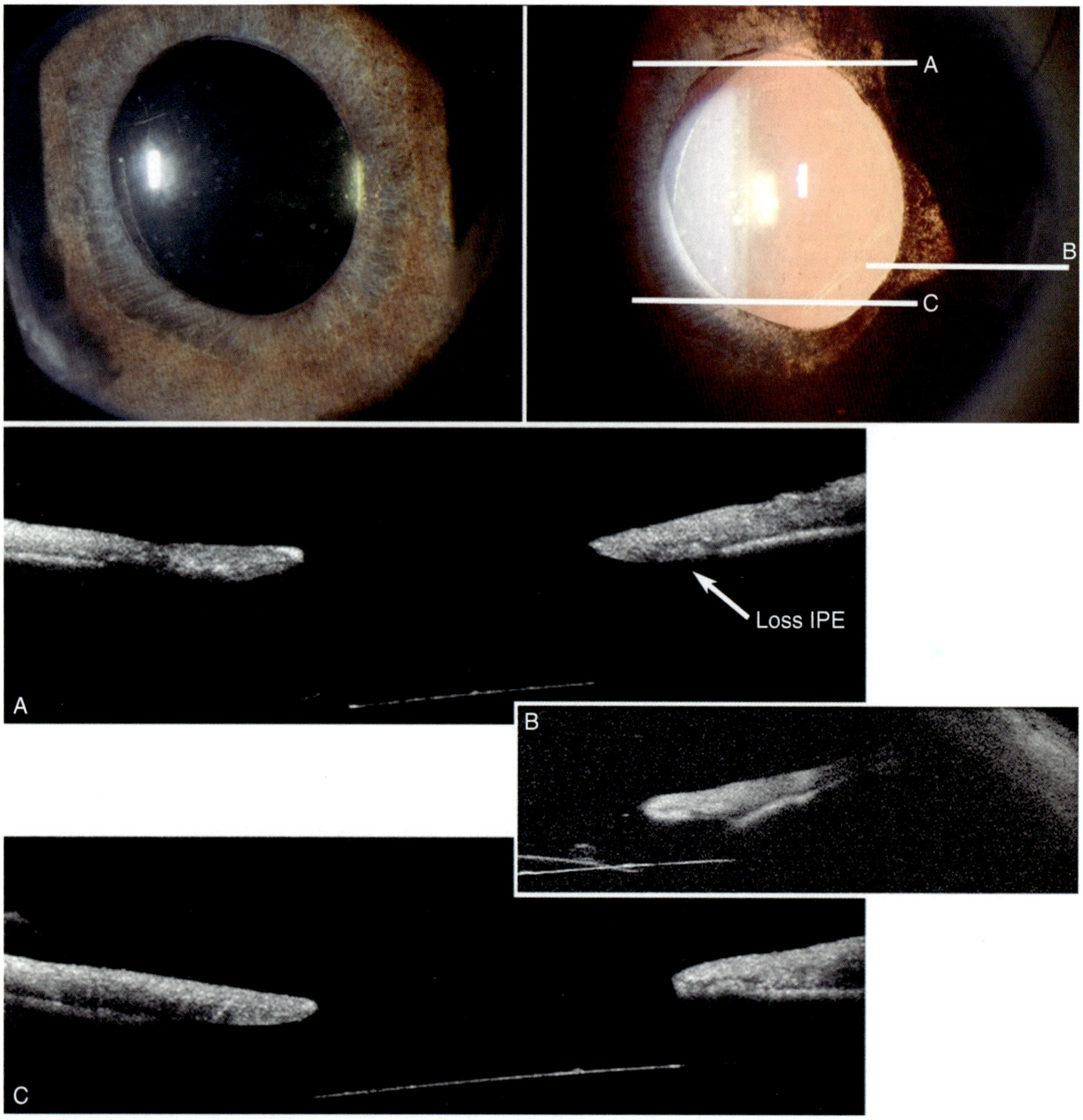

Fig. 9.15 Secondary iris atrophy and transillumination defect after radiation for diffuse iris melanoma. Composite photos showing a pseudophakic eye with discolored iris and transillumination defects four years after radiation and complete regression of ciliary body melanoma. AS-OCT images show thinning of the iris stroma and localized loss of the iris pigment epithelium that coincide with the areas of transillumination defect.

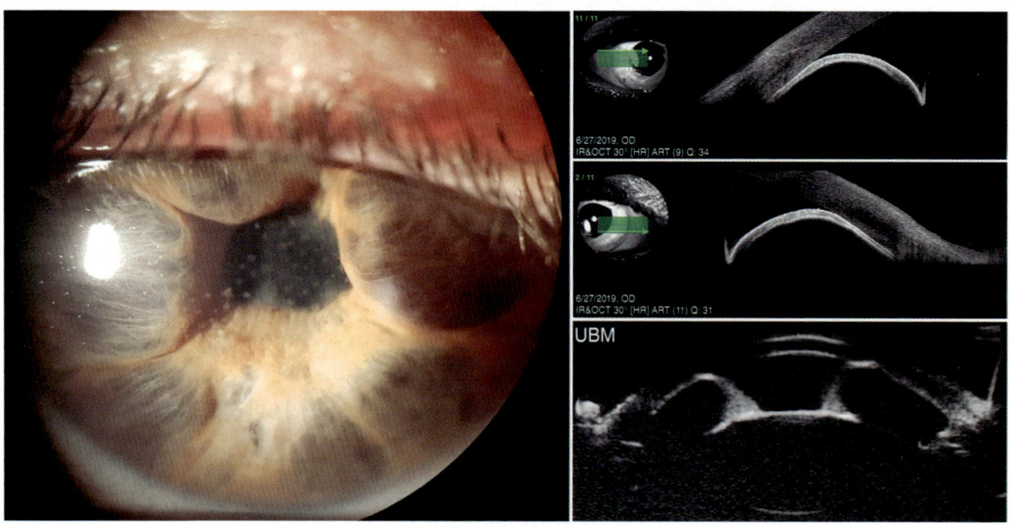

Fig. 9.16 Iris bombe. AS-OCT images showing the anterior iris bowing and occlusion of the anterior chamber angle (slit-lamp photograph and ultrasound biomicroscopy). (Courtesy Dra. Maria Sara Patrício, Hospital de Egas Moniz, Centro Hospitalar Lisboa Ocidental, Lisboa, Portugal.)

BIBLIOGRAPHY

Arslanturk Eren M, Gunduz AK, Gunduz OO. Evaluation of iris melanoma with anterior segment optical coherence tomography. *Turk J Ophthalmol*. 2017;47(4):231-234.

Augsburger JJ, Affel LL, Benarosh DA. Ultrasound biomicroscopy of cystic lesions of the iris and ciliary body. *Trans Am Ophthalmol Soc*. 1996;94:259-271; discussion 271-254.

Azuara-Blanco A, Spaeth GL, Araujo SV, Augsburger JJ, Terebuh AK. Plateau iris syndrome associated with multiple ciliary body cysts. Report of three cases. *Arch Ophthalmol*. 1996;114(6):666-668.

Bajwa A, Burstein E, Grainger RM, Netland PA. Anterior chamber angle in aniridia with and without glaucoma. *Clin Ophthalmol*. 2019;13:1469-1473.

Bianciotto C, Shields CL, Guzman JM, et al. Assessment of anterior segment tumors with ultrasound biomicroscopy versus anterior segment optical coherence tomography in 200 cases. *Ophthalmology*. 2011;118(7):1297-1302.

Broaddus E, Lystad LD, Schonfield L, Singh AD. Iris varix: report of a case and review of iris vascular anomalies. *Surv Ophthalmol*. 2009;54(1):118-127.

Georgalas I, Petrou P, Papaconstantinou D, Brouzas D, Koutsandrea C, Kanakis M. Iris cysts: a comprehensive review on diagnosis and treatment. *Surv Ophthalmol*. 2018;63(3):347-364.

Hau SC, Papastefanou V, Shah S, Sagoo MS, Restori M, Cohen V. Evaluation of iris and iridociliary body lesions with anterior segment optical coherence tomography versus ultrasound B-scan. *Br J Ophthalmol*. 2015;99(1):81-86.

Lewis RA, Merin LM. Iris flocculi and familial aortic dissection. *Arch Ophthalmol*. 1995;113(10):1330-1331.

Mori Y, Hashida N, Asao K, Maruyama K, Nishida K. Chronological observations of iris flocculi in a Japanese family with thoracic aortic aneurysm and dissections. *Case Rep Ophthalmol*. 2019;10(3):397-402.

Razzaq L, Emmanouilidis-van der Spek K, Luyten GP, de Keizer RJ. Anterior segment imaging for iris melanocytic tumors. *Eur J Ophthalmol*. 2011;21(5):608-614.

10 Abnormalities of the Angle

Monisha E. Nongpiur | Dan Eisenberg

I. INTRODUCTION

Anterior segment optical coherence tomography (AS-OCT) allows qualitative evaluation of the angles and anterior segment structures. The built-in and customized software can also facilitate precise quantitative and qualitative measurements of these structures. AS-OCT evaluation of the angle has several practical uses in routine clinical settings, such as evaluation of open versus closed angles in patients in whom gonioscopy may be difficult or in assessment of patients for consideration of phakic intraocular lens (pIOL).

The scleral spur is an important landmark usually used in the qualitative and quantitative evaluations of AS-OCT images. The scleral spur is the point where there is a change in curvature of the inner surface of the angle wall, often appearing as an inward protrusion of the sclera. It sometimes appears as a highly reflective region on AS-OCT (Fig. 10.1), though it may not be visualized in all eyes.

II. EVALUATION OF ANTERIOR CHAMBER ANGLES

Although gonioscopy is the gold standard for evaluating anterior chamber angles, AS-OCT can function as a supplementary diagnostic imaging tool in a wide range of clinical situations.

A. Qualitative Evaluation

The use of AS-OCT imaging has revolutionized our ability to evaluate the outflow angle. Before AS-OCT, gonioscopy and ultrasound biomicroscopy (UBM) were the only modalities available to clinicians. Gonioscopy provides an excellent 360-degree view of the angle but is dependent on both the examiner's skill and patient cooperation. Of note, gonioscopy may be insufficient to distinguish between classic pupil block iris bowing, anatomically thick iris, or phacomorphic lens resulting in angle narrowing. UBM can image the angle better than AS-OCT because the ultrasound energy can penetrate to

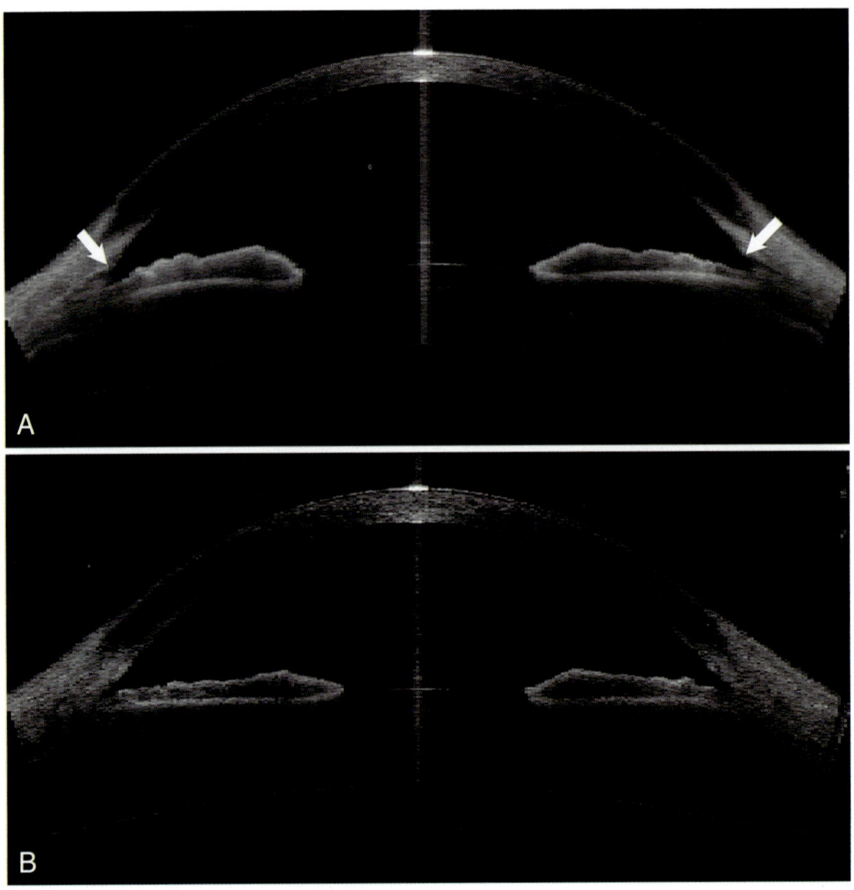

Fig. 10.1 AS-OCT of scleral spur. (A) AS-OCT image showing well-defined scleral spurs in which the *arrows* indicate the position of the scleral spur. (B) AS-OCT image with poorly defined scleral spurs.

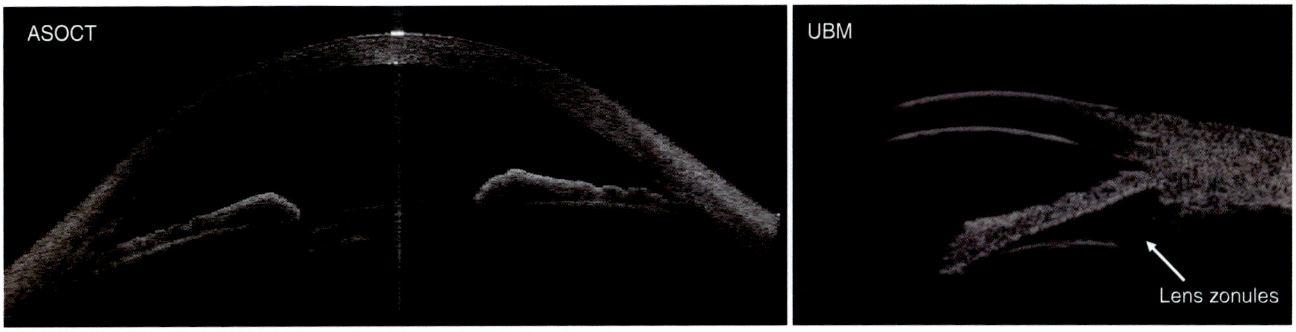

Fig. 10.2 AS-OCT vs UBM. UBM and AS-OCT images of the same eye showing the ability of the UBM to image structures posterior to the iris such as the ciliary body and lens zonules.

deeper structures posterior to the iris (Fig. 10.2); however, the contact nature of the procedure is a major limitation because it can induce discomfort for the patient and also can result in distortion of the angles as a result of inadvertent indentation. In addition, UBM relies on a skilled and experienced examiner to effectively use the device, which may not be available in all clinical settings.

> **CLINICAL PEARL**
>
> AS-OCT can be used to assess the angle in patients in whom gonioscopy is difficult or who may not be able to cooperate with a contact gonioscopy lens touching the eye. For example, in an extremely photophobic or touch-sensitive patient, AS-OCT offers a noncontact imaging modality to assess the angle to help the clinician decide on appropriate or necessary interventions.

Several features regarding the qualitative assessment of AS-OCT images include the following:

1. An angle is considered *closed* on AS-OCT when there is any contact between the iris and the angle wall anterior to the scleral spur (Fig. 10.3). It is important to remember that the definition of angle closure and the landmarks differ on gonioscopy and AS-OCT scans. An angle is considered closed in gonioscopy when the posterior trabecular meshwork is not visible. In contrast, on AS-OCT, an angle is considered closed when there is iridocorneal contact anterior to the scleral spur. This helps explain why the AS-OCT detects more closed angles than gonioscopy.
2. An angle is considered *narrow* when there is a narrow slit between the iris and anterior angle wall, but without contact between them (see Fig. 10.3).
3. AS-OCT also can be used to assess response to treatment. Fig. 10.4 shows angle widening after laser peripheral iridotomy (LPI), followed by lens extraction for the same patient. Lens extraction in patients with angle closure has the added benefit of reducing intraocular pressure (IOP).

> **CLINICAL PEARL**
>
> AS-OCT is an effective tool in the serial documentation of changes in anterior segment structures as a result of either intervention or the disease process. AS-OCT can be used to assess response to interventional treatments, such as laser peripheral iridotomy.

B. Quantitative Evaluation

The built-in semiautomated software of the AS-OCT machines (e.g., Visante OCT and Casia SS-OCT) facilitates measurements of the quantitative parameters of the angles, anterior chamber, iris, lens, and cornea (Fig. 10.5). For the quantitative assessment, prior identification of the scleral spur is necessary. The angle parameters include the angle opening distance, angle recess area, and trabecular iris space area. Anterior chamber parameters include measurements of the anterior chamber depth, width, area, and volume. The lens parameter is the lens vault; iris parameters include thickness, curvature, and area. The Casia SS-OCT software also allows measurement of the iridotrabecular contact index, quantifying the extent of angle closure across 360 degrees of the angles expressed as a percentage.

These measurements have both clinical and research utility. For example, quantitative measurement of the angles is an essential preoperative measurement before pIOL surgery. Although devices such as tomography can also measure the angle, AS-OCT offers surgeons an additional or supplemental angle measurement before pIOL surgery (see Chapter 12 for additional information regarding pIOLs). Smaller anterior chamber width, larger lens vault (Fig. 10.6), thicker iris (Fig. 10.7), and greater iris area are significantly associated with angle closure.

C. Physiologic Changes

AS-OCT can be used to assess dynamic changes in the anterior chamber angles. It has been shown that angle width generally decreases linearly with increasing pupil diameter, such as in mesopic and scotopic light conditions (Fig. 10.8). Differences in the angle width vary substantially among individuals depending on ambient light conditions.

> **CLINICAL PEARL**
>
> AS-OCT can highlight changes in the anterior chamber angle that occur in mesopic-scotopic versus photopic conditions. In dark light conditions, the angle width decreases secondary to increased pupil diameters. In bright light conditions, the angle width increases.

III. CLINICAL EXAMPLES OF ANTERIOR SEGMENT OPTICAL COHERENCE TOMOGRAPHY AND ANGLE PATHOLOGY

AS-OCT imaging is an important adjunctive tool that complements clinical assessment in evaluating the angles and visualization of the anterior segment structures in various pathologic conditions.

A. Narrow Angles and Laser Peripheral Iridotomy

A commonly encountered scenario in clinical practice is patients presenting with narrow angles at risk for angle-closure glaucoma. In addition to gonioscopy, AS-OCT can be used to

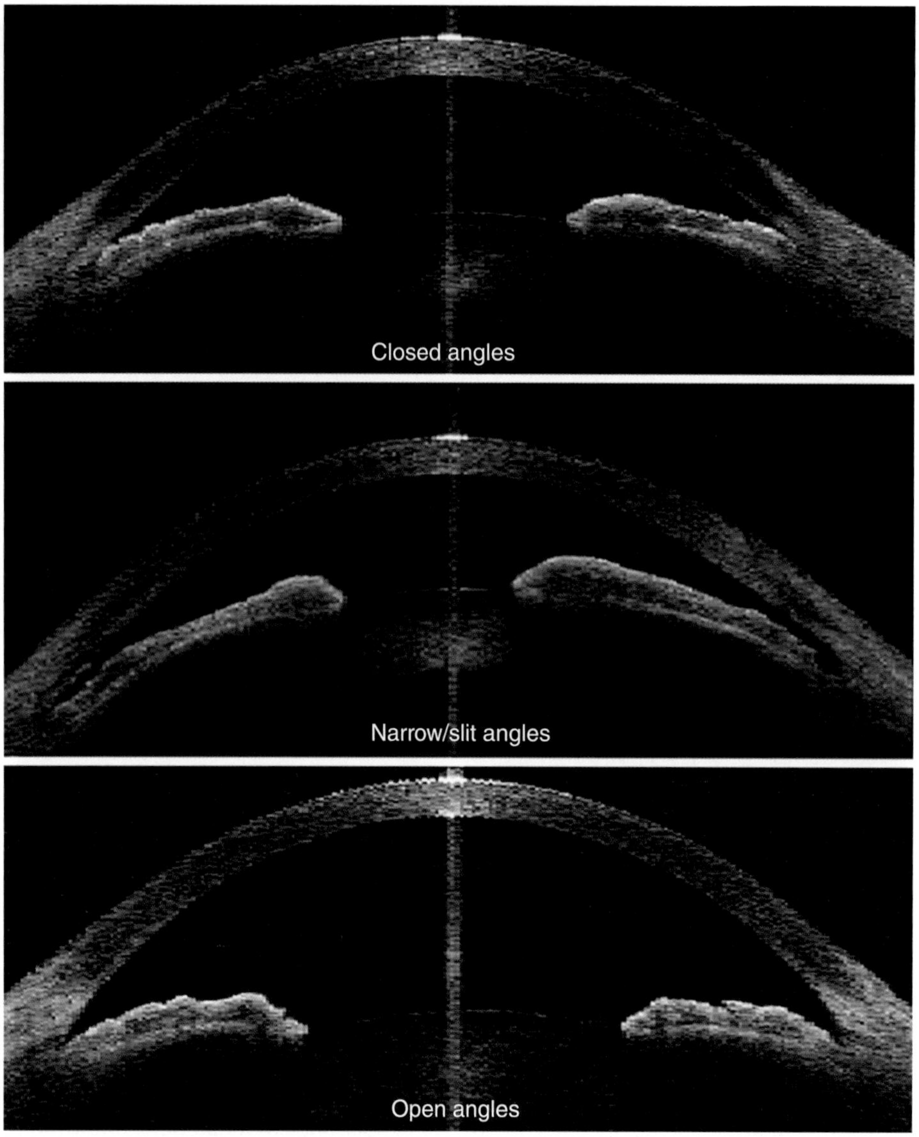

Fig. 10.3 AS-OCT of different angle depths. Qualitative assessment of anterior chamber angles.

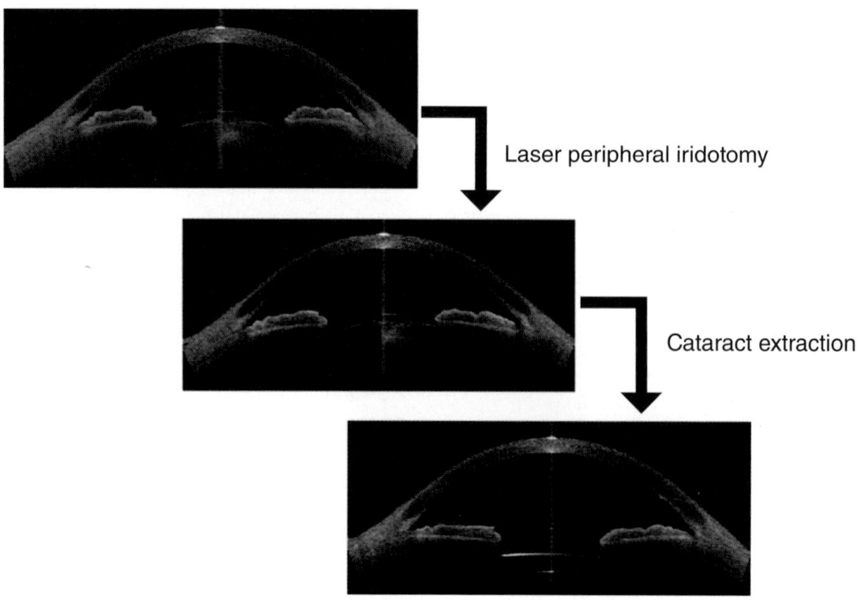

Fig. 10.4 Sequential AS-OCT after interventions. AS-OCT images showing response to treatment.

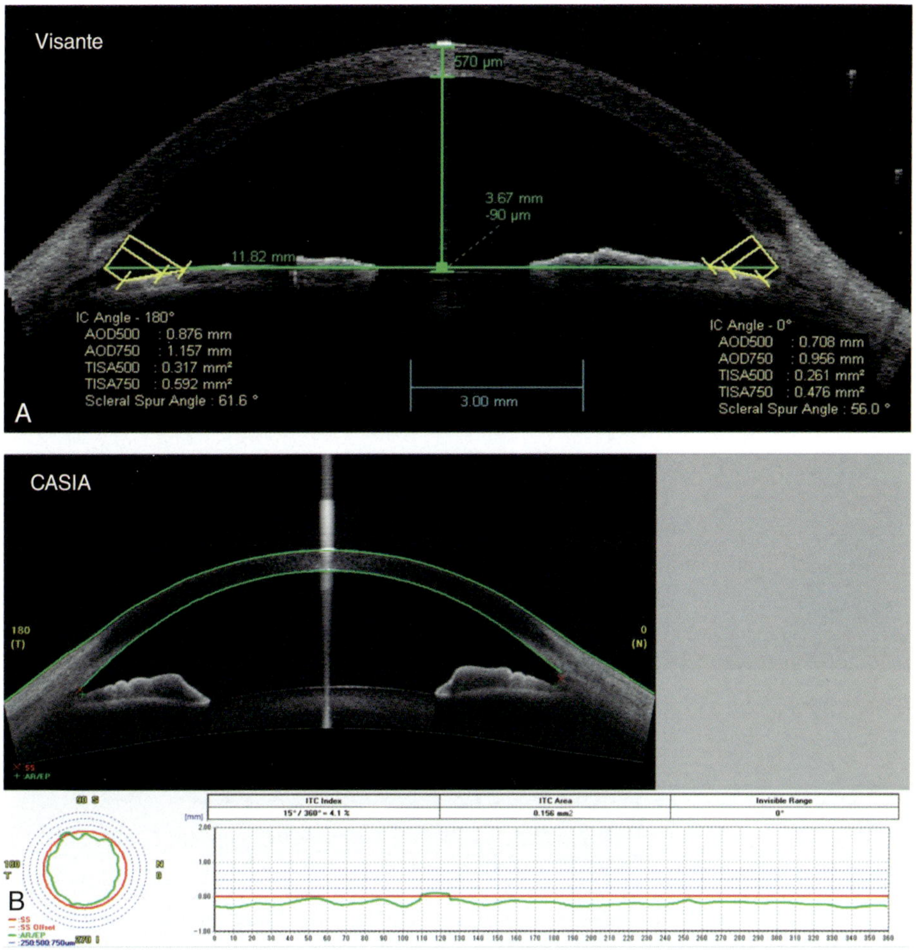

Fig. 10.5 Visante and Casia AS-OCT analyses. Built-in semiautomated software of the AS-OCT machines A, Visante OCT. B, Casia SS-OCT. (Courtesy Dr. Tin A Tunu.)

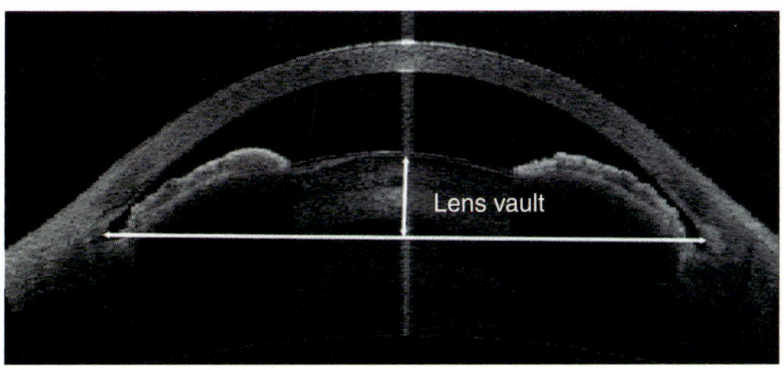

Fig. 10.6 AS-OCT enlarged lens vault. AS-OCT image showing an eye with a large lens vault.

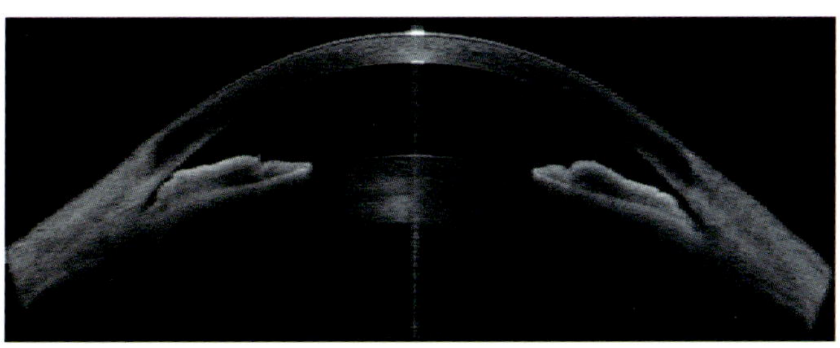

Fig. 10.7 AS-OCT of thick iris. AS-OCT image showing an eye with a thick iris.

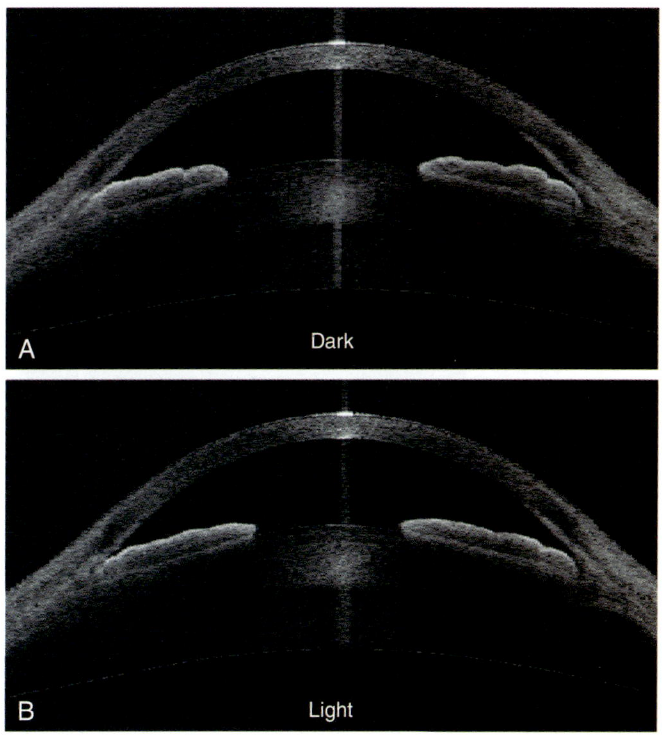

Fig. 10.8 AS-OCT dark vs light. AS-OCT imaging showing thicker peripheral iris and larger pupil in dark (A) compared with light (B) condition.

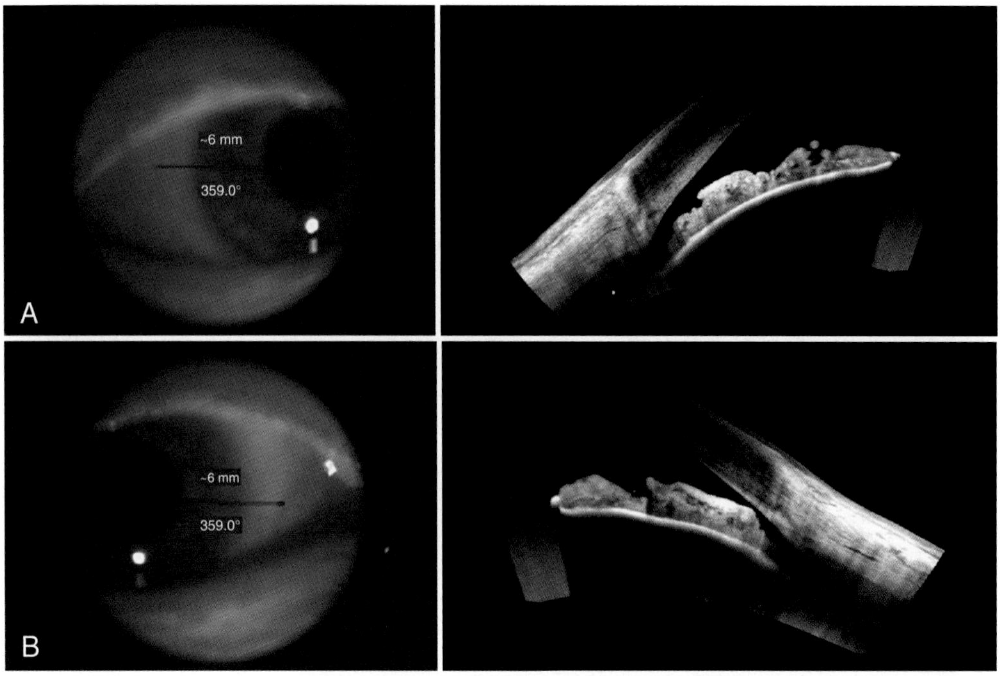

Fig. 10.9 AS-OCT narrow angle pre-LPI. AS-OCT highlights narrow angles temporally *(panel A)* and nasally *(panel B)* in the right eye of a patient before laser peripheral iridotomy.

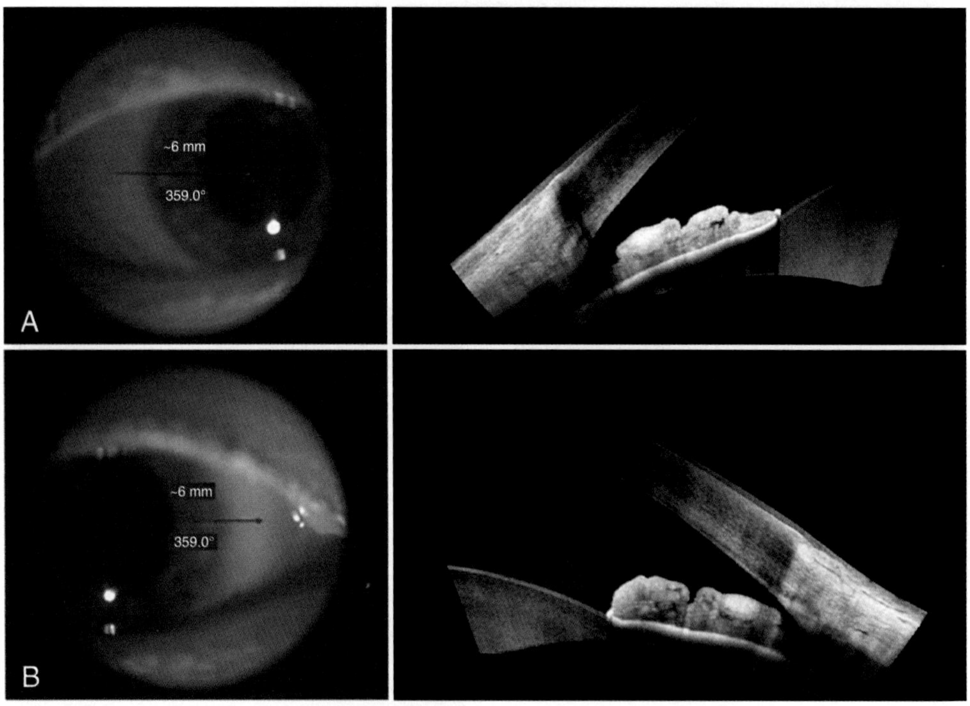

Fig. 10.10 AS-OCT narrow angle post-LPI. After laser peripheral iridotomy, there is a notable deepening of the temporal *(panel A)* and nasal *(panel B)* angle in the eye shown in Fig. 10.9.

better visualize the angle in suspect eyes (Fig. 10.9). After LPI (Fig. 10.10), AS-OCT can highlight the opening of the angle for clinical verification and for patient education regarding the effects of the procedure.

B. Subluxated Lens

Fig. 10.11 illustrates a patient with a markedly subluxated lens causing angle closure. Slit-lamp photographs of the patient in seated *(C)* and supine positions *(D)* are shown. The lens tips posteriorly when the patient is supine. A *and* B panels show the AS-OCT and UBM images, respectively, of the patient when in a supine position. Note the irregular depth of the anterior chamber in eyes with a subluxated lens (Fig. 10.12). These eyes need careful surgical management because of the potential risk for complications.

C. Iris Cysts

Slit-lamp biomicroscopy or gonioscopy can seldom detect iris and ciliary body cysts. These cysts can push the iris forward, resulting in secondary angle closure or pseudoplateau iris.

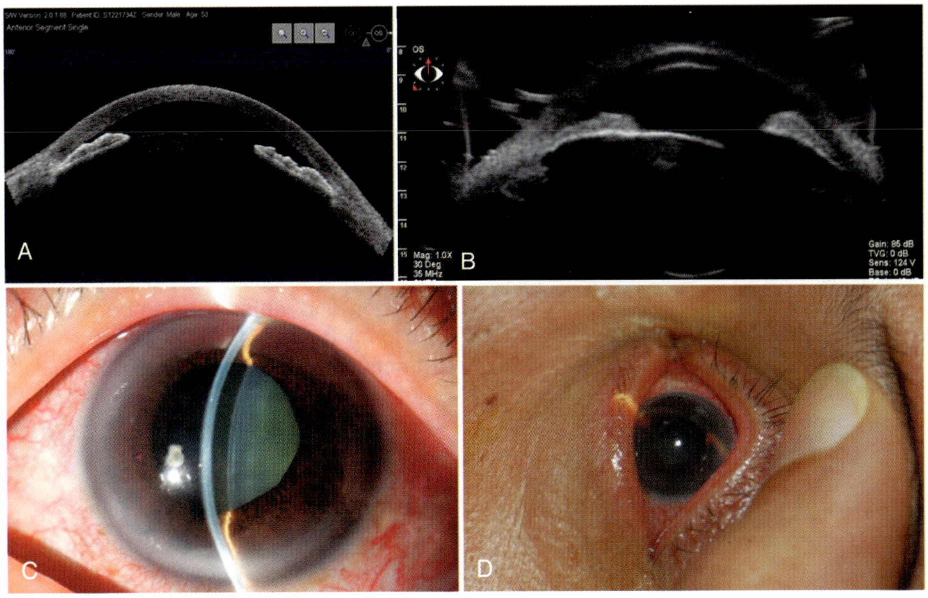

Fig. 10.11 AS-OCT and UBM of subluxated lens. Patient with subluxated lens on (A) AS-OCT and (B) UBM. Slit-lamp photography of patient in sitting up position (C) and supine (D).

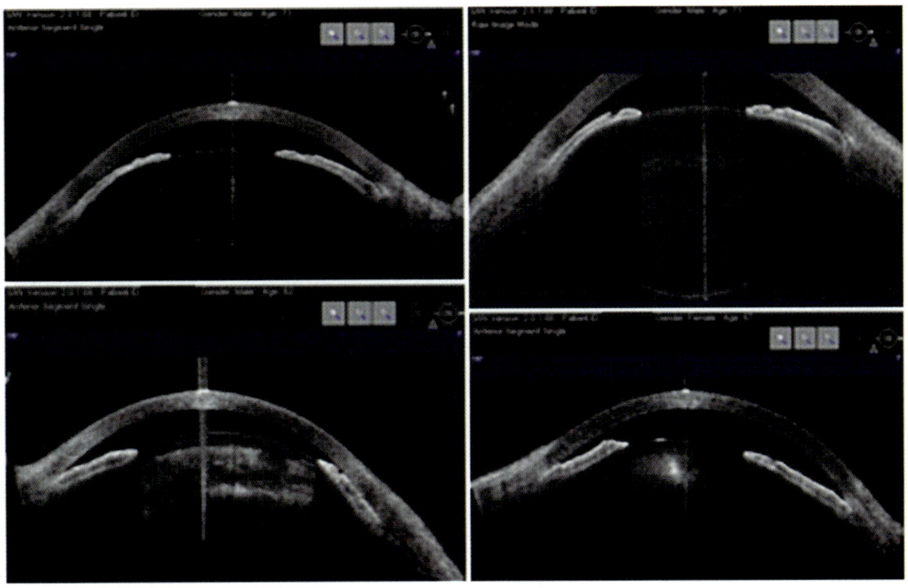

Fig. 10.12 AS-OCT subluxated lens examples. AS-OCT images of eyes with subluxated lens causing angle closure.

Although better visualized by UBM because they are often located in the middle-posterior iris, they also can be detected on AS-OCT scans (Fig. 10.13).

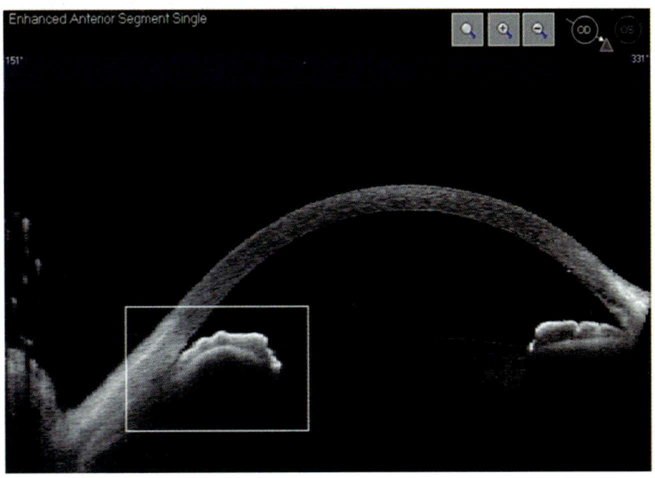

Fig. 10.13 AS-OCT of iris cyst. Iris cyst causing secondary angle closure.

D. Ciliochoroidal Effusion

Ciliochoroidal effusion (Fig. 10.14) is an abnormal accumulation of fluid in the suprachoroidal space secondary to an imbalance of pressure differentials. It is considered to play a significant role in the development of angle closure in some eyes. A higher prevalence of effusion has been observed in eyes with angle closure compared with those without it.

E. Acute Angle Closure as a Result of Large Lens Vault

Acute primary angle closure (APAC) is an ocular emergency with typical symptoms, such as acute onset of pain, tearing, and light sensitivity, and clinical signs on ocular examination. In addition to markedly elevated IOP, occludable drainage angles,

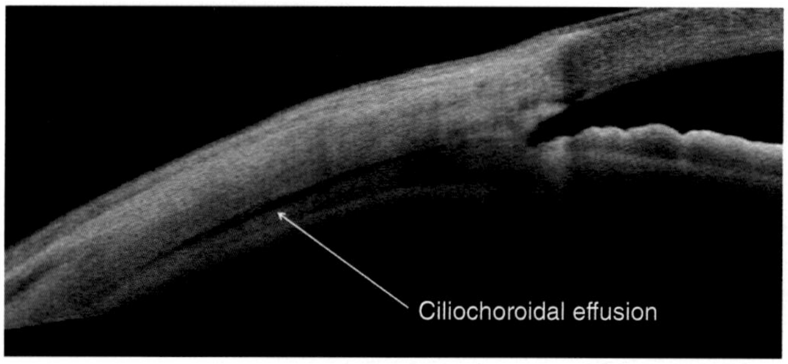

Fig. 10.14 AS-OCT of cilio-choroidal effusion. AS-OCT image showing ciliochoroidal effusion.

shallow anterior chambers, poorly reactive pupil, corneal edema, aqueous cells, and flare are also present in the anterior chamber. APAC is potentially blinding unless prompt treatment is administered to lower the elevated IOP. Some studies have found that eyes with previous attacks of APAC have larger lens vault than their fellow eyes. Fig. 10.15 shows the presence of a larger lens vault in an eye with previous APAC compared with the fellow eye.

F. Discernment and Treatment of Angle Closure Resulting from Pupil Block or Phacomorphic Lens

One of the benefits of the AS-OCT is the ability to differentiate the likely source of the narrow angles. The distinction between classic pupil block narrow angle and phacomorphic narrow angle is often impossible to appreciate with gonioscopy but may be readily determined with AS-OCT. Fig. 10.16 is an AS-OCT image that demonstrates a classic pupil block. Note the *red line* highlighting the anterior bowing of the iris. This bowing is caused by a pressure differential between the posterior and anterior chambers and is relieved with laser iridotomy. In the presence of a visually significant cataract, lens extraction may be performed as an initial treatment option.

On the other hand, Fig. 10.17 demonstrates a classic phacomorphic narrow angle. Note the *red line* in this image follows the contour of the lens. There is no or minimal space posterior to the iris, suggesting a negligible element of pupil block. Although LPI is considered the first line of treatment in eyes with primary angle closure, in these eyes, LPI may be ineffective in alleviating the narrow angles. Recently more clinicians have advocated for early lens extraction in these eyes, even in the absence of visually significant cataracts. The effectiveness of early lens extraction with intraocular lens implantation for the

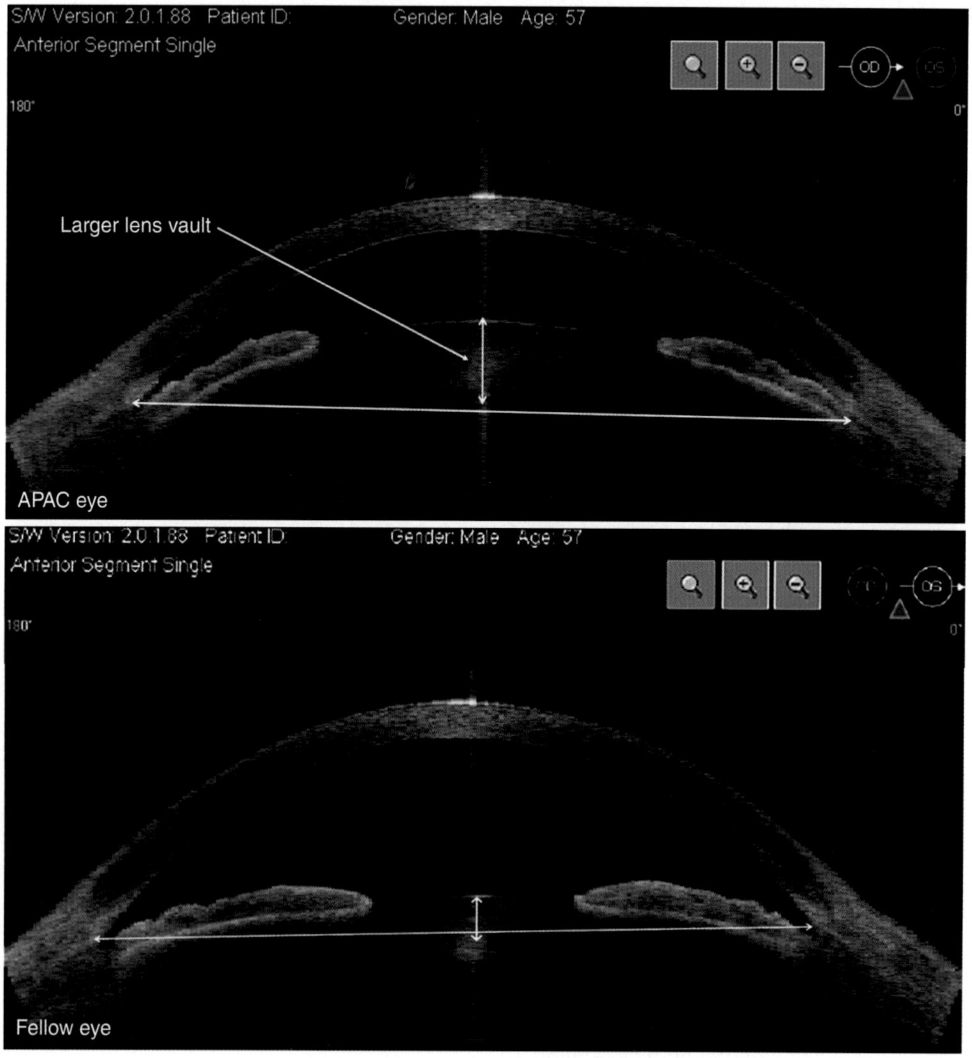

Fig. 10.15 AS-OCT spur to spur method for lens vault. Larger lens vault in an eye with acute primary angle closure (APAC) compared with the fellow eye.

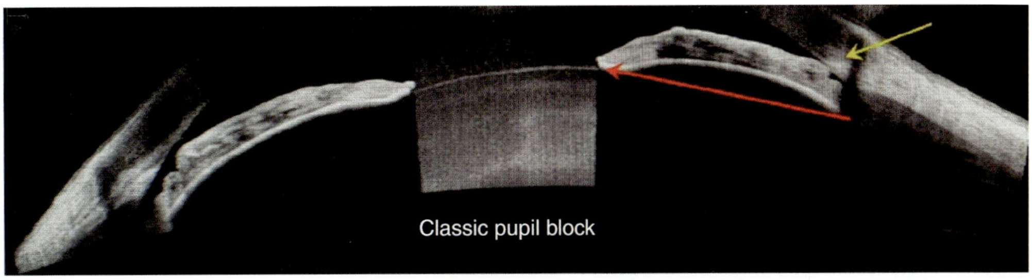

Fig. 10.16 AS-OCT lens contour method for narrow angle, classic pupil block. AS-OCT image that demonstrates classic pupillary block.

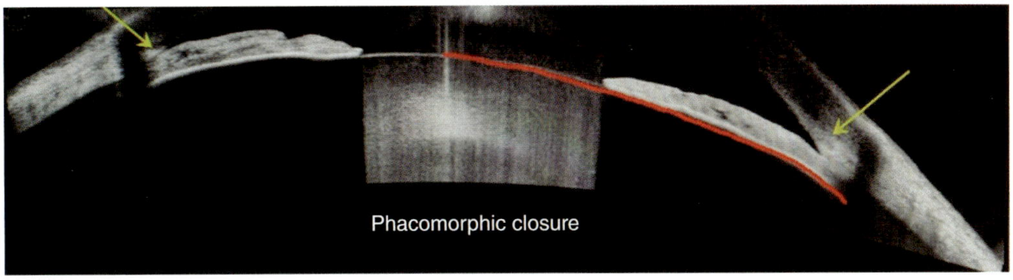

Fig. 10.17 AS-OCT lens contour method for phacomorphic narrow angle. An AS-OCT image that demonstrates classic phacomorphic narrow angle.

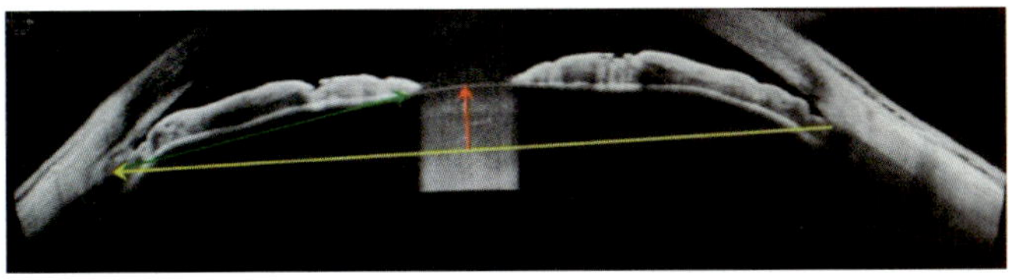

Fig. 10.18 AS-OCT lens contour method for mixed pupil block/ phacomorphic narrow angle. An AS-OCT image shows the presence of a mixed pupil block/phacomorphic narrow angle.

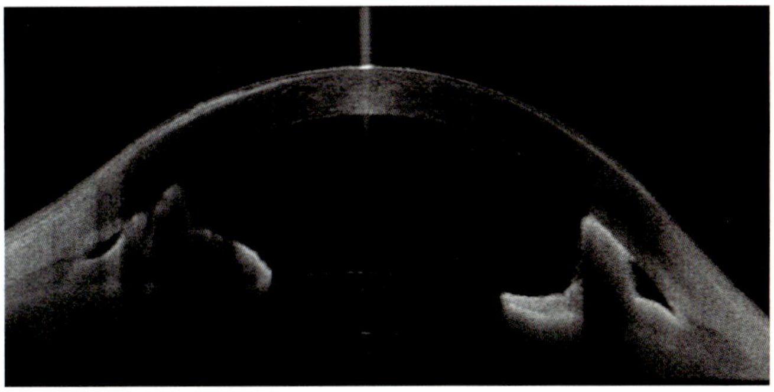

Fig. 10.19 AS-OCT with large peripheral anterior synechiae. Peripheral anterior synechiae.

treatment of primary angle-closure glaucoma (EAGLE) study, a randomized controlled trial, recommends early lens extraction in primary angle-closure glaucoma eyes or primary angle-closure eyes with elevated IOP (>30 mm Hg).

Furthermore, some eyes may exhibit the presence of a mixed pupil block/phacomorphic condition, as demonstrated in Fig. 10.18. The *green line* shows the moderate pupil bowing, and the *yellow line* (spur to spur) is a reference to estimate the amount of anterior lens vault *(red arrow).* The decision for the optimum treatment strategy would depend on several factors, including the visual acuity, IOP, cataract severity, and the presence and extent of peripheral anterior synechiae (PAS). Regardless of choice, all forms of narrow angle require either laser or surgical intervention. Topical therapies or observation may be harmfully insufficient in these eyes.

G. Evaluation of Peripheral Anterior Synechiae

PAS is the anterior adhesion of the peripheral iris to the anterior chamber angle (Fig. 10.19). PAS may be localized or broad and extensive. The high scan speed of swept source OCT (SS-OCT) technology facilitates circumferential imaging of the anterior chamber angles, including assessing the extent of PAS involvement. The PAS in AS-OCT can be discriminated from appositional closure with either dark-light imaging or reflectivity, where the reflectivity of PAS appears to be higher (hyperreflectivity) than that of apposition because PAS is essentially scar tissue. It is important to remember that indentation gonioscopy remains the gold standard to diagnose and quantify the extent of PAS. Phacoemulsification combined with goniosynechialysis (GSL) is effective in releasing synechial closure and reopening the angles compared with phacoemulsification alone. GSL involves manually separating the PAS from the trabecular meshwork using either a spatula or a microforceps.

H. Pigment Dispersion Syndrome

Pigment dispersion syndrome is characterized by the excessive release of pigments from the iris pigment epithelium throughout the anterior segment of the eye. The underlying mechanism is the presence of a concave iris contour, which causes rubbing of the posterior iris surface against the anterior lens zonules. The reverse pupillary block results in the concave iris configuration observed in these eyes (Fig. 10.20).

I. Iridocorneal Endothelial Syndrome and Essential Iris Atrophy

The linear scan of AS-OCT is the limiting feature for detecting iridocorneal endothelial syndrome in the angle, as iris process abnormalities are easily missed. Gonioscopy and standard slit-lamp biomicroscopy remain essential tools for accurate diagnosis, though AS-OCT can be used as an additional imaging modality in select cases. Fig. 10.21 shows the AS-OCT images of a young woman with essential iris atrophy and serial slit-lamp photographs of the progression of her iris atrophy.

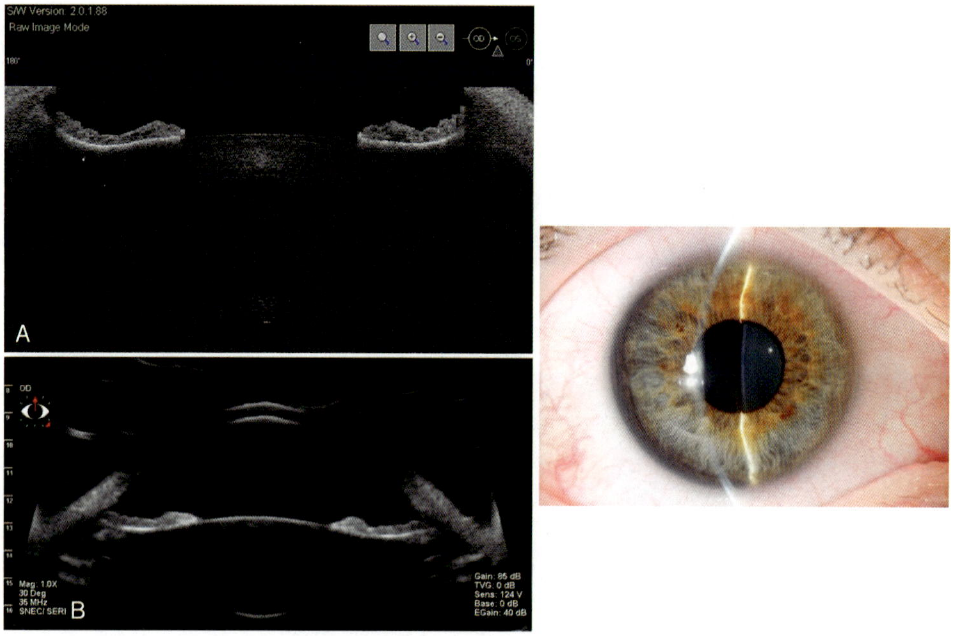

Fig. 10.20 AS-OCT and clinical photo of posterior iris bowing. An eye with pigment dispersion syndrome shows reverse pupillary block as viewed with (A) AS-OCT (B) and UBM.

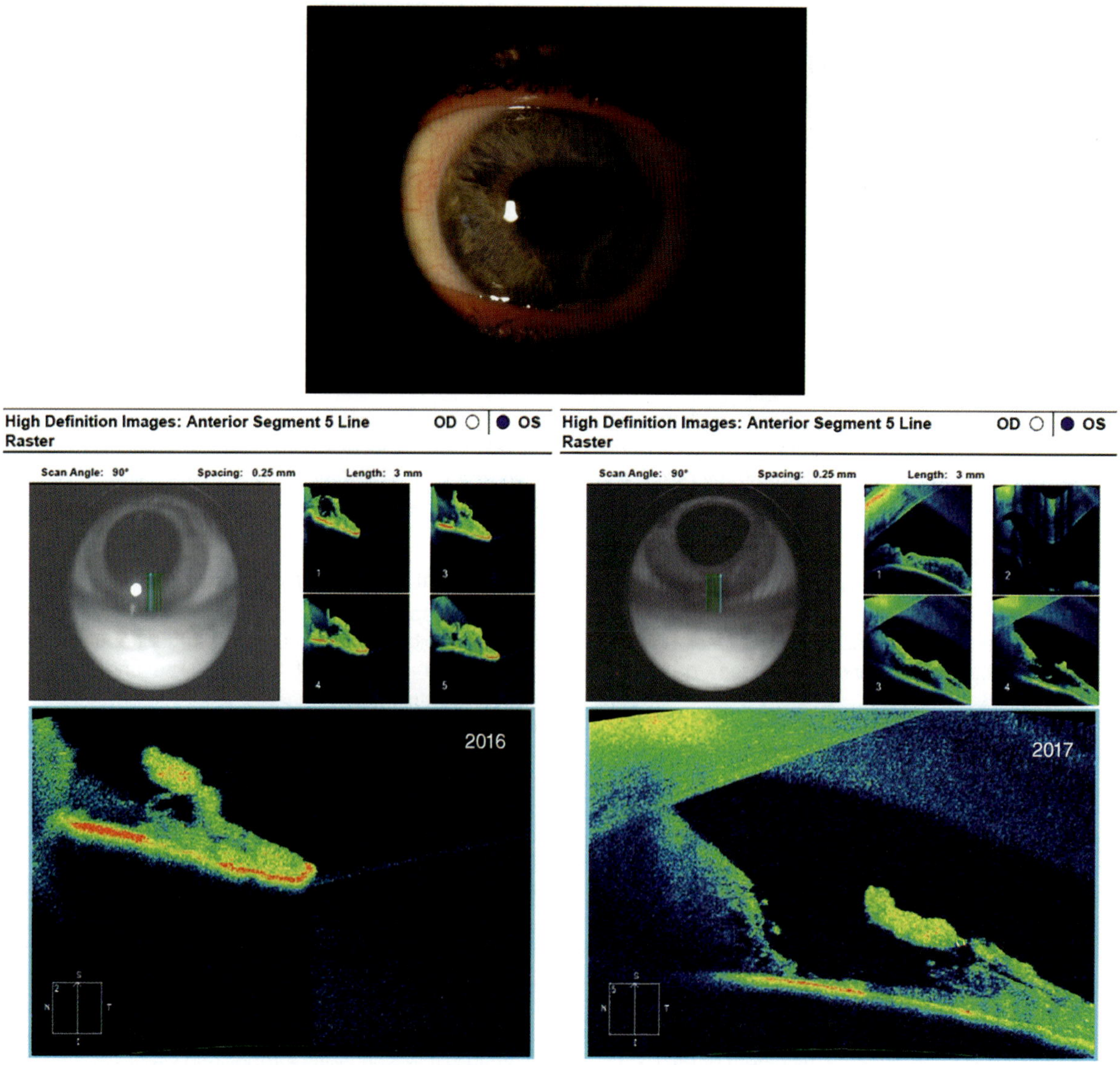

Fig. 10.21 AS-OCT and clinical photo of essential iris atrophy. Slit-lamp and AS-OCT images of an eye with essential iris atrophy.

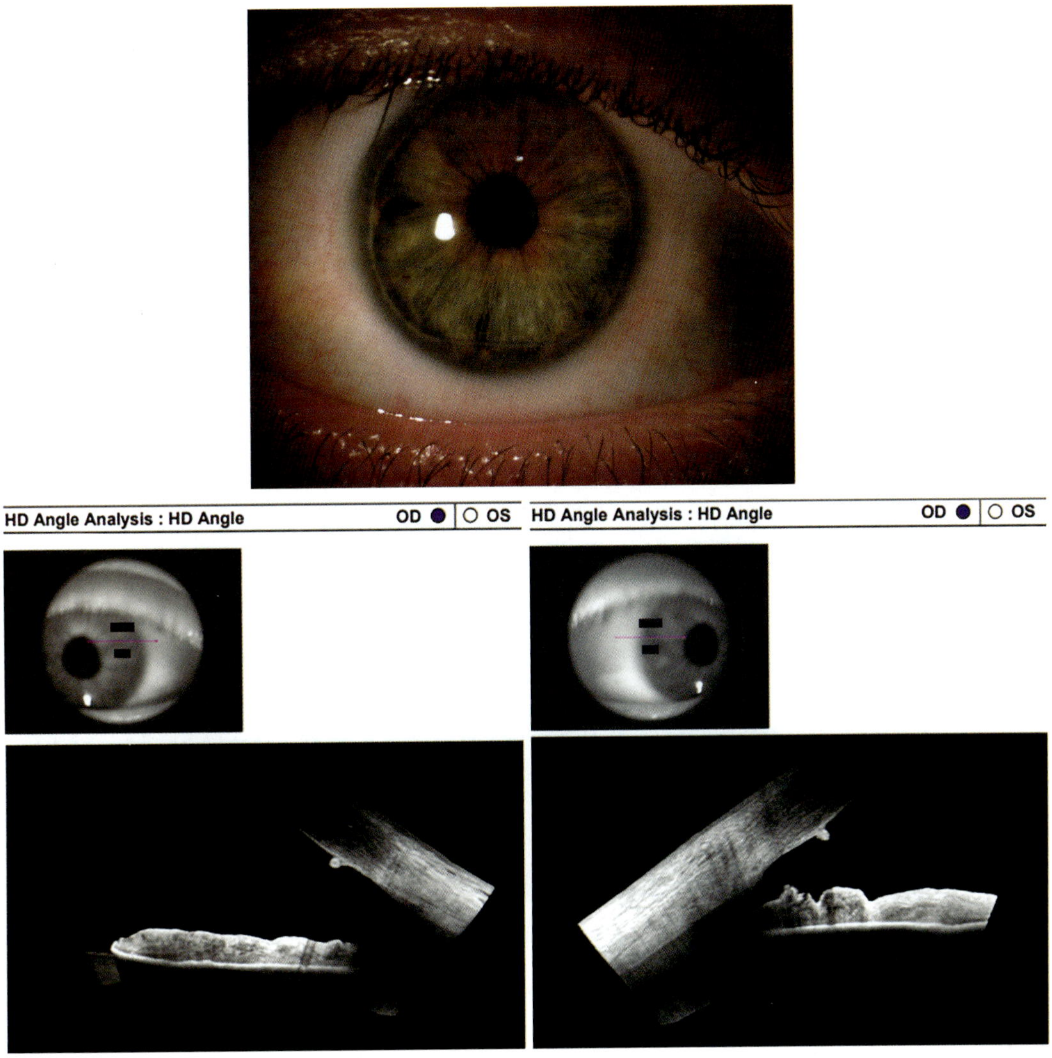

Fig. 10.22 AS-OCT and clinical photo of posterior embryotoxon. Posterior embryotoxon.

J. Posterior Embryotoxon

Fig. 10.22 presents images of a young man with classic posterior embryotoxon. The anterior location of the Schwalbe line is easily seen on AS-OCT

K. Imaging of Posttrabeculectomy Bleb Morphology

Posttrabeculectomy bleb morphology is an essential indicator of bleb function and possible future long-term success. AS-OCT imaging allows the assessment of internal bleb anatomy, which is otherwise not apparent on clinical examination, such as the total bleb height, bleb cavity, bleb wall thickness, scleral wall thickness, the position of the scleral flap relative to the sclera, presence or absence of hyporeflective subflap space, and patency or occlusion of the internal ostium (Fig. 10.23). Functioning blebs are characterized by the presence of internal fluid-filled cavities, low reflectivity of the bleb walls, and microcysts, whereas failed blebs have low bleb height, ostial occlusion, and the apposition of the scleral flap to its bed.

CLINICAL PEARL

In the surgical and postoperative management of glaucoma, AS-OCT complements clinical assessment because it allows visualization of the internal structures of the trabeculectomy bleb and minimally invasive glaucoma implants

L. Malignant Glaucoma**

Although a diagnosis of exclusion, malignant galucoma is a secondary angle-closure glaucoma that typically occurs in the early postoperative period after incisional ophthalmic surgery. On presentation, patients present with elevated IOP accompanied by a severely shallow peripheral and central anterior chamber, even if pseudophakic or in the presence of a patent peripheral iridotomy. Concurrently elevated posterior pressure and anterior rotation of the ciliary body is thought to be the likely mechanism.

The slit-lamp examination usually reveals an extremely shallow peripheral and central anterior chamber with variable iris appearance (Fig. 10.24, *panels A and B*). A B-scan should be obtained to rule out choroidal detachment and/or choroidal hemorrhage (see Fig. 10.24, *panel C*). AS-OCT (see Fig. 10.24, *panels D and E*) can be used to highlight salient features, such as iridocorneal touch, obscuration of the angle, and distortion of normal anterior chamber anatomy.

**The term "Aqueous Misdirection" is an older description based on what we now know is an incorrect mechanism. There is nothing being "misdirected". The more common and recent term is "Malignant Glaucoma" though that is also an incomplete description of the pathophysiological mechanism.

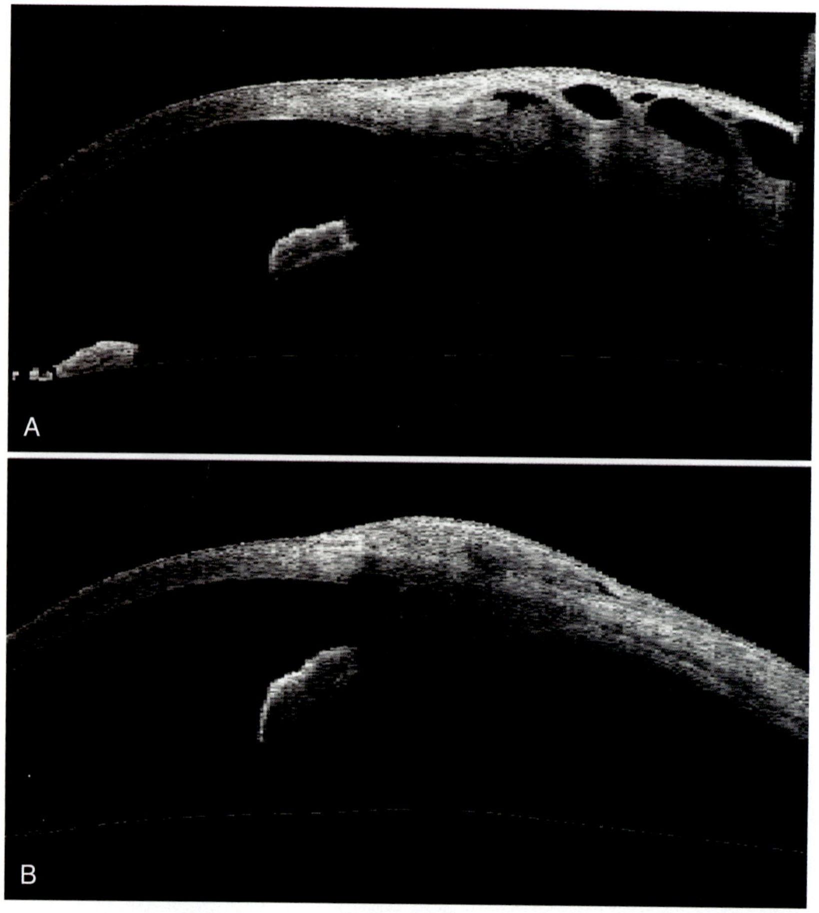

Fig. 10.23 AS-OCT of glaucoma bleb architecture, functioning versus failed. Posttrabeculectomy AS-OCT images show features of a filtering bleb (A) and failed bleb (B).

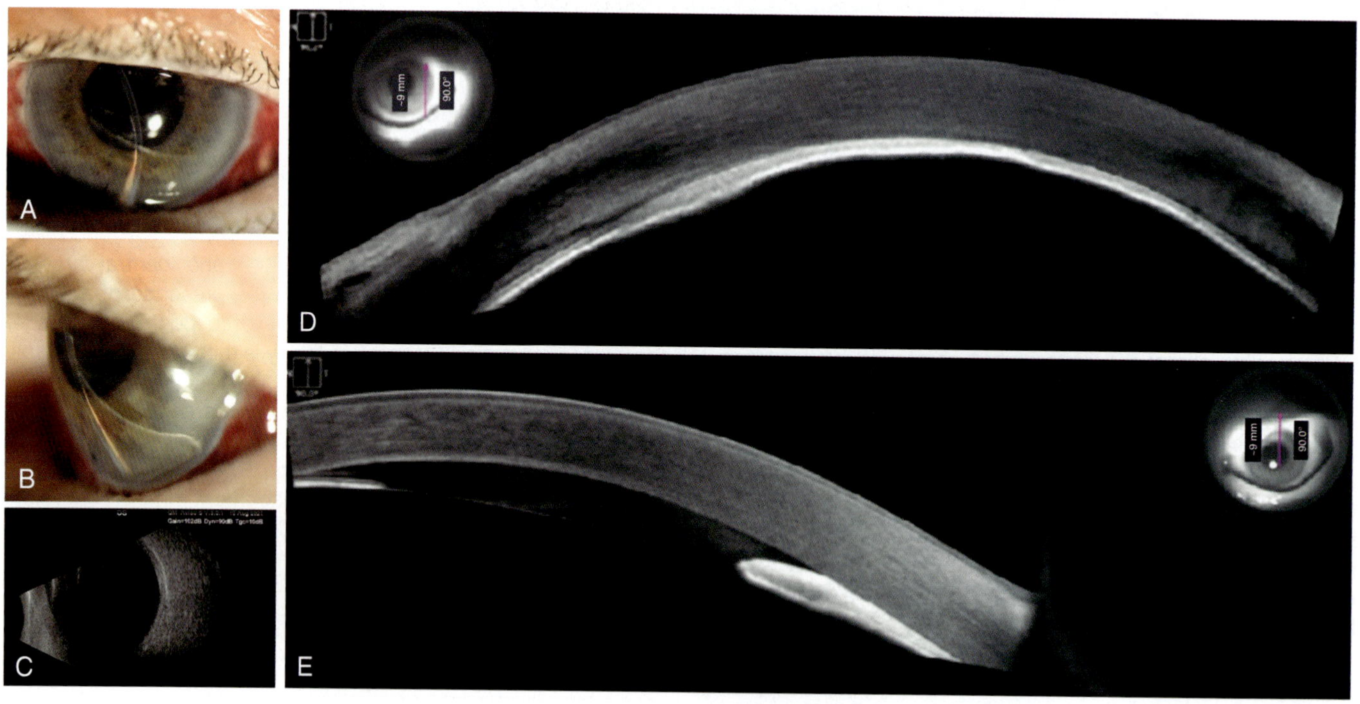

Fig. 10.24 AS-OCT of malignant glaucoma. Slit-lamp photographs *(panels A and B)* demonstrate an extremely narrow anterior chamber centrally and peripherally with multiple areas of iris-corneal touch. A B-scan *(panel C)* should be obtained to rule out presence of posterior segment pathologic conditions, such as choroidal hemorrhage or detachment. AS-OCT *(panels D and E)* can be used to confirm examination findings. Note the areas of central and peripheral iris-corneal touch, obscuration of the angle, and distortion of normal anterior chamber anatomy. (Courtesy Kamran M. Riaz, MD, Dean McGee Eye Institute, University of Oklahoma).

M. Glaucoma Drainage Devices

AS-OCT imaging allows clinicians to assess the position of the tube in relation to the surrounding tissues, patency, state of drainage, and presence of any tube-corneal or tube-iris touch.

BIBLIOGRAPHY

Azuara-Blanco A, Burr J, Ramsay C, et al. Effectiveness of early lens extraction for the treatment of primary angle-closure glaucoma (EAGLE): a randomised controlled trial. *Lancet*. 2016;388(10052): 1389-1397.

Hee MR, Izatt JA, Swanson EA, et al. Optical coherence tomography of the human retina. *Arch Ophthalmol*. 1995;113:325-332.

Izatt JA, Hee MR, Swanson EA, et al. Micrometer-scale resolution imaging of the anterior eye in vivo with optical coherence tomography. *Arch Ophthalmol*. 1994;112:1584-1589.

Kumar RS, Quek D, Lee KY, et al. Confirmation of uveal effusion in eyes with primary angle closure glaucoma: an ultrasound biomicroscopy study. *Arch Ophthalmol*. 2008;126:1647-1651.

Lai I, Mak H, Lai G, et al. Anterior chamber angle imaging with swept-source optical coherence tomography: measuring peripheral anterior synechia in glaucoma. *Ophthalmology*. 2013;120:1144-1149.

Moghimi S, Vahedian Z, Fakhraie G, et al. Ocular biometry in the subtypes of angle closure: an anterior segment optical coherence tomography study. *Am J Ophthalmol*. 2013;155:664–673, 673.e1.

Nolan WP, See JL, Chew PT, et al. Detection of primary angle closure using anterior segment optical coherence tomography in Asian eyes. *Ophthalmology*. 2007;114(1):33-39.

Nongpiur ME, He M, Amerasinghe N, et al. Lens vault, thickness, and position in Chinese subjects with angle closure. *Ophthalmology*. 2011;118:474-479.

Nongpiur ME, Sakata LM, Friedman DS, et al. Novel association of smaller anterior chamber width with angle closure in Singaporeans. *Ophthalmology*. 2010;117:1967-1973.

Quigley HA, Friedman DS, Congdon NG. Possible mechanisms of primary angle-closure and malignant glaucoma. *J Glaucoma*. 2003;12:167-180.

Sakai H, Morine-Shinjyo S, Shinzato M, et al. Uveal effusion in primary angle-closure glaucoma. *Ophthalmology*. 2005;112:413-419.

Sakata LM, Lavanya R, Friedman DS, et al. Comparison of gonioscopy and anterior segment ocular coherence tomography in detecting angle closure in different quadrants of the anterior chamber angle. *Ophthalmology*. 2008;115(5):769-774.

Sng CC, Aquino MC, Liao J, et al. Pretreatment anterior segment imaging during acute primary angle closure: insights into angle closure mechanisms in the acute phase. *Ophthalmology*. 2014;121:119-125.

Swanson EA, Izatt JA, Hee MR, et al. In vivo retinal imaging by optical coherence tomography. *Opt Lett*. 1993;18:1864-1866.

Tun TA, Baskaran M, Perera SA, et al. Swept-source optical coherence tomography assessment of iris-trabecular contact after phacoemulsification with or without goniosynechialysis in eyes with primary angle closure glaucoma. *Br J Ophthalmol*. 2015;99:927-931.

Wang B, Sakata LM, Friedman DS, et al. Quantitative iris parameters and association with narrow angles. *Ophthalmology*. 2010;117: 11-17.

11 Abnormalities of the Crystalline Lens and Intra-Ocular Lens

Abdelhalim A. Awidi | Kamran M. Riaz

I. IMAGING OF THE LENS USING AS-OCT

Although anterior segment optical coherence tomography (AS-OCT) can effectively image the ocular surface, cornea, anterior chamber, and angle, there may be limitations when acquiring images of the crystalline lens and zonules using existing AS-OCT technology and devices. The lens plane is inherently difficult to capture with most commercially available machines in a single, usable image. It is possible (and likely) that future developments in AS-OCT technology will improve imaging of the lens–intraocular lens (IOL) plane. Currently, clinicians can still image these structures using special lenses available with most AS-OCT devices. Alternatively, clinicians can simply modify existing posterior segment OCT devices to allow for anterior segment imaging. Pujari and Sharma described a simple yet elegant method of using a 20D lens with existing posterior segment OCT devices. This allows for multiple scans that can be reconstructed using computer software to obtain in-detail images from the ocular surface to the posterior capsule for diagnostic and management purposes.

II. TYPES OF CATARACTS

Cataracts refer to the opacification of the natural crystalline lens as a result of insults that disrupt the innate stability of crystalline lens proteins, thereby promoting aggregation of these proteins and altering the refractive index of the lens. Cataracts are a leading cause of preventable blindness globally, and age-related cataracts can be classified according to the location of the opacification, including nuclear, cortical, and posterior subcapsular cataracts.

Clinical examination and subjective patient complaints of decreased visual acuity remain the mainstay of diagnosis. Clinicians use both to determine a visually significant cataract and aid in surgical decision-making. Ancillary imaging, such as AS-OCT, is usually not required in routine diagnosis and management of cataracts. In most cases, the decision to proceed with cataract surgery is mutual by the surgeon and the patient.

In certain situations, AS-OCT may be helpful to the clinician both for diagnostic and management purposes. For example, objective assessment of cataract density and significance remains an emerging area of interest. The utility of AS-OCT for cataract evaluation has been described by several authors, such as using this technology to correlate with existing lens opacity classification system parameters. Other authors have additionally described using AS-OCT to quantify lens density as a measure of pixel units with high sensitivity and specificity. It is possible that as AS-OCT technology improves and its adoption increases among clinicians, its role in surgical decision-making may also increase correspondingly.

Intraoperatively, surgeons use AS-OCT during femtosecond laser–assisted cataract surgery (FLACS) for surgical planning; AS-OCT–derived images help plan and execute incisions of FLACS in the cornea, anterior capsule, and crystalline lens. Additionally, AS-OCT can help visualize the lens-zonular complex in unique circumstances, such as phacomorphic, zonule-deficient, and posterior polar cataracts. The information gained from AS-OCT may help surgeons with thoughtful surgical planning in these cases, including the potential need for concurrent vitreous management should complications arise in high-risk patients.

A. Nuclear Sclerotic Cataracts

Nuclear cataracts may develop as a result of long-term exposure to environmental insults (e.g., ultraviolet light, and such) causing oxidative damage and culminating in a hardened, brown crystalline lens, known as *nuclear sclerosis* (Fig. 11.1). Older age, smoking, and higher degrees of myopia play a vital role in the development of nuclear cataracts.

B. Cortical Cataracts

Cortical cataracts are caused by the opacification of outer edge lens fibers that surround the nucleus of the lens, forming wedge-shaped streaks commonly referred to as *cortical spokes* that appear hyperreflective on AS-OCT (Fig. 11.2). Vision is more prone to be affected after the progressive extension of the opacity from the periphery to the center of the lens. Patients usually complain of glare, halos around lights, and difficulty driving at night. Common risk factors associated with cortical cataracts include older age, higher hemoglobin A1c, lower socioeconomic status, hypertension, and smoking.

C. Posterior Subcapsular Cataracts

Posterior subcapsular (PSC) cataracts arise in the posterior cortex of the lens after degeneration and posterior migration of lens epithelial cells. They are commonly associated with a younger population and cause a rapid decline in vision. PSC cataracts may cause photophobia, halos, glare, and diminished vision in bright lights. PSC cataracts can arise secondary to diabetes, hypertension, uveitis, intraocular gas, and extended corticosteroid usage. They demonstrate a focal area of hyperreflectivity on AS-OCT, along with posterior capsule thickening and vacuolization (Fig. 11.3).

D. Mature Cataracts

Mature cataracts, including white, hypermature, and intumescent cataracts, remain a universal surgical challenge, primarily because of increased intralenticular pressure. A variety of preoperative clinical signs have been described, such as the presence of intralenticular fluid clefts, to help surgeons identify which eyes are at a higher risk for capsular compromise, including unwanted post-equatorial anterior capsule extension ("Argentinian flag" phenomenon) as a result of increased intralenticular pressure. Preoperative AS-OCT can be used in these cases to identify high intralenticular pressure so that surgeons can perform appropriate maneuvers, such as closed chamber needle aspiration, to reduce unwanted surgical risks (Fig. 11.4). Several classification

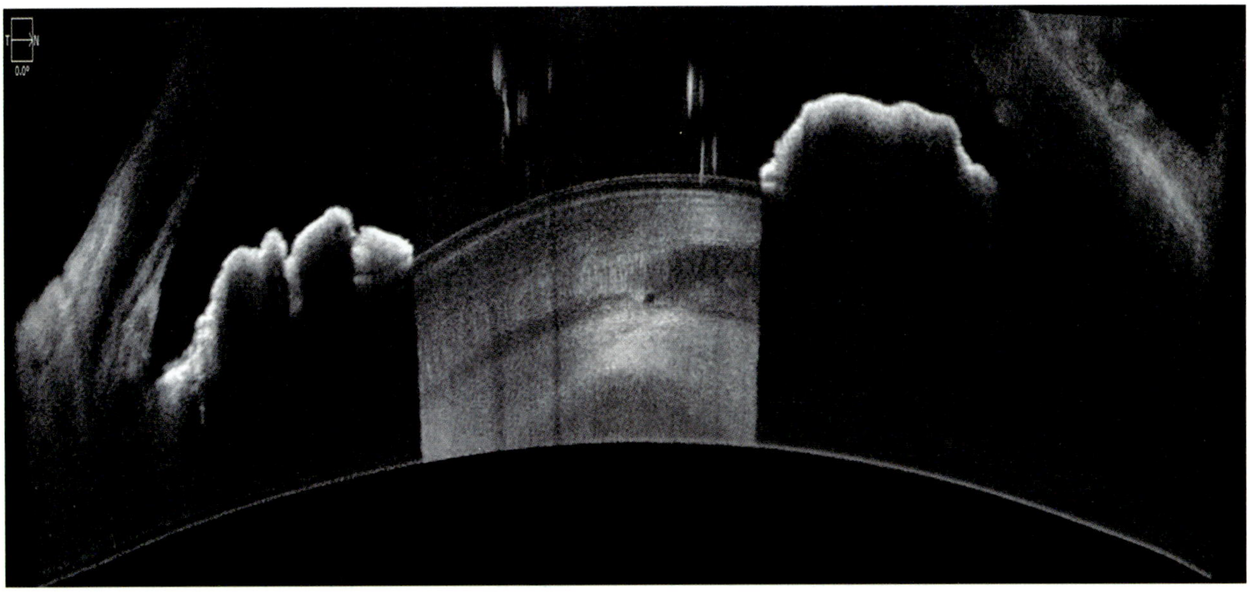

Fig. 11.1 A nuclear sclerotic cataract has areas of hyperreflectivity and hyporeflectivity on AS-OCT imaging. Note that only the lens's anterior half is visible in this frame with a single scan.

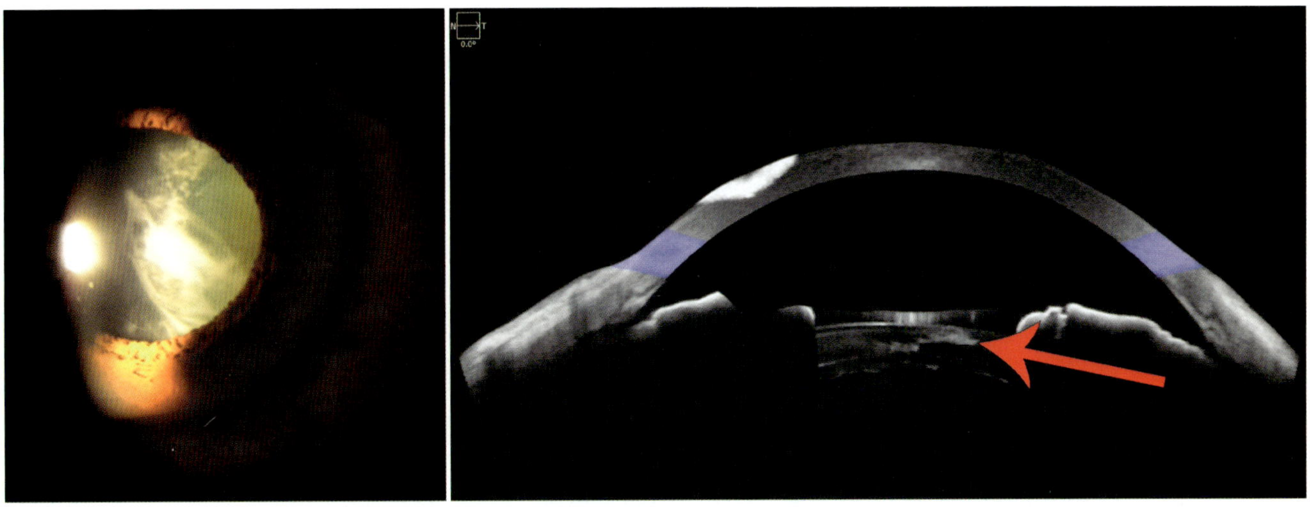

Fig. 11.2 Cortical cataracts are easily recognized by their wedge-shaped appearance on slit-lamp examination. AS-OCT can highlight the areas of cortical spoking, which appear as areas of intense hyperreflectivity *(arrow).*

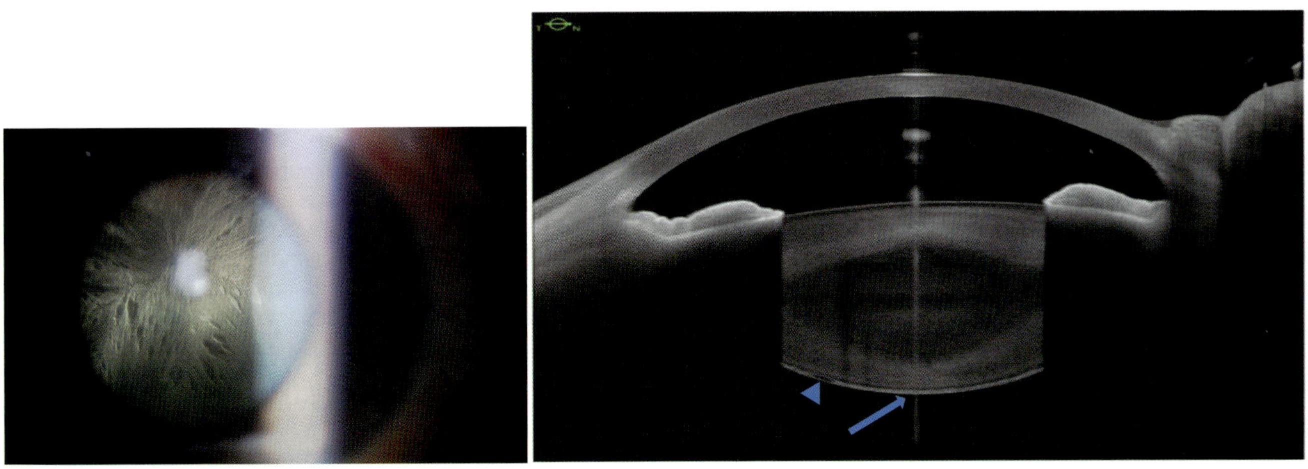

Fig. 11.3 Posterior subcapsular cataract. AS-OCT imaging of a posterior subcapsular cataract demonstrates posterior capsule thickening *(arrow)* along with areas of vacuolization *(arrowhead).* (Courtesy Hiroshi Enaida, MD, PhD, Department of Ophthalmology, Saga University, Saga, Japan.)

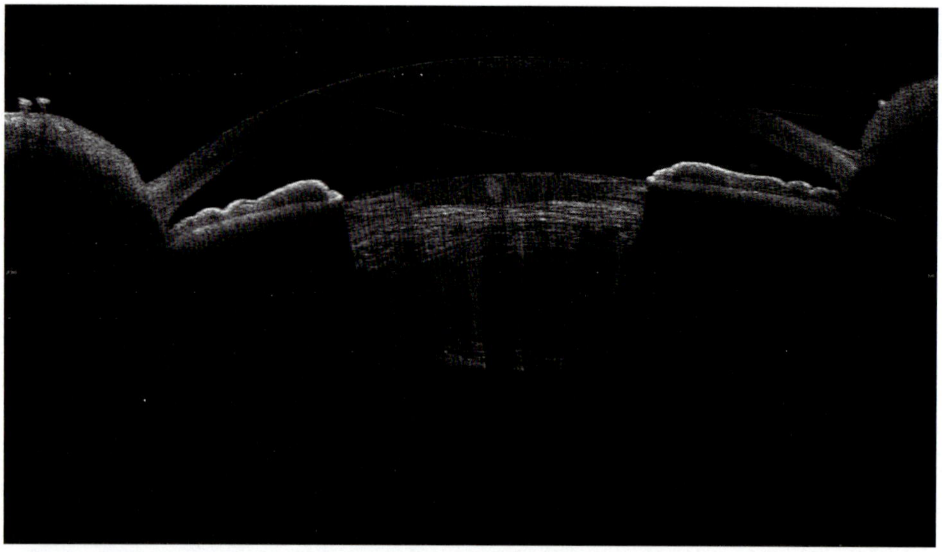

Fig. 11.4 AS-OCT image of a senile mature cataract shows the intumescent nature of the cataract with anteriorly accumulated liquified lens matter. There is evidence of increased intralenticular pressure. Intraoperative rhexis-related complications, such as rhexis extension, are high. Surgical maneuvers to decrease the risk for rhexis extension can be appropriately planned preoperatively. (Courtesy Amar Pujari, MD, Dr. Rajendra Prasad Centre for Ophthalmic Sciences, All India Institute of Medical Sciences [AIIMS], New Delhi, India.)

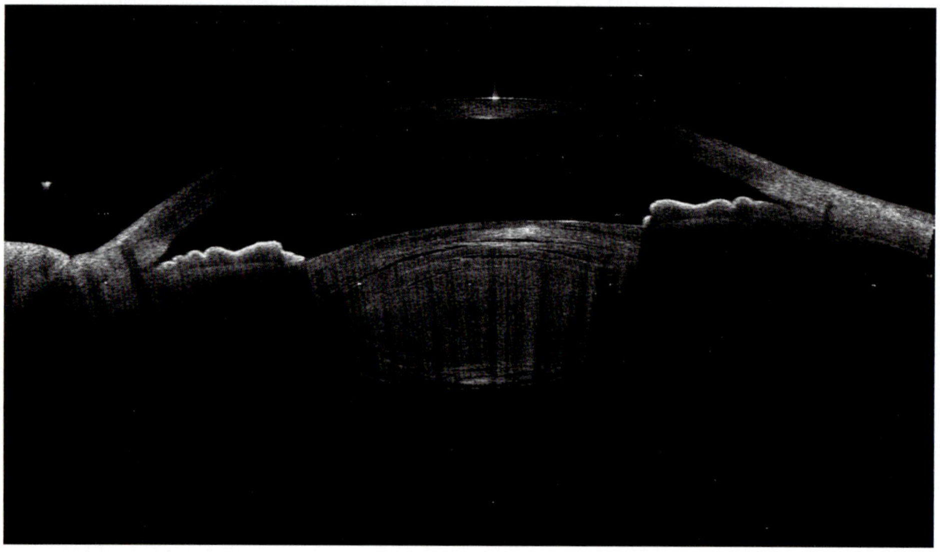

Fig. 11.5 AS-OCT of another senile mature cataract reveals the homogenously hyperintense lens matter. In addition, the lamellar separation along the anterior and posterior cortex can be visualized. However, there is no frank collection of liquified lens material here. While there are fewer risks related to rhexis extension, the lens will be hard to fragment, and appropriate surgical maneuvers, such as increased ultrasound energy, mechanical disassembly of the cataract, or planned extracapsular extraction, can be utilized. (Courtesy Amar Pujari, MD, Dr. Rajendra Prasad Centre for Ophthalmic Sciences, All India Institute of Medical Sciences [AIIMS], New Delhi, India.)

systems, including those by Pujari and Sharma, have been described in the literature. Increased areas of hyporeflectivity seen on AS-OCT represent areas of liquefaction and potentially increased intralenticular pressure.

CLINICAL PEARL

AS-OCT can be used preoperatively in cases of mature cataracts to assess the presence and extent of increased intralenticular pressure by identifying areas of hyporeflectivity within the lens. Surgeons can then exercise appropriate surgical maneuvers to decrease the risk of capsular compromise, including unwanted post-equatorial anterior capsule extension (Argentinian flag sign).

In another variant of mature cataract, lamellar separation and increased density of the nucleus and cortex can be appreciated both on slit-lamp and AS-OCT examination (Fig. 11.5). Of surgical importance, AS-OCT can demonstrate the lack of increased intralenticular pressure in these cataracts. Surgical removal of the cataract itself remains a separate challenge.

A rare complication associated with mature cataracts is phacomorphic glaucoma, in which the size of the cataract increases significantly, causing shallowing of the anterior chamber and secondary angle closure. AS-OCT can aid in visualizing the distended lens and obtaining measurements of the anterior chamber (Fig. 11.6). The information from AS-OCT can supplement the slit-lamp examination, gonioscopy,

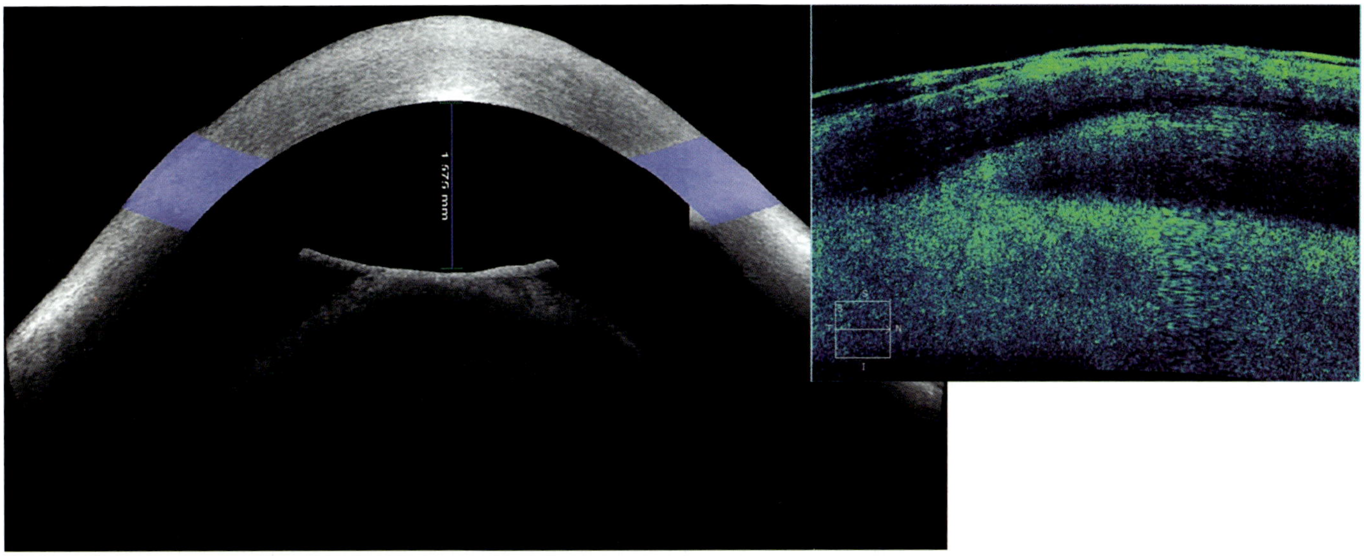

Fig. 11.6 Phacomorphic glaucoma. AS-OCT can be used to appreciate phacomorphic glaucoma, with distention of the lens capsule appearing as an exaggerated convexity in both swept-source AS-OCT and HD-OCT imaging. These types of cataracts are surgical emergencies that warrant urgent cataract removal for visual rehabilitation and intraocular pressure control.

and optical biometry measurements. For example, the anterior chamber depth (ACD) obtained on AS-OCT can be correlated with ACD measurements obtained by optical biometry. As another example, a cloudy cornea in some cases of phacomorphic glaucoma may make gonioscopy difficult; AS-OCT can better visualize and measure the size of the anterior chamber angle. Ultimately, phacomorphic glaucoma is a surgical emergency that warrants prompt cataract extraction for visual rehabilitation and control of intraocular pressure.

E. Subluxated Cataracts

Subluxated cataracts may occur both secondary to and independent of ocular trauma. These cataracts can have different appearances based on patient positioning. In the usual upright position, subluxated cataracts appear similar to intumescent and/or phacomorphic cataracts with features of increased lens convexity and anterior chamber shallowing. When the patient is supine, the cataract shifts posteriorly, and the anterior chamber expands considerably. In some cases, significant subluxation of the lens can cause secondary angle closure (Fig. 11.7). Because many of these cases are surgical emergencies, the amount of subluxation, including posterior shifting in the supine position, can help the surgeon preoperatively evaluate lens-zonular integrity and plan the surgical approach accordingly.

F. Traumatic Cataracts

High variability of lenticular changes may occur due to traumatic injury, including intralenticular and zonular changes. Historically, clinical examination was used with diagnostic imaging, such as ultrasound biomicroscopy (UBM), to visualize cataract changes, such as anterior/posterior capsule violation, and help guide surgical planning. AS-OCT may similarly be used with higher sensitivity for visualizing posterior capsule rupture compared with UBM (Fig. 11.8 and 11.9).

G. Posterior Polar Cataracts

Posterior polar cataracts (PPCs) are surgically challenging given the high incidence of concurrent posterior capsule deficiency and violation underlying the posterior opacity. The posterior capsule in PPCs may be fully intact, partially deficient, or lacking in these eyes. Clinical examination alone may be insufficient to fully assess and appreciate posterior capsule integrity. Several authors have previously reported using AS-OCT to enhance clinical examination findings with variable observations regarding the AS-OCT findings and encountered intraoperative pathologic issues. AS-OCT can be especially helpful in determining the presence of posterior capsule violation (Fig. 11.10) or its absence (Fig. 11.11). Pujari and Sharma have described the importance of both "capsule" and "contour" features of PPCs on AS-OCT to assess posterior capsule integrity better.

CLINICAL PEARL

AS-OCT can be used in cases of posterior polar cataracts (PPCs) to evaluate the integrity of the posterior capsule. As many PPCs may have concurrent posterior capsule violation (or even absence), preoperative imaging can help surgeons with surgical planning, including advanced planning for vitreous management or combined surgical case with a vitreoretinal surgeon. Therefore patients with PPCs can be appropriately counseled preoperatively about the level of risk with the proposed cataract surgery and the need for additional surgery based on these findings.

III. TYPES OF IMPLANTABLE LENSES

A. Phakic Intraocular Lens

Phakic IOLs (pIOLs) are indicated as an alternative to corneal refractive surgery, especially in cases of thin corneas, correction of pathologic myopia, moderate to severe ocular surface disease, large mesopic-scotopic pupil size, and corneal disease in which laser refractive surgery incurs undesirable risks (e.g., forme-fruste corneal ectatic disease, corneal scarring, and such). pIOLs are most commonly used for patients with high refractive errors because these patients take longer to recover visually, have poor refractive predictability, and have a higher risk of developing corneal ectasia after laser refractive surgery. pIOLs offer a reversible treatment that avoids alteration of the cornea and is not limited by the patient's corneal thickness

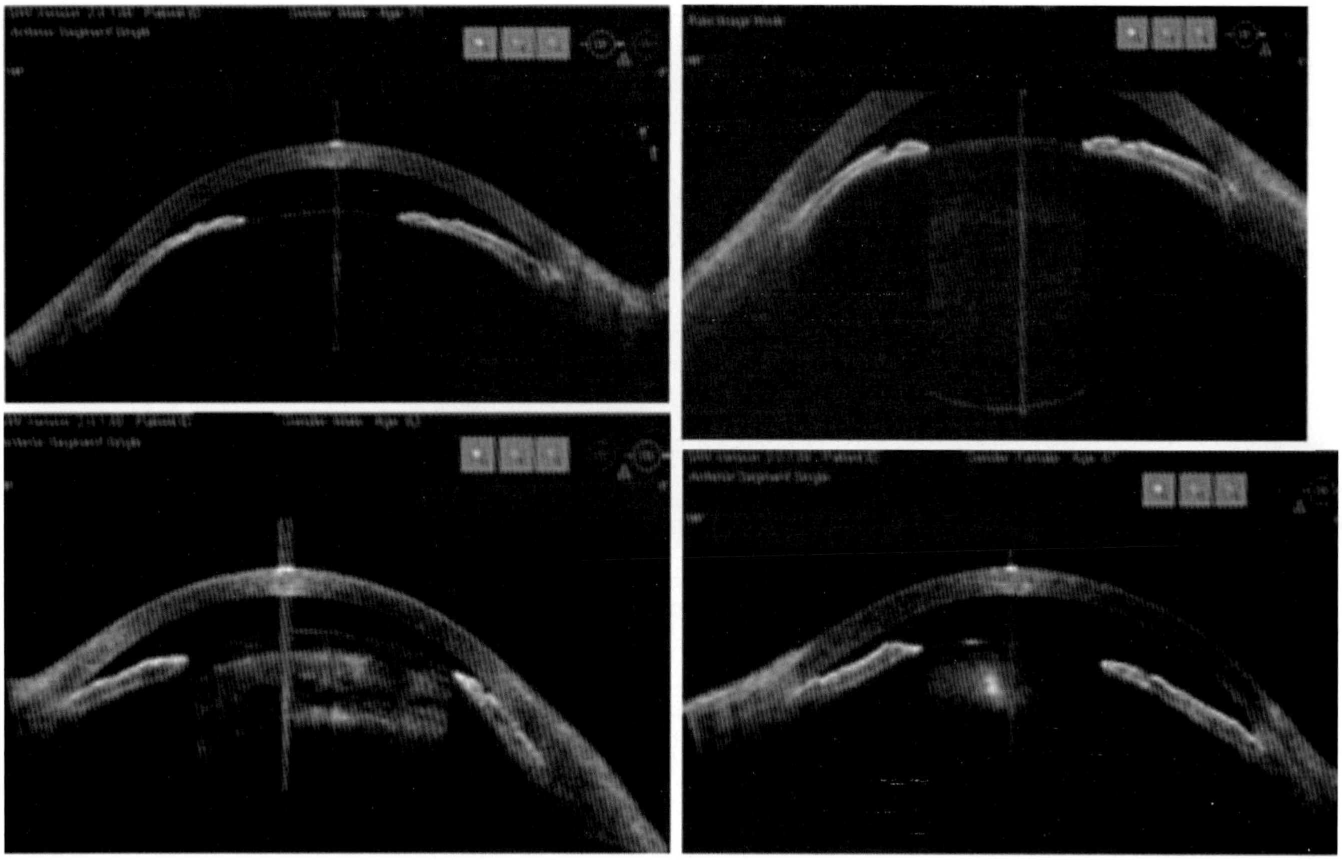

Fig. 11.7 In severe cases of subluxated cataracts, secondary angle closure may occur. Prompt surgical intervention may be required, including peripheral iridotomy or lens extraction.

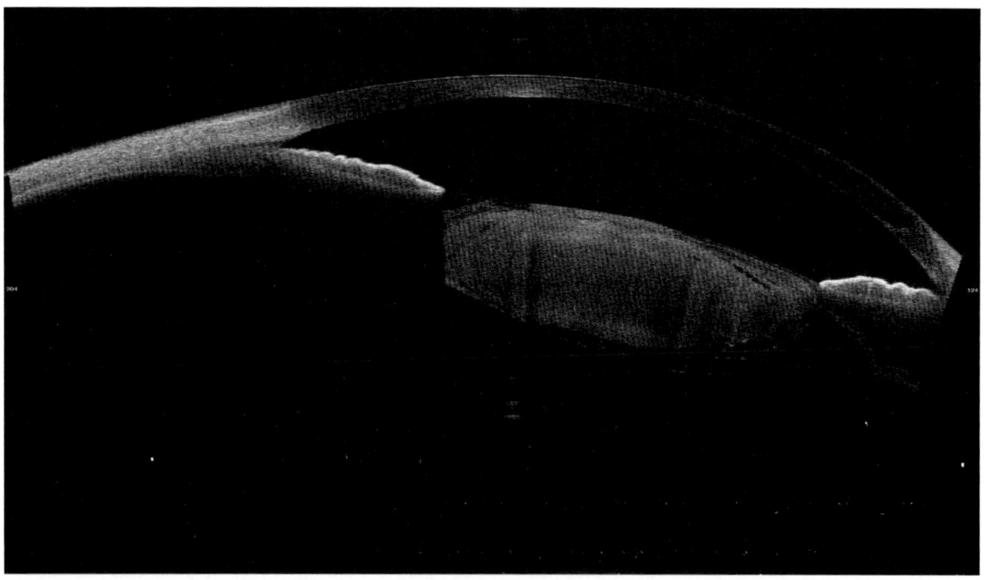

Fig. 11.8 AS-OCT of a posttraumatic cataract demonstrates a partially absorbed lens. The posterior capsule is intact, and the lens is homogenously opaque with a collection of liquefied material along the anterior and posterior capsules. (Courtesy Amar Pujari, MD, Dr. Rajendra Prasad Centre for Ophthalmic Sciences, All India Institute of Medical Sciences [AIIMS], New Delhi, India.)

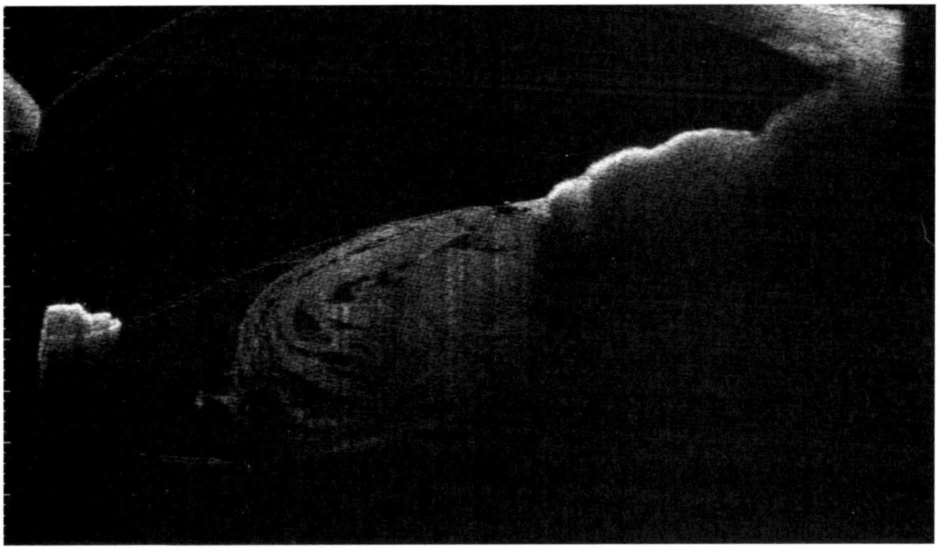

Fig. 11.9 AS-OCT of another traumatic cataract highlights distorted lens anatomy with a large proportion of liquefied lens material. Additionally, the lens shows prominent intralenticular cavitations with an eccentric collection of residual lens material. The posterior capsule appears to be intact. (Courtesy Amar Pujari, MD, Dr. Rajendra Prasad Centre for Ophthalmic Sciences, All India Institute of Medical Sciences [AIIMS], New Delhi, India.)

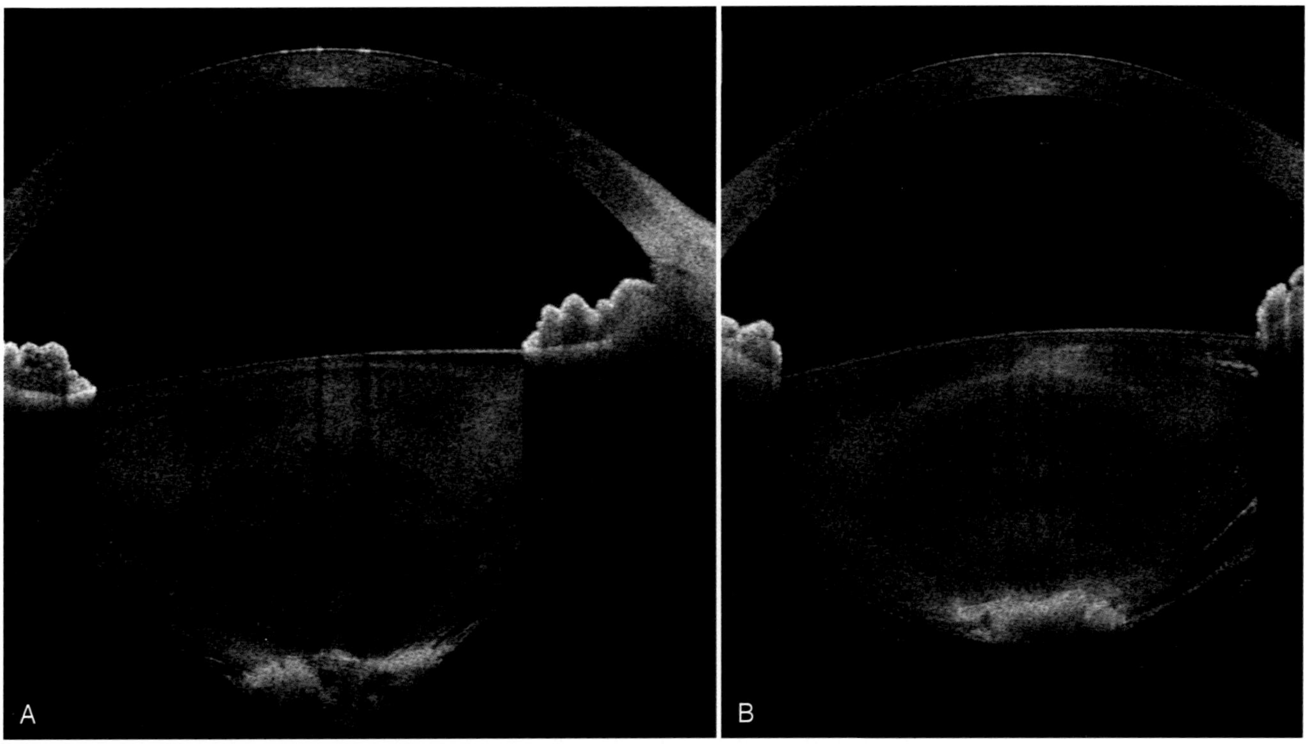

Fig. 11.10 AS-OCT of a posterior polar cataract (PPC). *Panel A* demonstrates dehiscence of the posterior capsule immediately beneath the opacity with an associated herniation of lens material into the anterior vitreous space. This deficient morphology resembles a cone shape with posterior bowing toward the vitreous space. In *panel B,* this PPC demonstrates a deficient posterior capsule beneath the lens opacity with an excavation anteriorly into the posterior lens substance, opposite of the conical morphology seen in *panel A*. This morphology demonstrates a moth-eaten–like configuration. The surgical approach for both cases should include appropriate planning for vitreous management during cataract surgery because of the posterior capsule deficiency and/or dehiscence. (Courtesy Amar Pujari, MD, Dr. Rajendra Prasad Centre for Ophthalmic Sciences, All India Institute of Medical Sciences [AIIMS], New Delhi, India.)

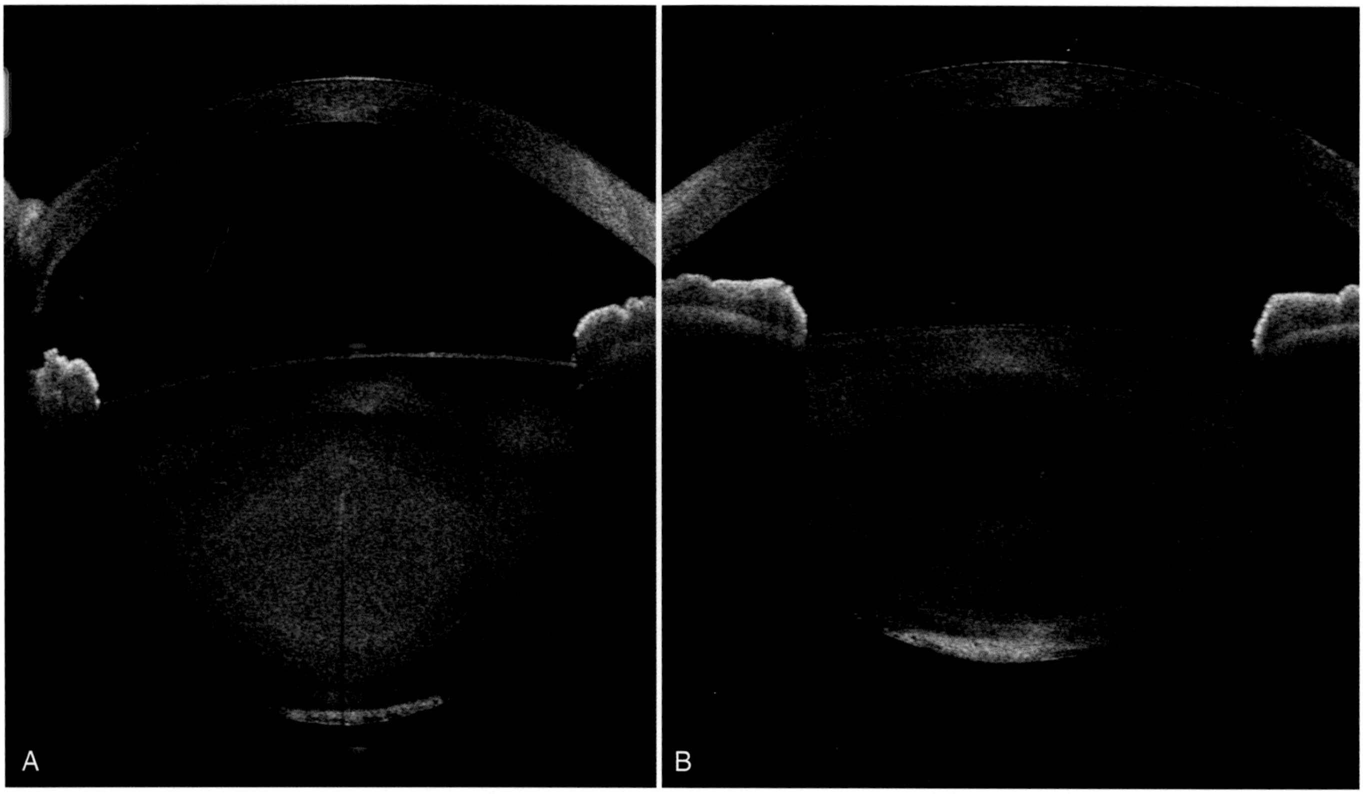

Fig. 11.11 AS-OCT of a posterior polar cataract (PPC). *Panel A* reveals an intact posterior capsule. Between the opacity and the posterior capsule, there are multiple hypoechoic or echolucent areas present. These spaces are likely to help with easier separation of the posterior opacity intraoperatively during hydrodissection. There is a low risk for vitreous prolapse in this case. In *panel B,* this PPC again demonstrates an intact posterior capsule. However, there are no appreciable hypoechoic or echolucent areas between the opacity and the posterior capsule, as seen in *panel A.* This appearance may cause variable difficulty separating the last fragment from the capsule. Vitreous management may be necessary in this case. (Courtesy Amar Pujari, MD, Dr. Rajendra Prasad Centre for Ophthalmic Sciences, All India Institute of Medical Sciences [AIIMS], New Delhi, India.)

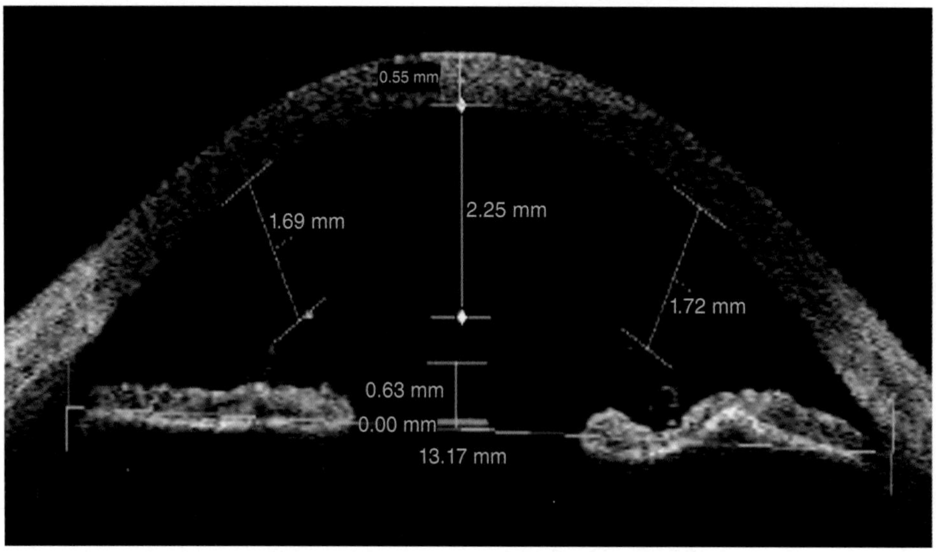

Fig. 11.12 Appearance of a well-placed iris-claw lens on AS-OCT. (Courtesy Helena P. Filipe, MD, Universidade de Lisboa, Lisboa, Portugal.)

status. Commonly encountered pIOLs include iris-claw pIOLs (Fig. 11.12), angle-supported pIOLs, implantable collamer lenses (ICLs), and toric variants of each.

Candidacy for pIOL during the preoperative examination requires several important anatomic measurements, including but not limited to ACD greater than 3.0 mm, anterior chamber angle of grade 3 or greater, and endothelial cell density requirements (variable with age). Along with corneal topography and tomography, AS-OCT can be used preoperatively for quantifying ACD and anterior chamber angle values to identify appropriate candidates and screen out poor surgical candidates.

In the United States, collamer ICLs (Staar Surgical, Monrovia, California, United States) are the only posterior chamber phakic IOL approved by the US Food and Drug Administration to treat myopia. A key component of surgical success is the space ("vault") between the posterior surface of the pIOL and the anterior surface of the crystalline lens. An acceptable pIOL vault is between 250 and 750 μm, or around 100% of the corneal thickness, for which AS-OCT can be helpful to evaluate and quantify (Fig. 11.13). Patients with a low vault have a greater risk of developing lens opacifications postoperatively, typically the anterior subcapsular subtype (anterior subcapsular cataract) (Fig. 11.14). This occurs due to chronic mechanical trauma between the pIOL and the crystalline lens. On the other hand, patients with a high vault may have an increased risk for corneal endothelial cell loss and pupillary block glaucoma (Fig. 11.15). The creation of peripheral iridotomies before an ICL implant can help minimize the risk for pupillary block. AS-OCT also can be used for serial monitoring in patients with suboptimal vaulting to help guide decision-making for continued observation or removal of the pIOL.

CLINICAL PEARL

AS-OCT can be used for serial monitoring in phakic IOL (pIOL) patients with suboptimal vaulting. For example, if a patient demonstrates progressive narrowing of pIOL vaulting with increasing ASC opacity, the clinician may recommend removal of the pIOL before the development of visually significant cataract and/or pupillary block. Similarly, a progressively increasing vault may help guide the surgeon to recommend the removal of the pIOL to avoid endothelial cell damage and secondary angle closure.

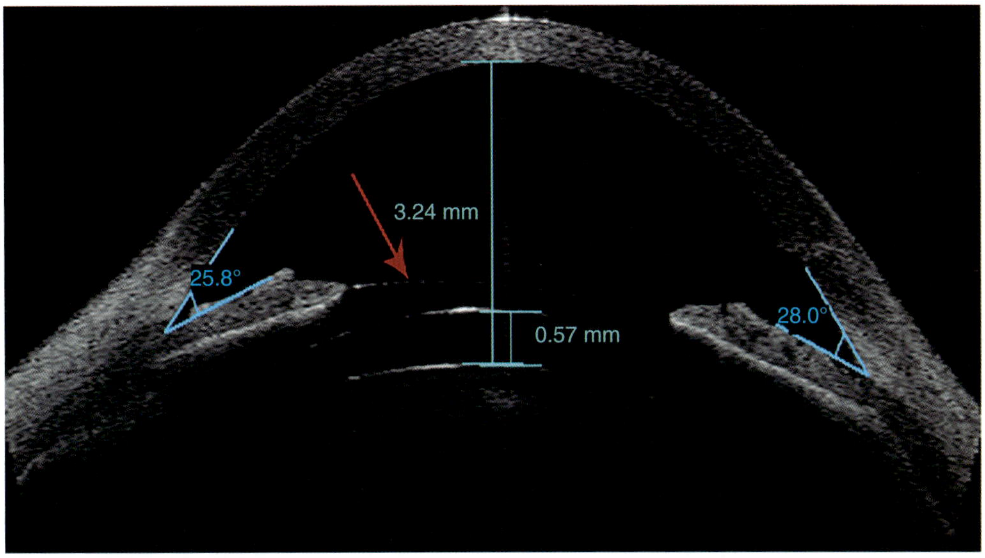

Fig. 11.13 AS-OCT can be used to assess the location of phakic intraocular lenses (pIOLs) after placement. The *red arrow* indicates the anterior aspect of the pIOL. The caliper measurement feature can be used to quantify the distance between the pIOL and the anterior lens capsule, as well as the anterior chamber angle. The vault in this patient is approximately 570 microns, indicating an appropriate space between the posterior surface of the pIOL and the anterior surface of the crystalline lens. (Courtesy Kraig Bower, MD, Wilmer Eye Institute, Baltimore, Maryland, United States.)

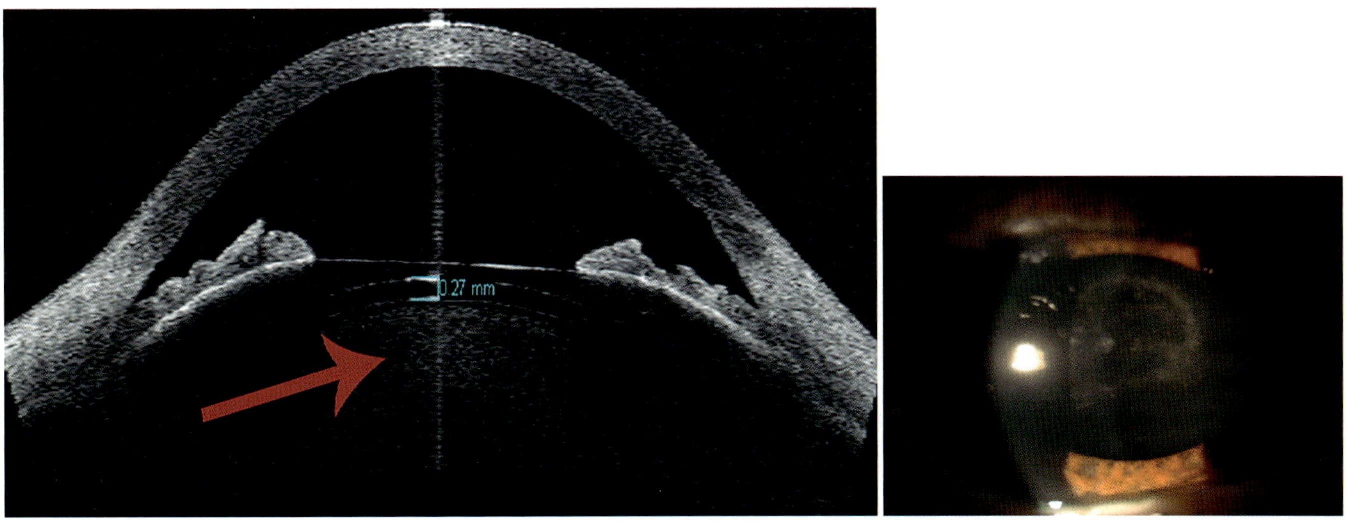

Fig. 11.14 Low vault with anterior subcapsular cataract formation with implantable collamer lens. In this patient, AS-OCT can be used to measure less-than-ideal vaulting of approximately 270 microns between the phakic intraocular lens and the anterior capsule of the crystalline lens. An anterior subcapsular cataract is also seen as an area of increased hyperreflectivity in the anterior aspect of the crystalline lens *(arrow)*, confirming the lens changes seen on slit-lamp examination. (Courtesy Kraig Bower, MD, Wilmer Eye Institute, Baltimore, Maryland, United States.)

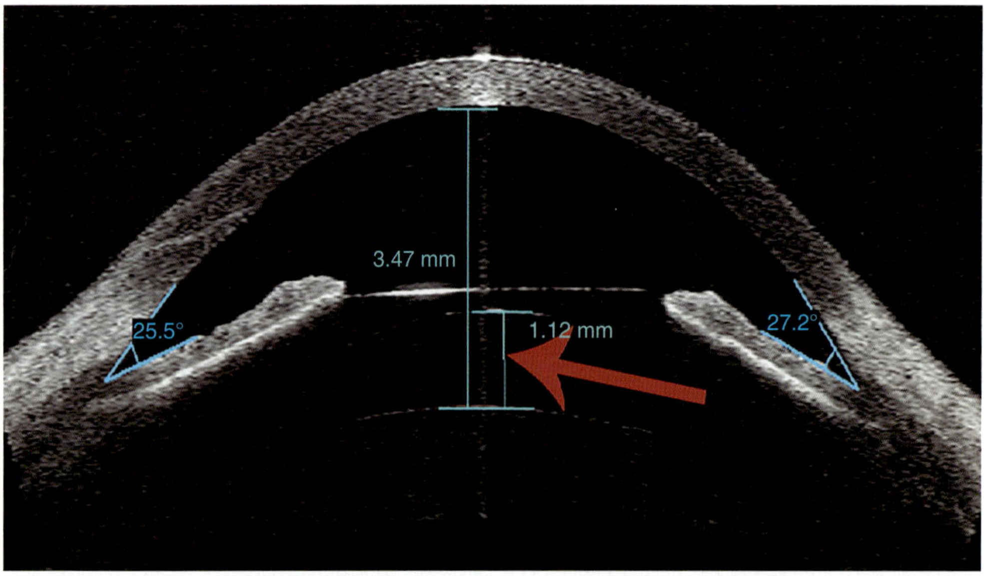

Fig. 11.15 Implantable collamer lens (ICL) with undesirable high vault. AS-OCT demonstrates an extremely high vault (approximately 1120 microns) between the ICL and the anterior lens capsule *(arrow)*. In such eyes, the effective anterior chamber depth is decreased, thereby increasing the risk for secondary angle closure, increased intraocular pressure, and endothelial cell loss. (Courtesy Kraig Bower, MD, Wilmer Eye Institute, Baltimore, Maryland, United States.)

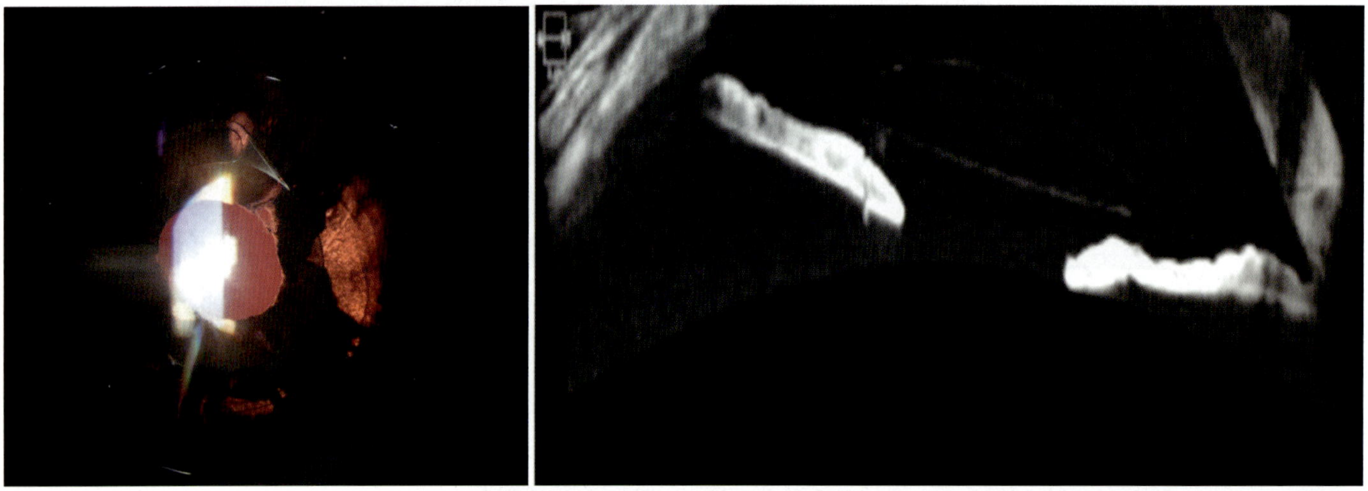

Fig. 11.16 Appearance of anterior chamber intraocular lens (ACIOL). The slit-lamp photograph shows a well-centered ACIOL in the presence of multiple iris defects secondary to complicated surgery. On AS-OCT, the convex-plano shape of the ACIOL is observed anterior to the iris.

B. Pseudophakic Intraoperative Lens

Most surgeons will place the IOL in the capsular bag during routine cataract surgery because this is the most physiologic and stable position. Although the clinical examination is usually sufficient to confirm the proper location of the IOL, ancillary imaging, such as UBM and AS-OCT, can be used to visualize IOL centration and planarity in certain cases. The previously described technique for using a 20D lens affixed to a posterior segment OCT device may be necessary to improve the visualization of the deeper lens-zonule-capsule structures.

In complex cases where anterior capsular support is unsatisfactory or deficient, placement of the IOL in a location other than the intracapsular space, such as the sulcus or anterior chamber, may be necessary. Various techniques for IOL fixation in cases of aphakia, such as iris fixation and scleral fixation (both with and without sutures), have been described. Anterior chamber IOLs (ACIOLs) also can be considered for such eyes. They may be a reasonable option, especially with carefully measured placement, and for surgeons who lack experience with IOL fixation techniques (Fig. 11.16). Complications of ACIOL implants include uveitis-glaucoma-hyphema (UGH) syndrome, increased intraocular pressure (IOP), macular edema, and pseudophakic bullous keratopathy (PBK).

For patients with aphakia, scleral-fixated IOL (SFIOL) surgery has recently become a popular method for ACIOL placement. SFIOL fixation can be performed in several ways, including suture-fixation, glue-assisted techniques, and transconjunctival intrascleral haptic fixation (Yamane technique). SFIOL surgery avoids surgical manipulation of the iris, a highly vascularized tissue unsuitable for long-term device fixation.

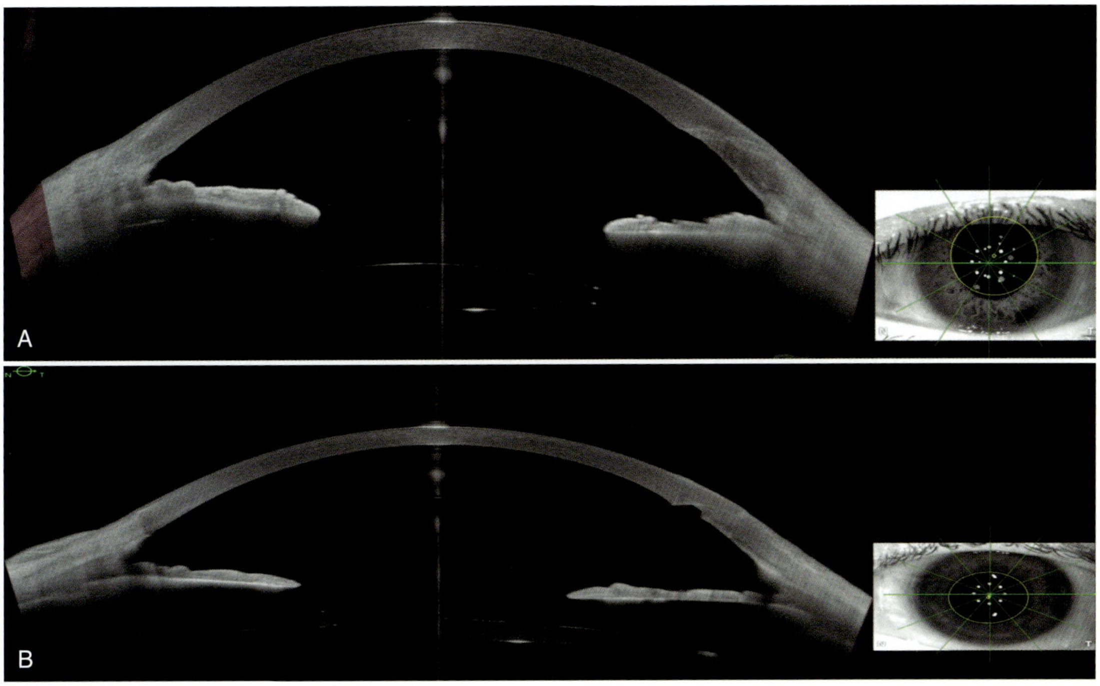

Fig. 11.17 AS-OCT can assess the position, decentration, and tilt of scleral-fixated IOLs (SFIOLs). *Panel A* demonstrates an SFIOL with good centration and minimal tilt. *Panel B* demonstrates an SFIOL with slight decentration and mild tilt. (Courtesy Matthew Ohr, MD, and Mairghread Casey, MD, Ohio State University, Columbus, Ohio, United States.)

AS-OCT also can be used to evaluate SFIOLs to assess centration and tilt with accuracy similar to that of UBM. Fig. 11.17 demonstrates an SFIOL with good centration and minimal tilt *(panel A)* contrasted with an SFIOL with mild to moderate tilt *(panel B)*. In Fig. 11.18, AS-OCT can help visualize a decentered Gore-Tex suture–fixated eyelet-haptic IOL (Envista, Bausch and Lomb, Tampa, Florida, United States). Clinicians can use this information to determine a course of treatment.

C. Iris-Clip Intraoperative Lens

Although mainly of historical relevance, various early-model IOLs were introduced between 1950 and 1970. Several anterior chamber and pupil-supported IOLs, such as the Choyce Mark VIII and Mark IX, were among the earliest IOLs used after cataract surgery. Although innovative, these early IOLs had numerous problems, including UGH syndrome, PBK, and IOL dislocation.

Iris-clip IOLs used haptics to encircle or ensnare the iris anteriorly and posteriorly. Interestingly, these early iris-clip IOLs used metallic haptics, contributing to many postoperative problems. These types of IOLs included the Binkhorst, Worst, and Fyodorov (aptly named the "Sputnik IOL" due to its appearance resembling the historically famous satellite). In modern ophthalmic practice, these iris-clip IOLs may be decreasingly encountered over time.

The Binkhorst IOL had a design involving a pair of horseshoe-shaped haptics that clipped the iris anterior and posteriorly in a "paperclip" manner. Because of this configuration, the Binkhorst IOL was prone to anterior or posterior dislocation after pupil dilation. Thus it is vital never to dilate the eyes of these patients if encountered clinically. These patients were often placed on chronic miotic agents to prevent this complication. On AS-OCT imaging (Fig. 11.19), this IOL can be seen with its optic anterior to the iris. Even with the anterior segment lens attachment, the metallic clip-style haptics are barely noticeable.

IV. POSTOPERATIVE COMPLICATIONS OF CATARACT SURGERY

Although complication rates after cataract surgery have been significantly reduced in recent years, possible complications include posterior capsule opacification (PCO), IOL dislocation, anterior capsule phimosis, and capsular block syndrome. Features of these conditions on AS-OCT are noted in the following section.

A. Posterior Capsule Opacification

PCO is the most common complication after cataract surgery, with incidence rates between 5% and 50%. It frequently arises due to the proliferation of lens epithelial cells at the anterior lens capsule that eventually infiltrate the posterior capsule and induce secondary vision loss. Clinical examination, especially with dilation, is usually sufficient to detect PCO; on AS-OCT, PCO appears as an area of hyperreflectivity immediately posterior to the IOL optic (Fig. 11.20).

In some instances, a robust PCO can form years later if a significant amount of cortex is not removed during the initial cataract surgery. In Fig. 11.21, the patient presented with progressive vision loss after cataract surgery 10 years previously. The PCO is readily observed on the slit-lamp examination; on AS-OCT, the residual cortex can be observed with a profound expansion of the intact posterior capsule.

Creating a posterior capsulotomy with a neodymium-doped yttrium aluminum garnet (Nd:YAG) laser is the preferred treatment of choice for visually significant PCO but carries infrequent risks with it, such as retinal detachment, cystoid macular edema, and floaters. AS-OCT can be used to demonstrate improved clarity of the posterior aspect of the IOL optic after a successful YAG capsulotomy (Fig. 11.22).

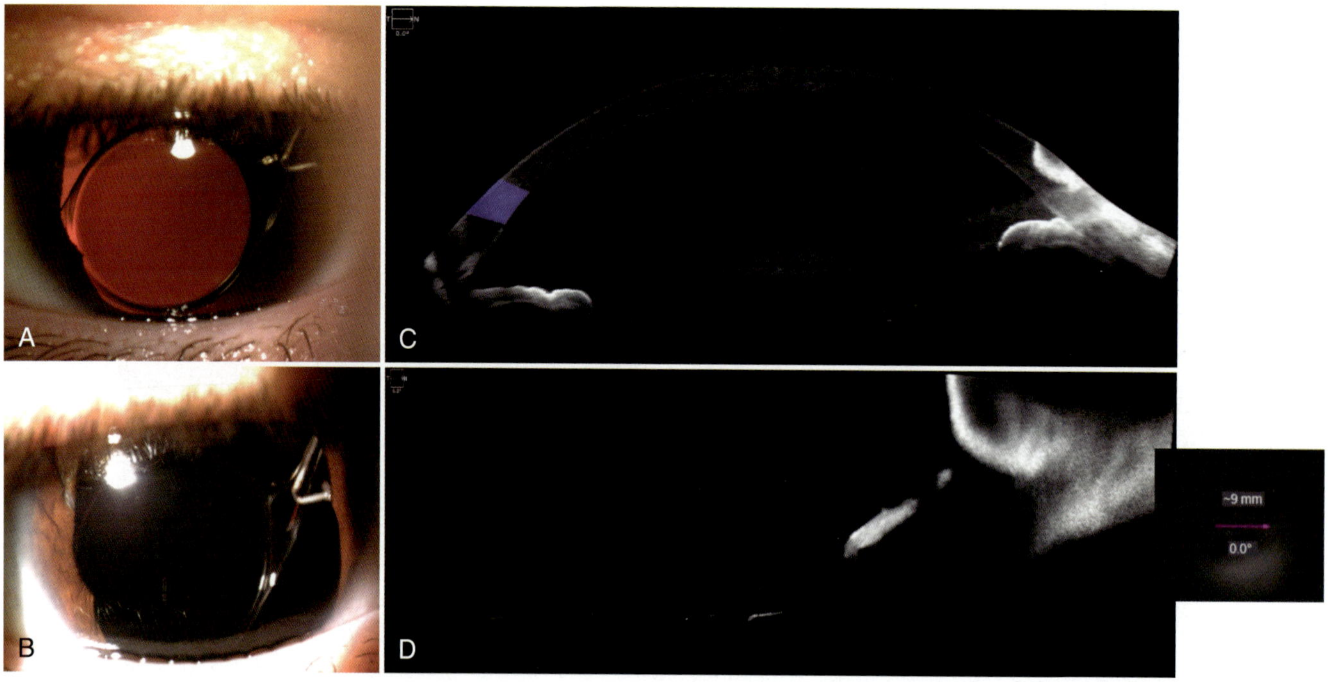

Fig. 11.18 Decentration of scleral-fixated intraocular lens (SFIOL). Slit-lamp photographs *(panels A and B)* demonstrate Gore-Tex suture looping through the eyelet of a single-piece acrylic IOL (Envista, Bausch and Lomb, Tampa, Florida, United States) used for SFIOL surgery. The SFIOL is temporally decentered. AS-OCT *(panel C)* shows the temporally decentered IOL. Gore-Tex suture is seen looped through the eyelet of the IOL in a higher magnification view *(panel D)* on AS-OCT.

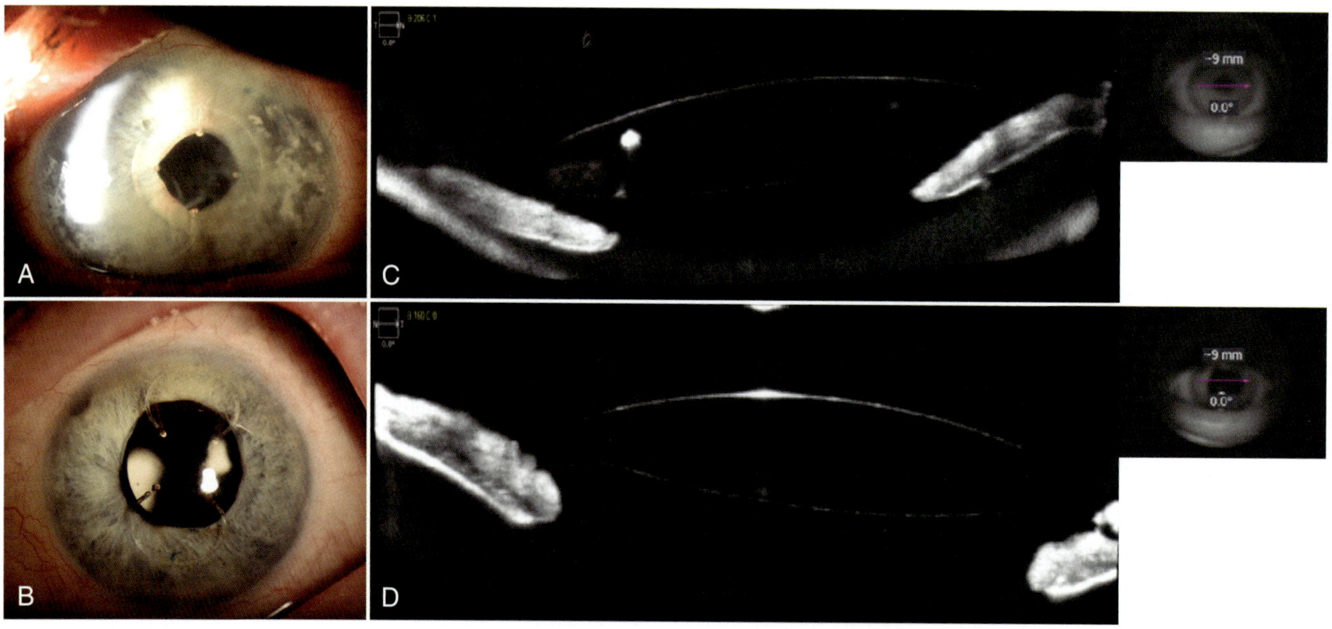

Fig. 11.19 Binkhorst iris-clip intraocular lens (IOL). Slit-lamp images of the right eye *(panel A)* and left eye *(panel B)* demonstrate the optic of the IOL anterior to the iris, along with the two anterior horseshoe-haptics clipping the IOL. The two posterior horseshoe haptics are not visible in the image. Of note, the right eye had long-standing chronic inflammation secondary to retinal detachment after the iris-clip placement, which led to glaucoma and band keratopathy, the latter of which is noticeable in the cornea of the right eye and obscuring some details of the IOL and the haptics. AS-OCT images of the right *eye (panel C)* and left eye *(panel D)* show the optic anterior to the iris. Other than a prominent reflection noted in *panel C*, the metallic haptics are unremarkable.

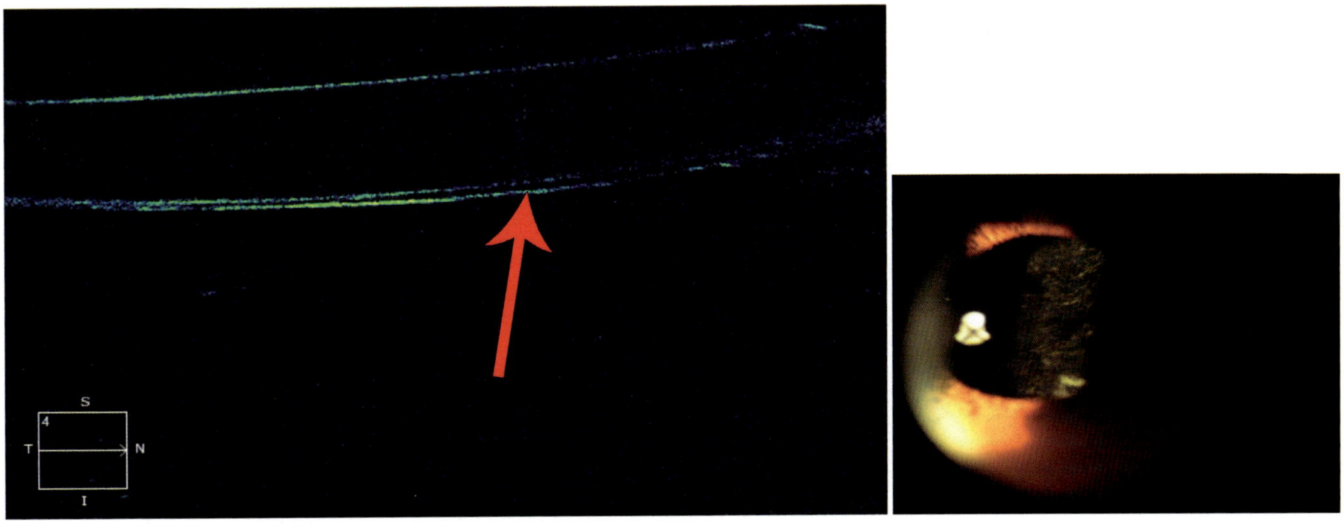

Fig. 11.20 Posterior capsule opacification (PCO). Although the clinical examination is usually sufficient to confirm proper intraocular lens (IOL) placement and the presence of PCO, AS-OCT can identify IOL components and the presence of an intact capsule. PCO can be appreciated as an area of increased hyperreflectivity immediately posterior to the IOL *(arrow)*.

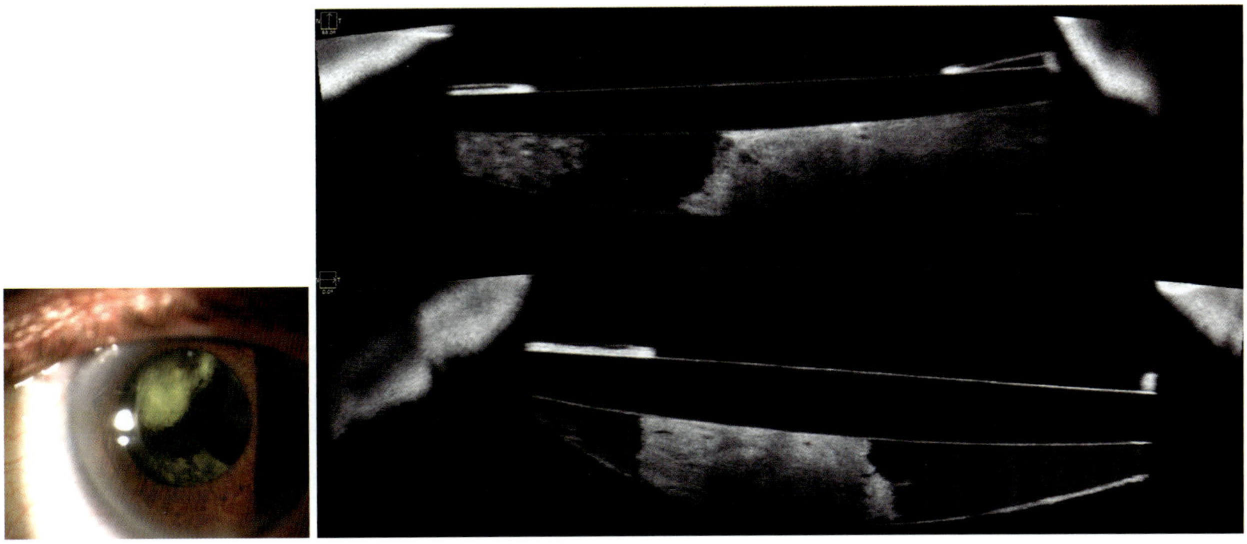

Fig. 11.21 Retained cortex at the time of initial cataract surgery. The retained cortex can cause significant PCO with associated capsular distention. AS-OCT delineates the area of PCO admixed with retained cortex posterior to the intraocular lens.

B. Malpositioned Intraocular Lens

Malpositioned IOLs, including intracapsular, sulcus, and iris/scleral-fixated IOLs, can be grouped into three categories (see Figs. 11.17 and 11.18):

- IOL shift (or IOL displacement): a longitudinal shift of the IOL, either away from or toward the cornea. This is the most important of the malpositioned IOL errors and mainly causes a hyperopic or myopic shift respectively.
- IOL decentration: a lateral shift of the IOL perpendicular to the line of sight (visual axis).
- IOL tilt: a rotational tilt of the IOL around the line of sight (visual axis).

The latter two unwanted IOL positions can induce undesirable spherical and cylindrical refractive errors. In many cases, the clinical examination is equivocal and may be compounded by poor visualization due to concomitant pathologic conditions, such as corneal edema and poor dilation. Diagnostic imaging, such as UBM and AS-OCT, can visualize IOL position better and help the clinician decide whether conservative management is sufficient or surgical intervention is needed. For example, if a patient with a single-piece IOL with square edges presents with recurrent UGH syndrome, AS-OCT may help determine if a displaced or tilted IOL is causing mechanical iris chafing. In such cases, surgical removal of the IOL is recommended with the placement of a rounded-edge three-piece IOL or other IOL fixation strategy.

CLINICAL PEARL

Several innovative surgical techniques have been introduced for the scleral fixation of IOLs in eyes without capsular support. One possible limitation of these techniques is the potential for undesirable IOL tilt and decentration that can induce significant spherical and astigmatic refractive errors postoperatively. Although assessment of IOL decentration can be easily detected on slit-lamp examination, IOL tilt may be harder to detect. Imaging such as AS-OCT or UBM can help identify and quantify the decentration or tilt in cases with unexpected postoperative refractive errors.

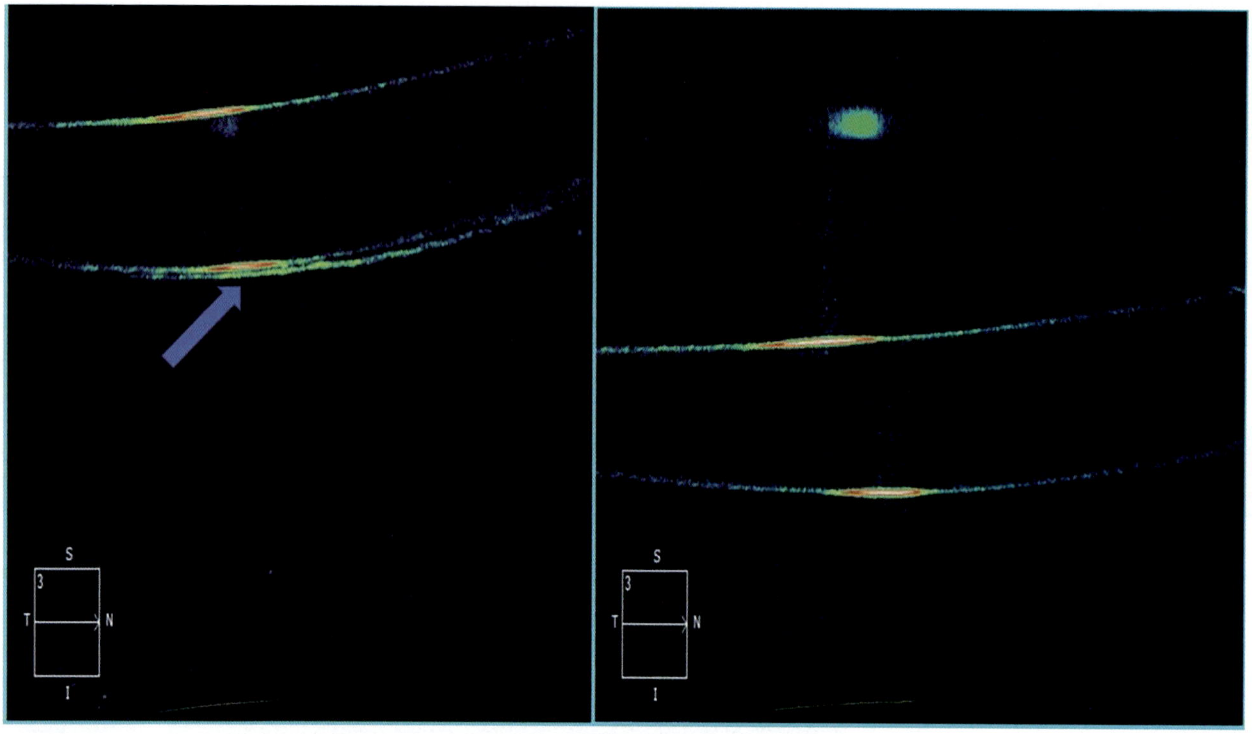

Fig. 11.22 Posterior capsule opacification (PCO). In most cases, PCO is readily detectable on clinical examination, especially on postdilation slit-lamp examination of the intraocular lens (IOL)-capsular bag complex. The PCO *(left panel)* on AS-OCT is seen as a dense, hyperreflective area immediately posterior to the IOL *(blue arrow)*. After YAG capsulotomy *(right panel)*, the PCO is no longer present, and only the reflectivity of the IOL remains.

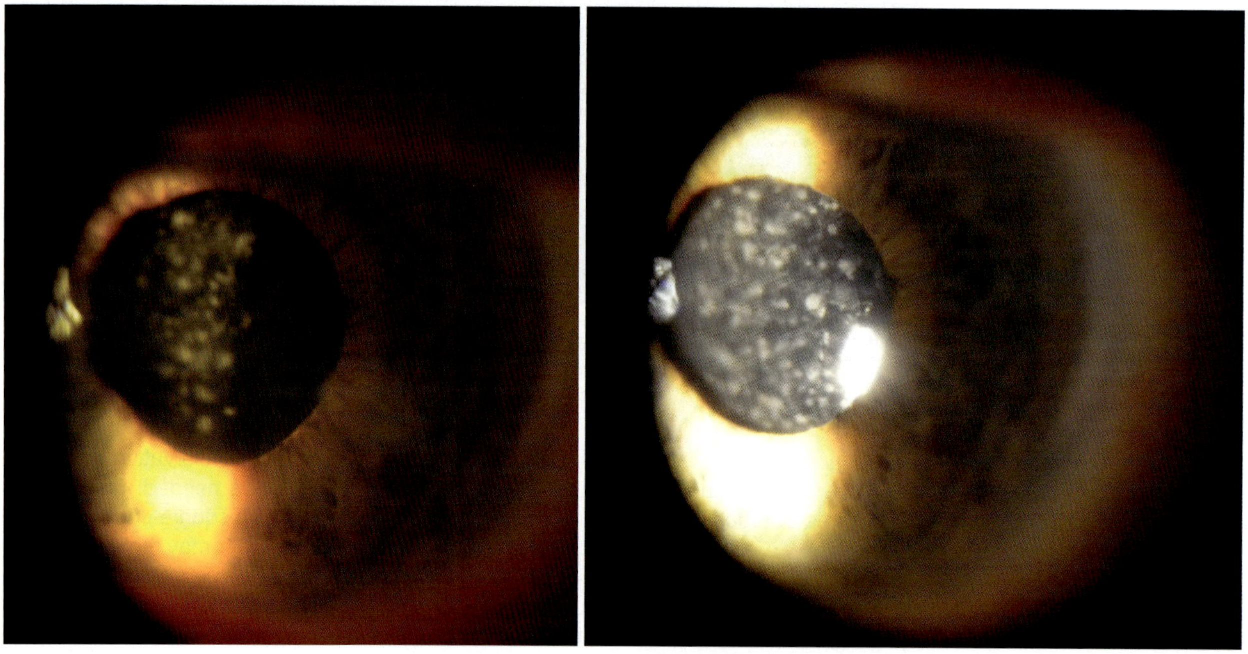

Fig. 11.23 Slit-lamp photographs of mild to moderate anterior capsule debris *(left panel)* and moderate debris with associated anterior capsule opacification *(right panel)*.

C. Anterior Capsule Debris and Opacification

Prolonged or excessive postoperative inflammation, such as in cases of dense cataracts and concurrent uveitis, may lead to an accumulation of inflammatory deposits on the anterior optic (Figs. 11.23 and 11.24). The majority of these have a negligible effect on visual acuity. In rare cases, YAG removal of these deposits or IOL exchange may be necessary.

D. Anterior Capsule Phimosis

Anterior capsular phimosis may occur in cases in which postoperative inflammation, fibrosis, and subsequent contraction, especially in the presence of a small capsulorhexis, can encroach and negatively affect the visual axis (Fig. 11.25). Although the clinical examination is usually sufficient to diagnose this condition, AS-OCT can highlight the extent of the

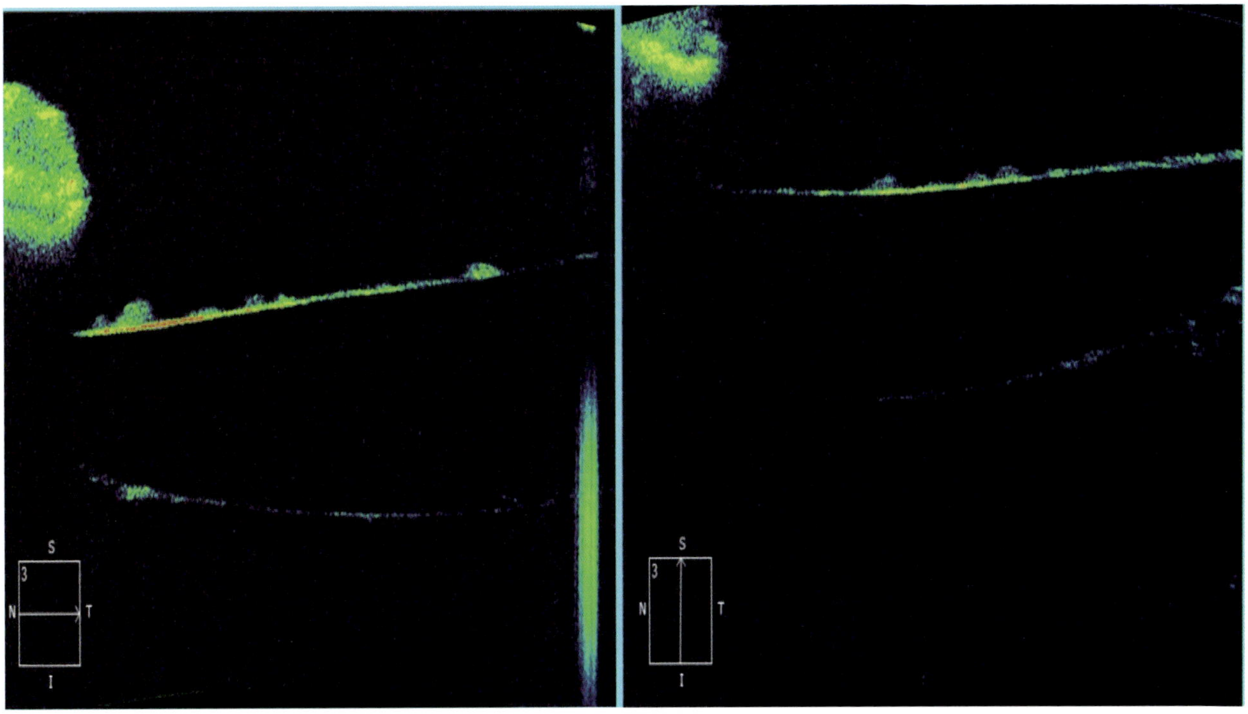

Fig. 11.24 AS-OCT images of anterior capsule debris in horizontal view *(left panel)* and vertical view *(right panel).*

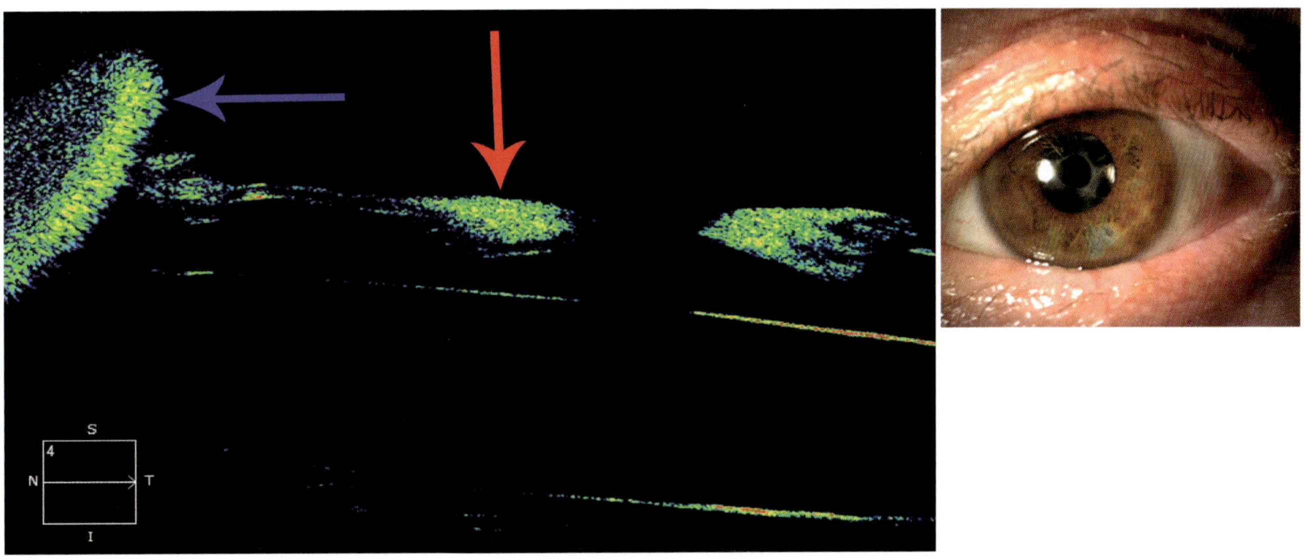

Fig. 11.25 AS-OCT image of anterior capsule phimosis. The iris is indicated with a *blue arrow.* The *red arrow* indicates the area of fibrotic contraction of the anterior capsule remnants.

phimotic changes, including the integrity of surrounding structures such as the iris, zonules, and ciliary body. This information may help guide surgeons toward continued observation or surgical intervention. Long-term anterior capsular phimosis can cause zonular laxity or dehiscence, which may cause IOL mispositioning. Risk factors associated with anterior capsular phimosis include a small diameter capsulorhexis, uveitis, zonular weakness or laxity, pseudoexfoliation syndrome, and advanced age.

E. Capsular Block Syndrome

Capsular block syndrome (CBS) can occur after cataract surgery. Classically, CBS is due to a small (<4 mm) capsulorhexis in the presence of retained viscoelastic material. This likely creates an osmotic gradient that draws fluid into the normally minuscule space between the posterior IOL optic and the posterior capsule. With circumferential adherence between the anterior capsule and the anterior IOL optic, fluid accumulates in this space. This pushes the IOL forward, causing a myopic shift, increased IOP, and low-grade inflammation.

Slit-lamp examination characteristically demonstrates a small rhexis such that its edges may be visible even in an undilated pupil. A thin-slit technique may help the examiner visualize a milky, turbid fluid behind the IOL, along with a notable gap between the posterior optic and posterior capsule. The IOL may appear to be highly luminescent with distention of the capsular

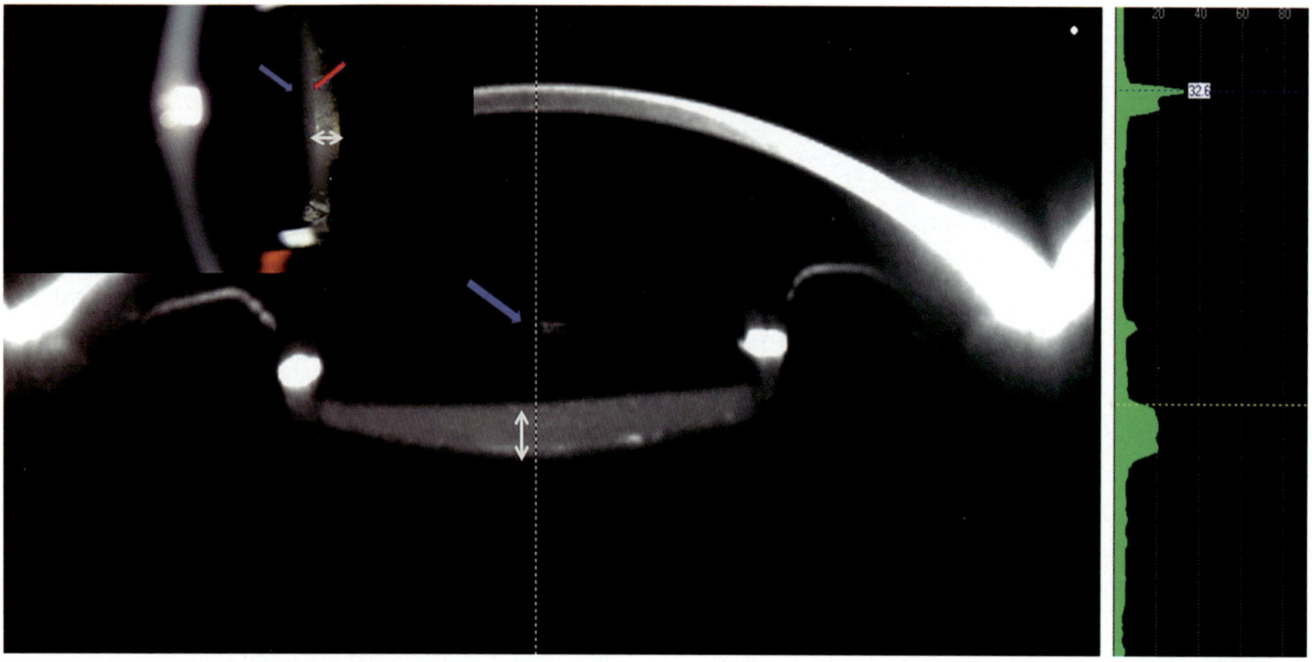

Fig. 11.26 Capsular block syndrome (CBS). CBS can be seen at the slit-lamp *(top left panel)* as a posterior distention of the capsular bag *(double white arrow).* Scheimpflug imaging can be used to visualize CBS changes. The posterior distention is seen as an area of slightly increased reflectivity *(double white arrow).* The *blue arrow* denotes the anterior surface of the intraocular lens (IOL), and the *red arrow* denotes the posterior surface of the IOL. (Image Credit: Dilraj S. Grewal, MD, Duke University, Durham, NC, USA.)

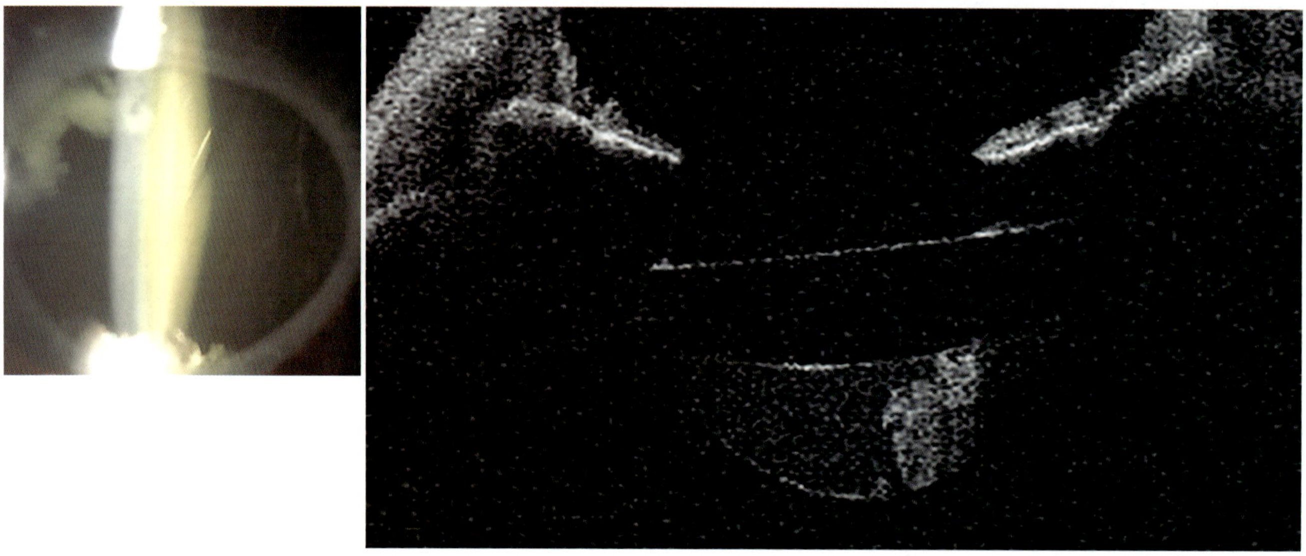

Fig. 11.27 Capsular block syndrome (CBS). CBS may cause the intraocular lens (IOL) to appear extremely bright on examination *(left photograph)* Whitish-turbid material can be seen behind the IOL, causing fluid to accumulate between the IOL and the posterior capsule. AS-OCT may be extremely helpful in visualizing the anterior shift of the IOL caused by milky/turbid fluid behind the IOL, causing posterior capsule distention. (Left photograph courtesy William Trattler, MD, Miami, Florida, United States; right AS-OCT image courtesy Dilraj Grewal, MD, Duke University, Chapel Hill, North Carolina, United States.)

bag. Because CBS is a rare condition, clinical examination may be equivocal for correct diagnosis (Fig. 11.26). AS-OCT may help visualize the turbid fluid behind the anteriorly shifted IOL complex in such cases (Fig. 11.27).

Careful examination with IOP control and intraocular inflammation management may be sufficient for early cases of CBS (one–four days postoperatively). YAG capsulotomy or surgical disruption of the posterior capsule may be diagnostic and therapeutic for late and more severe cases.

V. SUMMARY

This chapter highlights the use of AS-OCT in diagnosing and managing cataracts, a commonly encountered condition in modern ophthalmic practice. A detailed description of using AS-OCT to diagnose cataracts, including the appearance of various cataract types, is provided. Subtopics presented in the chapter include information for presurgical planning and postsurgical management, including IOL complications.

Additionally, AS-OCT imaging offers accurate measurements of anterior chamber structures and can aid the surgeon in surgical decision-making with phakic IOLs. AS-OCT can help clinicians assess preoperative risk factors or pathologies that may cause intraoperative and postoperative complications. Postoperatively, AS-OCT imaging can help evaluate the location of IOLs, highlighting any findings that may have been missed on clinical examination.

ACKNOWLEDGMENT

The authors would like to thank Yassine J. Daoud, MD, for his assistance in preparing this chapter.

BIBLIOGRAPHY

Almalki S, Abubaker A, Alsabaani NA, Edward DP. Causes of elevated intraocular pressure following implantation of phakic intraocular lenses for myopia. *Int Ophthalmol*. 2016;36(2):259-265.

Casey M, Karl MD, Roberts CJ, Ohr M. Comparison of scleral-fixated intraocular lens position measured with anterior segment swept-source OCT and ultrasound biomicroscopy. *Invest Ophthalmol Vis Sci*. 2020;61(7):2564.

Chan TC, Li EY, Yau JC. Application of anterior segment optical coherence tomography to identify eyes with posterior polar cataract at high risk for posterior capsule rupture. *J Cataract Refract Surg*. 2014;40:2076-2081.

Dhami A, Dhami AS, Singh H, Dhami GS. Role of anterior segment optical coherence tomography for safer management of mature white cataracts. *J Cataract Refract Surg*. 2019;45:480-484.

Hyun J, Lim DH, Eo DR, Hwang S, Chung ES, Chung TY. A comparison of visual outcome and rotational stability of two types of toric implantable collamer lenses (TICL): V4 versus V4c. *PLoS One*. 2017;12(8):e0183335.

Kymionis GD, Diakonis VF, Liakopoulos DA, Tsoulnaras KI, Klados NE, Pallikaris IG. Anterior segment optical coherence tomography for demonstrating posterior capsular rent in posterior polar cataract. *Clin Ophthalmol*. 2014;8:215-217.

Michael R, Bron AJ. The ageing lens and cataract: a model of normal and pathological ageing. *Philos Trans R Soc Lond B Biol Sci*. 2011;366(1568):1278-1292.

Panthier C, de Wazieres A, Rouger H, Moran S, Saad A, Gatinel D. Average lens density quantification with swept-source optical coherence tomography: optimized, automated cataract grading technique. *J Cataract Refract Surg*. 2019;45(12):1746-1752.

Pujari A, Sharma N. The emerging role of anterior segment optical coherence tomography in cataract surgery: current role and future perspectives. *Clin Ophthalmol*. 2021;15:389-401.

Raj SM, Vasavada AR, Johar SR, Vasavada VA, Vasavada VA. Post-operative capsular opacification: a review. *Int J Biomed Sci*. 2007;3(4):237-250.

Schmidinger G, Lackner B, Pieh S, Skorpik C. Long-term changes in posterior chamber phakic intraocular collamer lens vaulting in myopic patients. *Ophthalmology*. 2010;117(8):1506-1511.

Sugar A, Rapuano CJ, Culbertson WW, et al. Laser in situ keratomileusis for myopia and astigmatism: safety and efficacy: a report by the American Academy of Ophthalmology. *Ophthalmology*. 2002;109(1): 175-187.

Tabatabaei SA, Soleimani M, Etesali H, Naderan M. Accuracy of swept source optical coherence tomography and ultrasound biomicroscopy for evaluation of posterior lens capsule in traumatic cataract [published online ahead of print, 2020 Apr 2]. *Am J Ophthalmol*. 2020;216:55-58.

Truscott RJ. Age-related nuclear cataract-oxidation is the key. *Exp Eye Res*. 2005;80(5):709-725.

Vrensen G, Willekens B. Biomicroscopy and scanning electron microscopy of early opacities in the aging human lens. *Invest Ophthalmol Vis Sci*. 1990;31(8):1582-1591.

Wong AL, Leung CK, Weinreb RN, et al. Quantitative assessment of lens opacities with anterior segment optical coherence tomography. *Br J Ophthalmol*. 2009;93(1):61-65.

SECTION 5

Surgery and Associated Complications

12 Refractive Surgery

Nakul Shekhawat | Kraig Bower

Anterior segment optical coherence tomography (AS-OCT) can be a valuable ancillary tool for several functions in refractive surgery including preoperative patient selection, postoperative evaluation, and monitoring for complications. Specific conditions and example images are shown in this chapter. Discussion of specific treatments for each of these conditions is beyond the scope of this chapter.

I. LASER IN-SITU KERATOMILEUSIS

A. Normal Flap

Laser in-situ keratomileusis (LASIK) is one of the most common refractive surgery procedures performed in the world. Because LASIK requires creation of a flap before ablation of the underlying stromal bed, AS-OCT can be used to visualize flap depth, diameter, and location. During preoperative evaluation and planning for refractive surgery, AS-OCT can be used to measure corneal thickness and predict residual stromal bed thickness with greater precision than Scheimpflug tomography or ultrasound pachymetry. After uncomplicated LASIK, a normal LASIK flap interface will show a mild linear hyperreflectivity (Fig. 12.1). AS-OCT also can be used to evaluate several flap-related complications and interface abnormalities that may otherwise be difficult to discern using slit-lamp examination. Along with slit-lamp photography, AS-OCT can be used to more objectively monitor for subtle clinical changes by measurement of lesion location, size, and signal intensity.

B. LASIK Flap Complications

I. MACROSTRIAE

LASIK flap striae can occur as a result of misalignment of the flap immediately after ablation, "wrinkling" of the flap because of a mismatch between the flap stroma and the underlying ablated stromal bed, or shifting of the flap position postoperatively

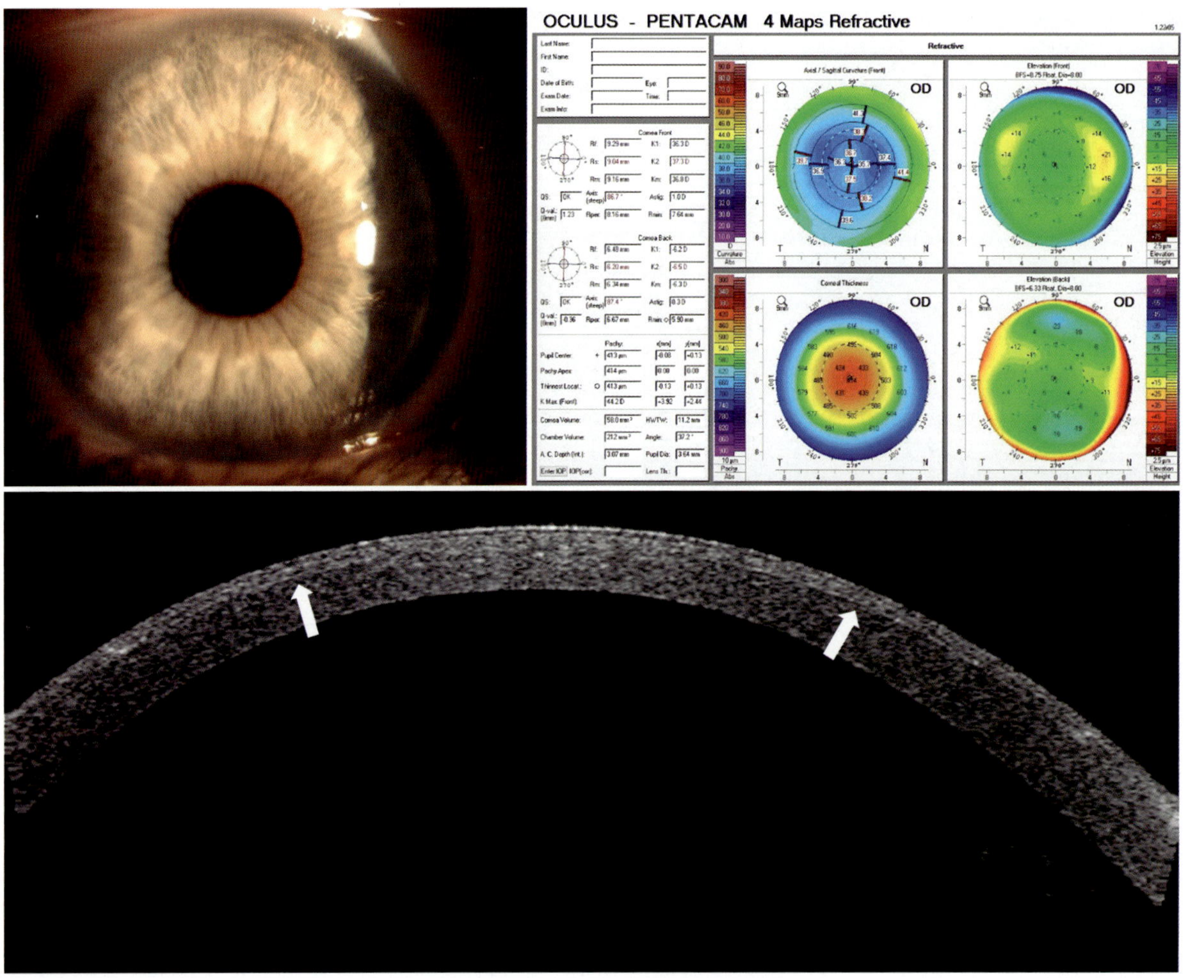

Fig. 12.1 Normal LASIK flap.

secondary to eye rubbing or trauma. Microstriae (not pictured here) are visible only on retro-illumination and typically do not affect visual acuity. Macrostriae are more readily visible on slit-lamp examination and may affect patients' vision because of reduced visual acuity, induced astigmatism, diplopia, or glare (Figs. 12.2 and 12.3). Fig. 12.2 shows an AS-OCT image of a dislocated flap with hyperreflectivity within the interface *(red arrows),* and areas of missing flap and exposed stroma appear thinner relative to the surrounding cornea *(white arrows).* Fig. 12.3 shows a free cap with macrostriae and epithelial ingrowth. The *red arrows* show where the keratome surfaced during loss of suction, with the cut extending through the Bowman layer and leading to subepithelial

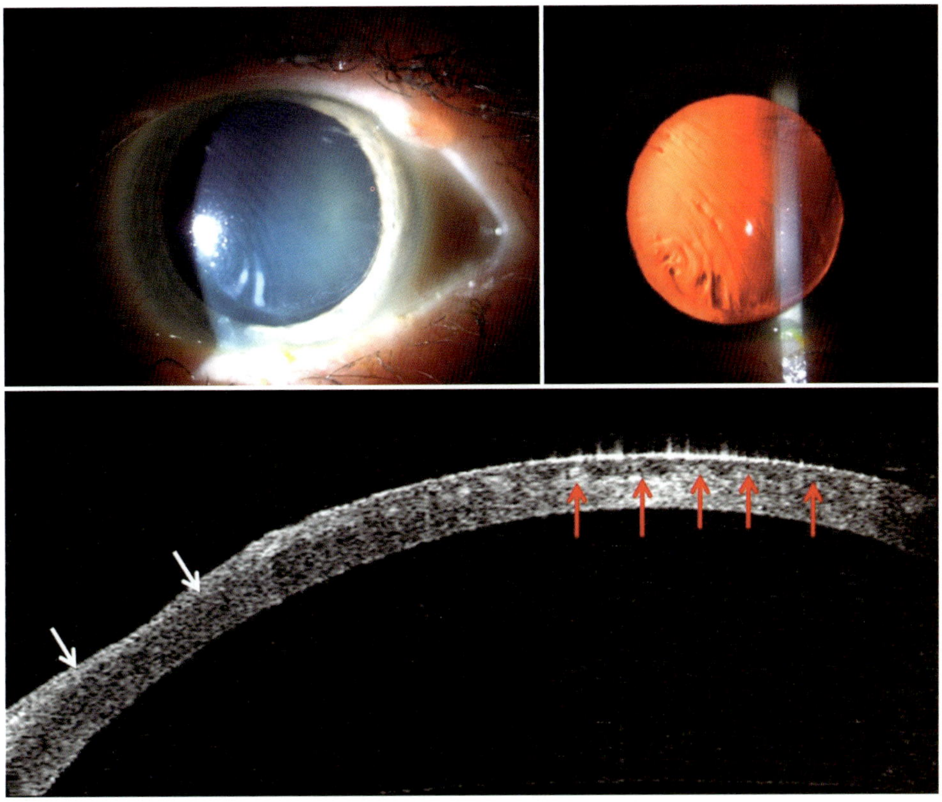

Fig. 12.2 LASIK flap dislocation with macrostriae.

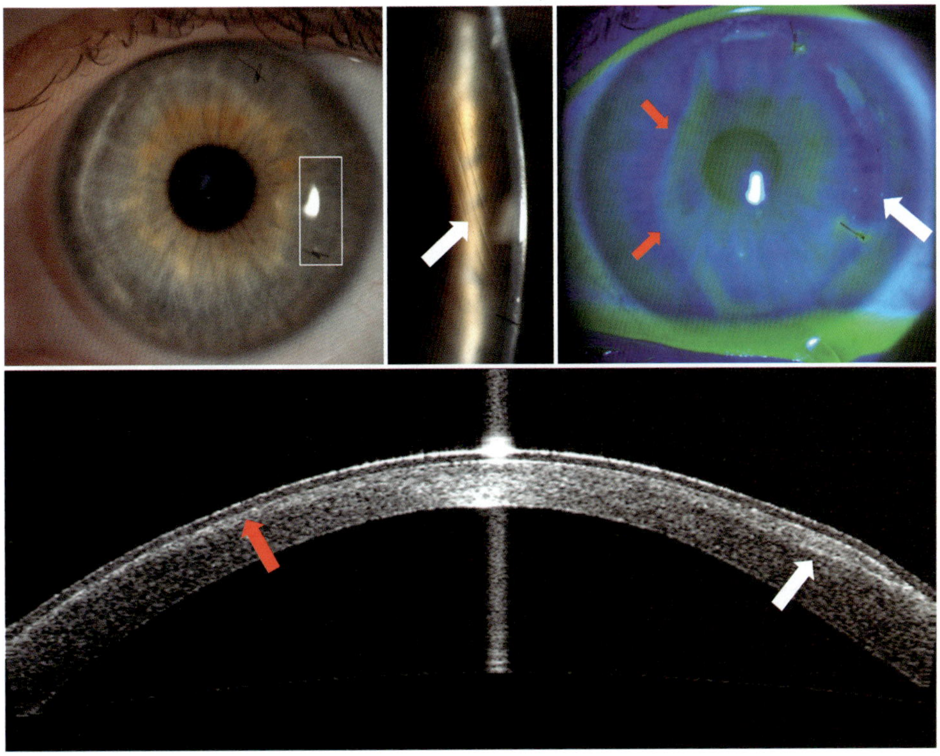

Fig. 12.3 LASIK free cap with macrostriae and epithelial ingrowth.

haze. The *white arrows* point to hyperreflective areas of epithelial ingrowth. There is a bandage contact lens in place. AS-OCT also can help identify flap macrostriae; although these striae can sometimes be difficult to visualize at the slit-lamp without careful retro-illumination, such contour abnormalities are more readily observed on AS-OCT imaging because of variability in flap thickness, hyperreflectivity within the flap, and in some cases local alterations of overall corneal thickness relative to surrounding cornea *(white arrow).*

Fig. 12.4 shows a patient nine months after traumatic LASIK flap dislocation of the right eye (thumbnail injury). Uncorrected visual acuity is 20/50 and best corrected acuity with manifest refraction + 1.25 + 1.00 × 038 was 20/30-2. On examination she had inferotemporal flap dislocation with macrostriae and epithelial ingrowth (*top left* slit-lamp photograph—*asterisk* shows ingrowth under flap striae). The macrostriae are easily highlighted with fluorescein stain/cobalt blue filter *(top center).* There is irregular astigmatism (Tomography axial keratometry image t*op right* and anterior elevation map below that.)

The corneal OCT *(bottom)* shows the epithelial ingrowth in the interface *(red arrows)* and the macrostriae *(white arrows).* The *red asterisk* corresponds to the *red asterisk* in the slit-lamp photograph.

II. INTERFACE DEBRIS

Although a minimal amount of meibum in the flap interface is not uncommon immediately after LASIK, persistent interface debris could be visually significant or predispose to infection. AS-OCT can be used to visualize interface debris and objectively monitor for changes over time. This is particularly useful when there is concern for interface debris leading to infection. In such situations, AS-OCT permits high-resolution monitoring for worsening haze or infiltrates. Fig. 12.5 shows a flap tear in a patient that suffered blunt trauma while gardening. A triangular portion of the flap was folded inward, leaving vegetable foreign body material incarcerated within the flap interface and a triangular area of exposed stromal bed that had filled in with epithelium by the time of presentation. On AS-OCT, the abnormal "double interface" is visible as two hyperreflective lines, indicating three distinct planes of stromal tissue (residual stromal bed, original LASIK flap, and traumatically folded LASIK flap in-between). The retained vegetable foreign body material appears as a hyperreflective deposit within the interface. This patient underwent careful epithelial debridement, removal of the retained foreign body material, and repositioning of the triangular folded flap and achieved 20/25 range contact lens–corrected visual acuity.

III. DIFFUSE LAMELLAR KERATITIS

Diffuse lamellar keratitis (DLK) is an inflammation within the LASIK flap interface that typically occurs within the first 24 to 72 hours postoperatively but can also occur months or years later. DLK can manifest as focal gray-white colored granular interface material (grade 1), gray-white granular material located diffusely throughout the interface (grade 2), diffuse and confluent granular material with associated conjunctival injection (grade 3), and the aforementioned presentation with central corneal haze and striae (grade 4). In chronic or severe cases, sterile keratolysis can occur starting at the flap edges. AS-OCT can help visualize interface inflammatory debris and flap melt (Fig. 12.6). Interface debris from DLK will appear as abnormally hyperreflective material *(white arrow)* above the flap *(white asterisk).* The flap edge is thickened and hyperreflective because of ongoing inflammation. Flap melt is occurring secondary to this inflammation and is evidenced by the sharply demarcated

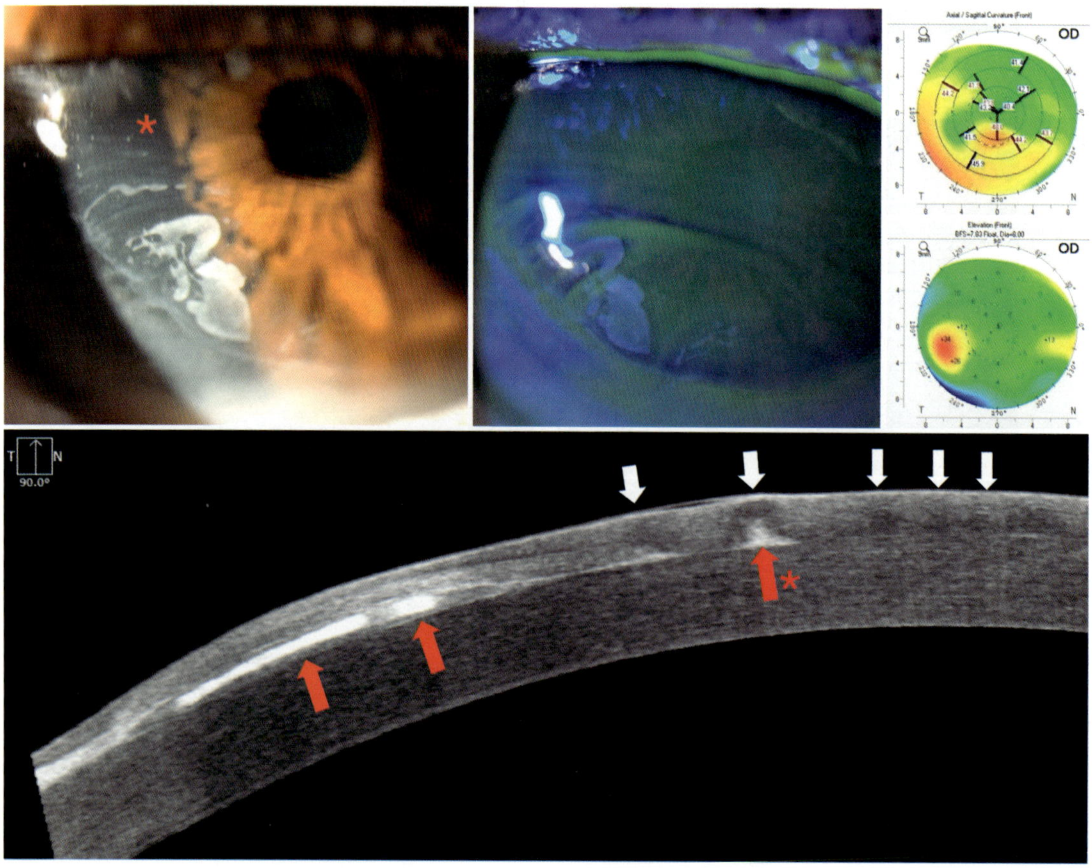

Fig. 12.4 Traumatic macrostriae and epithelial ingrowth.

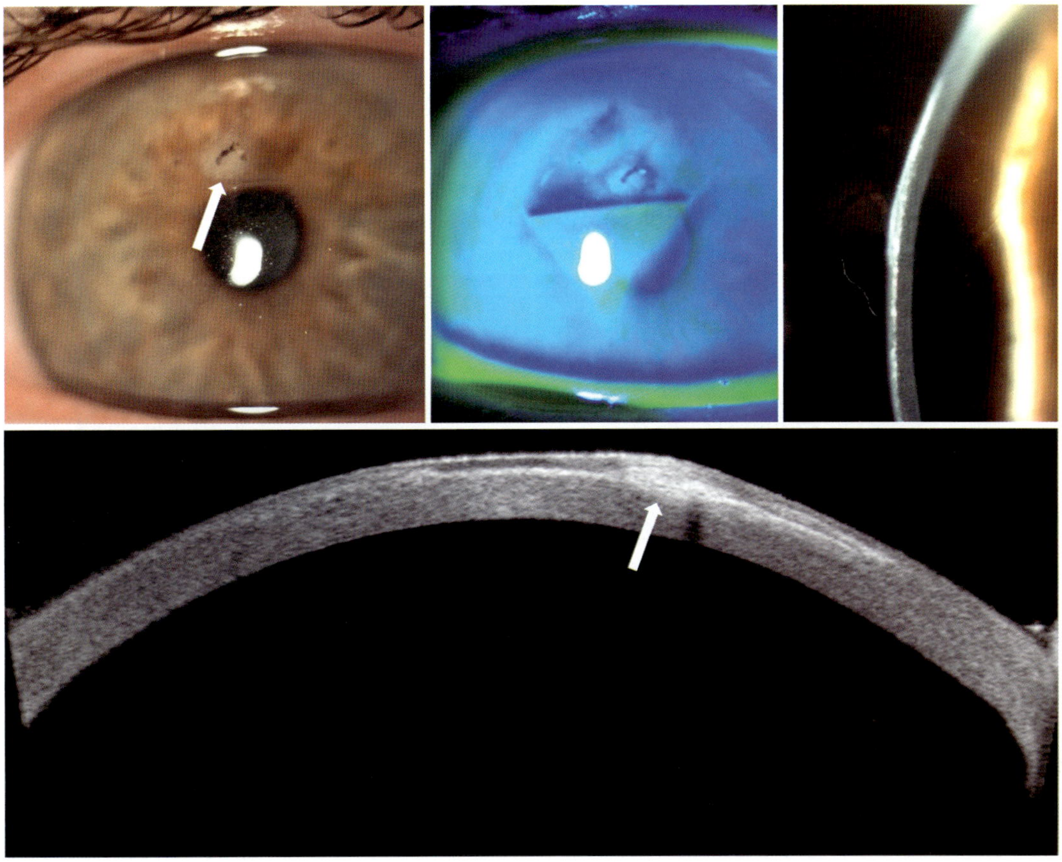

Fig. 12.5 Triangular flap tear with retained vegetable foreign body material.

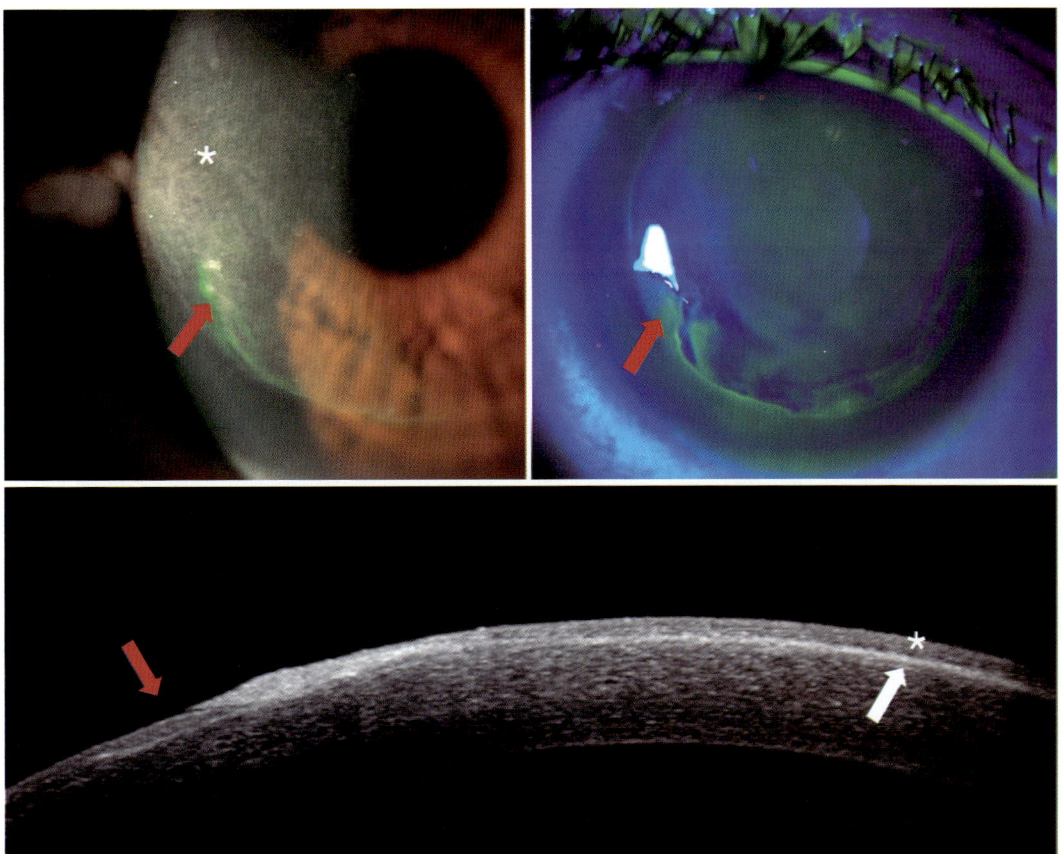

Fig. 12.6 Chronic DLK and flap melt.

flap edge. In some cases, surrounding epithelium will hypertrophy to fill in the area of flap melt, and this is visible as normoreflective material that appears distinct from the hyperreflective flap or the stromal bed *(red arrow)*.

IV. EPITHELIAL INGROWTH

Epithelial ingrowth into the flap interface can occur weeks to years after LASIK. The condition can involve a faint one to two mm border of epithelium just within the flap edge (grade 1), well-defined clusters or nests of epithelial cells within a limited area (grade 2), more diffuse area of epithelial clusters or nests (grade 3), and/or associated flap melt (grade 4). Serial AS-OCT imaging can help monitor for extension of epithelial ingrowth past the flap edge (Fig. 12.7) and toward the central cornea (Fig. 12.8). Fig. 12.8 shows a horseshoe flap tear that resulted in epithelial ingrowth. The *red arrows* indicate stromal scarring and epithelial

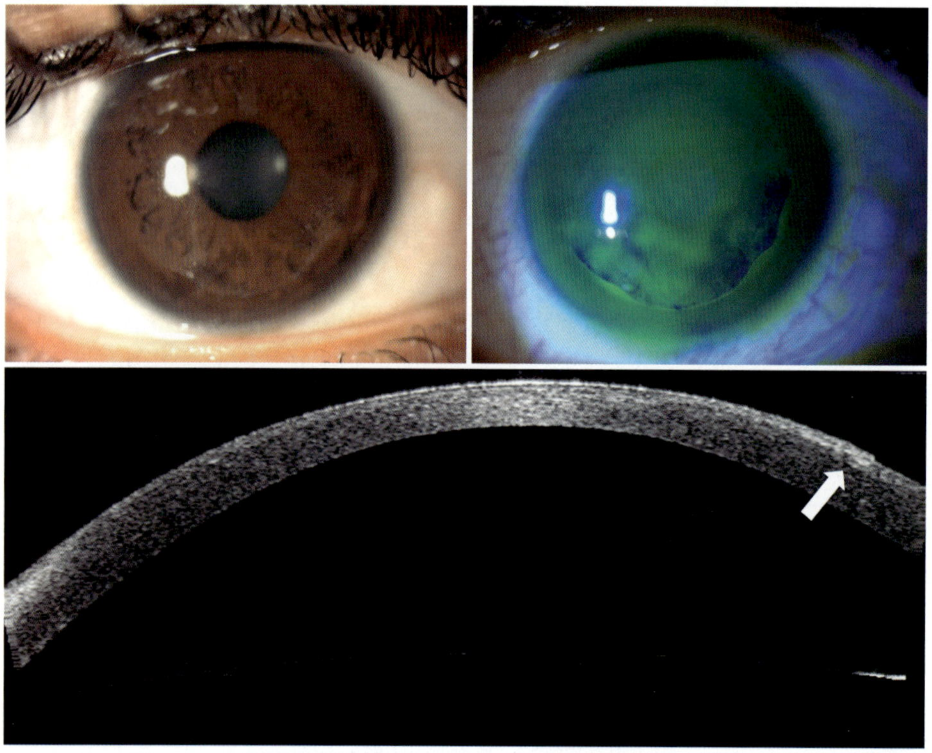

Fig. 12.7 Epithelial ingrowth with LASIK flap melt.

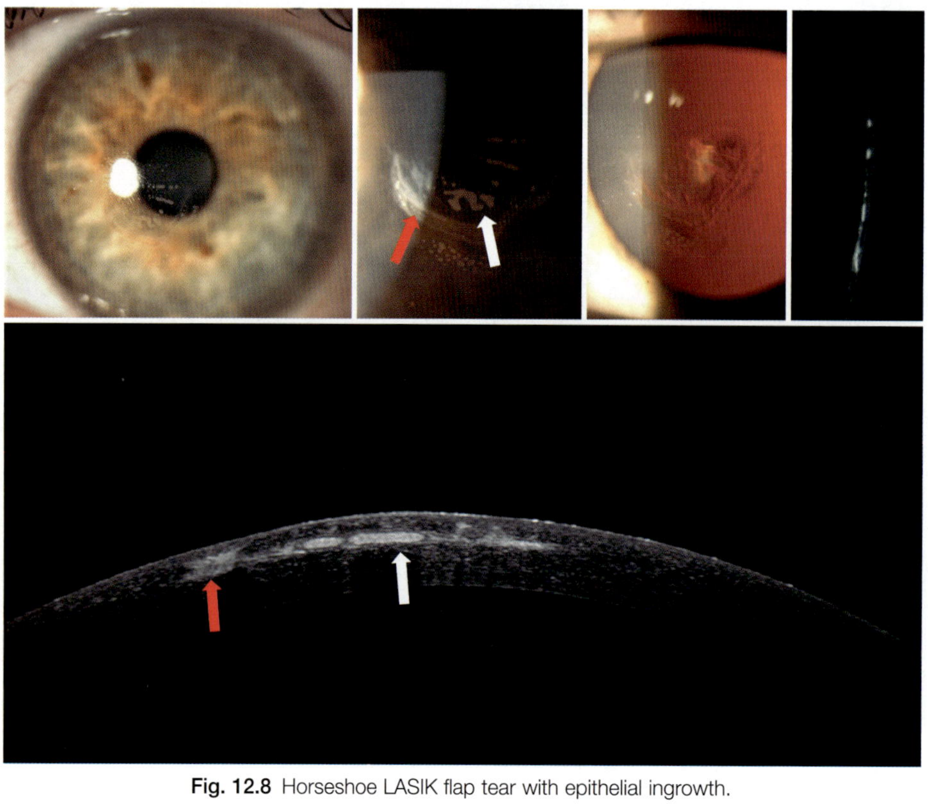

Fig. 12.8 Horseshoe LASIK flap tear with epithelial ingrowth.

fill-in within a gap where the torn flap did not completely realign with the stromal bed. The *white arrows* indicate epithelial nests which appear as multiple, well-demarcated hyperreflective deposits within the interface. AS-OCT is also a sensitive means for detecting subtle and early flap melt (see Figs. 12.6 and 12.7), which will show a thinned or missing overlying LASIK flap, an intact underlying stromal bed, and an irregular anterior corneal contour in the area of melt. Fig. 12.9 shows the dense clusters of epithelium in the LASIK flap. The *blue arrows* show retraction of the LASIK flap seen on the slit-lamp with scarring and the corresponding hyperreflective area on AS-OCT. The *red arrows* slow the line of demarcation between the epithelial ingrowth and normal flap stroma, and the *white arrows* show the dense nests of epithelial cells in the LASIK flap with the very dense hyperreflective areas seen on the AS-OCT image. Figs. 12.10 and 12.11 show a dense cluster of epithelial ingrowth and the corresponding

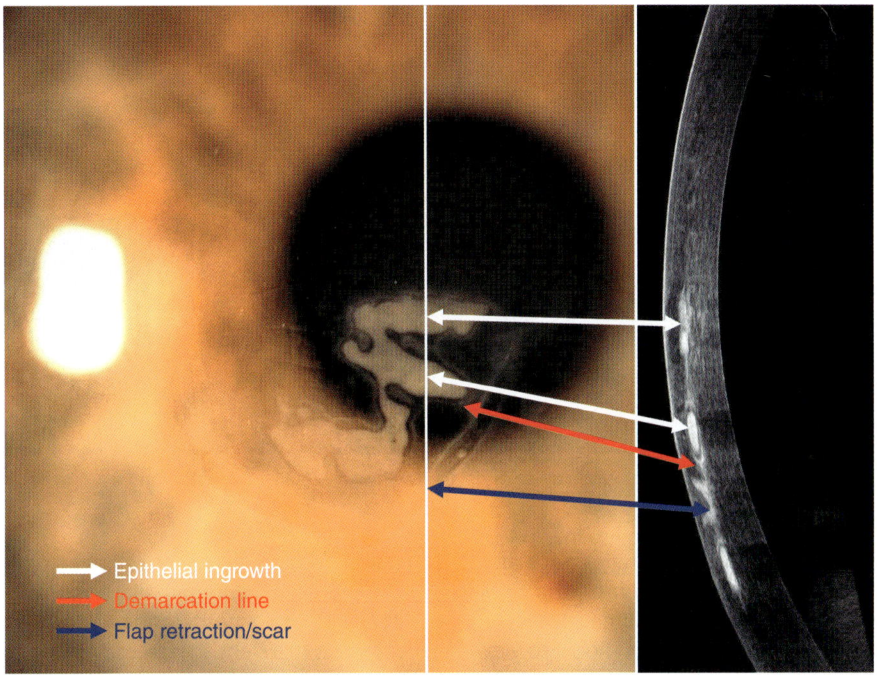

Fig. 12.9 Epithelial ingrowth with demarcation line and flap retraction/scar.

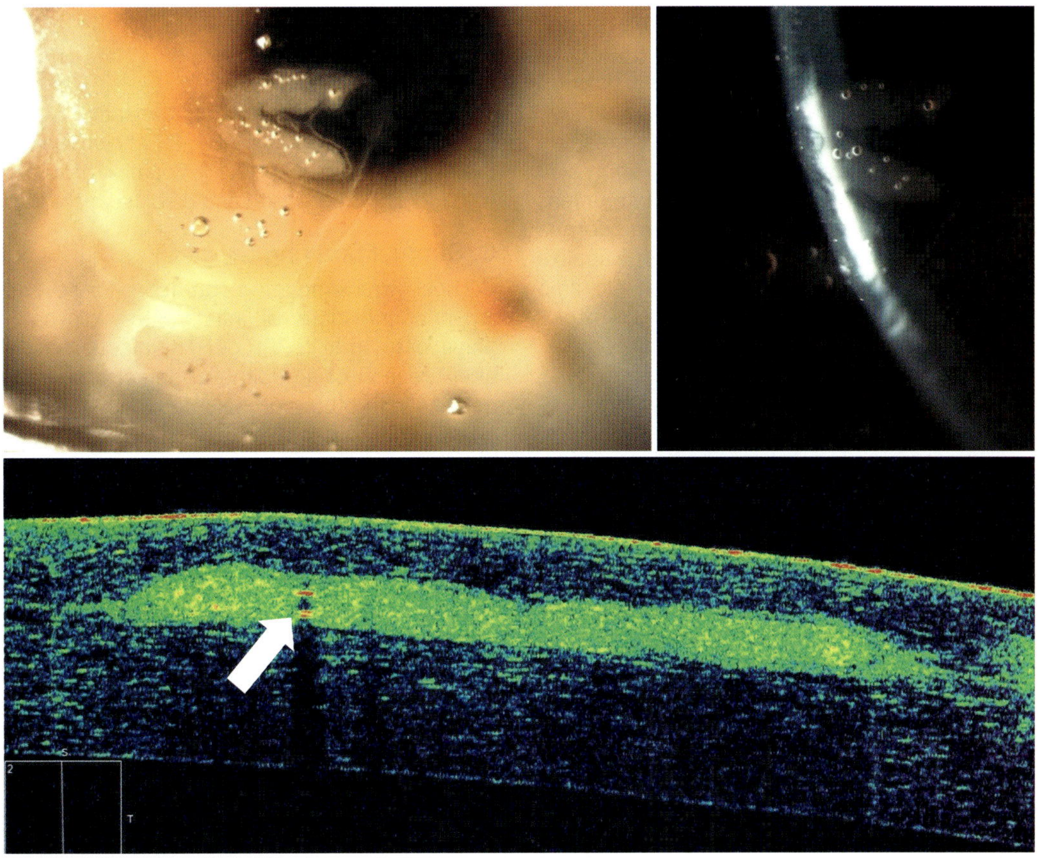

Fig. 12.10 YAG laser treatment of epithelial ingrowth.

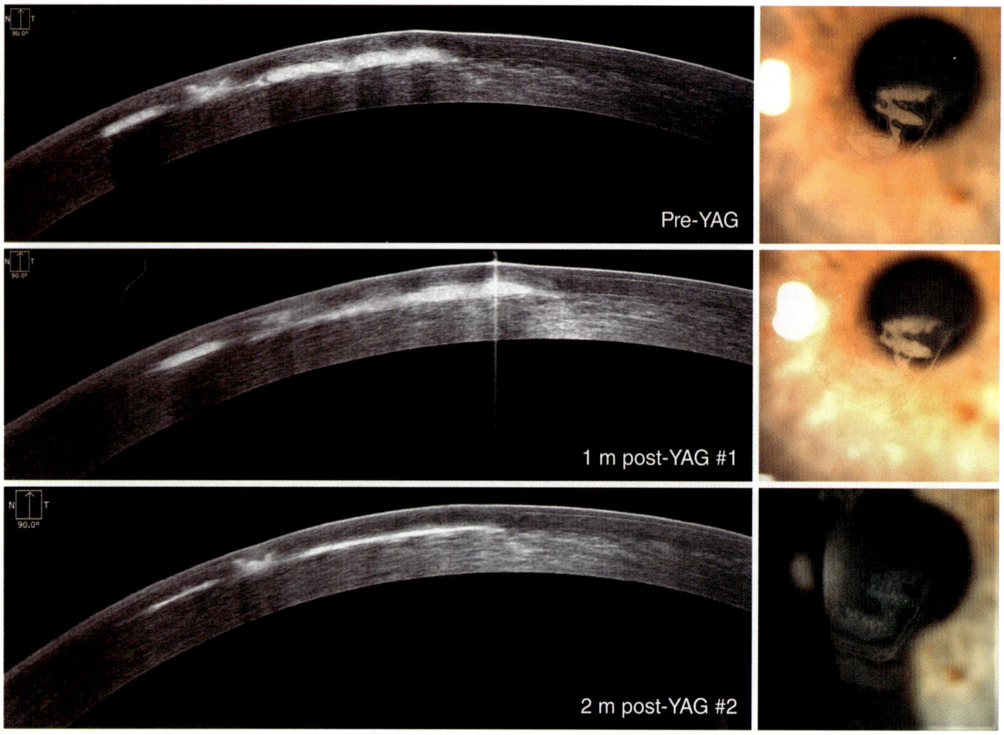

Fig. 12.11 Regression of epithelial ingrowth after YAG laser treatment.

normalization of these cells one and two months after YAG laser treatment. The epithelial cells appear *dense green* on the color image and *dense white* on the black and white. Sometimes more details can be seen on the color image, but it often helps to view both the color and black and white images.

V. PRESSURE-INDUCED STROMAL KERATITIS

Pressure-induced stromal keratitis is an easily missed condition in which steroid-induced elevation in intraocular pressure causes fluid accumulation within the LASIK flap interface. Small accumulations of interface fluid can be difficult to visualize on slit-lamp examination. Intraocular pressure measurements taken over the area of fluid accumulation also can be artificially low, masking the underlying problem unless intraocular pressure is measured in the peripheral cornea outside the area of fluid accumulation. AS-OCT can visualize interface fluid accumulation much more readily than slit-lamp examination (Fig. 12.12) and can also help monitor for fluid resolution. Interface fluid appears as a discrete hyporeflective line.

II. PHOTOREFRACTIVE KERATECTOMY

Surface ablation procedures such as photorefractive keratectomy (PRK) are commonly performed for refractive correction, but they can lead to complications such as haze, subepithelial fibrosis, and stromal scarring. Although slit-lamp evaluation and photography are useful for subjectively evaluating the size and density of these opacities, AS-OCT can help more objectively track changes over time. AS-OCT can also identify depth of involvement and guide surgical planning if further ablation or stroma removal is indicated.

A. Haze

Subepithelial haze commonly occurs within a few weeks after PRK, peaks at 3 months, and tends to regress with no visual effects in the majority of patients. On slit-lamp examination, haze classically exhibits a reticular pattern, whereas AS-OCT will show a linear subepithelial hyperreflectivity with varying diameter and thickness depending on severity (Figs. 12.13 through 12.15). Dense haze may be visually significant enough to require treatment with epithelial debridement and application of mitomycin-C (see Figs. 12.13 and 12.14). For dense haze, surface ablation with phototherapeutic keratectomy (PTK) is also a treatment option (see Fig. 12.15).

B. Subepithelial Fibrosis

Subepithelial fibrosis can occur beneath a LASIK flap or after surface ablation procedures. AS-OCT shows linear hyperreflectivity at the level of fibrosis (Fig. 12.16). Location of fibrosis on AS-OCT can help monitor progression and guide surgical planning.

C. Stromal Scarring

Corneal stromal scarring can occur for several reasons including prior infectious or inflammatory disease, corneal dystrophies, or trauma. In PRK or PTK, infectious keratitis can develop after creation of an epithelial defect and lead to stromal scarring. As with other corneal infections, AS-OCT can be used to qualitatively evaluate density of scarring and objectively evaluate anatomic changes such as scar size, depth, and location and any stromal thinning (Fig. 12.17). These parameters are helpful when deciding whether to treat scarring with superficial keratectomy, laser ablation, deep anterior lamellar keratoplasty, or penetrating keratoplasty.

III. PHOTOTHERAPEUTIC KERATECTOMY

Depending on lesion depth, corneal opacities such as granular dystrophy (Figs. 12.18 and 12.19) and surface irregularities such as anterior basement membrane dystrophy (Figs. 12.20 and 12.21) can be treated with epithelial debridement, laser surface ablation procedures such as PTK, lamellar keratoplasty, or penetrating keratoplasty. Slit-lamp examination can be subjective

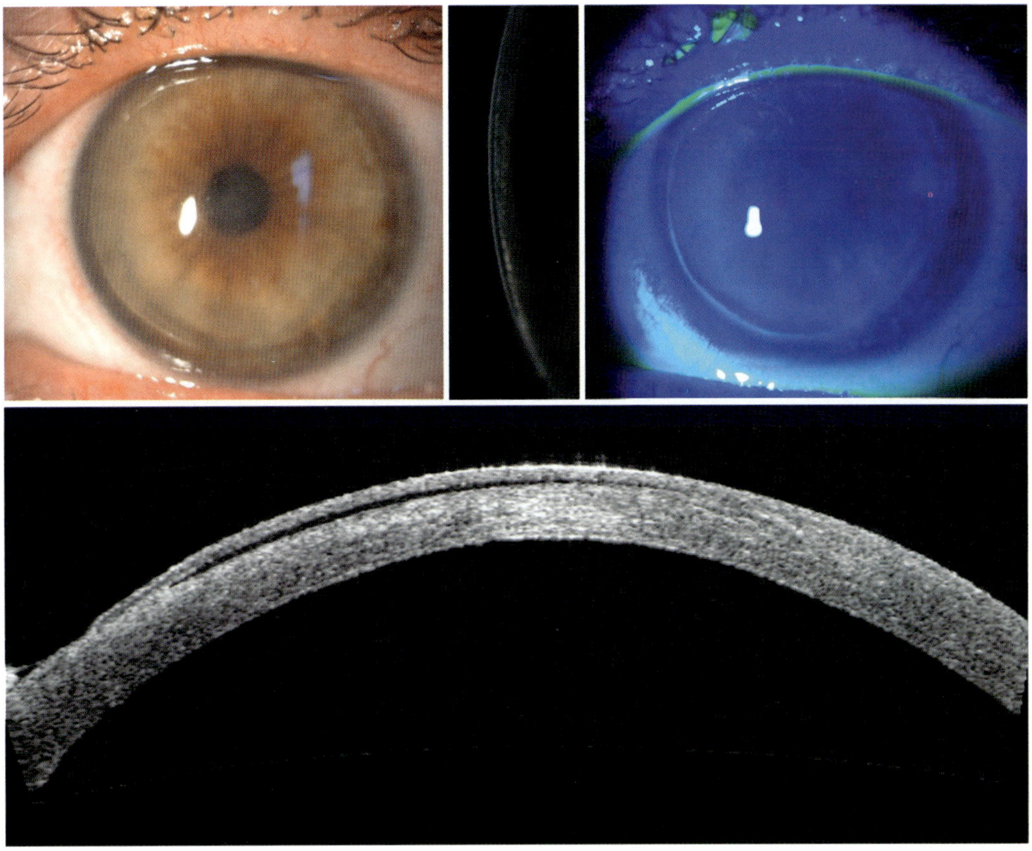

Fig. 12.12 Pressure-induced stromal keratitis.

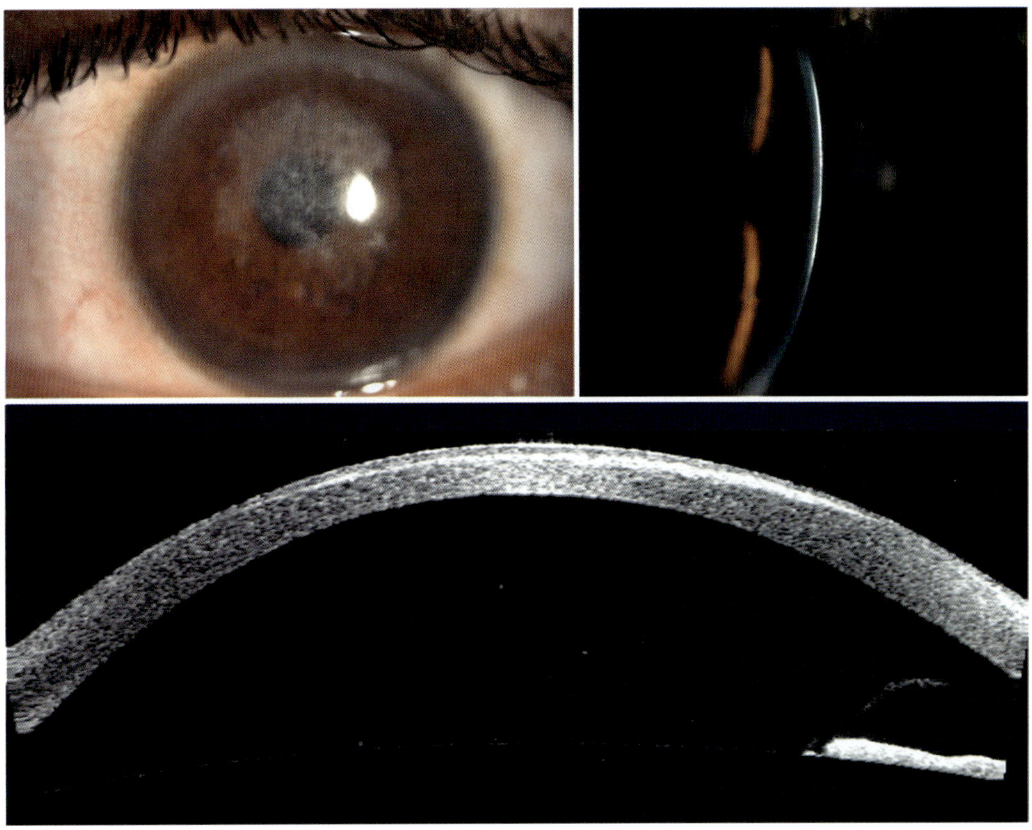

Fig. 12.13 Post–photorefractive keratectomy haze.

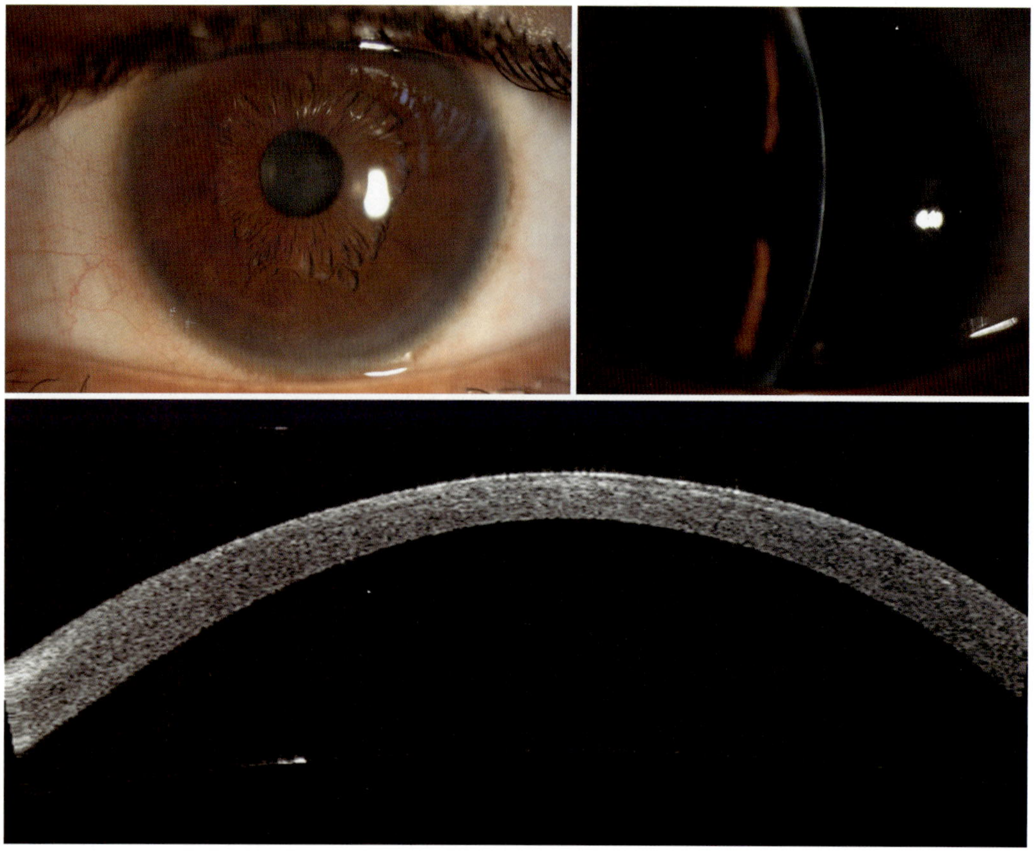

Fig. 12.14 Post–photorefractive keratectomy haze 3 months after epithelial debridement and application of mitomycin-C.

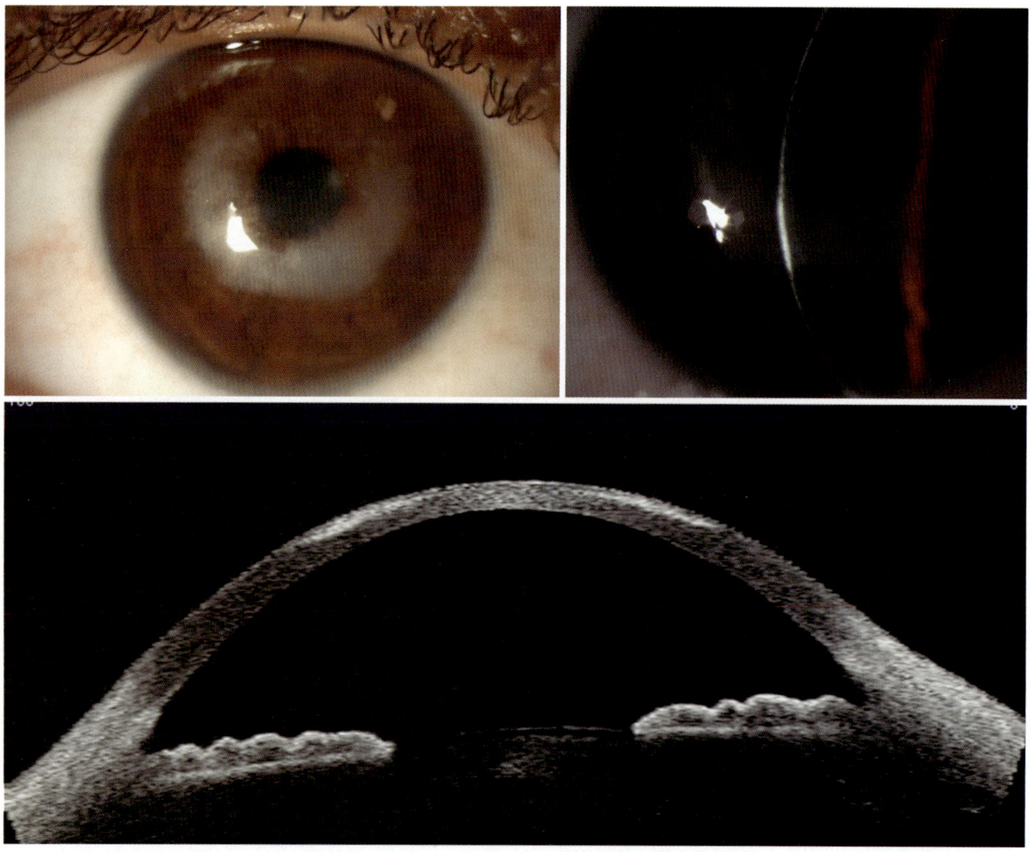

Fig. 12.15 Severe post–photorefractive keratectomy haze treated with phototherapeutic keratectomy.

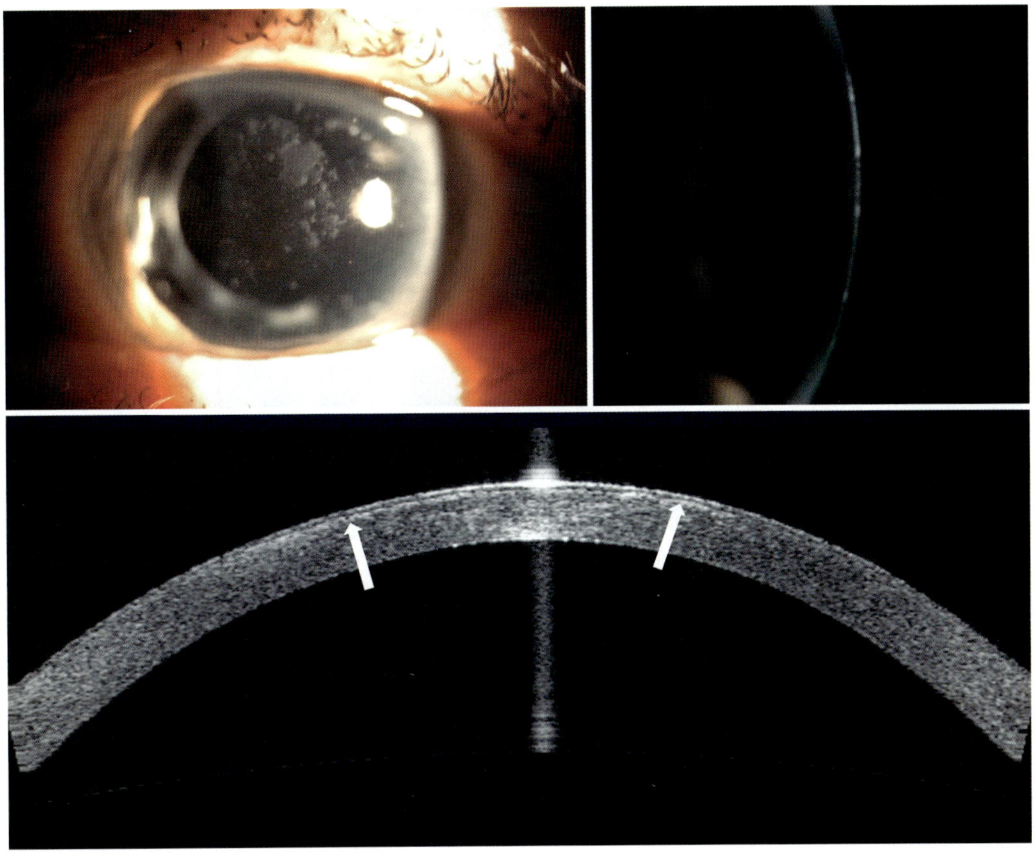

Fig. 12.16 Post-LASIK subepithelial fibrosis.

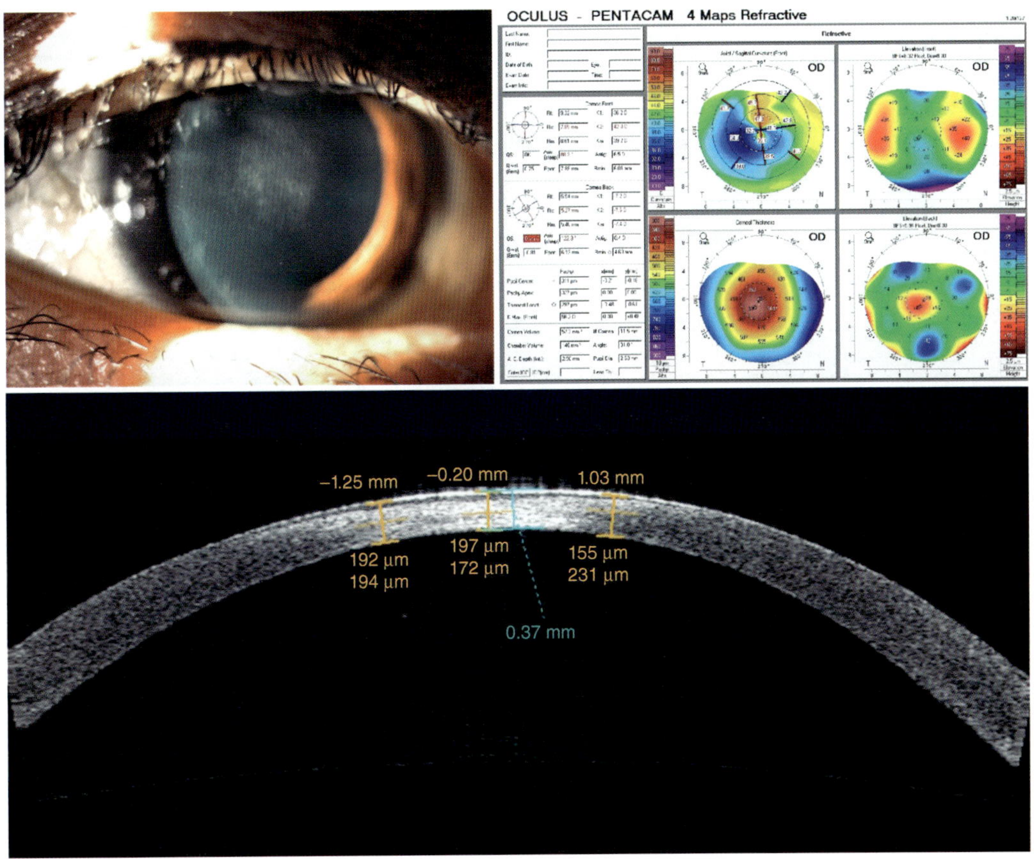

Fig. 12.17 Corneal scarring and thinning from infectious keratitis after post–photorefractive keratectomy.

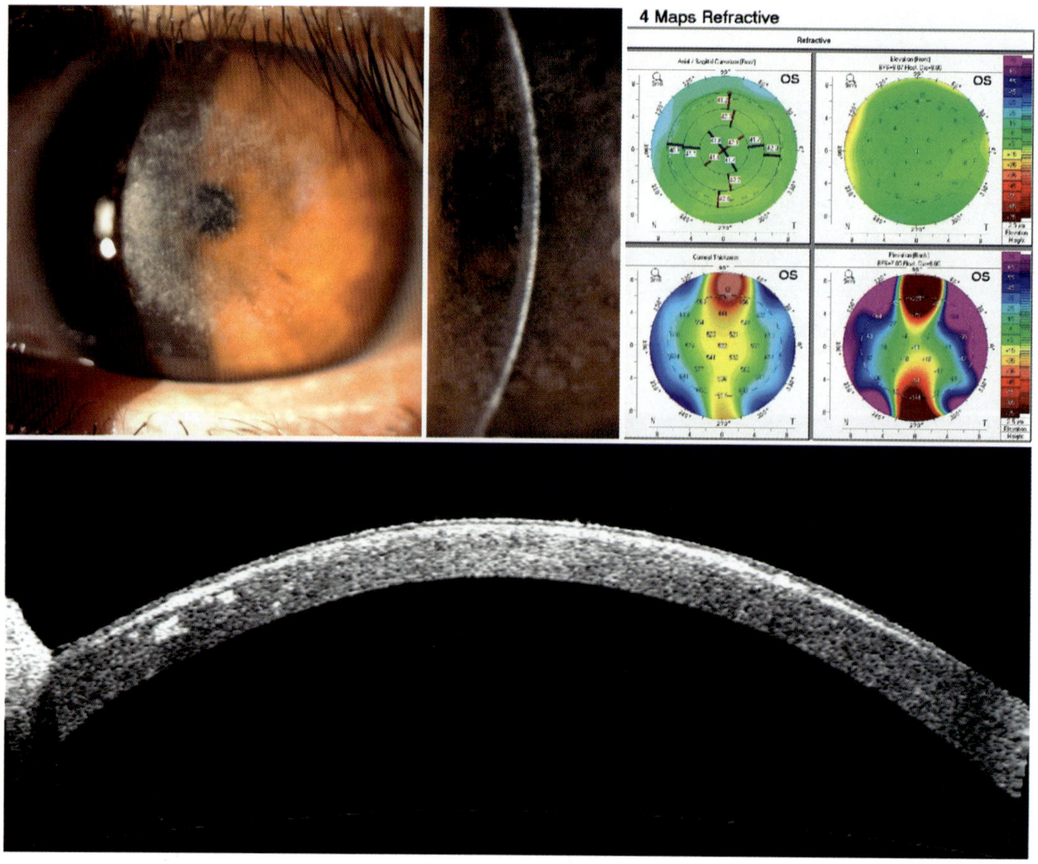

Fig. 12.18 Phototherapeutic keratectomy for granular dystrophy (preoperative).

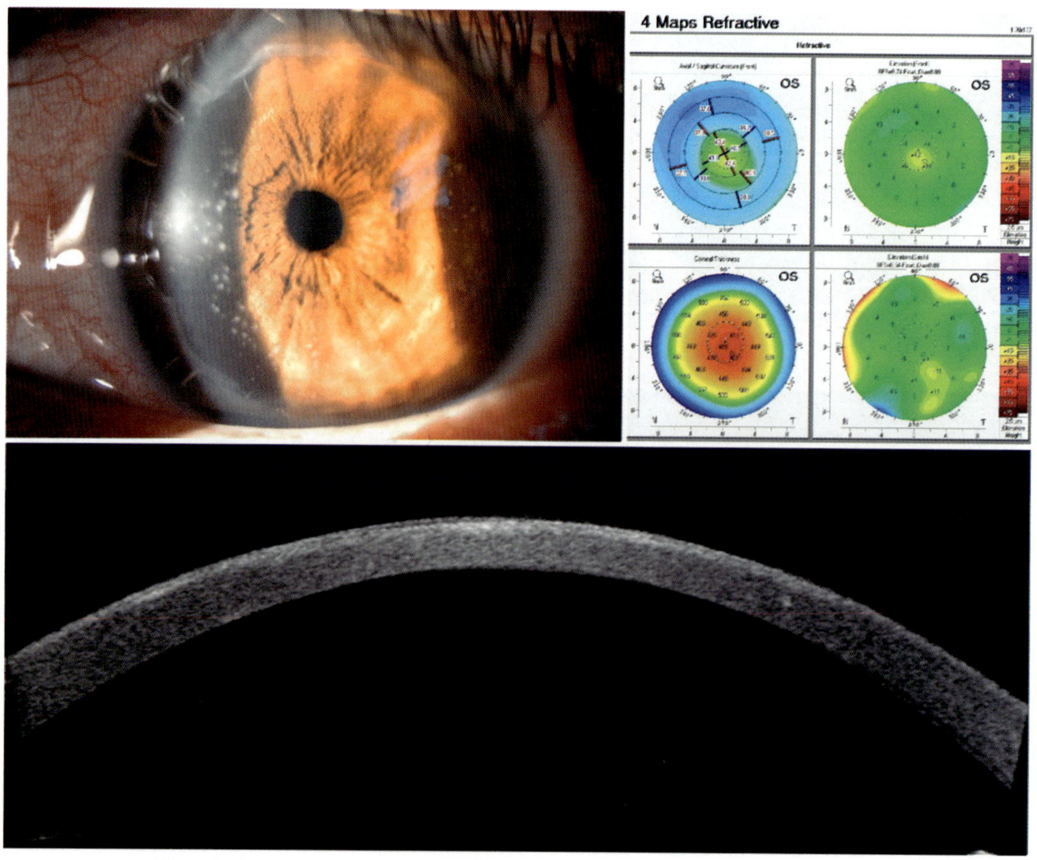

Fig. 12.19 Phototherapeutic keratectomy for granular dystrophy (postoperative).

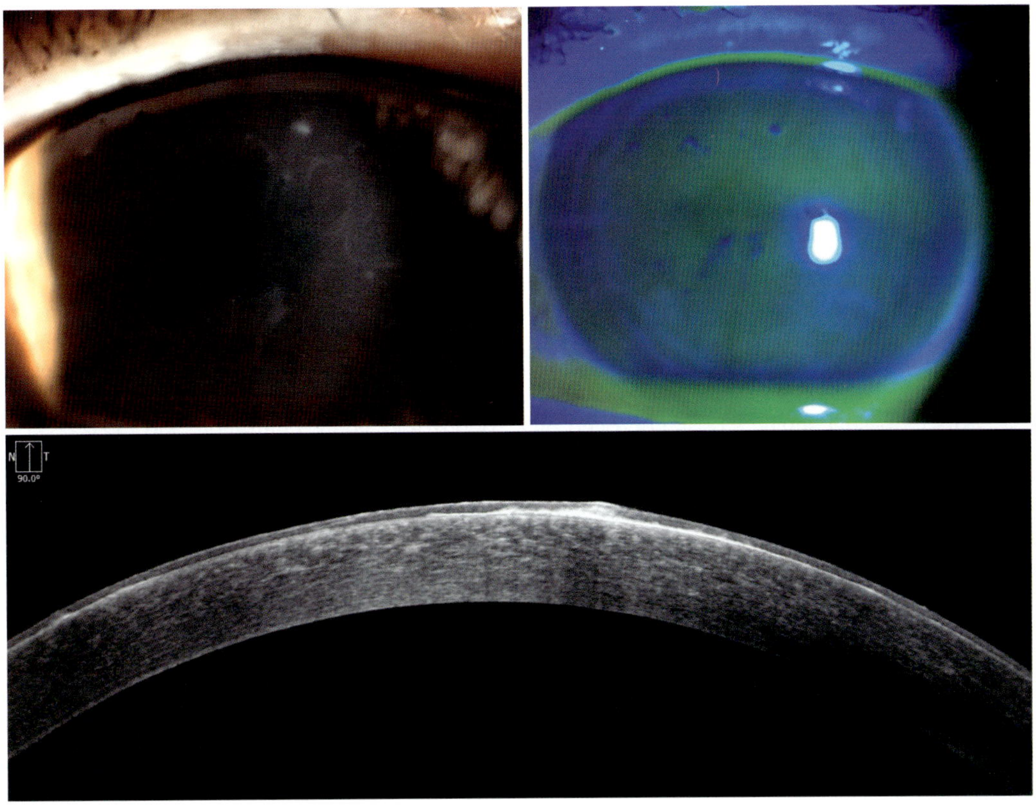

Fig. 12.20 Phototherapeutic keratectomy for visually significant anterior basement membrane dystrophy (preoperative).

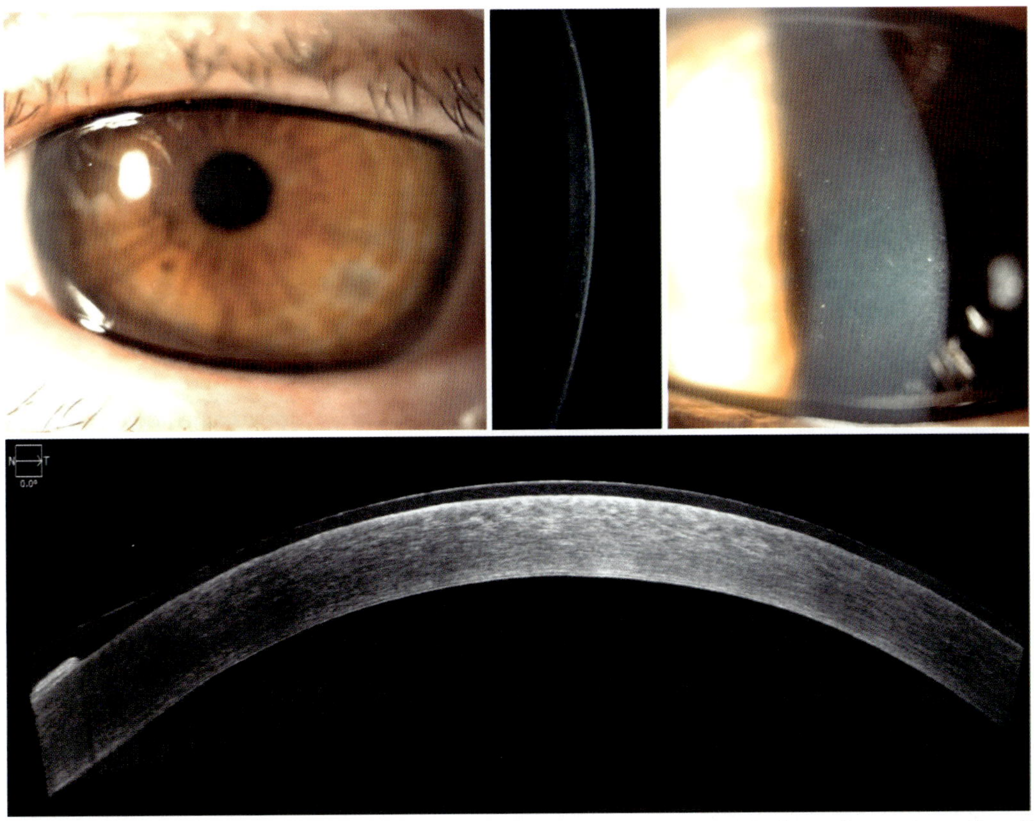

Fig. 12.21 Phototherapeutic keratectomy for visually significant anterior basement membrane dystrophy (immediate postoperative with overlying bandage contact lens).

depending on the examiner. To permit more objective monitoring of patients with corneal opacities, slit-lamp photography is recommended when feasible. However, even the appearance of corneal opacities on slit-lamp photography can vary significantly depending on depth of focus, light exposure, and camera settings. AS-OCT is an increasingly useful tool to precisely quantify lesion depth and guide surgical planning. Even in the absence of surgery, AS-OCT can also help objectively monitor changes in depth, dimensions, and density of media opacities over time. Fig. 12.18 shows preoperative AS-OCT of a patient with granular dystrophy. Fig. 12.19 shows the postoperative AS-OCT after the patient underwent PTK. After laser ablation, the anterior stromal hyperreflective hyaline deposits are reduced in size, particularly in the central cornea, leading to improvement in best corrected visual acuity. PTK is approved by the US Food and Drug Administration (FDA) for treatment of anterior basement membrane dystrophy (ABMD), and it is a viable treatment option for patients with recurrent erosions due to lesions involving the visual axis. Fig. 12.20 shows a preoperative AS-OCT image of a patient with ABMD associated with recurrent erosions. AS-OCT shows hyperreflective subepithelial ridges with overlying abnormalities in epithelial contour, providing much more detailed insights about the extent and depth of ABMD involvement than would be apparent on slit-lamp examination. Fig. 12.21 shows the same patient after PTK. The subepithelial contour is essentially smooth, and a bandage contact lens covers the cornea with a good tear meniscus.

IV. CORNEAL INLAYS AND ONLAYS

AS-OCT can be used to precisely evaluate depth, centration, and tilt of corneal inlays and onlays as part of postoperative evaluation. OCT imaging also can be used to qualitatively assess complications such as implant malposition and implant-associated haze, scarring, infiltrate, and keratolysis.

A. Kamra and Raindrop Corneal Inlay

Corneal inlays such as Kamra (AcuFocus) and Raindrop (ReVision Optics) have been used to treat presbyopia. The Kamra inlay is typically implanted in the nondominant eye and uses small-aperture optics with a pinhole-like effect to increase the depth of focus, improving intermediate and near visual acuity and alleviating symptoms of presbyopia. The Kamra corneal inlay has a diameter of 3.8 mm and a central aperture of 1.6 mm. The implant is inserted into a lamellar pocket created using a femtosecond laser. AS-OCT can be used to measure inlay depth and verify centration. Fig. 12.22 shows a decentered Kamra inlay that was subsequently removed. When implanted, the Kamra inlay material blocks signal to the posterior stroma. After removal, the Kamra inlay can leave mid-stromal scars that are seen as linear hyperreflective changes (Fig. 12.23).

The Raindrop corneal inlay was FDA approved in 2016 for implantation in the nondominant eye for the correction of presbyopia; however, the FDA recommended that surgeons no longer implant the inlay in late 2018 because of a high rate of central corneal haze. Many patients have elected to have the Raindrop removed due to the risk of visually significant corneal scarring.

Fig. 12.24 shows that of a 51-year-old woman with a remote history of LASIK with enhancement, and more recently in 2018 repeat enhancement and placement of a Raindrop corneal inlay for presbyopia in the right eye. Six months before presentation she had yet another enhancement in the right eye and two subsequent procedures to remove "skin cells" from under the flap. She presented for a second opinion with complaints of "hazy"

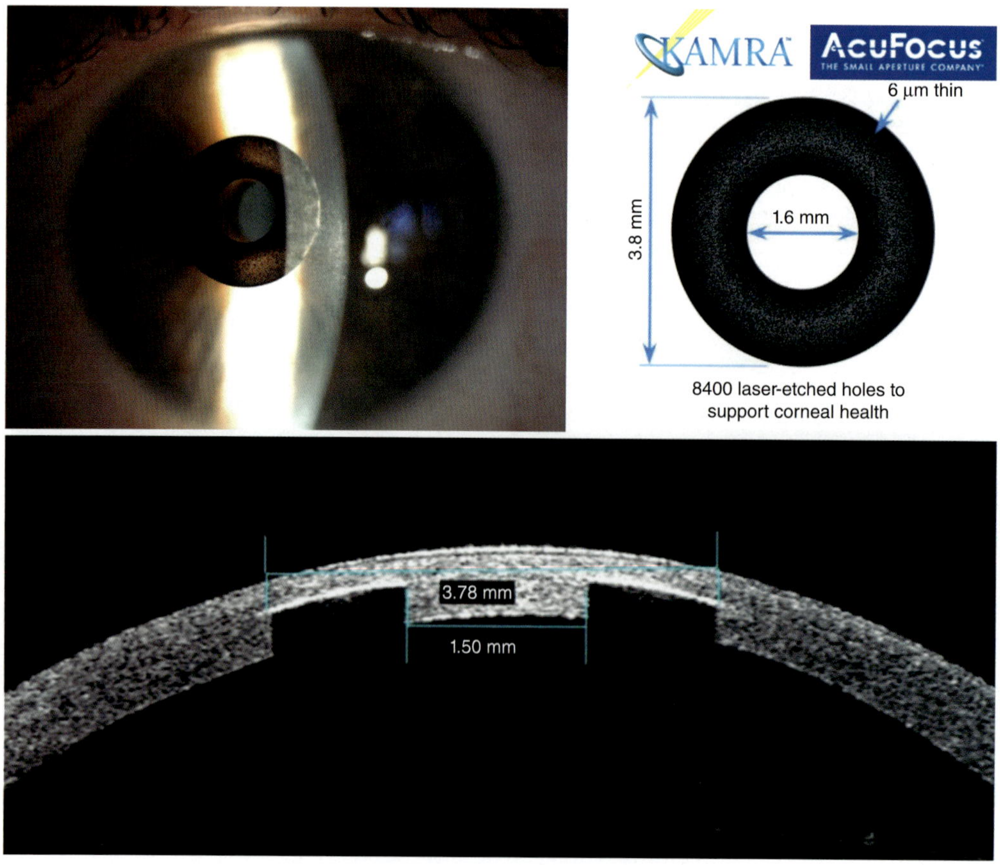

Fig. 12.22 Decentered Kamra Inlay.

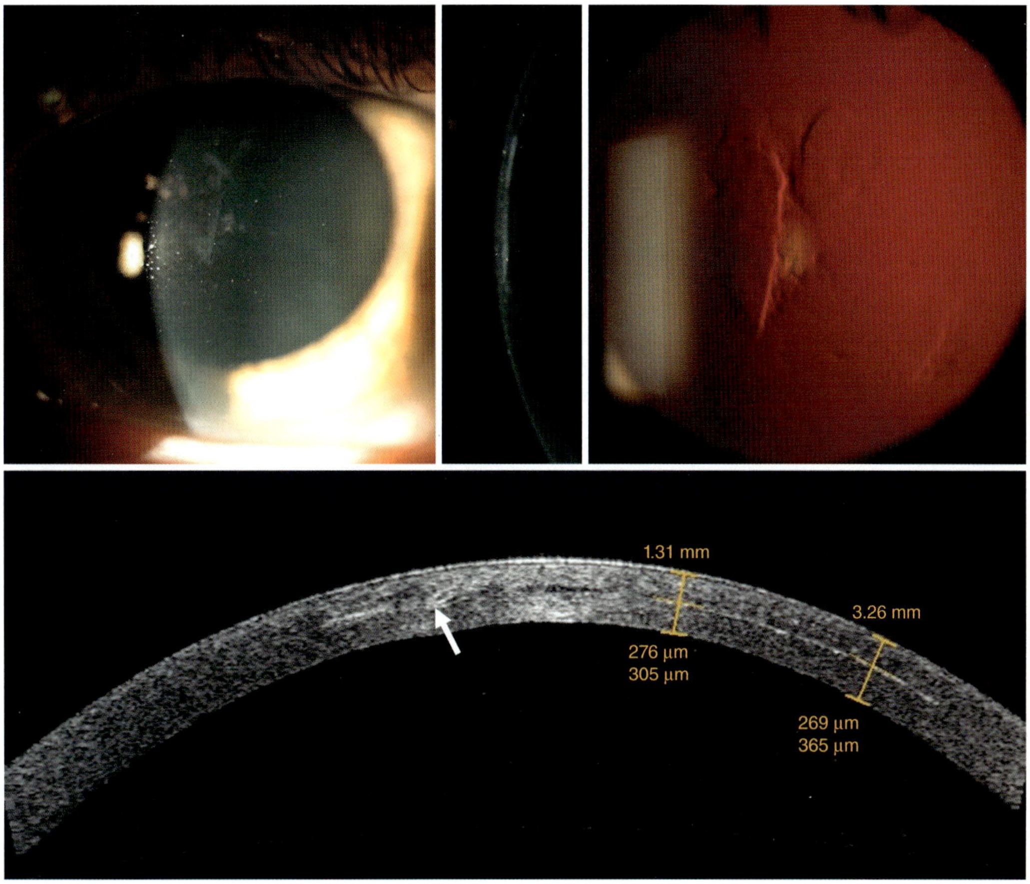

Fig. 12.23 Corneal scar from Kamra inlay.

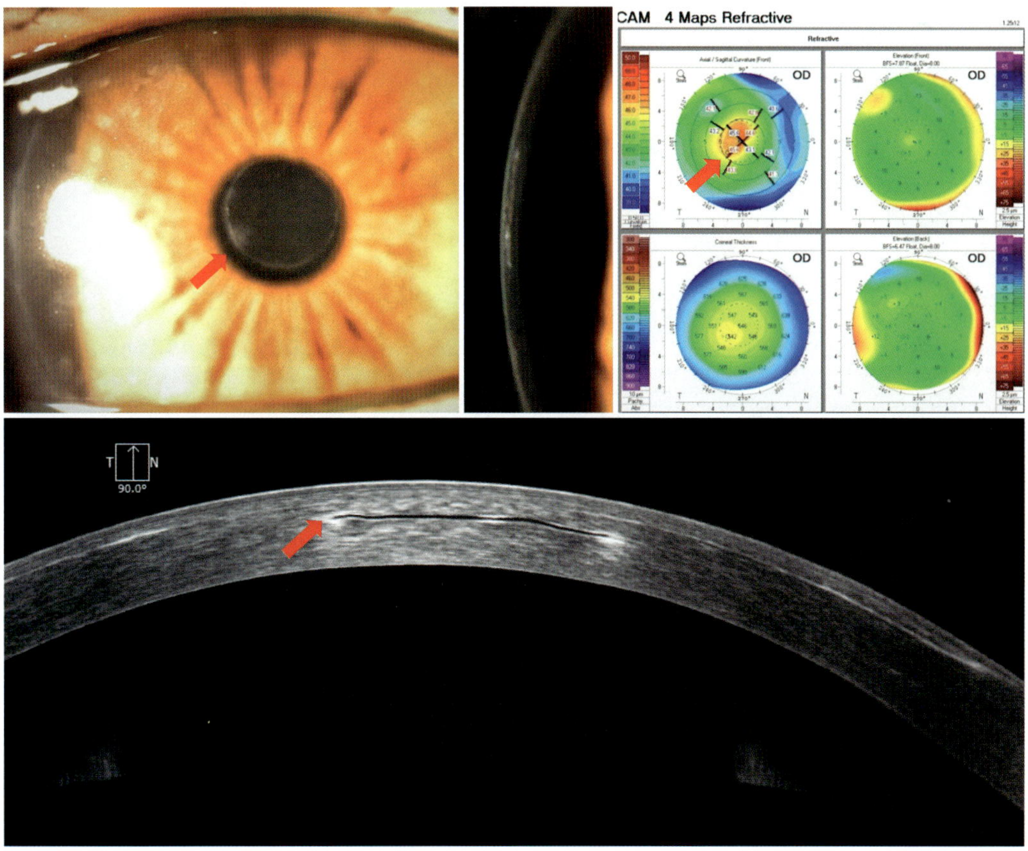

Fig. 12.24 Raindrop corneal inlay.

vision, glare disability, tearing, photophobia, and foreign bodies, all in the right eye. She was aware of the FDA recall of the Raindrop and wanted hers removed.

Uncorrected acuity in the right eye was 20/60 distance, J1 at near. With manifest refraction—1.25 + 0.25 × 180—her distance acuity improved to 20/30 but no better. Slit-lamp examination of the right eye showed the Raindrop inlay with surrounding opacity/scarring. There was also flap fibrosis with epithelial ingrowth superonasally and irregularity of the flap edge temporally. The epithelium was intact.

Fig. 12.24 shows the Raindrop inlay in the anterior stroma and corresponding topographic changes. There is scarring at the edge of the inlay *(red arrows)*. Corneal topography *(top right)* shows abnormal central elevation consistent with hyperopic ablation as well as the inlay *(red arrow)*.

Fig. 12.25 depicts the same patient with history of LASIK and removed Raindrop inlay, with slit-lamp photographs above and AS-OCT below showing superonasal flap fibrosis *(white arrows)* and epithelial ingrowth *(red arrows)*.

In Fig. 12.26, in the same patient, the Raindrop inlay is inserted into a pocket deep to the LASIK flap. *White arrows* show *(a)* epithelial thickness approximately 50 μm; *(b)* flap thickness approximately 120 to 130 μm; and *(c)* Raindrop pocket depth 240 to 250 μm. The entrance to the Raindrop pocket is clearly visible *(red arrow)*.

Melting of the temporal flap edge is observed. The *solid green arrow* shows the corresponding areas on the slit-lamp photograph *(top)* and the AS-OCT *(bottom)*. The *dashed green arrow* shows the edge of the stromal bed, over which the epithelium has hypertrophied to fill in the gap where the flap edge is missing.

Fig. 12.27 shows the same patient three months postoperatively. The Raindrop inlay has been removed, but there is still mild stromal scarring *(red arrows)*. Although the superonasal ingrowth is gone, flap fibrosis/scarring in that region remains *(inset, white asterisks)*. The temporal flap/pocket edge is comparable to preoperatively, with no further flap melting or new epithelial ingrowth *(white arrows)*. The patient has 20/30 uncorrected distance acuity and with manifest refraction −1.00 + 0.50 × 165 she corrects to 20/20+. Her symptoms are resolved, and ironically the patient's only complaint was of her worsened near vision (J4).

B. Intacs

Intacs ring segments are used to treat keratectasia and associated astigmatism. In some cases, Intacs insertion improves corneal contour enough to enable contact lens wear in patients with severe keratectasia who might not otherwise have been contact lens candidates. Intacs can also be combined with corneal collagen cross linking (CXL) to provide additional structural support to prevent ectasia progression. On AS-OCT, normally implanted Intacs ring segments appear as hyporeflective elliptical or octagonal spaces at the level of midstroma with no blockage of signal posterior to the segment (Fig. 12.28). Implantation of the ring segments within a stromal pocket can be technically challenging; AS-OCT can be used to verify depth of segment implantation (see Fig. 12.28). OCT can also help better characterize deposits or opacities within the Intacs channel (Fig. 12.29). Finally, AS-OCT can precisely ascertain location, severity, and progression of segment malposition or extrusion (Fig. 12.30).

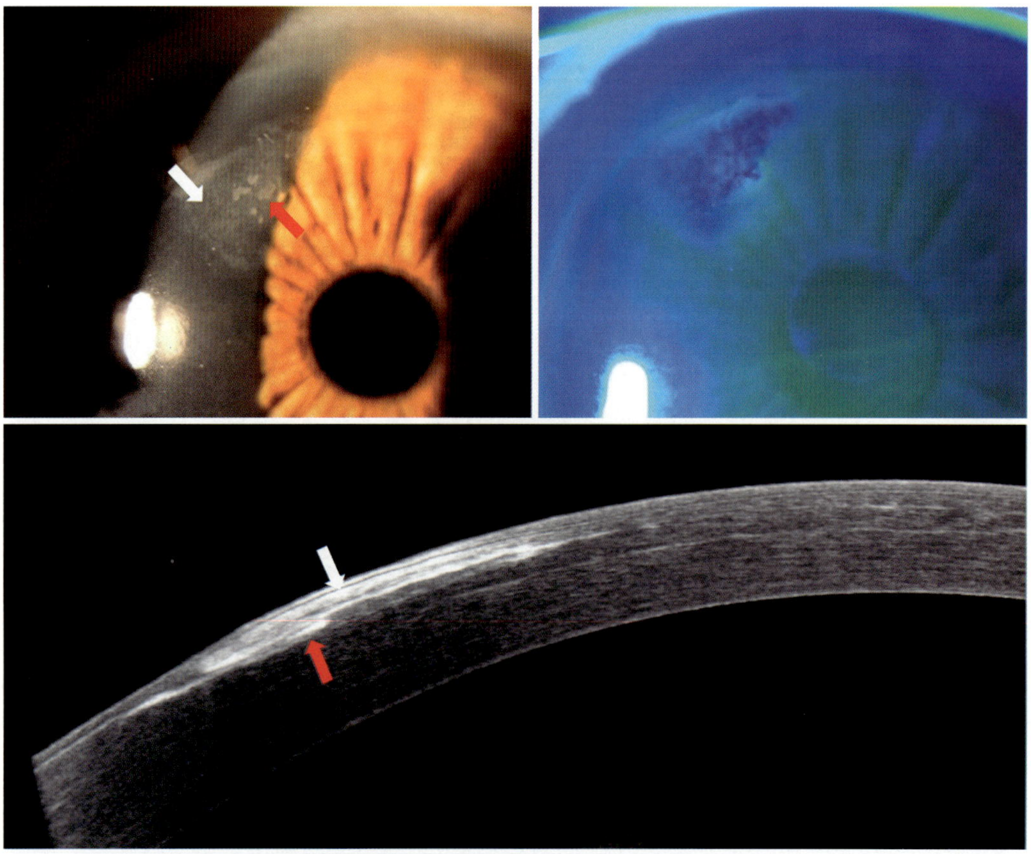

Fig. 12.25 Raindrop corneal inlay. Same patient, with slit-lamp photographs above and AS-OCT below showing superonasal flap fibrosis *(white arrows)* and epithelial ingrowth *(red arrows)*.

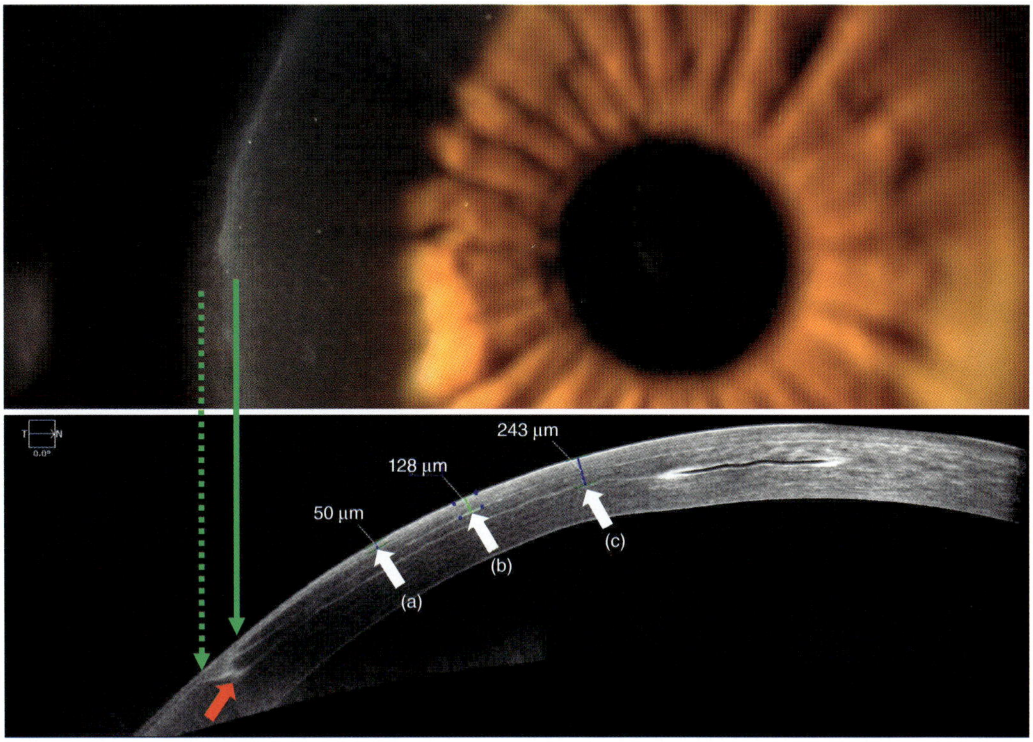

Fig. 12.26 Raindrop corneal inlay. In this patient the Raindrop inlay is inserted into a pocket deep to the LASIK flap. *White arrows* show *(a)* epithelial thickness ~50 μm; *(b)* flap thickness ~120 to 130 μm; and *(c)* Raindrop pocket depth 240 to 250 μm. The entrance to the Raindrop pocket is clearly visible *(red arrow).* There is melting of the temporal flap edge. The *solid green arrow* shows the corresponding areas on the slit-lamp photograph *(top)* and the AS-OCT *(bottom).* The *dashed green arrow* shows the edge of the stromal bed, over which the epithelium has hypertrophied to fill in the gap where the flap edge is missing.

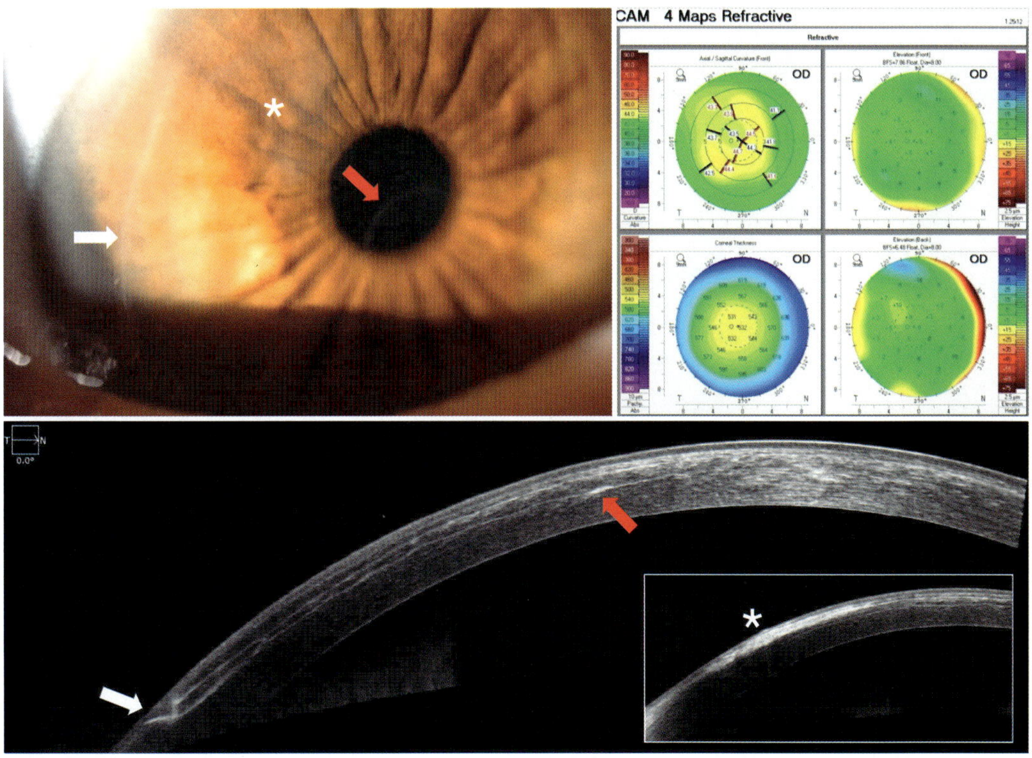

Fig. 12.27 Raindrop corneal inlay. Patient three months postoperatively. The Raindrop inlay is removed, but there is still mild stromal scarring *(red arrows).* Although the superonasal ingrowth is gone, flap fibrosis/scarring in that region remains *(inset, white asterisks).* The temporal flap/pocket edge is comparable to preoperatively, with no further flap melting or new epithelial ingrowth *(white arrows).* The patient has 20/30 uncorrected distance acuity and with manifest refraction –1.00 + 0.50 × 165 she corrects 20/20+. Her symptoms are resolved, and she only complains of her worsened near vision (J4).

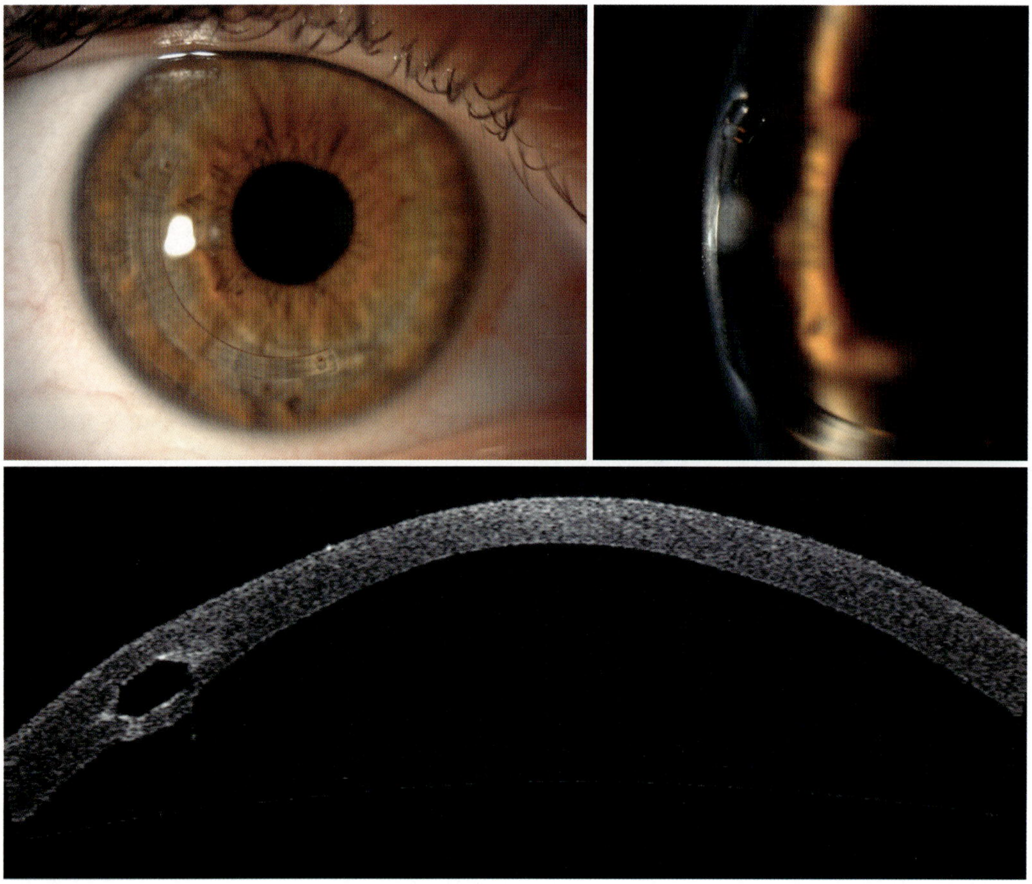

Fig. 12.28 Normal Intacs ring segment.

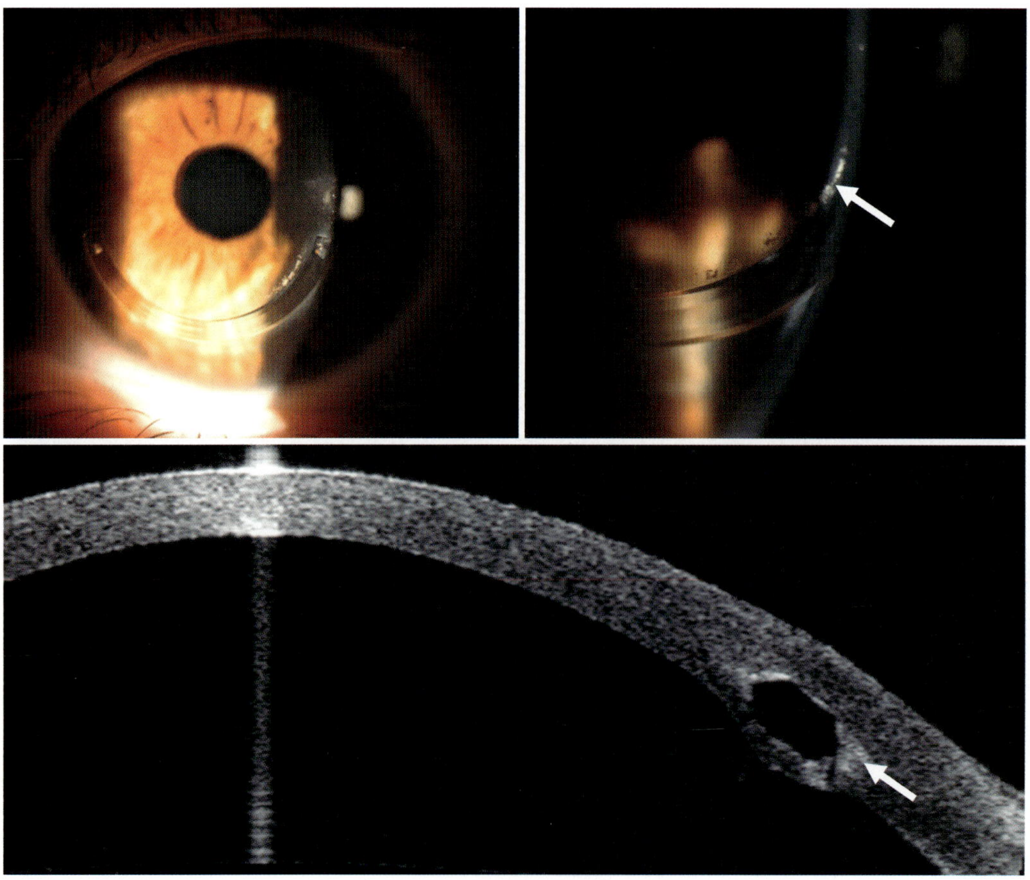

Fig. 12.29 Intacs channel deposits.

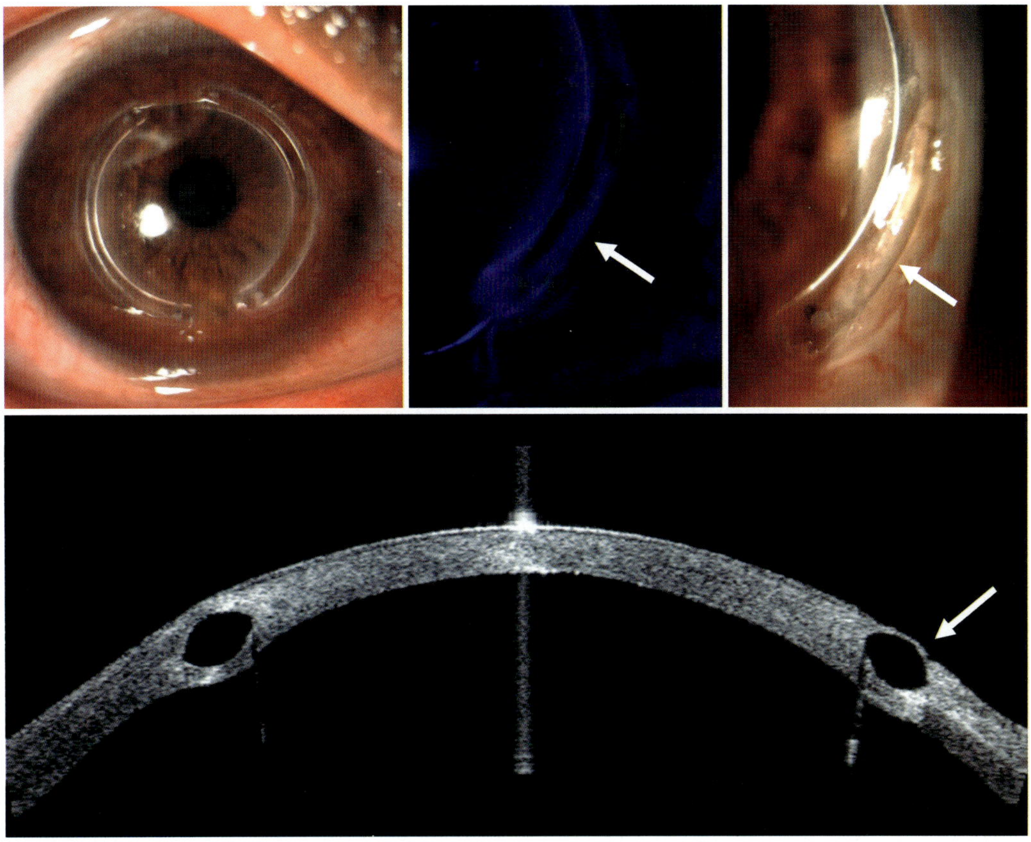

Fig. 12.30 Eroded and extruding Intacs ring segment.

C. Epikeratoplasty

Epikeratoplasty, also called *onlay lamellar keratoplasty* or *epikeratophakia* when performed in aphakic patients, involves suturing of a donor stromal lenticule onto the recipient cornea. The procedure was developed in the mid-20th century and has largely been replaced by laser refractive surgery and secondary intraocular lens insertion techniques. However, epikeratoplasty is still occasionally performed for treatment of severe ectasia or high refractive error that cannot be corrected with refractive surgery. Complications include decreased best corrected visual acuity and irregular astigmatism. AS-OCT shows a faint interface line between donor and host stroma, although with stromal remodeling over time the two tissue layers can become more difficult to differentiate (Figs. 12.31 and 12.32).

V. CORNEAL COLLAGEN CROSS LINKING

Corneal CXL is an FDA-approved therapy that has transformed treatment of progressive keratectasia, greatly reducing the need for keratoplasty in conditions such as keratoconus and postrefractive ectasia. In the classic Dresden protocol, CXL involves saturation of deepithelialized corneal stroma with riboflavin, followed by irradiation with ultraviolet A light at 370 nm for 30 minutes. Irradiating riboflavin leads to formation of covalent bonds between stromal collagen fibrils, thereby strengthening the biomechanical rigidity of the cornea, reducing risk of ectasia progression, and in many cases leading to some flattening of corneal curvature. The procedure's effects largely occur in the anterior 300 microns of the stroma, and irradiation of the endothelium should be avoided because of the risk of toxicity and corneal edema. Preoperative pachymetry should be used to confirm stromal thickness of at least 400 microns, and AS-OCT can be useful for this purpose. If the stromal thickness is less than desired, contact lens–assisted CXL can be performed to reduce risk of endothelial damage (Fig. 12.33). In the early postoperative period, AS-OCT imaging often shows an area of anterior stromal haze and an indistinct hyperreflective demarcation line between cross-linked anterior stroma and deeper stroma (Fig. 12.34). These changes typically disappear after several weeks to months. Potential complications of CXL include infectious keratitis after epithelial debridement, non-healing epithelial defects, persistent stromal haze, sterile or infectious stromal infiltrates, endothelial toxicity, and failure to prevent ectasia progression.

VI. PHAKIC INTRAOCULAR LENSES

Phakic intraocular lenses can be implanted in the anterior segment to correct refractive error, particularly among patients who are not good candidates for refractive surgery. Appropriate patient and lens selection, based on biometric parameters and verification of appropriate lens positioning is critical to achieve good refractive outcomes and avoid complications. AS-OCT can serve a critical role in precisely evaluating phakic intraocular lens position relative to other anterior segment structures.

The Visian implantable collamer lens is inserted in the ciliary sulcus in phakic patients to correct refractive error. AS-OCT can help measure lens vault in normal cases (Fig. 12.35) and abnormal cases such as shallow vault (Fig. 12.36), steep vault (Fig. 12.37), or lens decentration or tilt (Fig. 12.38). AS-OCT can also help characterize complications of malposition such as

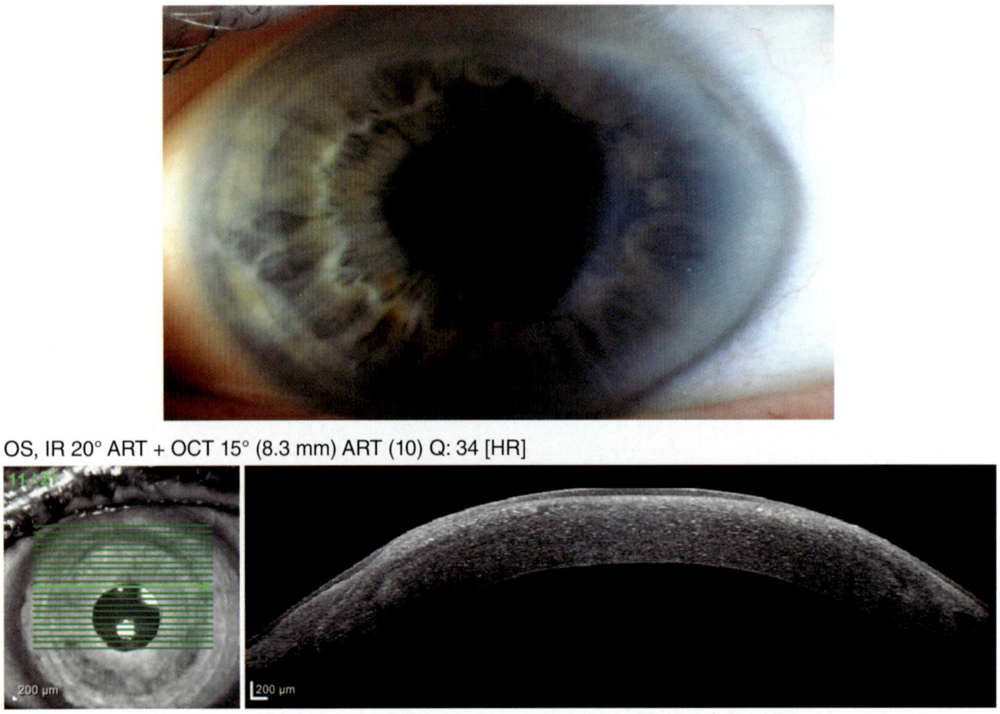

Fig. 12.31 Epikeratophakia.

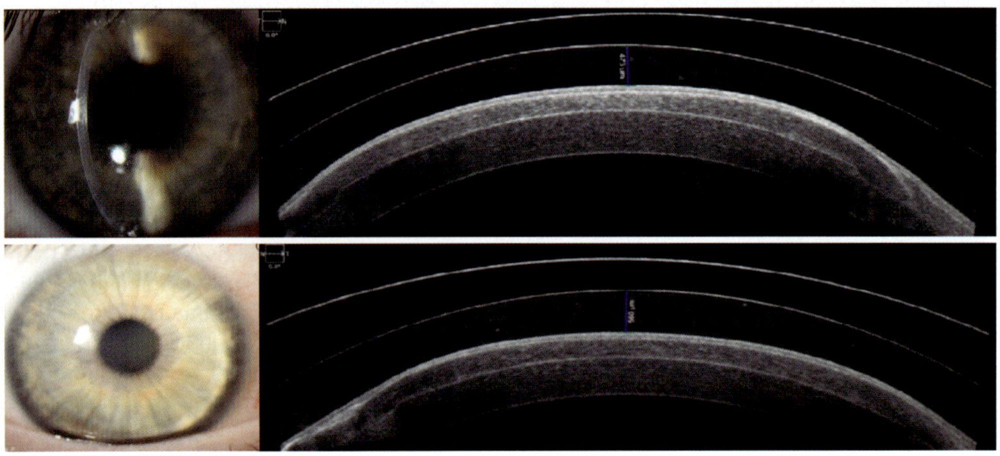

Fig. 12.32 Epikeratophakia.

anterior subcapsular cataract (Fig. 12.39), corneal endothelial damage, lens-iris chafing causing uveitis or ocular hypertension, pupillary block (Fig. 12.40), and malignant glaucoma (Fig. 12.41). In the latter example, serial anterior chamber depth measurements by AS-OCT helped verify normalization of anatomic structures to preoperative levels over time.

The Artiflex and Verisyse phakic intraocular lenses are iris-fixated and must achieve sufficient vault to prevent iris chafing or pupillary block. Fig. 12.42 shows well-centered Artiflex phakic intraocular lens with appropriate vault, while Fig. 12.43 shows a dislocated Verisyse phakic intraocular lens with significant decentration and tilt.

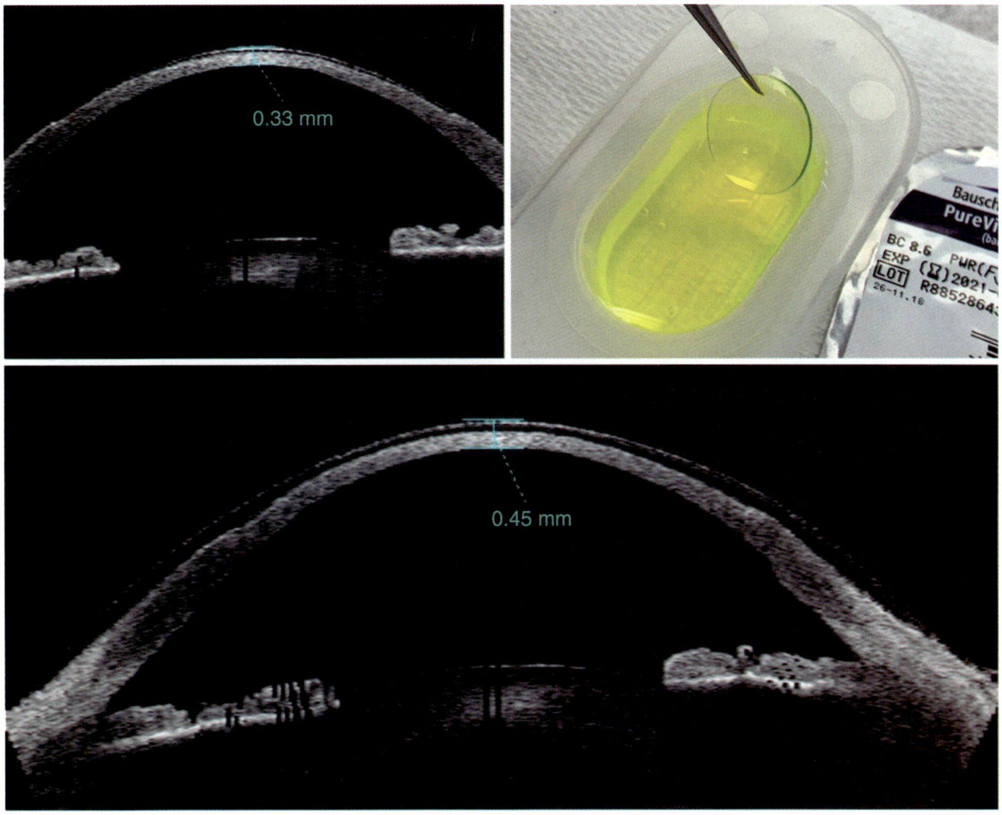

Fig. 12.33 Contact lens–assisted corneal collagen cross linking.

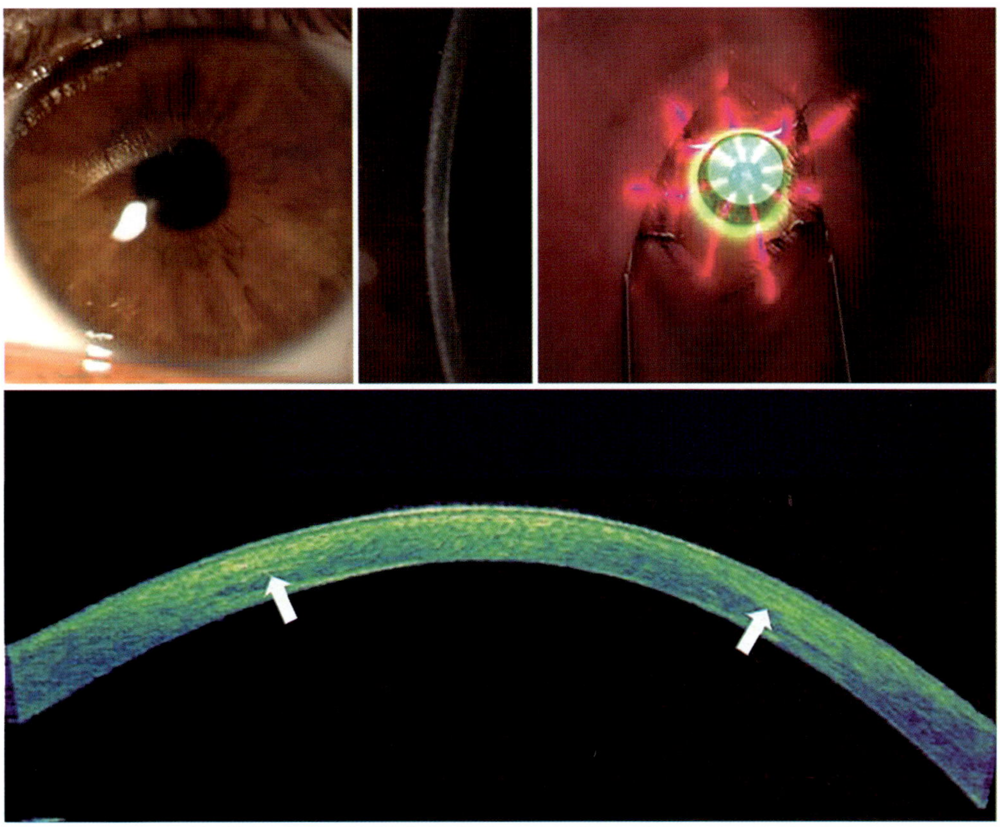

Fig. 12.34 Demarcation line after corneal collagen cross linking.

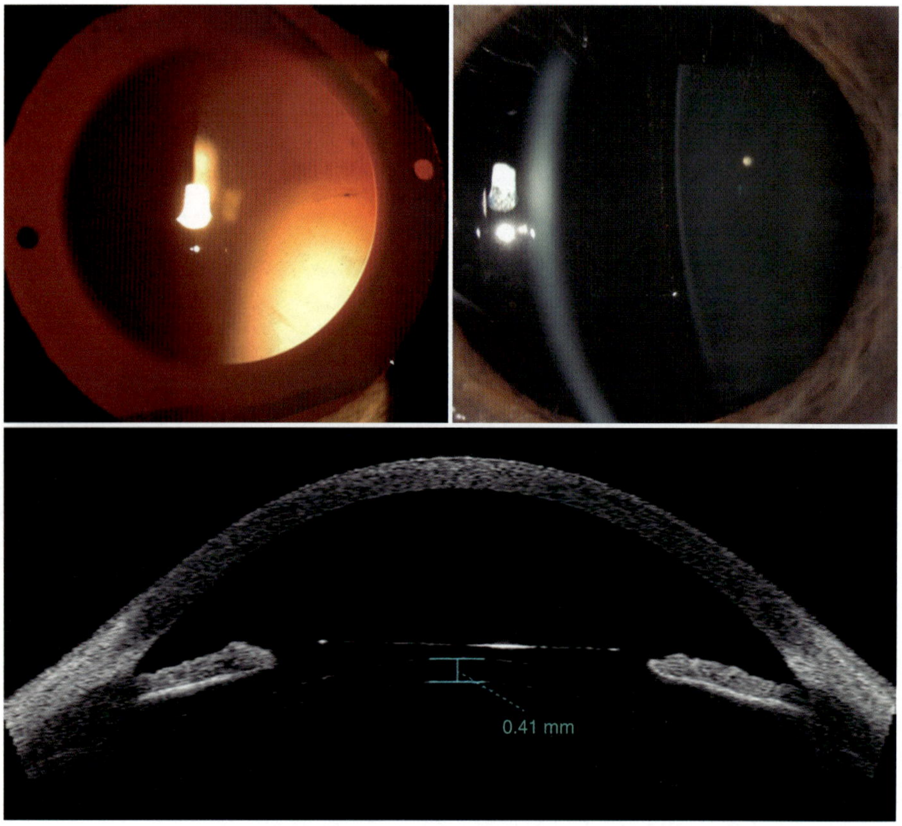

Fig. 12.35 Visian ICL with normal vault.

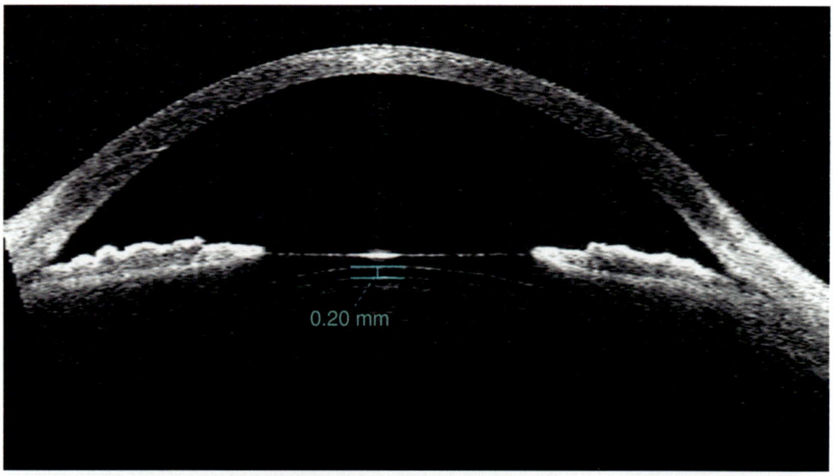

Fig. 12.36 Visian ICL with shallow vault.

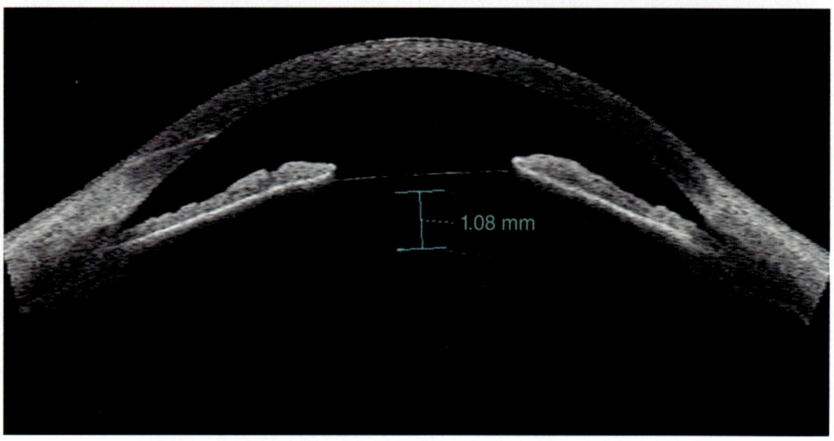

Fig. 12.37 Visian ICL with steep vault and iris contact.

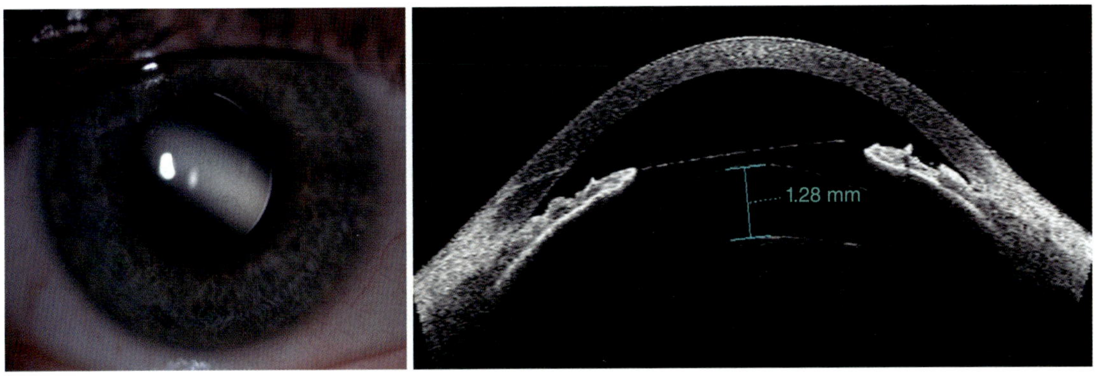

Fig. 12.38 Visian ICL with steep vault, decentration, and tilt.

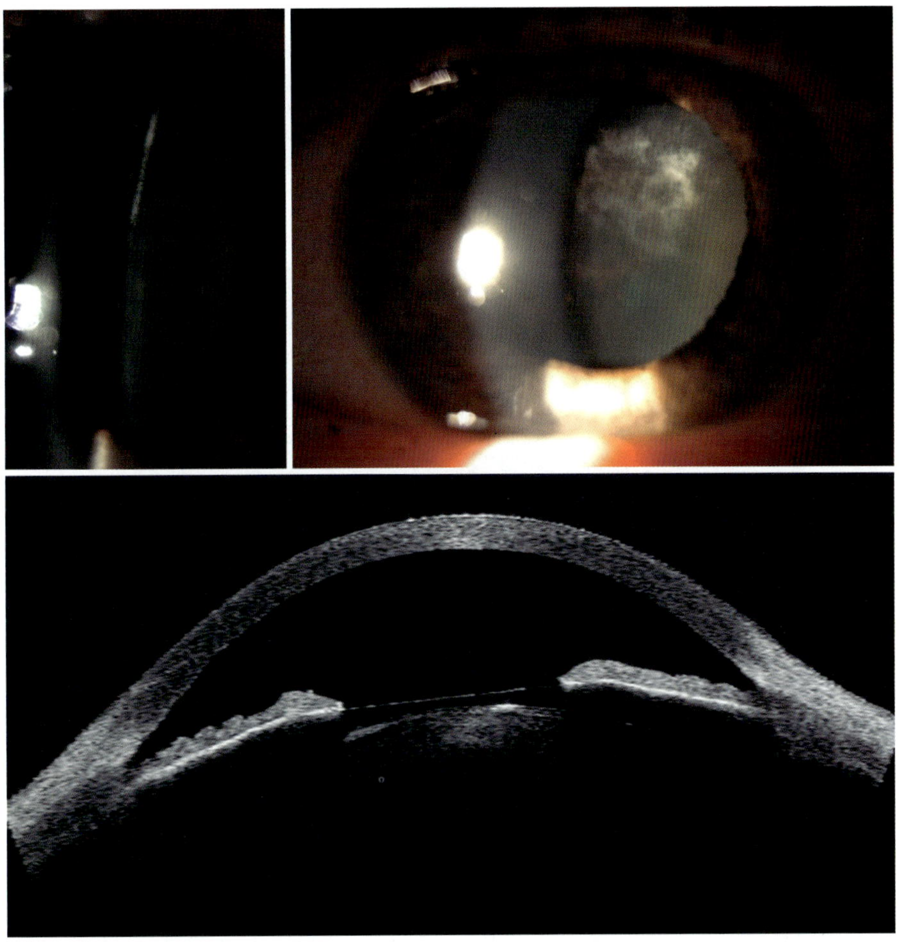

Fig. 12.39 Visian ICL with flat vault and associated anterior subcapsular cataract.

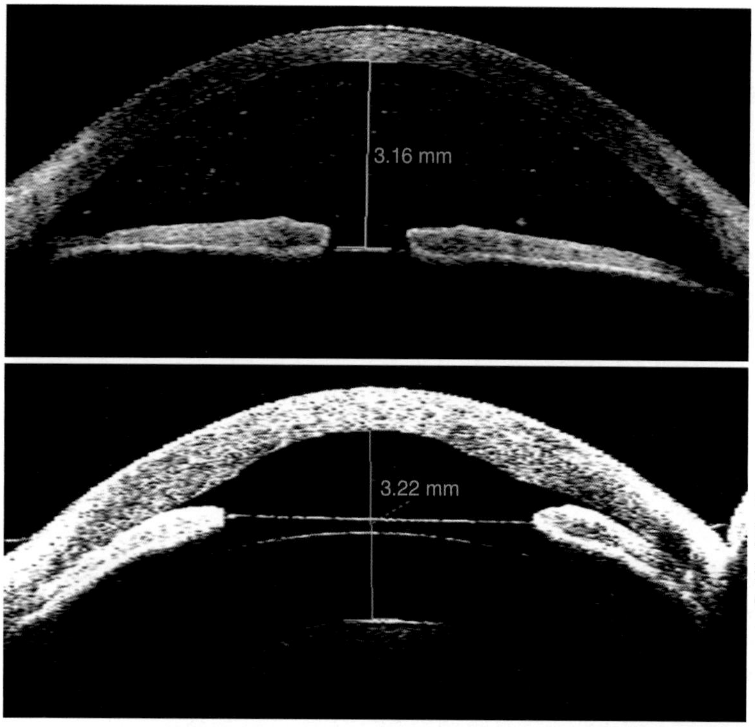

Pre-operative image showing normal anterior chamber

Visian ICL shows angle closure from pupillary block. The line shows the distance from endothelium to anterior capsule.

Fig. 12.40 Visian ICL with pupillary block.

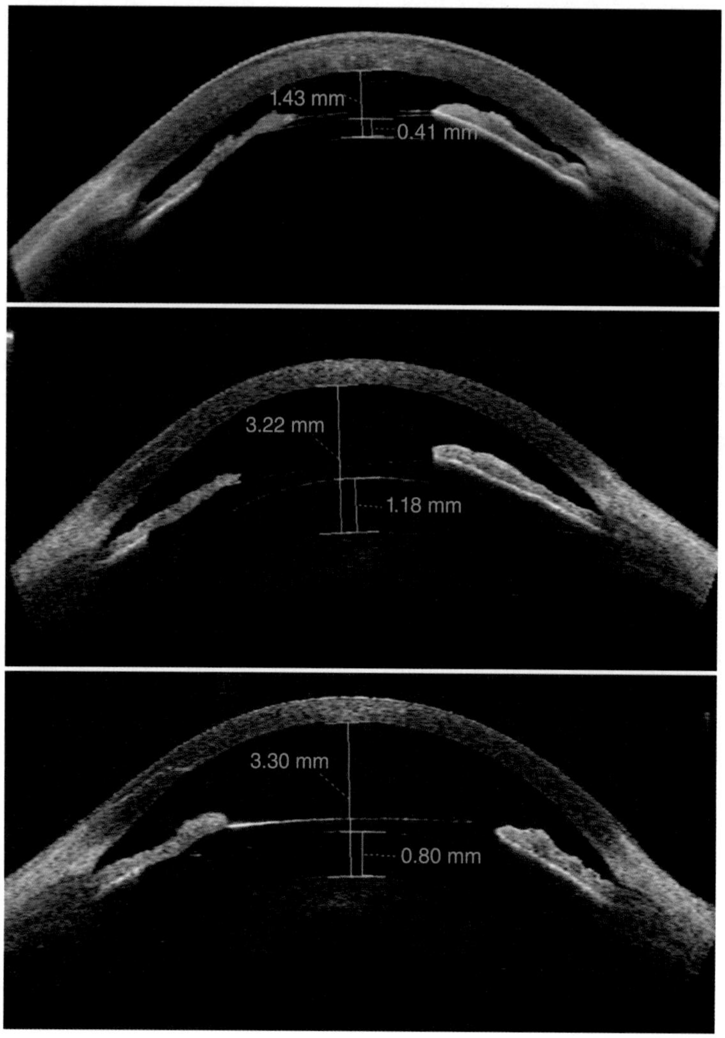

Fig. 12.41 ICL with malignant glaucoma at postoperative day one, week one, and month one.

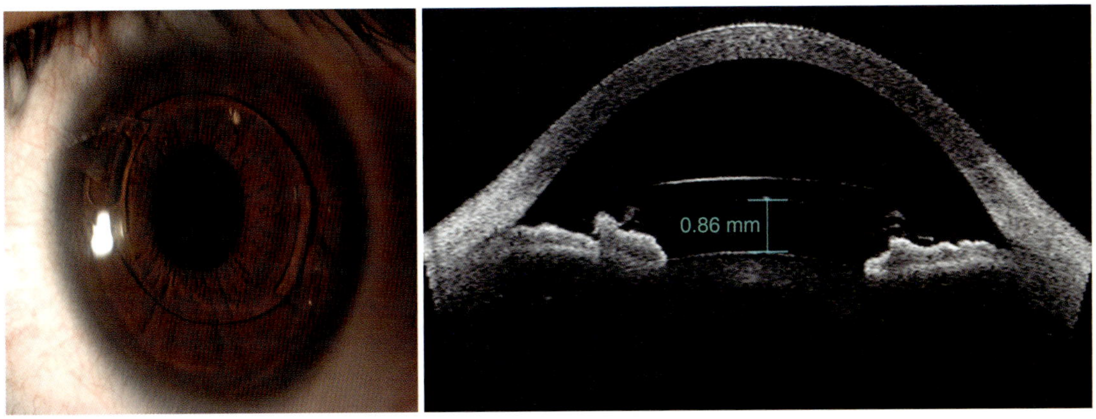

Fig. 12.42 Artiflex phakic intraocular lens.

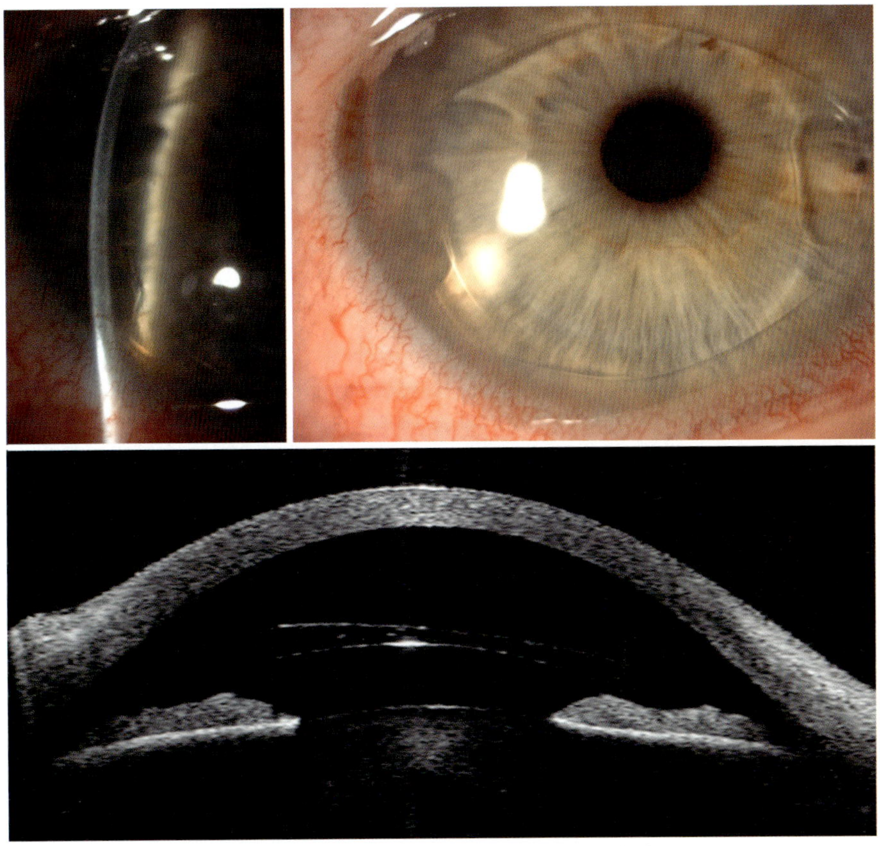

Fig. 12.43 Dislocated Verisyse phakic intraocular lens.

BIBLIOGRAPHY

1. Ang M, Baskaran M, Werkmeister RM, et al. Anterior segment optical coherence tomography. *Prog Retin Eye Res*. 2018;66:132-156.
2. Kanski J, Bowling B. Cornea. In: *Kanski's Clinical Ophthalmology: A Systematic Approach*. 8th ed. London, UK: Saunders Ltd; 2016:167-238.
3. Krachmer JH, Mannis MJ, Holland EJ. *Cornea: Fundamentals, Diagnosis and Management*. 3rd ed. Cincinnati, OH: Mosby; 2011.
4. Koide T, Daito M. Effects of various collagen crosslinking techniques on mechanical properties of collagen film. *Dent Mater J*. 1997;16(1):1-9.

13 Use of Intraoperative AS-OCT in Corneal Transplant Surgery

Samir Jabbour | Albert Jun

I. INTRODUCTION

With advancements in anterior segment optical coherence tomography (AS-OCT) technology, intraoperative OCT (iOCT) devices are now available for use during ophthalmic surgery. The advantage of iOCT is its ability to provide surgeons with precise, real-time visualization of the cornea and anterior segment. This can be especially advantageous in situations in which corneal edema and scarring may preclude surgeons' view, especially with longer duration surgeries. This chapter will focus on the use of iOCT during corneal transplant surgery, focusing on partial-thickness procedures. The next chapter will discuss the use of AS-OCT for postoperative management of patients after corneal transplant surgery.

II. DESCEMET STRIPPING AUTOMATED ENDOTHELIAL KERATOPLASTY

Descemet stripping automated endothelial keratoplasty (DSAEK) is the most commonly used endothelial keratoplasty (EK) technique worldwide for surgical rehabilitation of corneal endothelial disease, including but not limited to Fuchs endothelial dystrophy (FED), pseudophakic bullous keratopathy (PBK), and endothelial failure after penetrating keratoplasty (PKP). DSAEK involves replacing the diseased host endothelium and Descemet membrane (DM) with a donor tissue comprising endothelium, DM, and posterior stroma with thickness ranging from 30 to 150 μm.

A potentially common complication after DSAEK is postoperative graft dislocation, especially with thinner DSAEK grafts (ultrathin DSAEK, sub50-DSAEK, and nano-thin DSAEK). Residual graft-host interface fluid is known to be a main contributor to postoperative graft detachments. Multiple techniques, including sweeping and venting incisions, have been described to address interface fluid.

CLINICAL PEARL

Intraoperative OCT (iOCT) can be useful in qualifying and quantifying interface fluid. It allows for easy monitoring of the interface while different maneuvers are employed. The iOCT also improves visualization of the anterior chamber in eyes with opaque corneas, allowing easier graft positioning.

Figs. 13.1 to 13.5 demonstrate the use of iOCT during DSAEK surgery. In Fig. 13.1, there is a prominent fold in the inferior aspect of the DSAEK graft after placement of the air bubble seen in the surgical microscope view, which is also readily seen in the iOCT view. After unfolding of the graft, residual interface fluid was found at the temporal edge of the graft (Fig. 13.2). The small area of interface fluid could be easily missed with the surgical microscope. External tapping and sweeping maneuvers can be used to smooth out the graft and ensure proper anatomic adherence (Fig. 13.3). Although the graft appears to be well apposed to the posterior surface of the host cornea through the surgical microscope, there are notable areas of residual interface fluid seen on iOCT. External sweeping with gentle pressure in a centrifugal fashion can help evacuate interface fluid (Fig. 13.4). After sweeping, the iOCT can be used to determine appropriate positioning of the DSAEK graft in real-time (Fig. 13.5).

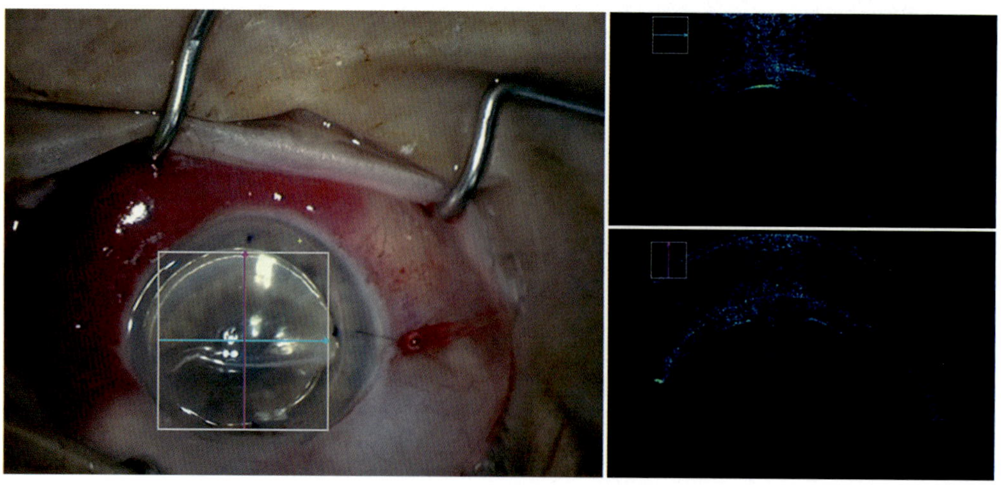

Fig. 13.1 Prominent inferior fold noted in the Descemet stripping automated endothelial keratoplasty graft both in the surgical microscope view and on iOCT. (Courtesy Michael Mimouni, MD, University of Toronto, Toronto, Canada.)

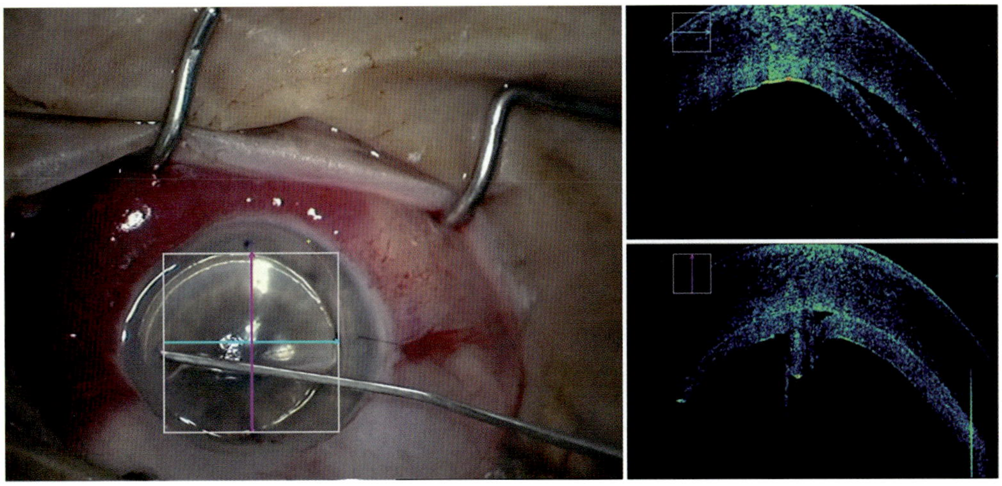

Fig. 13.2 External tapping and unfolding maneuvers used to ensure proper graft apposition. Note in the horizontal view *(top right panel)* that the graft appears to be attached centrally with peripheral non-adherence. In the vertical view *(bottom right panel),* there is a prominent fold. (Courtesy Michael Mimouni, MD, University of Toronto, Toronto, Canada.)

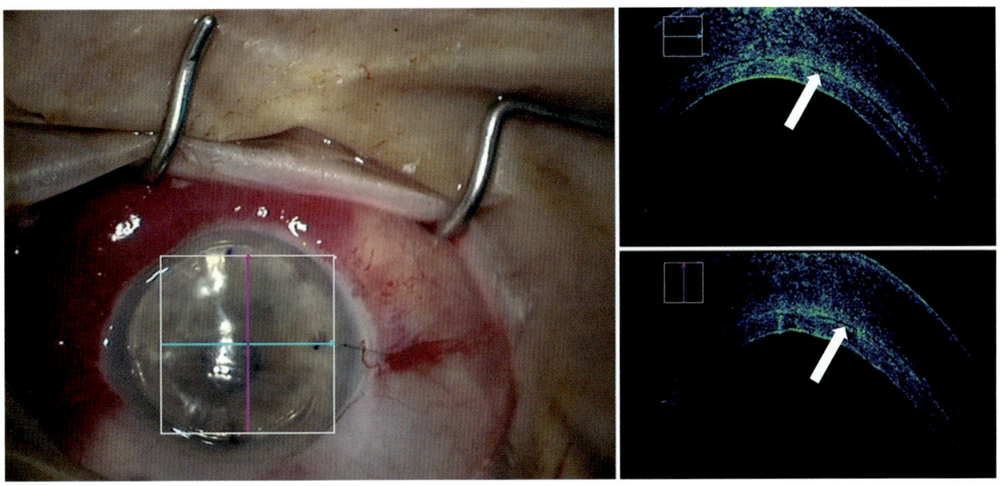

Fig. 13.3 After successful tapping and sweeping maneuvers, the DSAEK lenticule is shown with good apposition to the host posterior stromal surface. Both the horizontal *(top right panel)* and vertical *(bottom right panel)* views of the iOCT confirm good graft apposition. A small amount of interface fluid is still present *(arrow)* as areas of optically empty spaces between the host cornea and DSAEK graft. (Courtesy Michael Mimouni, MD, University of Toronto, Toronto, Canada.)

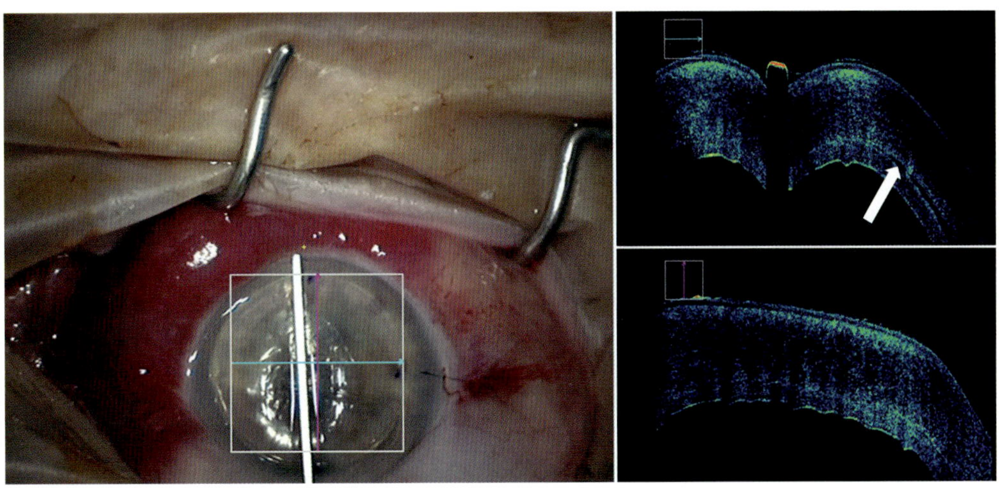

Fig. 13.4 External sweeping in a centrifugal fashion (peripheral sweeping) used to push interface fluid to the peripheral edges and outside the graft. In the *top right panel,* iOCT shows corneal dimpling from the external pressure applied by the cannula with movement of fluid to the peripheral aspect of the graft *(white arrow).* (Courtesy Michael Mimouni, MD, University of Toronto, Toronto, Canada.)

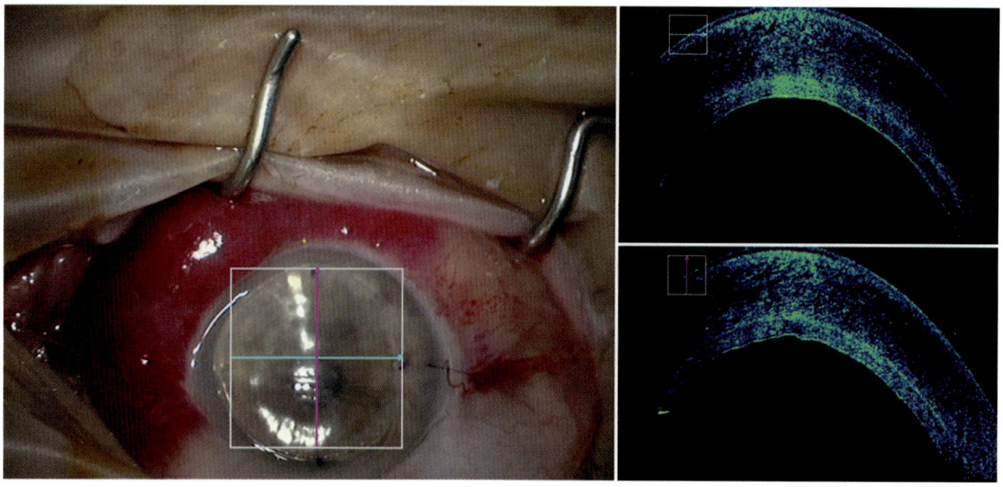

Fig. 13.5 After sweeping maneuvers, iOCT is used to check graft apposition and ensure absence of interface fluid. (Courtesy Michael Mimouni, MD, University of Toronto, Toronto, Canada.)

III. DESCEMET MEMBRANE ENDOTHELIAL KERATOPLASTY

Descemet membrane endothelial keratoplasty (DMEK) consists of selective, 1:1 replacement of host DM and endothelium. It can offer superior recovery of visual acuity compared with DSAEK. DMEK tissue is thinner than DSAEK (approximately 10–15 μm thickness). During surgery, this thin tissue has a natural tendency to roll up into a scroll configuration with "endothelium side-out." Additionally, the tissue is transparent, making it difficult to visualize during surgery, unless ophthalmic dyes (e.g., trypan blue) are used to stain the tissue. These inherent properties contribute to the technical challenges associated with DMEK.

DMEK is a "no-touch technique"; therefore conventional surgical techniques involve injection of the naturally scrolled tissue in the eye followed by a sequence of "tapping and pinning" maneuvers on the corneal surface, injecting intracameral balanced salt solution, and shallowing the anterior chamber to help with unscrolling of the graft. The tissue is extremely fragile; thus visualization at the surgical microscope can be challenging, especially in the presence of cloudy and edematous corneas.

iOCT can facilitate DMEK surgery by determining whether the graft is in the proper orientation. In Fig. 13.6, iOCT can be used to ascertain the scroll's natural "endothelium side-out" configuration, in which the scroll lumen opening should be facing up toward the host stroma before unfolding. In this configuration, the graft can be tapped along the long axis for opening, unfolding, and eventual positioning. Once partially unfolded, graft orientation can be confirmed by inspecting for the presence of upward curling, indicating an appropriate "endothelium-side down" orientation (Fig. 13.7). Similar to DSAEK, after insertion of air/gas, the iOCT can help ensure proper DMEK graft apposition and determine the presence of interface fluid (Fig. 13.7).

CLINICAL PEARL

Intraoperative OCT (iOCT) can be especially useful in DMEK surgery to assess proper scroll orientation. Confirmation of appropriate scroll orientation can assure the surgeon that untapping/opening maneuvers can be subsequently performed so that the graft can open in the desired orientation.

IV. DEEP ANTERIOR LAMELLAR KERATOPLASTY

Deep anterior lamellar keratoplasty (DALK) is a surgical procedure for selectively replacing the corneal stroma to restore transparency and curvature for stromal diseases with a healthy endothelium. Despite the obvious advantages of no endothelial rejection and increased graft survival, DALK has been slow to adopt because of its highly technical nature and slower visual outcomes compared with PKP when the DM is not exposed. Compared with PKP, DALK is more technically challenging because it requires careful dissection of the stroma close to the DM, avoiding any inadvertent perforations.

Given the comparable long-term visual outcomes to PKP, current practice aims to bare the DM-endothelium or to leave behind as little residual stroma as possible (≤80 μm) to optimize visual recovery. There are a variety of DALK techniques (e.g., peeling off, hydrodissection, layer-by-layer manual dissection, big bubble, viscodissection, and air-visco bubble) that can be used to achieve this. The most popular is the big bubble technique described by Anwar and colleagues in which air is injected in the posterior stroma close to the DM, creating a "big bubble" that permits easier removal of the overlying stroma. Three types of big bubbles have been described. A type 1 big bubble involves separation of the deep stroma (anteriorly) and Dua's layer (posteriorly). A type 2 big bubble involves complete separation between the Dua's layer (anteriorly) and the host DM (posteriorly). A type 3, or mixed, big bubble occurs when the above two coexist, usually with a complete type 1 and a partial type 2 big bubbles. Manual dissection is another popular technique and can be performed from the sclera (Melles technique) or from the cornea after partial trephination of the host tissue.

Because the DALK procedure relies heavily on the surgeon finding the appropriate location within the posterior corneal stroma, the iOCT is particularly useful because it allows real-time, detailed assessment of the depth within the cornea for surgical manipulations, allowing for more precise and predictable dissection.

The iOCT can help determine the depth of the initial partial trephination, an important first step for both manual dissection and big bubble techniques. In Fig. 13.8, iOCT shows a partial trephination at approximately 80% depth.

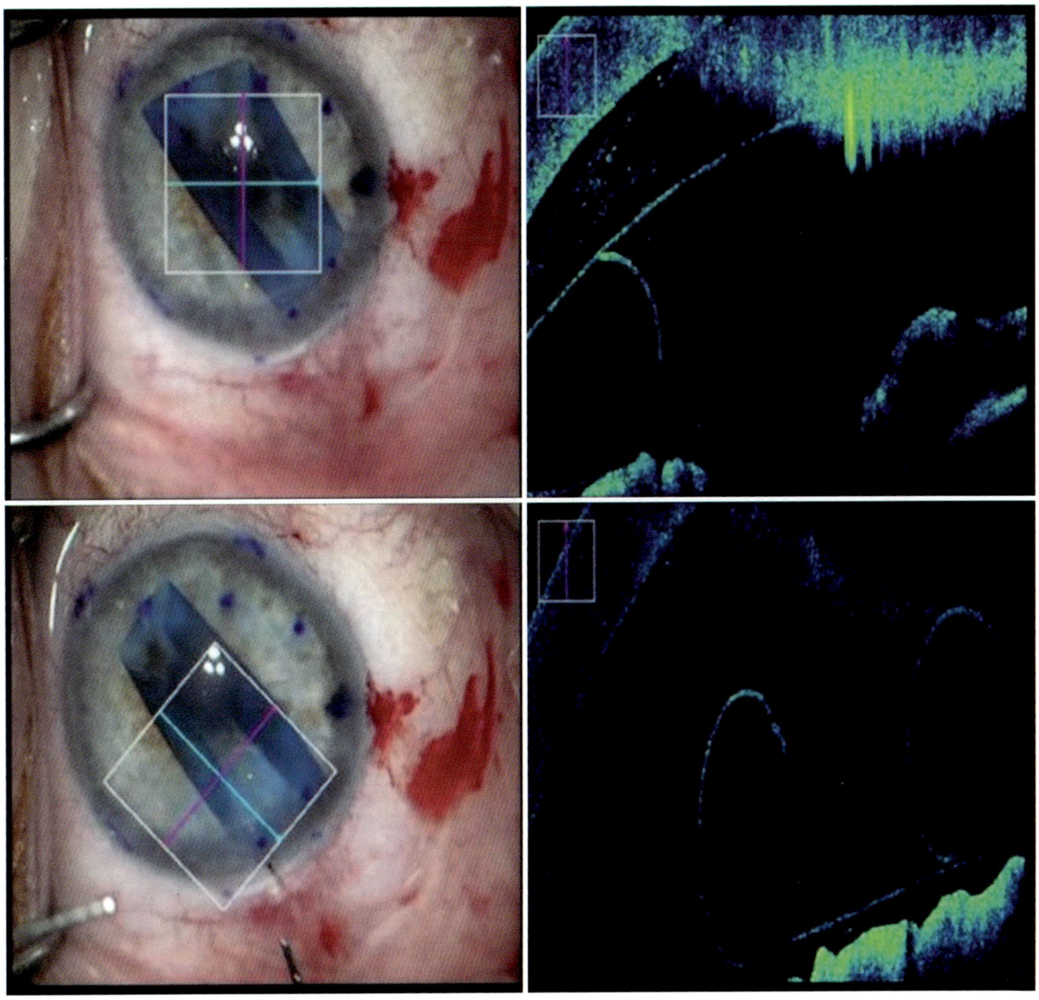

Fig. 13.6 In the surgical microscope view, the DMEK graft has been inserted into the anterior chamber. In the iOCT view, the DMEK graft is noted to be in the proper orientation wherein the scroll opening is facing the stroma *(top right panel)*. (Reprinted with permission from Brian Cost, Jeffrey M. Goshe, Sunil Srivastava, Justis P. Ehlers, Intraoperative Optical Coherence Tomography–Assisted Descemet Membrane Endothelial Keratoplasty in the DISCOVER Study, American Journal of Ophthalmology, Volume 160, Issue 3, 2015, Pages 430-437.)

After partial trephination, air can be forcefully injected into the deep stroma to create the big bubble. The iOCT is a useful tool in approximating the depth of cannula placement to ensure close proximity to DM. However, it is important to note that shadowing of the OCT signal from the metallic cannula prevents imaging posterior to it (Fig. 13.9). Thus once the tract within the deep stroma is established, the cannula can be removed to allow iOCT assessment of the residual stroma behind the tract.

CLINICAL PEARL

Intraoperative OCT (iOCT) is particularly useful in deep anterior lamellar keratoplasty (DALK) procedures to orient the surgeon before attempting the big bubble and confirmation of the bubble after intrastromal air injection.

The iOCT can also facilitate visualization of the big bubble once formed. This is characterized by a concave, optically empty space with a hyperreflective thin floor comprising the pre-Descemet layer (Dua layer) and DM for type I bubbles (Fig. 13.10). In a case of a type II bubble, a thinner floor comprising only DM can sometimes be appreciated. Type II bubbles are more prone to perforation during surgery.

Once the overlying stroma is carefully dissected, a thin posterior layer of the pre-Descemet layer and DM is noted (Fig. 13.11), on which an endothelium-stripped donor cornea can be sutured in position.

In the manual dissection DALK technique, the iOCT can allow detailed assessment of the residual posterior stroma and guide dissection to the appropriate depth (Fig. 13.12). Several consecutive planes can be established until the appropriate depth is achieved.

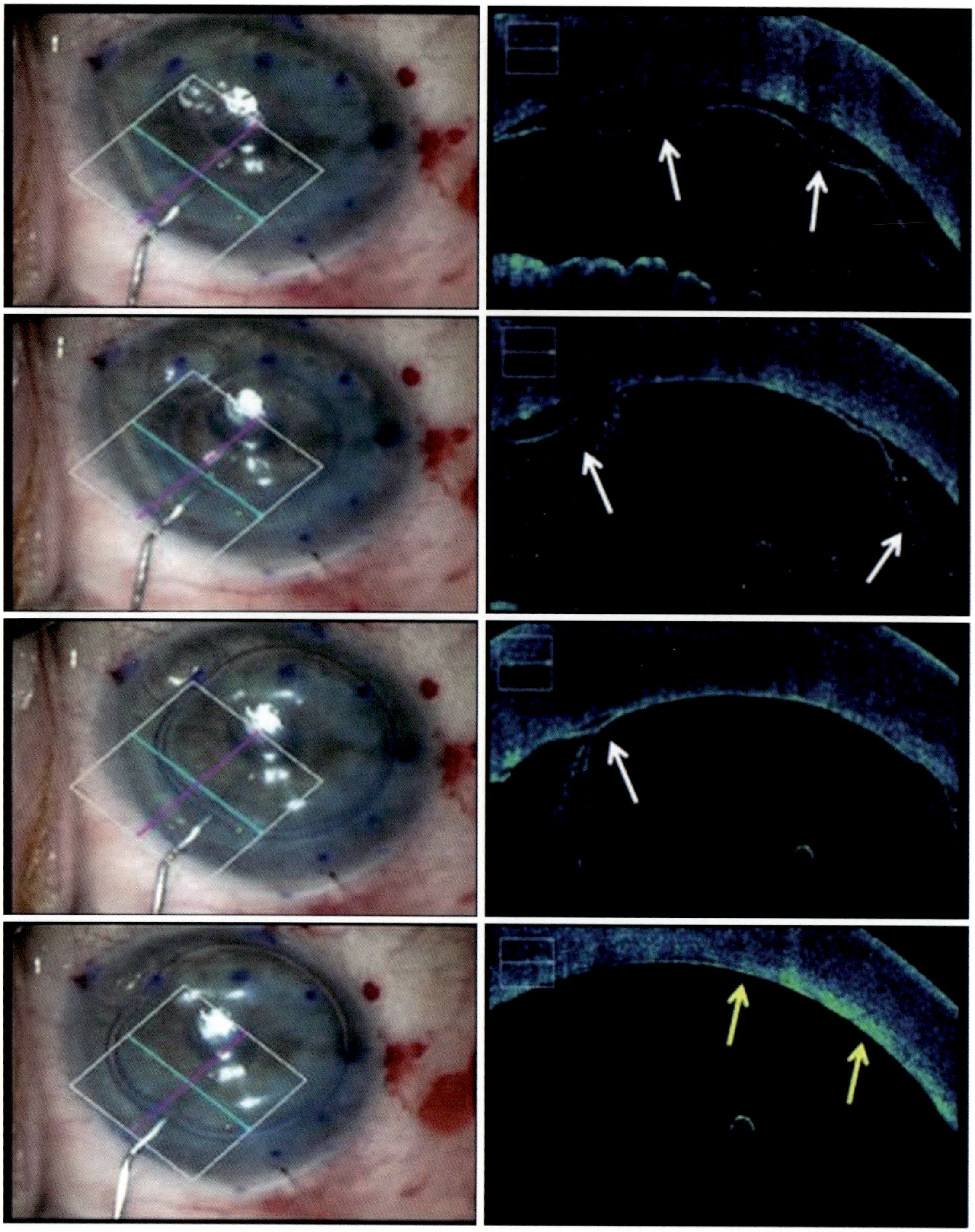

Fig. 13.7 The graft appears to be in the proper position in the surgical microscope view. In the iOCT view *(top right panel)*, there is slight "upward curling" of the unfolded tissue, which is an indication that the graft is in the proper orientation. However, there is a considerable amount of interface fluid (optically empty space between the DMEK graft and host cornea) as these images are taken prior to anterior chamber air/gas injection. After injection of air/gas *(middle right panels)*, iOCT can be used to assess graft apposition and determine the presence of interface fluid. The microscope view suggests good attachment of the DMEK graft, but the iOCT views confirm this, which makes it very useful in cases of corneal edema or poor surgical view. In the bottom right panel, no interface fluid is present, confirming the complete attachment of the DMEK graft. (Reprinted with permission from Brian Cost, Jeffrey M. Goshe, Sunil Srivastava, Justis P. Ehlers, Intraoperative Optical Coherence Tomography–Assisted Descemet Membrane Endothelial Keratoplasty in the DISCOVER Study, American Journal of Ophthalmology, Volume 160, Issue 3, 2015, Pages 430-437.)

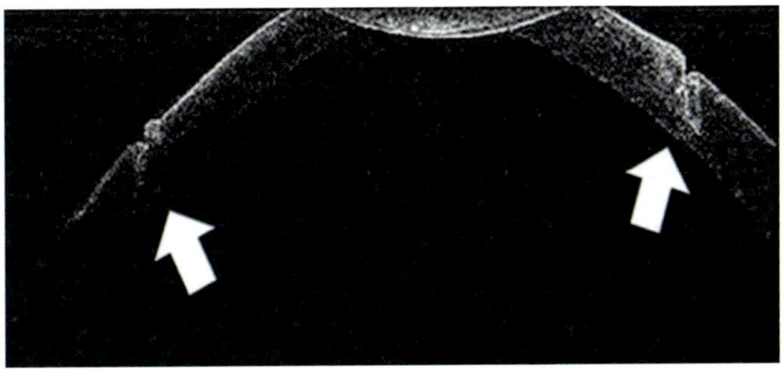

Fig. 13.8 iOCT used to check the amount of partial trephination before injection of air for the big bubble. In this case there is approximately 80% depth trephination *(arrows).* (Courtesy Philipp Steven, University of Cologne, Cologne, Germany.)

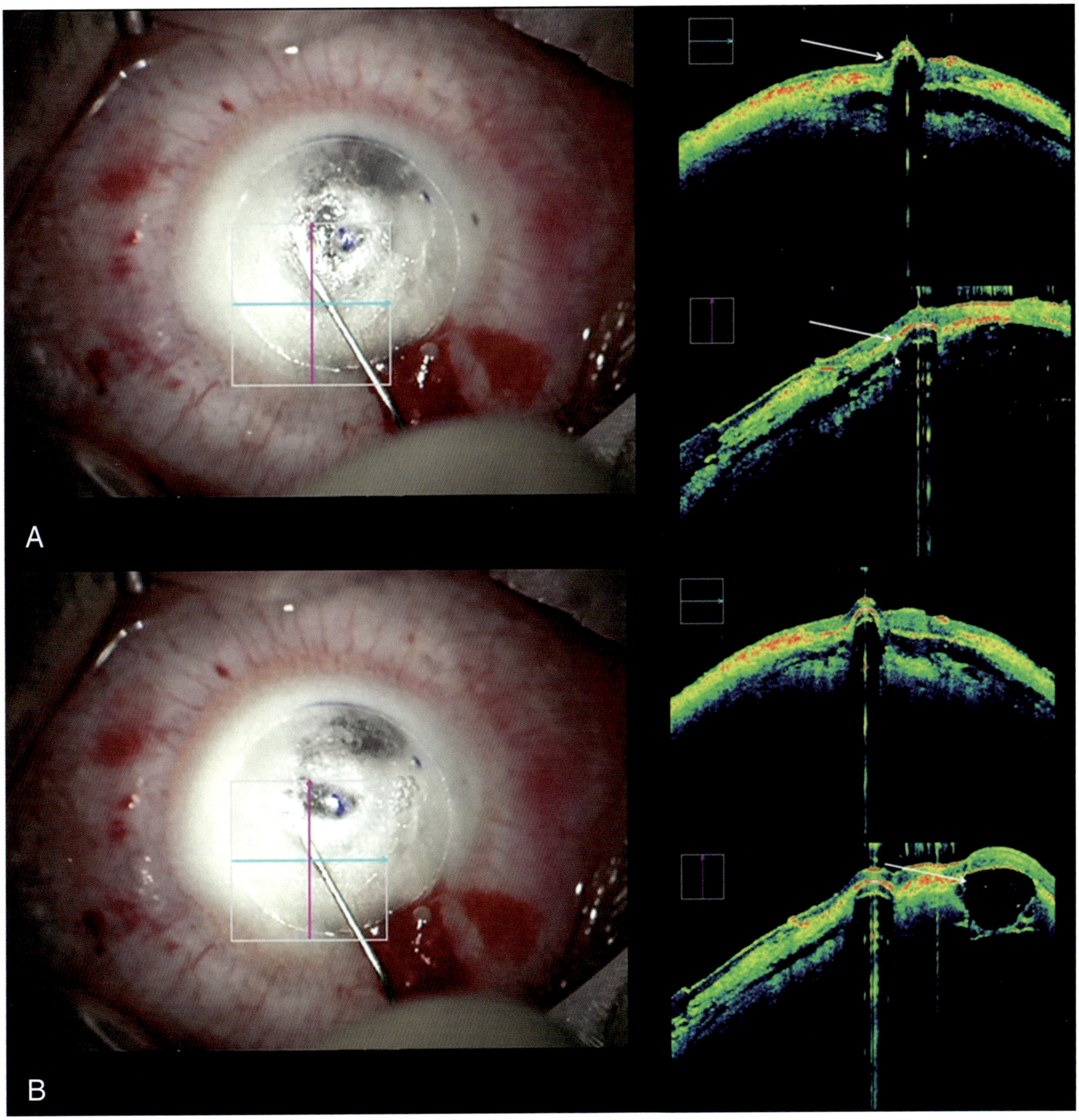

Fig. 13.9 The iOCT view shows the metallic cannula in the deep posterior stroma after injection of air to create a big bubble. (Image Credit: Stefan Lang, Albert-Ludwigs-University of Freiburg, Freiburg, Germany. Reprinted with permission from Lang, S. et al. Indications for intraoperative anterior segment optical coherence tomography in corneal surgery. Published in: International Ophthalmology (Springer). 2020. Oct: 40(10): 2617-2625.)

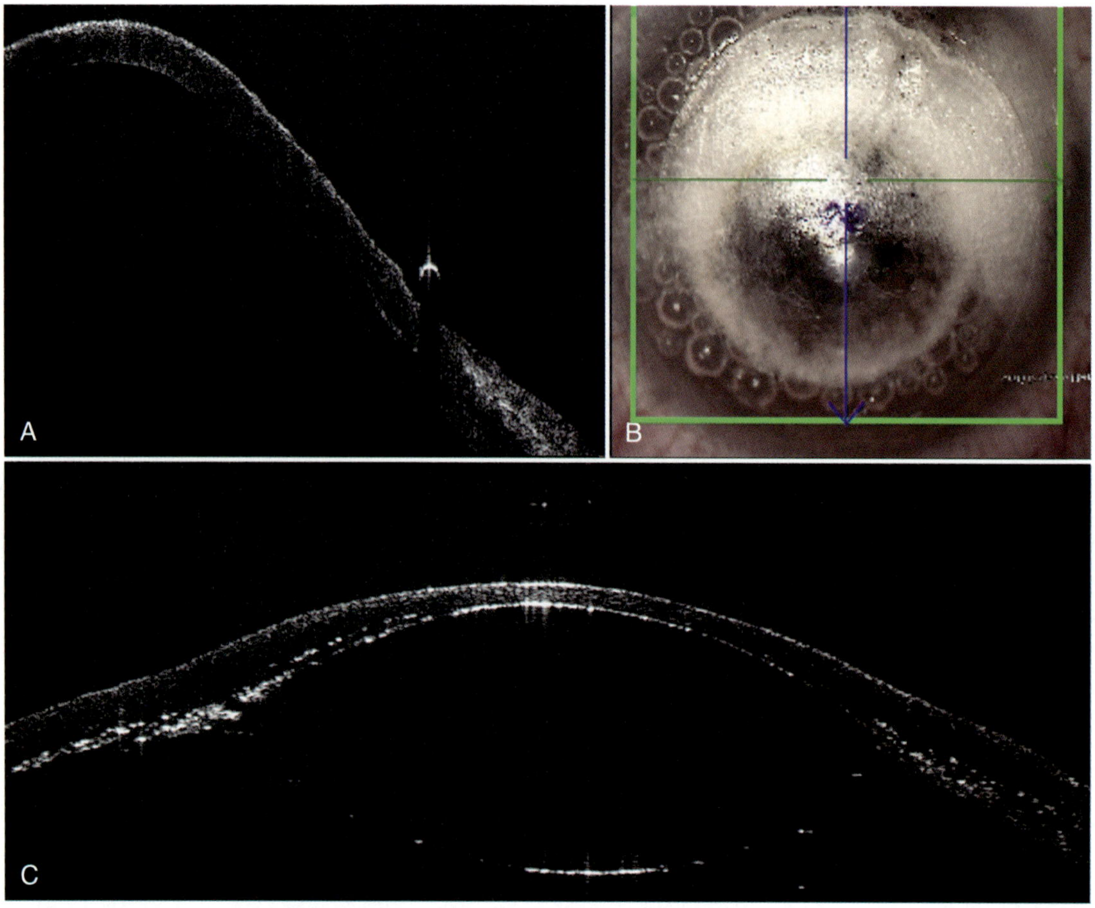

Fig. 13.10 Appearance of a type I big bubble immediately after air injection during deep anterior lamellar keratoplasty. Through the surgical microscope view *(panel B),* it can be difficult to confirm the presence of a successful big bubble. With iOCT, the bubble can be seen as an optically empty space between the posterior stroma and pre-Descemet layer (concave appearance with increased hyperreflectivity). (Image Credit: James Myerscough, Southend University Hospital, Southend, UK. Reprinted with permission from James Myerscough, Asaf Friehmann, Massimo Busin, Didier Goor,Successful Visualization of a Big Bubble during Deep Anterior Lamellar Keratoplasty using Intraoperative OCT, Ophthalmology, Volume 126, Issue 7, 2019, Page 1062, © Elsevier.)

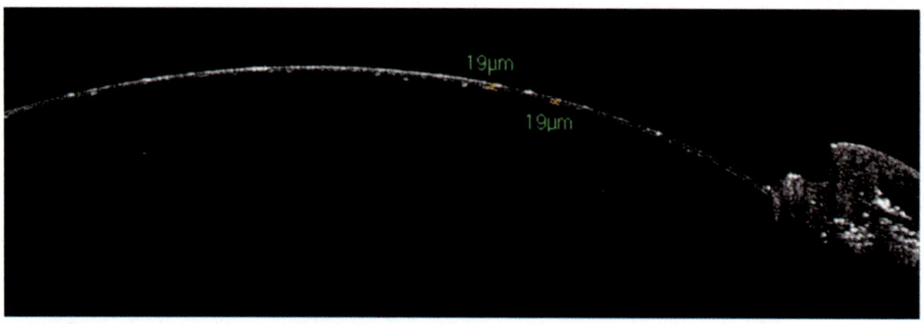

Fig. 13.11 Appearance on iOCT of bare Descemet membrane after successful big bubble formation and dissection of overlying stroma in deep anterior lamellar keratoplasty. (Image Credit: Laura De Benito-Llopis, Singapore National Eye Center, Singapore. Reprinted with permission from Benito-Llopis, et al - Intraoperative Anterior Segment Optical Coherence Tomography: A Novel Assessment Tool during Deep Anterior Lamellar Keratoplasty, American Journal of Ophthalmology 2014; 157:334-341 Figure 1 © Elsevier.)

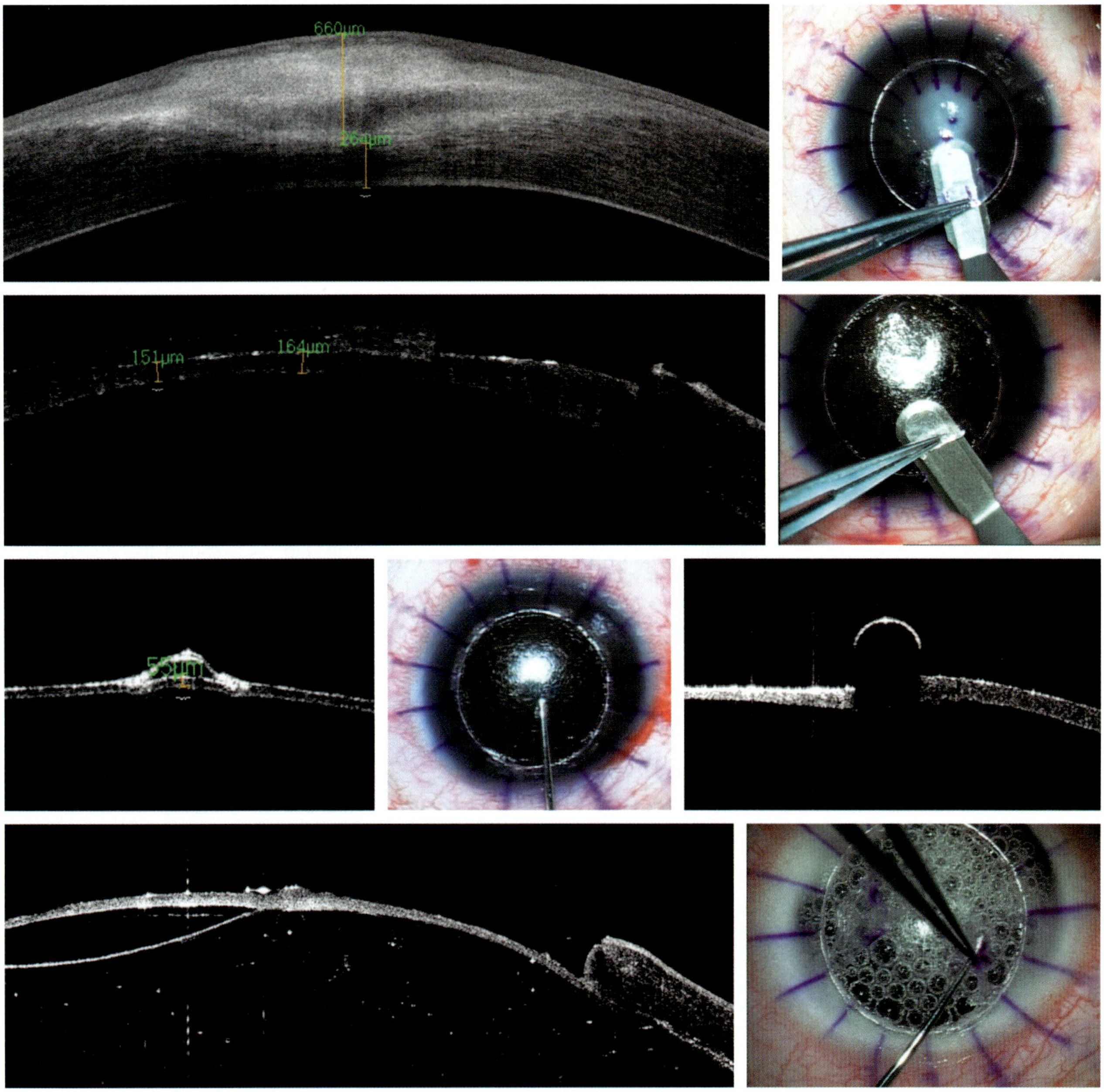

Fig. 13.12 Appearance on iOCT of residual stroma following manual dissection. (Image Credit: Laura De Benito-Llopis, Singapore National Eye Center, Singapore. Reprinted with permission from Benito-Llopis, et al - Intraoperative Anterior Segment Optical Coherence Tomography: A Novel Assessment Tool during Deep Anterior Lamellar Keratoplasty, American Journal of Ophthalmology 2014; 157:334-341 Figure 1 © Elsevier.)

BIBLIOGRAPHY

1. Anwar M, Teichmann KD. Deep lamellar keratoplasty: surgical techniques for anterior lamellar keratoplasty with and without baring of Descemet's membrane. *Cornea*. 2002;21(4):374-383.
2. De Benito-Llopis L, Mehta JS, Angunawela RI, Ang M, Tan DT. Intraoperative anterior segment optical coherence tomography: a novel assessment tool during deep anterior lamellar keratoplasty. *Am J Ophthalmol*. 2014;157(2):334-341.e3.
3. Lang SJ, Heinzelmann S, Böhringer D, Reinhard T, Maier P. Indications for intraoperative anterior segment optical coherence tomography in corneal surgery. *Int Ophthalmol*. 2020;40(10):2617-2625.
4. Muijzer MB, Soeters N, Godefrooij DA, van Luijk CM, Wisse RPL. Intraoperative optical coherence tomography-assisted descemet membrane endothelial keratoplasty: toward more efficient, safer surgery. *Cornea*. 2020;39(6):674-679.
5. Myerscough J, Friehmann A, Busin M, Goor D. Successful visualization of a big bubble during deep anterior lamellar keratoplasty using intraoperative OCT. *Ophthalmology*. 2019;126(7):1062.
6. Steven P, Le Blanc C, Lankenau E, et al. Optimising deep anterior lamellar keratoplasty (DALK) using intraoperative online optical coherence tomography (iOCT). *Br J Ophthalmol*. 2014;98(7):900-904.

14 Use of Anterior Segment Optical Coherence Tomography (AS-OCT) in Postoperative Management of Full-Thickness Penetrating Keratoplasty and Lamellar Keratoplasty

Joseph H. Jeffrey | Albert Y. Cheung

I. INTRODUCTION

The postoperative mangement of keratoplasties is crucial to ensuring long-term visual rehabilitation and graft longevity. While clinical slit lamp examination and certain ancillary imaging (ie. topography, keratometry, specular microscopy) have traditionally been used postoperatively, anterior segment optical coherence tomography (AS-OCT) can provide additional helpful information to manage these patients. This can be particularly helpful when clinical examination is difficult or equivocal. This chapter will highlight specific uses of AS-OCT for penetrating keratoplasty and partial-thickness lamellar keratoplasty procedures.

II. USE OF AS-OCT AFTER PENETRATING KERATOPLASTY

Penetrating keratoplasty (PKP) continues to be performed by corneal surgeons for a variety of conditions, including but not limited to, corneal ectasias (e.g., keratoconus, pellucid marginal degeneration, etc.), corneal scarring, intractable corneal infections, and failed previous PKP. Though clinical examination is usually sufficient after PKP surgery to determine the integrity of the graft-host junction, anterior segment optical coherence tomography (AS-OCT) can be used in select cases. Fig. 14.1 shows AS-OCT images of a patient after uneventful PKP. The host corneal rim is seen in the periphery as a slightly thickened and irregular area, whereas the donor corneal button is compact and located centrally.

In certain cases, the PKP may dehisce from the graft-host junction in the early postoperative period as a result of trauma or chronic eye rubbing. Fig. 14.2 shows the AS-OCT appearance of an area of nasal dehiscence at the graft-host junction. Depending on the clinical setting, such cases usually warrant a return to the operating room for placement of additional sutures.

III. USE OF AS-OCT AFTER ANTERIOR LAMELLAR KERATOPLASTY

Technical challenges associated with lamellar keratoplasty procedures, especially deep anterior lamellar keratoplasty (DALK), were previously discussed in Chapter 13. In any lamellar

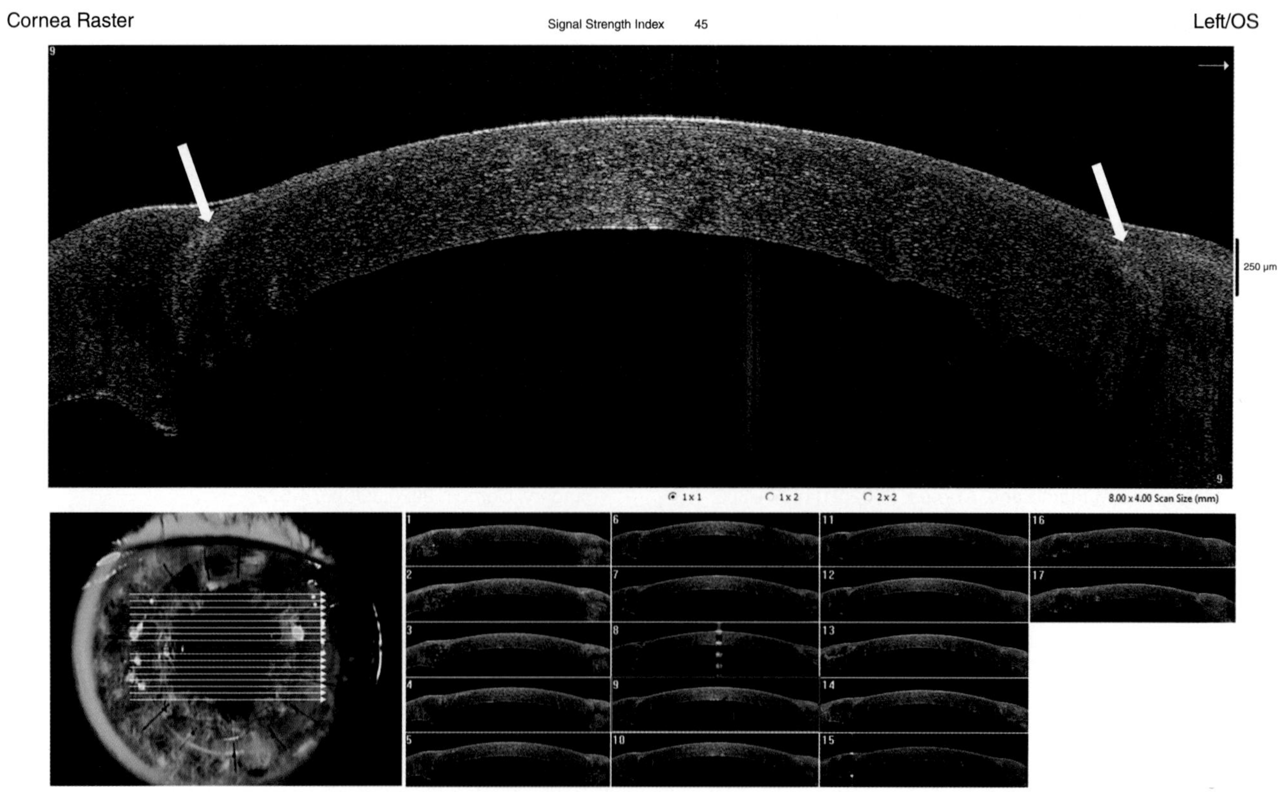

Fig. 14.1 Postoperative AS-OCT of a patient after uneventful penetrating keratoplasty. The host cornea is seen in the periphery and is slightly thickened compared with the compact, central donor corneal button. The graft-host junction can be appreciated as a hyperreflective line *(arrows)*. (Courtesy Parag Majmudar, MD, Rush University, Chicago, Illinois, United States.)

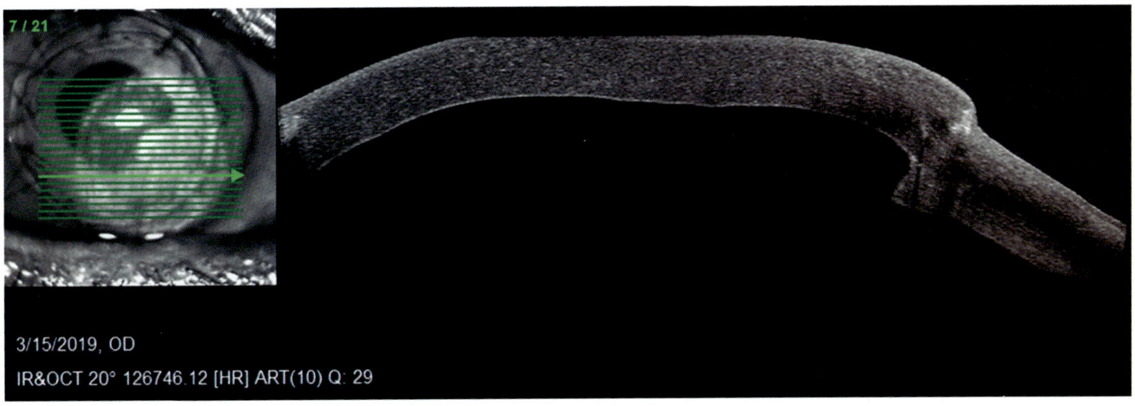

Fig. 14.2 AS-OCT image of wound slippage at the nasal graft-host junction after penetrating keratoplasty. Note the irregular, anterior elevation of the donor button above the graft-host junction

surgery, determining the position and layer of pathologic conditions is vital. Preoperatively, identifying the level of scarring or whether Descemet membrane (DM) is fully intact can help the surgeon plan whether a "big bubble" technique is prudent compared with a manual approach (i.e., areas of posterior scarring may influence the surgeon to forgo a big bubble and start with manual dissection to minimize risk for DM rupture).[1] Postoperatively, AS-OCT can be used to assess and manage adverse postoperative outcomes.

Fig. 14.3 displays four different AS-OCT images that demonstrate the varying residual stromal bed thicknesses based on several different DALK techniques. In *panel A,* a successful big bubble and stromectomy left behind an intact recipient DM-endothelium complex. It is difficult to discern between the donor and host interface. *Panel B* demonstrates a minimally thickened residual bed (minimal stromal layers with DM and endothelium) after an air-visco bubble technique that separated at a very deep intrastromal layer. In *panel C,* manual dissection achieved a uniform and deep stromectomy with a thin (≤80 μm) stromal residual bed. *Panel D* shows another manual dissection with a significantly thicker stromal residual bed (>80 μm) compared with *panel C;* this procedure was more in the anterior lamellar keratoplasty range and not a true DALK. Current practice aims to bare DM-endothelium or to leave behind as little residual stroma as possible (≤ 80 μm, as this amount of stroma appears to be equivalent to PKP visually at 2 years postoperatively) to optimize visual recovery.[2]

CLINICAL PEARL

Postoperative AS-OCT can be used after DALK to measure the amount of residual host stroma left behind, especially when using manual dissection techniques.

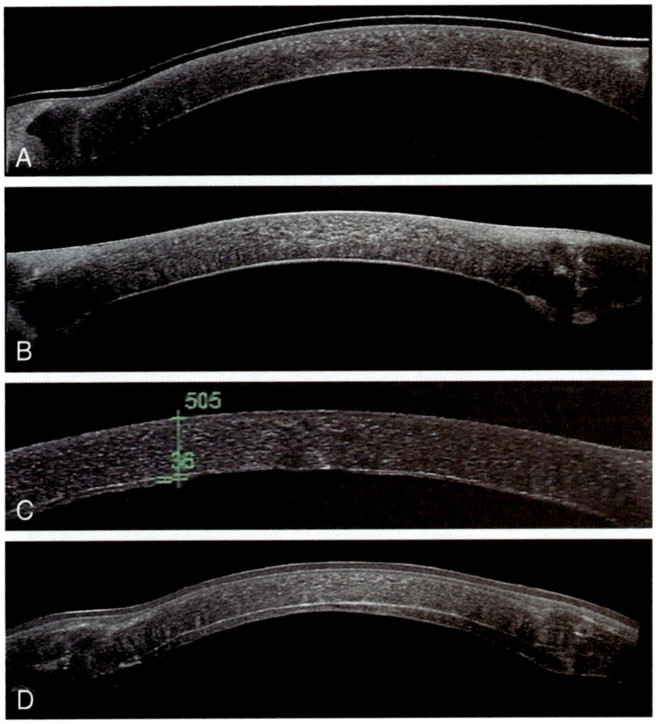

Fig. 14.3 Four different AS-OCT images after deep anterior lamellar keratoplasty surgery. *Panel A* displays postoperative images after a successful type I big bubble, removal of host stroma, and transplantation of a donor button onto the host Descemet membrane (DM)-endothelium bed. It is difficult to discern a demarcation between the host and donor tissues. *Panel B* displays postoperative images after air-visco bubble technique. There is minimal residual host stromal bed along with the DM-endothelium complex. In *panel C,* manual dissection (layer-by-layer technique) was performed, leaving behind a very thin residual stromal bed. In *panel D,* manual dissection left behind a significant amount of host stroma. (Courtesy of Enrica Sarnicola, Caterina Sarnicola, and Vincenzo Sarnicola.)

Postoperatively, AS-OCT can help detect or confirm certain complications such as double anterior chamber, graft haze/scarring, graft dehiscence, DM folds, interface debris, and recurrence of pathologic findings in the graft. Additionally, AS-OCT allows measurement of the residual stromal bed thickness. Of note, early postoperative measurements overestimate the thickness because of postoperative edema; this usually improves and stabilizes over the following months. If the residual bed is significantly thicker than 80 μm and not uniform, a repeat DALK may be warranted to improve visual acuity if current vision is unsatisfactory.[3]

Formation of a double anterior chamber typically results from an intraoperative DM perforation and is evident early in the postoperative course. In such cases, there is fluid between the donor graft and the residual recipient bed. Fig. 14.4 demonstrates a postoperative double anterior chamber with detached DM and endothelium (denoted by the *arrows*) with overlying corneal edema in *panel A* and the accompanying slit-lamp photograph. After injection of intracameral air with face-up positioning, there was resolution of the DM-endothelium detachment with subsequent improvement in corneal edema *(panel B).* A corresponding slit-lamp photograph demonstrates the double anterior chamber.

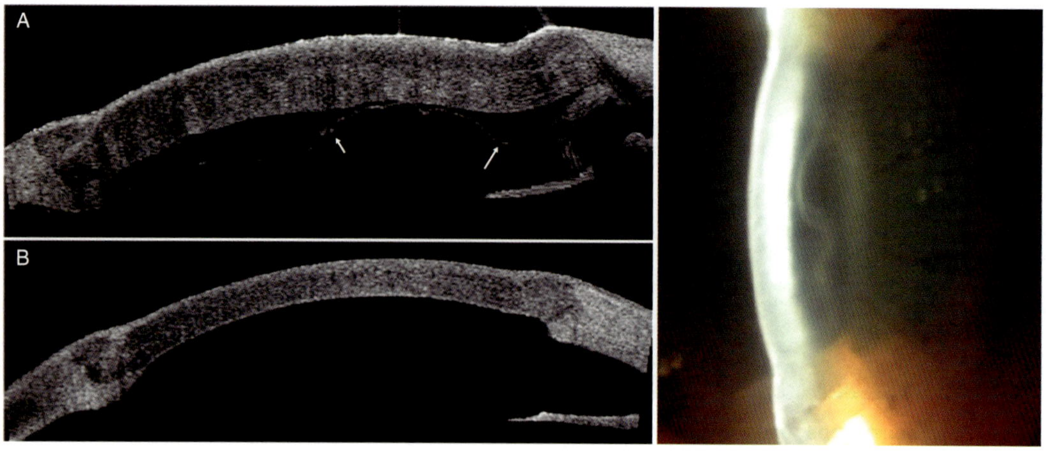

Fig. 14.4 Double anterior chamber. A double anterior chamber after deep anterior lamellar keratoplasty can be readily seen at the slit lamp as a wavy, undulating layer of Descemet membrane (DM)-endothelium detached from the corneal graft *(arrows)*. AS-OCT can be used *(panel A)* to visualize the amount of interface fluid and areas of DM-endothelium separation. After injection of intracameral air, the detached DM-endothelium complex is well apposed to the overlying tissue *(panel B)*. (Courtesy of Enrica Sarnicola, Caterina Sarnicola, and Vincenzo Sarnicola.)

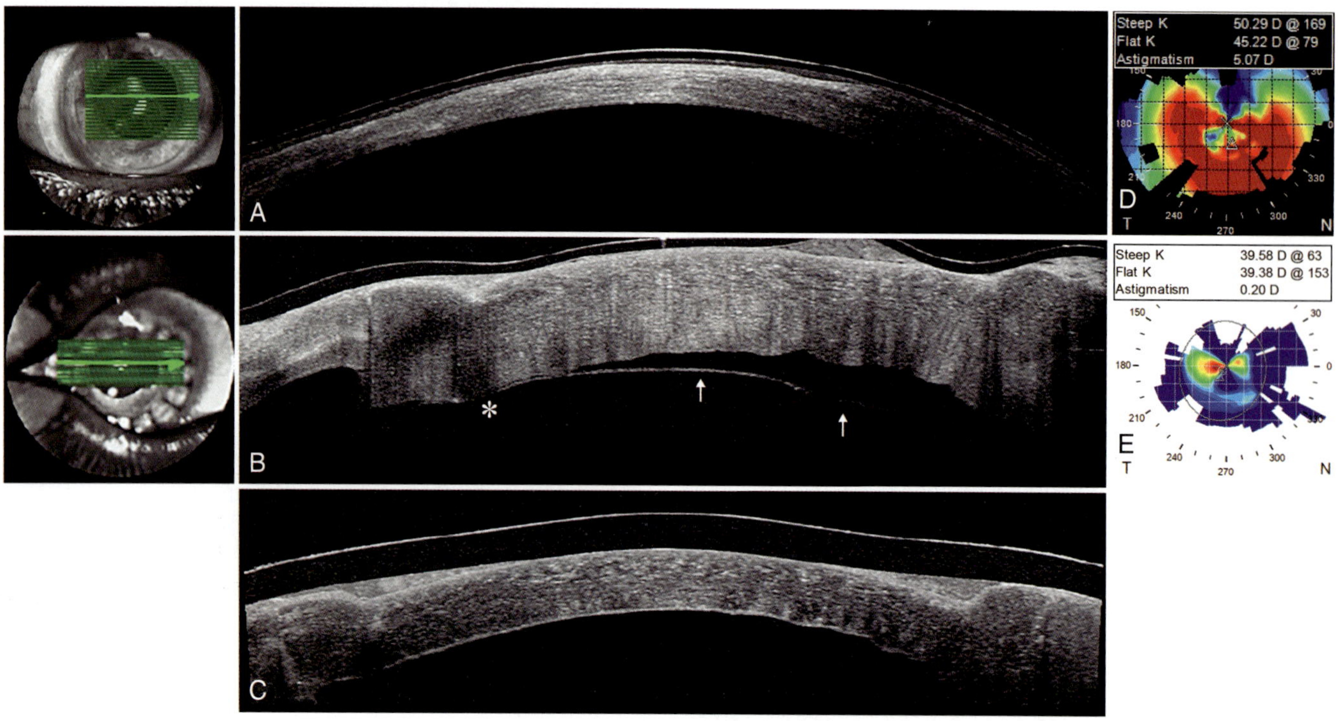

Fig. 14.5 Keratoconus and stromal scarring secondary to herpetic infection. Preoperatively, the patient had keratoconus and stromal scarring secondary to herpetic infection *(panel A)*. After deep anterior lamellar keratoplasty (DALK) *(panel B)*, detachment of the Descemet membrane (DM)-endothelium *(arrows)* causing a double anterior chamber was noted. Notably, there were areas of DM attachment *(asterisk)*, which guided the surgeon to safely enter in this location for injection of intracameral air. After successful injection, the DM-endothelium complex is well apposed to the overlying cornea *(panel C)*. Preoperative and postoperative topographies demonstrate the improvement in irregular nature and degree of astigmatism (*panels D and E*, respectively).

CLINICAL PEARL

Although a double anterior chamber may be apparent on postoperative examination, AS-OCT can be quite helpful in discerning details obscured by corneal edema or other factors (e.g., tarsorrhaphy, amniotic membrane). The extent and location of the double anterior chamber can easily be outlined by AS-OCT. Areas of shallow detachment can be distinguished from larger detachments, and relationships between the detachment and other pertinent anterior chamber structures can be visualized. This can assist the surgeon in how to best approach the rebubbling (descemetopexy) in terms of where to enter the anterior chamber and where the cannula or needle may have a greater risk for dangerously touching endothelium.

Fig. 14.5 shows another example of a double anterior chamber. Preoperatively, this eye had stromal scarring and thinning secondary to herpes simplex virus and keratoconus *(panel A)*. A postoperative AS-OCT *(panel B)* highlights the double anterior chamber with detached DM and endothelium (denoted by the *arrows*) with overlying corneal edema. The asterisk *(*)* denotes the area where DM is attached, which was difficult to determine in the setting of a tarsorrhaphy and markedly edematous cornea. AS-OCT after injection of air *(panel C)* shows resolution; the paracentesis was made based on where the AS-OCT had noted attached DM to decrease the risk for DM-endothelium

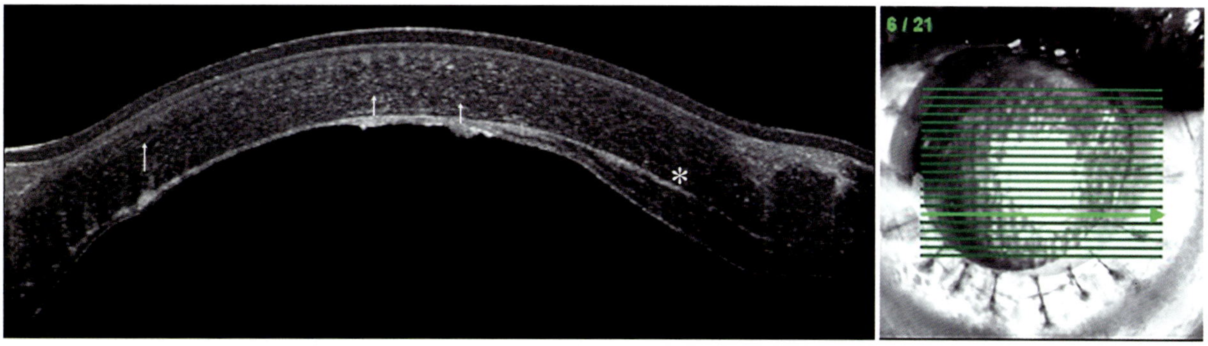

Fig. 14.6 Intraoperative rupture during manual dissection in deep anterior lamellar keratoplasty (DALK). The donor corneal tissue was sutured uneventfully. Postoperatively, there is an irregular contour as a result of a significantly thick residual host stromal bed *(asterisk)*. Additionally, there are areas of inert debris *(arrows)* in the graft-host interface. These can be observed without surgical intervention, especially if not visually significant.

damage. Preoperative and postoperative topographies demonstrate the improvement in irregular nature and degree of astigmatism *(panels D and E,* respectively).

Fig. 14.6 demonstrates an inferior cut seen on AS-OCT through the graft after a DM rupture that occurred from manual dissection during DALK. Note the irregular contour resulting from the thick residual bed *(asterisk)* that was left behind inferiorly. There is also inert debris *(arrows)* seen in the interface.

DM folds can result from redundancies in DM, potentially when there is a donor-recipient curvature disparity when the recipient bed is much steeper than that of the donor. Other identified risk factors may include recipient age older than 20.5 years, duration of keratoconus disease more than 5.5 years, and possibly shorter axial length.[4] Residual folds also can be seen after resolution of a combined big bubble types I and II.

In Fig. 14.7, preoperative AS-OCT demonstrates stromal scarring and apical thinning/ectasia secondary to keratoconus *(panel A)*. After manual dissection DALK, a double anterior chamber resulted from an interoperative DM rupture peripherally. After injection of air, there was a persistent double anterior chamber *(panel B)* with multiple areas of nonattachment of DM. After the second injection of air, there was near resolution of the double anterior chamber *(panel C),* although because of the donor-recipient curvature disparity, a residual fold *(asterisk)* resulted *(panel D)*. The fold is highlighted on the slit-lamp photographs *(panels E and F)*. Preoperative topography demonstrates the steep recipient *(panel G),* and postoperative topography (before suture removal) illustrates the much flatter postoperative keratometry readings *(panel H)*.

CLINICAL PEARL

Redundancies in the Descemet membrane (DM) can occur from a donor-recipient curvature disparity, especially if the recipient bed is much steeper than that of the donor. Conversely, if the recipient bed is significantly flatter than that of the donor, the recipient bed may appear taut. These two scenarios of donor-recipient curvature disparity may be accompanied by a double anterior chamber in the setting of DM rupture and can be identified on AS-OCT. If this is recalcitrant to rebubbling, the recipient bed may be cut to repair the curvature disparity and avoid a PKP.[5]

Although different surgeons have varying protocols as to the ideal time for suture removal after DALK, if corneal sutures loosen or are removed early, there may be graft dehiscence or wound slippage at the graft-host junction. Fig. 14.8 demonstrates wound slippage at the graft-host junction. *Panel A* shows AS-OCT images of an intact graft-host junction 6 months after manual dissection DALK. Six months later (12 months postoperatively), the patient came in with a foreign body sensation for 1 month (presumably from rubbing her eye overnight). There were four consecutive sutures along the graft-host junction that had broken, with resultant wound slippage seen on AS-OCT *(panel B)* and slit-lamp photograph *(panel C)*. This was treated with a wound revision. In another example (after big bubble DALK), the AS-OCT of the graft-host junction identifies where there was graft dehiscence while removing a suture 11 months after surgery. The wound was revised with replacement of three sutures; however, one suture broke with subsequent mild graft slippage seen on AS-OCT *(panel D)* and slit-lamp photographs *(panels E and F)*.

With its clear advantages and improved surgical techniques, DALK will likely be used increasingly more frequently. AS-OCT can be a crucial component for both the preoperative workup and postoperative follow-up to manage these surgical patients.

IV. USE OF AS-OCT IN SELECT CASES OF CORNEAL TRANSPLANT SURGERY

Although a lamellar patch graft can be used to restore corneal integrity, a double anterior chamber may form postoperatively secondary to Descemet rupture, retained ophthalmic viscoelastic device, or adherent/incarcerated iris. AS-OCT may aid in discerning these details. Fig. 14.9 displays images from a patient who underwent a lamellar patch graft to treat a corneal perforation in a prior PKP plagued with recurrent herpes simplex keratitis *(panel A)*. The high magnification view over the area of the lamellar patch graft highlights the small Descemet membrane detachment *(panel B)*. AS-OCT taken at two levels of the patch graft demonstrates the small double anterior chamber *(panels 1 and 2)*. Notably, in *panel 2,* AS-OCT demonstrates an area of iris still adherent to the previously perforated area that was not readily seen on clinical examination. Two weeks later, there was resolution of the double anterior chamber without additional intervention *(panel C)*. Repeat AS-OCT shows a well-apposed DM-endothelium complex to the overlying corneal tissue.

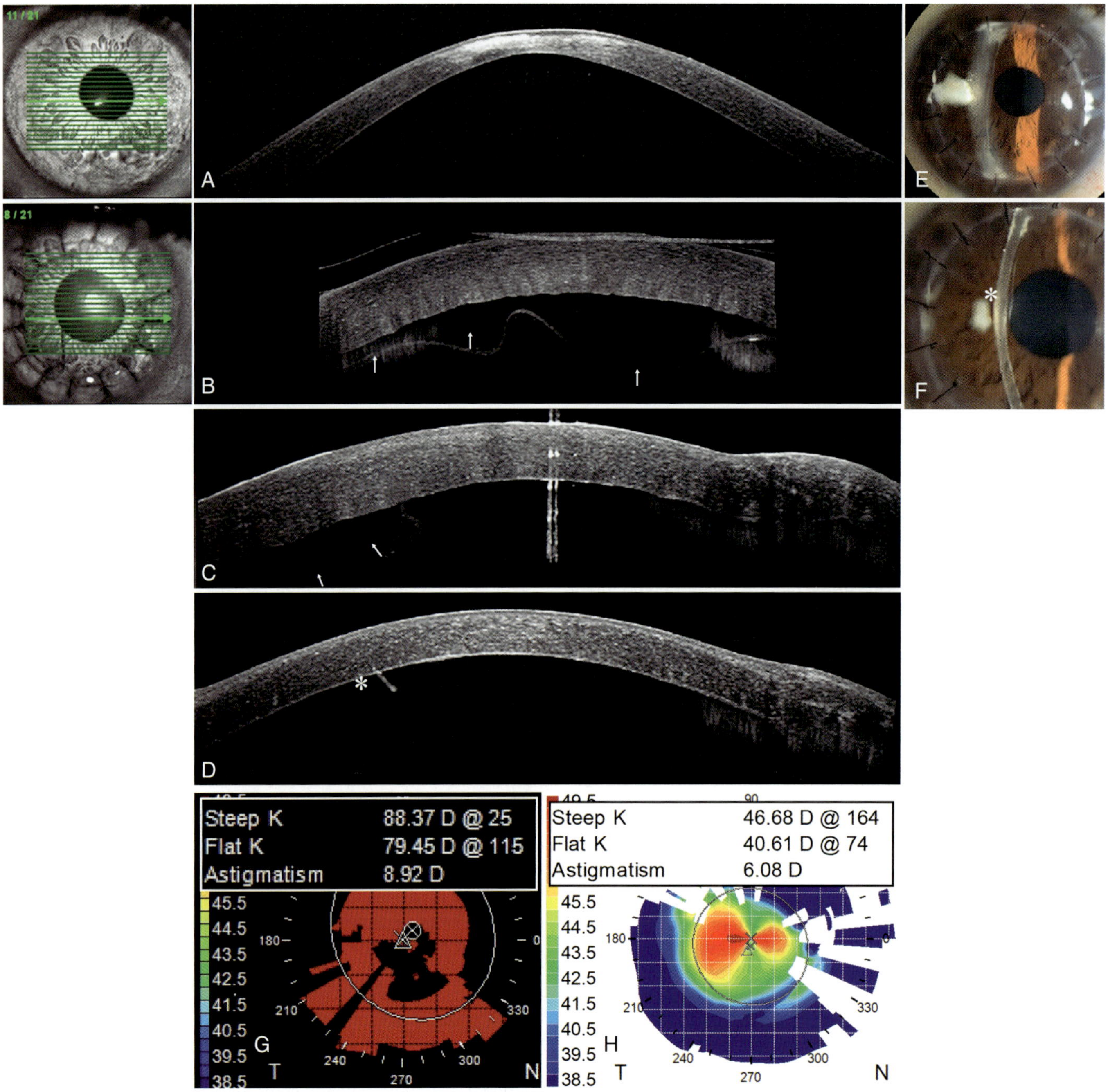

Fig. 14.7 Preoperative AS-OCT images of a keratoconus patient with significant stromal scarring *(panel A).* After manual dissection deep anterior lamellar keratoplasty (DALK), a double anterior chamber was noted *(panel B)* with multiple areas of nonattached Descemet membrane (DM) *(arrows).* After several injections of intracameral air, the detachment resolved *(panel C),* though a residual DM fold was noted because of significant donor-recipient disparity *(panel D, asterisk).* This fold is also seen on clinical examination at the slit lamp *(panels E and F).* Preoperative topography demonstrates the steep recipient *(panel G),* and postoperative topography illustrates significantly flatter keratometry readings *(panel H).*

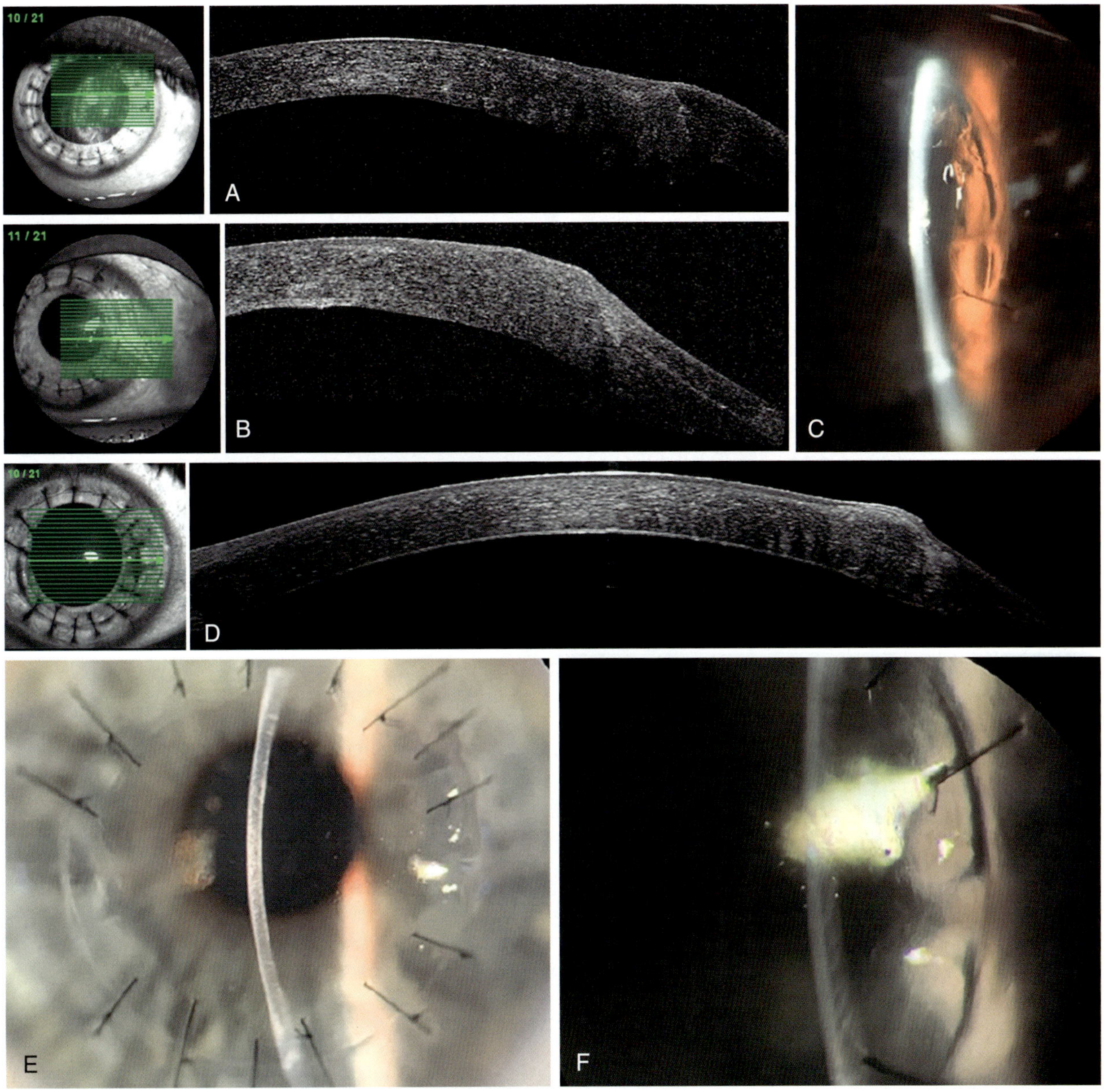

Fig. 14.8 Wound slippage after deep anterior lamellar keratoplasty (DALK) at the graft-host junction. *Panel A* shows an AS-OCT image of a well-apposed DALK taken at the 6-month postoperative visit. In *panel B* (taken approximately 1 year postoperatively), the patient presented with 1-month history of foreign body sensation and eye rubbing. Clinical examination revealed four broken sutures at the graft-host junction. Repeat AS-OCT shows wound slippage at the graft-host junction, which was also seen at the slit-lamp *(panel C).* In another patient who underwent big bubble DALK, an inadvertent graft dehiscence occurred after suture removal approximately 11 months after surgery *(panel D).* After wound revision, there is still a mild, persistent graft-host junction slippage present *(panels E and F).*

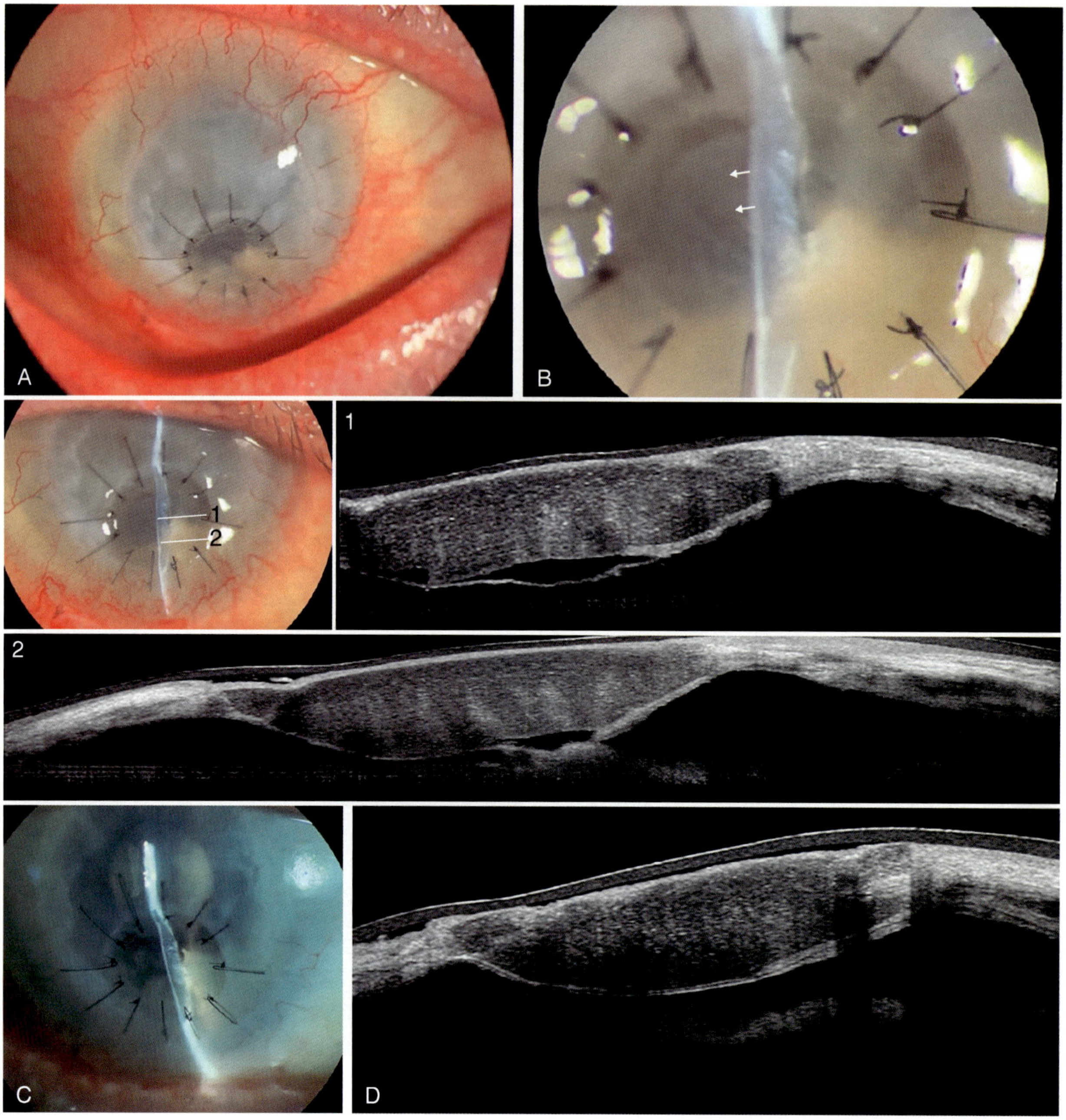

Fig. 14.9 Lamellar patch graft for corneal perforation. A patient with prior penetrating keratoplasty (PKP) underwent a lamellar patch graft because of corneal perforation from recalcitrant herpes simplex keratitis *(panel A).* High magnification of the patch graft revealed a Descemet membrane (DM)-detachment and the presence of a double anterior chamber. AS-OCT images *(panels 1 and 2)* taken over the patch graft confirmed areas of DM detachment with other areas of DM attachment. The decision was made to observe at this time. Two weeks later, the detachment resolved without additional intervention *(panel C).* Repeat AS-OCT *(panel D)* demonstrates good apposition of the DM-endothelium complex to the overlying corneal tissue.

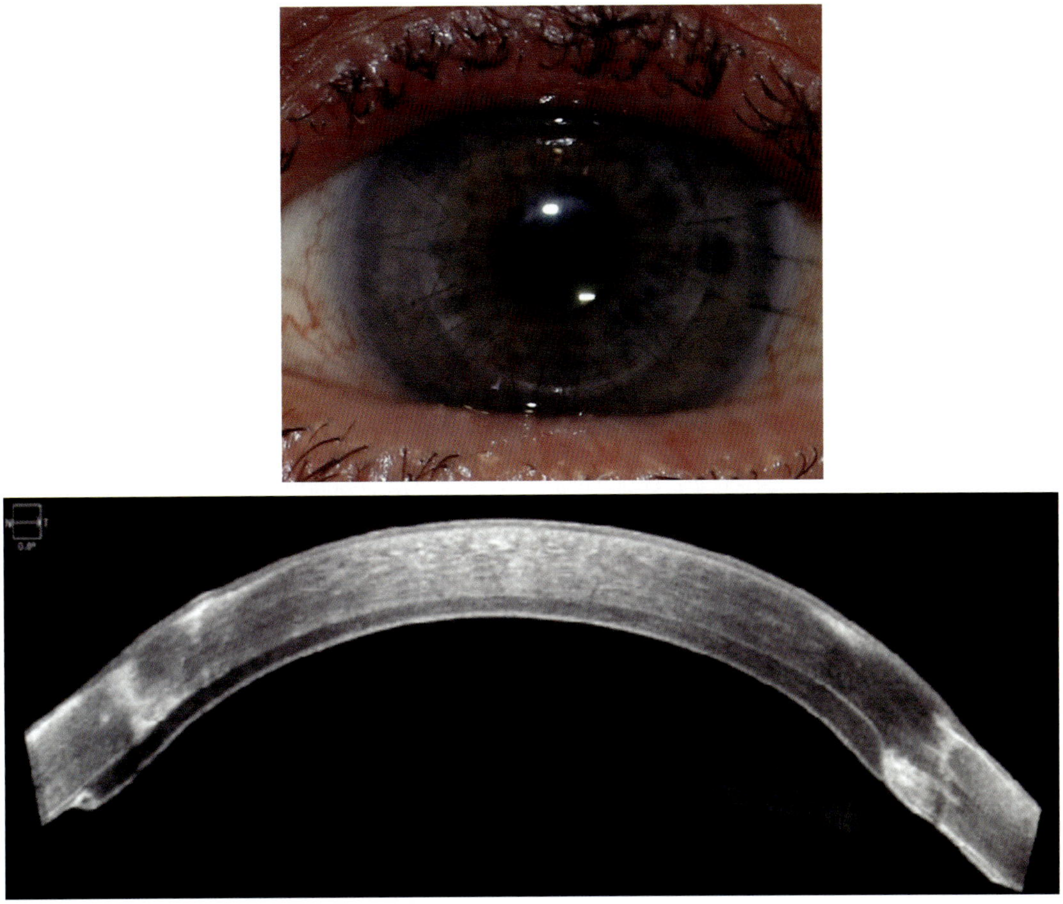

Fig. 14.10 Descemet stripping automated endothelial keratoplasty (DSAEK). Appearance of a DSAEK performed underneath a preexisting penetrating keratoplasty (PKP) graft that experienced endothelial failure. AS-OCT can be used to confirm good apposition of the DSAEK graft to the overlying PKP.

CLINICAL PEARL

AS-OCT can help confirm the level of scarring, infectious keratitis, blood vessels, or debris and whether the pathologic findings are located in the interface (potential space). For certain pathologic conditions (e.g., stromal dystrophies), recurrence of deposits in the graft may be confirmed with AS-OCT. Furthermore, the posterior contour can be evaluated for uniformity and irregularity.

Patients with graft failure after PKP because of endothelial dysfunction may undergo an endothelial keratoplasty procedure (DSAEK or DMEK) under the existing PKP. In such cases, there is a benefit in maintaining the "healthy," anterior portion of the PKP and replacing only the underlying endothelium. Fig. 14.10 displays images from a patient who underwent a DSAEK for endothelial failure in a long-standing PKP. Slit-lamp examination and AS-OCT confirm good apposition of the DSAEK graft underneath the overlying PKP.

BIBLIOGRAPHY

1. Ozmen MC, Yesilirmak N, Aydin B, Ceylanoglu KS, Atalay HT, Akata F. Prediction of descemet membrane perforation during deep anterior lamellar keratoplasty in patients with keratoconus with stromal scar. *Eye Contact Lens*. 2018;44(suppl 2):S176-S179.
2. Sarnicola E, Sarnicola C, Cheung AY, Holland EJ, Sarnicola V. Surgical corneal anatomy in deep anterior lamellar keratoplasty: suggestion of new acronyms. *Cornea*. 2019;38(4):515-522.
3. Sarnicola C, Sarnicola E, Cheung AY, Panico E, Panico C, Sarnicola V. Deep anterior lamellar keratoplasty (DALK) after previous anterior lamellar keratoplasty (ALK) to improve the visual outcomes. *Cornea*. 2021;40(5):613-617.
4. Li X, Zhao Y, Chen H, Li Y, Hong J, Xu J. Clinical properties and risk factors for descemet membrane folds after deep anterior lamellar keratoplasty in patients with keratoconus. *Cornea*. 2019;38(10):1222-1227.
5. Sarnicola E, Sarnicola C, Cheung AY, Panico E, Panico C, Sarnicola V. Total or subtotal full thickness recipient bed cut to repair donor-recipient curvature disparity in cases of DM rupture with manual DALK. *Eur J Ophthalmol*. 2020;30(5):1172-1178. doi:10.1177/1120672120932833.
6. Nanavaty MA, Vijjan KS, Yvon C. Deep anterior lamellar keratoplasty: a surgeon's guide. *J Curr Ophthalmol*. 2018;30(4):297-310.

15 Use of AS-OCT in Postoperative Management of Endothelial Keratoplasty

Kendrick Wang | Divya Srikumaran

I. INTRODUCTION

The original gold standard for surgical treatment of corneal endothelial dysfunction was full-thickness corneal transplants, also known as *penetrating keratoplasty (PKP)*. However, advances in partial-thickness transplant techniques, particularly endothelial keratoplasty (EK), offer advantages to PKP. Compared with PKP, EK procedures offer patients faster recovery, improved visual outcomes, and lower rates of rejection and infection. Although there are many EK procedures, such as pre-Descemet endothelial keratoplasty, this chapter will primarily discuss the two most popular EK procedures: Descemet stripping (automated) endothelial keratoplasty (DS[A]EK) and Descemet membrane endothelial keratoplasty (DMEK). DSEK donor tissue contains corneal stroma, Descemet membrane (DM), and endothelium, whereas DMEK donor tissue contains only DM and endothelium.

The use of anterior segment optical coherence tomography (AS-OCT) during EK procedures intraoperatively was previously discussed in Chapter 13. This chapter will primarily focus on the use of AS-OCT to allow for surgeons to visualize the transplanted EK graft and monitor the clinical course in post-EK eyes.

II. USE OF AS-OCT IN POST-DSEK EYES

A. Normal Postoperative Appearance

In an eye that has had uncomplicated DSEK surgery, it is usually possible to visualize the donor graft attached on the posterior corneal surface on clinical examination alone. AS-OCT can be used to confirm these clinical findings. Because the implanted graft is approximately 50 to 150 microns thick, there is an appreciable difference in reflectivity of the donor graft and the host stroma making the graft easy to visualize (Fig. 15.1). A prominent "line of attachment" can be seen between the donor lenticule and the host stroma, and the increased hyperreflectivity of the donor endothelium can be appreciated.

Serial AS-OCT postoperative measurements after DSAEK can demonstrate a progressive improvement in graft clarity and decreasing corneal thickness. In Fig. 15.2, AS-OCT of a routine, well-adherent DSAEK graft is shown in an eye 1 week postoperatively. The graft tissue, indicated by the *red arrow,* can be seen attached to the host cornea. Increased corneal thickness after DSEK is a sign of corneal edema, which can be an indicator of graft detachment, graft rejection, or endothelial failure. Immediately after surgery, there may be variable amounts of corneal edema apparent on clinical examination; however, this should decrease with time postoperatively. In the presence of persistent corneal edema, corneal thickness (as measured by pachymetry) can be significantly increased.

Pachymetry of the same eye shown in Fig. 15.2 can be seen in Fig. 15.3. Although the overall corneal thickness after DSEK can be expected to be slightly increased given the additional thickness of the donor graft tissue, a significant increase in corneal thickness can be a sign of corneal edema and graft separation or failure. In this patient, note the significant improvement

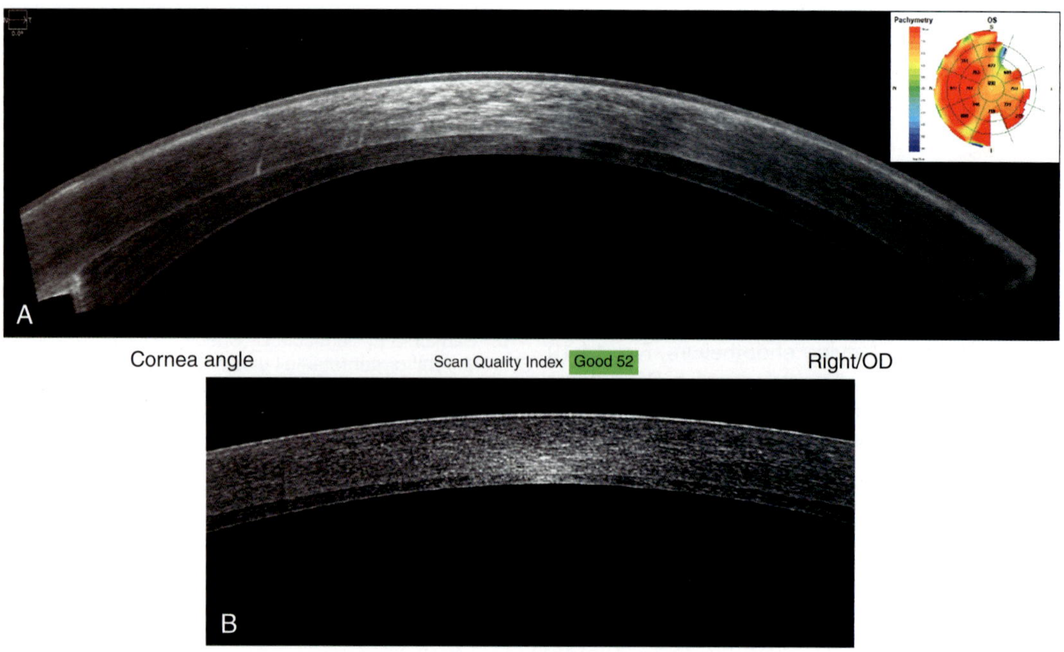

Fig. 15.1 Appearances of two well-attached Descemet stripping automated endothelial keratoplasty (DSAEK) grafts with two different devices in two different patients. In *panel A,* accompanying pachymetry obtained from the AS-OCT device is displayed.

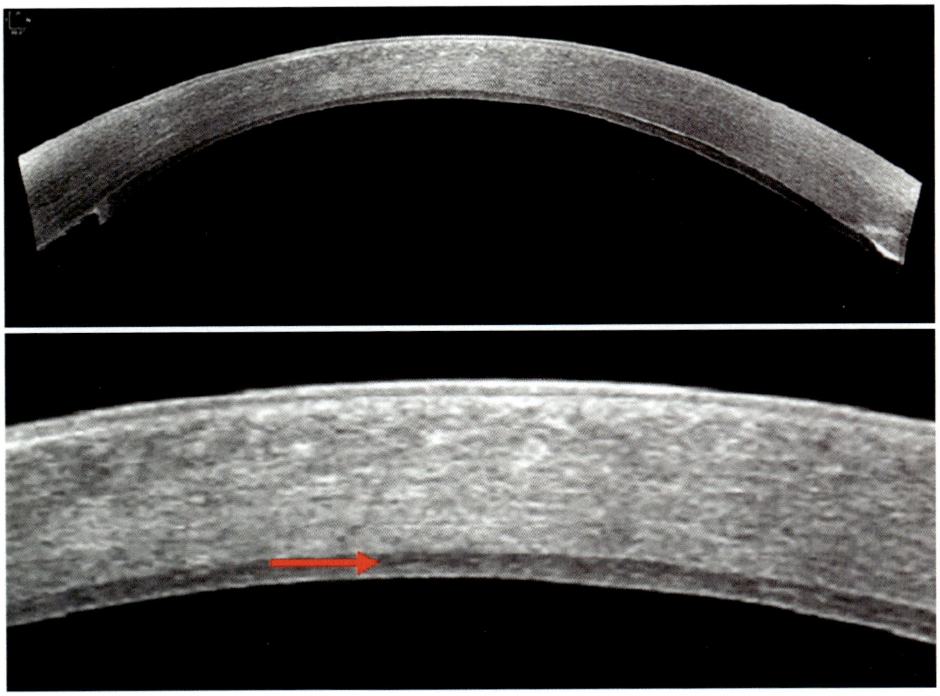

Fig. 15.2 Normal attached Descemet stripping automated endothelial keratoplasty (DSAEK) graft visualized with AS-OCT. The red arrow highlights the graft tissue.

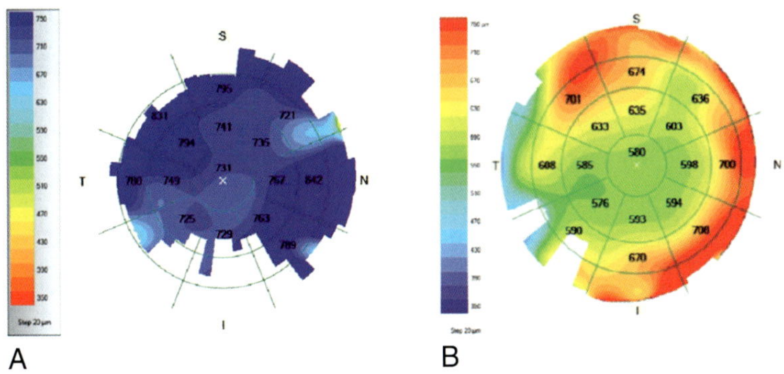

Fig. 15.3 Pachymetry at 1 day (*panel A*) after Descemet stripping endothelial keratoplasty (DSEK) and 1 week (*panel B*) after DSEK of the same eye measured using AS-OCT.

(nearly 150 microns) in corneal thickness between postoperative day 1 and postoperative week 1.

B. Partial and Full Detachments

DSEK procedures may encounter complications such as graft detachments, dislocations, rejection, and failure. DSEK detachments can be either partial or complete. Although slit-lamp examination is sufficient for detection of most instances of graft detachment, other cases may be difficult to assess, especially in the presence of significant corneal edema. In these cases, AS-OCT is a useful tool to help assess the extent of detachments. This can help guide the surgeon if rebubbling is needed.

Fig. 15.4 shows a partially detached DSAEK lenticule. This patient had a shallow nasal detachment that was readily seen on clinical examination and further accentuated on AS-OCT. Such detachments likely will benefit from a "rebubble" procedure to promote graft adherence.

In other cases, the detachment may be very subtle, especially if in a focal or peripheral area and obscured by overlying edema. Fig. 15.5 shows an example of a patient who had a shallow nasal detachment of the DSAEK graft with relatively preserved central attachment. These cases may be observed with close follow-up, depending on other clinical findings, to allow for spontaneous reattachment. However, superior areas of detachment, worsening edema, and involvement of the central visual axis are all indications for relatively urgent intervention with rebubbling.

CLINICAL PEARL

AS-OCT can be used to confirm the presence or absence of DSEK/DSAEK graft detachment, especially in cases in which the overlying corneal edema may obscure clinical examination at the slit lamp. Based on the type of detachment and its location, clinicians can choose to observe or intervene as necessary with rebubble and/or repositioning interventions.

Complete (total) DSEK detachments will always require surgical intervention. A complete DSEK detachment, seen in Fig. 15.6, resolved after a rebubble procedure performed at the

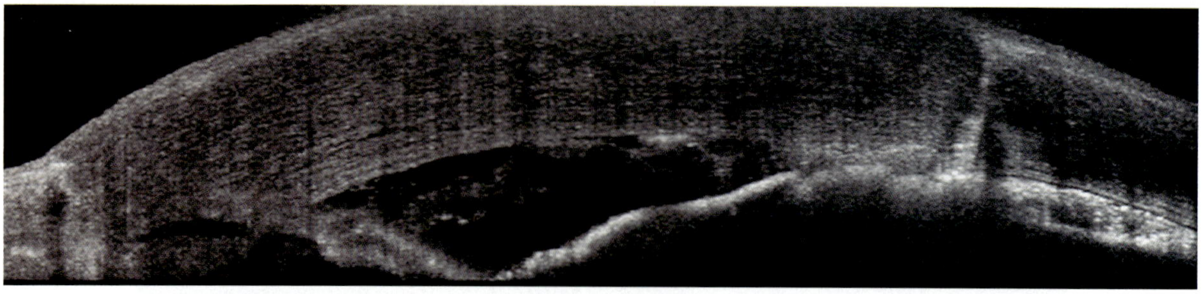

Fig. 15.4 Partially detached Descemet stripping automated endothelial keratoplasty (DSAEK) seen on AS-OCT at postoperative day 3. (Courtesy Dr. Christian Berry, MD, and Dr. Kamran Riaz, MD, Dean McGee Eye Institute, Oklahoma City, Oklahoma, United States.)

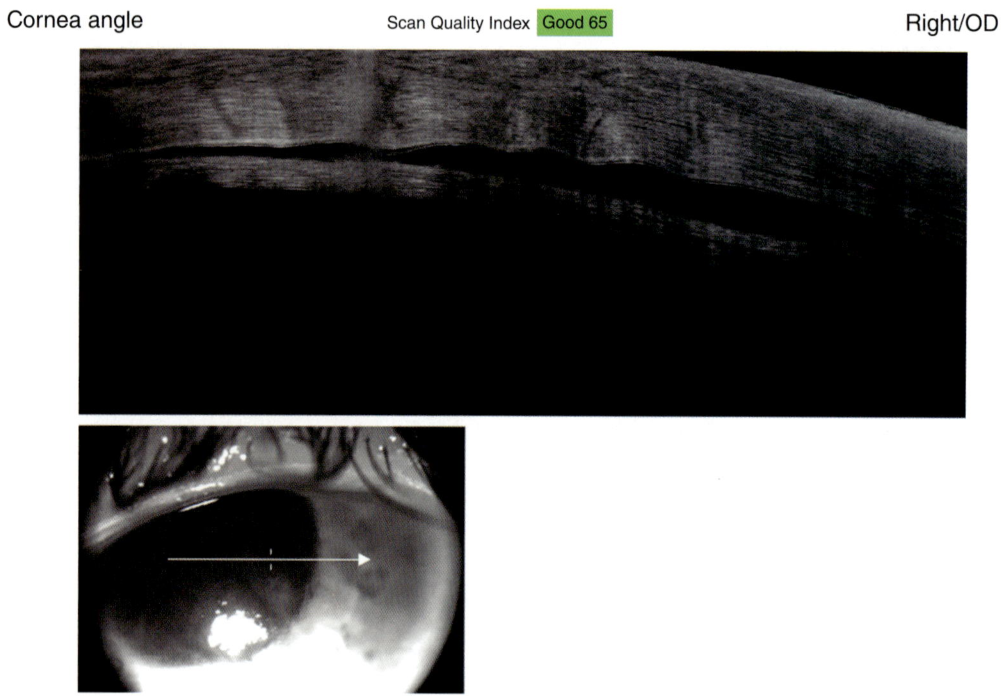

Fig. 15.5 Shallow nasal detachment of Descemet stripping automated endothelial keratoplasty (DSAEK) graft. Note the relatively good adherence of the central portion of the graft. The arrow indicates the orientation and location of the AS-OCT scan.

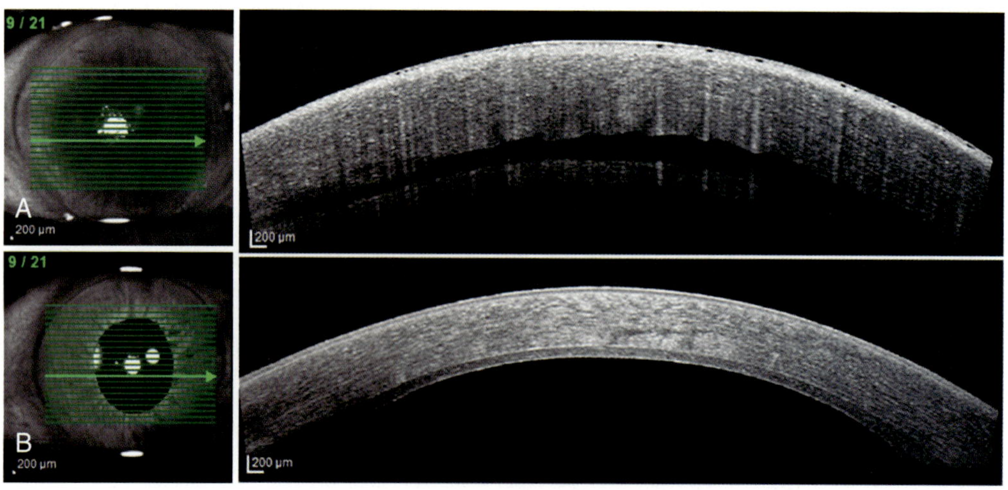

Fig. 15.6 Complete Descemet stripping endothelial keratoplasty (DSEK) detachment before (*panel A*) and after rebubbling procedure (*panel B*). Note the line of attachment that can be readily observed after the rebubble procedure. (Courtesy Dr. Albert Cheung, Eastern Virginia Medical School, Norfolk, Virginia, United States.)

slit lamp. Note the line of attachment that can be readily observed after the rebubble procedure.

CLINICAL PEARL

When rebubble procedures are performed, AS-OCT can be used to confirm reattachment of the DSEK/DSAEK lenticule. This can be especially helpful to show patients as a "before and after" image to demonstrate the success of the postoperative intervention.

C. Dislocated Lenticules

Detached grafts can also become dislocated or decentered, which can be visualized on AS-OCT. In Fig. 15.7 note the combination of detachment and dislocation of the DSAEK graft. In these cases, rebubbling will not be sufficient because the graft has decentered. Repositioning in the operating room with additional maneuvers, such as increased air fill, use of SF6 gas, or anchoring sutures, may be required in complex eyes such as aphakic eyes, prior vitrectomy, and/or the presence of glaucoma drainage devices.

D. Graft Failure

Despite its lower incidence in post-DSAEK eyes compared with post-PKP eyes, graft failure can occur. In these cases, the overall corneal thickness is significantly increased because of impaired endothelial cell function. Focal and regional variations in graft thickness may also be appreciated through the use of AS-OCT, and this may represent the origin of where the graft rejection/failure is most severe or initiated. Fig. 15.8 represents an eye in which the DSAEK graft failed; note the slightly increased thickness of the central portion of the graft *(panel A)* compared with the significantly increased thickness in the superior aspect of the graft *(panel B)*. Fig. 15.9 displays the significant differences in corneal thickness between the central aspect of the graft *(panel A)* compared with the superior portion of the graft *(panel B)*. Nonsurgical management with intensive topical, injectable, and/or systemic steroids may be tried. Ultimately, some patients may require a repeat EK procedure if medical therapy is unsuccessful.

III. USE OF AS-OCT IN POST-DMEK EYES

DMEK grafts are much thinner than DSEK/DSAEK lenticules because they are composed only of DM and endothelium. DMEK grafts are extremely thin (approximately 10–15 microns); therefore AS-OCT is exquisitely suited for precise visualization of the DMEK tissue, especially in cases when the clinical examination to ascertain attachment is equivocal.

A. Normal Postoperative Appearance

Fig. 15.10 shows an AS-OCT image of a well-healing eye 1 month after DMEK. The graft can be seen attached to the host cornea with good apposition. Note that this eye also has stromal hyperreflectivity from chronic long-standing edema as a result of Fuchs endothelial dystrophy before DMEK surgery.

Similar to post-DSEK eyes, corneal thickness in post-DMEK eyes will progressively decrease as the eye continues to heal and stromal edema improves. The pachymetry measurement feature in some AS-OCT devices can again be used for serial measurements of corneal thickness. Fig. 15.11 displays pachymetry measurements obtained with AS-OCT in the eye from Fig. 15.10 at 1 week *(panel A)* and 1 month after DMEK *(panel B)*; note the overall improvement in corneal thickness between the measurements indicating good function of the donor endothelium. Also note the overall thickness of the cornea

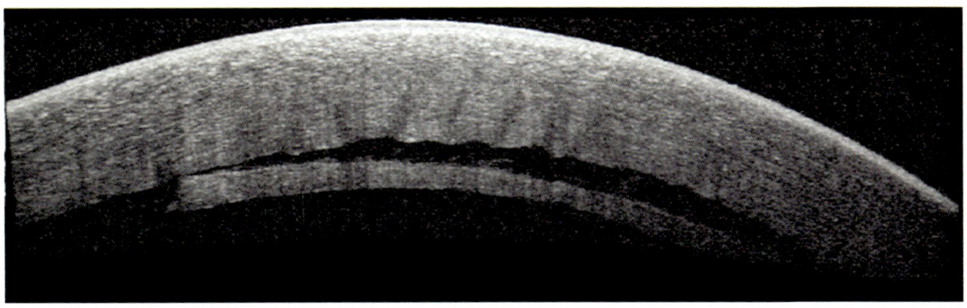

Fig. 15.7 Detached and dislocated Descemet stripping automated endothelial keratoplasty (DSAEK) graft. (Courtesy Dr. Christian Berry MD and Dr. Kamran Riaz MD, Dean McGee Eye Institute, Oklahoma City, Oklahoma, United States.)

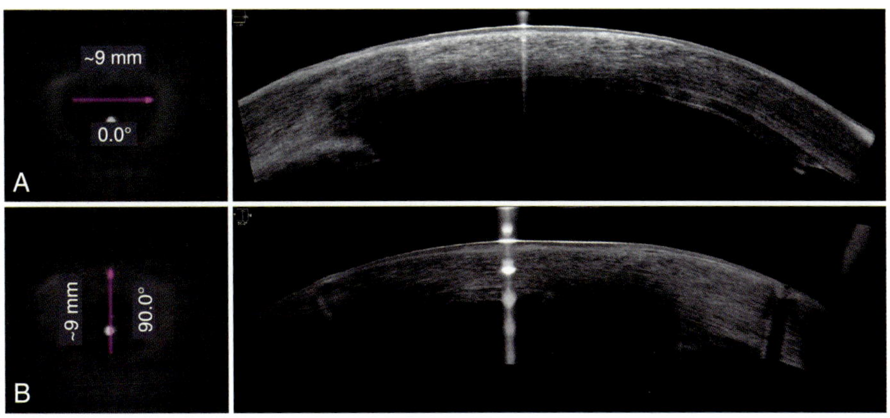

Fig. 15.8 A failed Descemet stripping automated endothelial keratoplasty (DSAEK) graft. *Panel A* shows a central horizontal OCT slice demonstrating slightly increased central graft thickness. *Panel B* shows a central vertical OCT slice demonstrating significantly increased thickness of the graft worsening from inferior to superior.

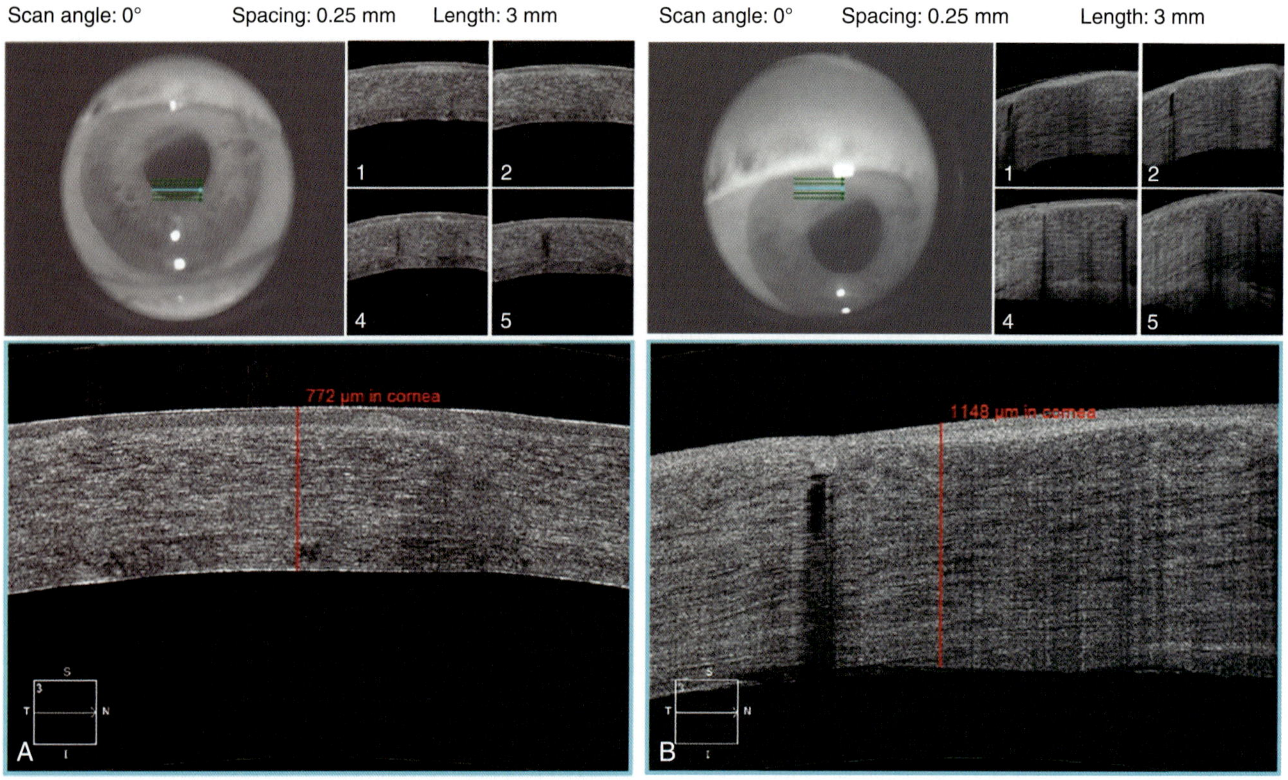

Fig. 15.9 Focal severity of Descemet stripping automated endothelial keratoplasty (DSAEK) graft failure can be seen by differences in corneal thickness among various locations of the graft. There is increased corneal thickness of the superior aspect of the graft *(panel B)* compared with the central aspect of the graft *(panel A)*, which increases the suspicion for a superior origin of graft failure.

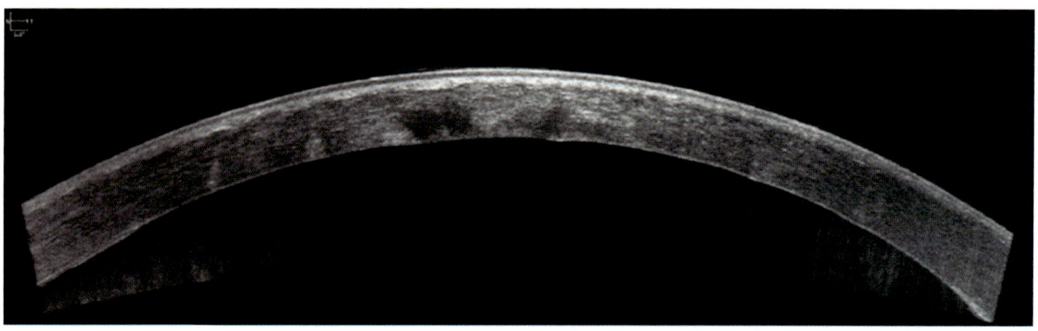

Fig. 15.10 Normal attached Descemet membrane endothelial keratoplasty (DMEK) graft visualized at 1 month after surgery using AS-OCT in a patient who had chronic long-standing edema from Fuchs endothelial dystrophy.

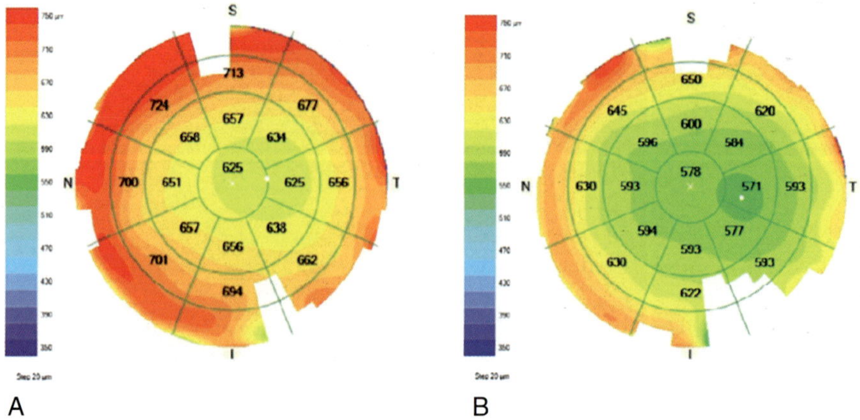

Fig. 15.11 Pachymetry measurement of corneal thickness in the same eye as Fig. 15.10 at 1 week (*panel A*) and at 1 month (*panel B*) after Descemet membrane endothelial keratoplasty (DMEK).

in *panel B* is thinner than the cornea shown in Fig 15.3, *panel B*; this is due to the thinner donor graft in the former compared to the thicker donor graft in the latter.

In addition to AS-OCT, specular microscopy allows for cell counts of the endothelium and can help be an indicator of graft health and success (Fig. 15.12). An expected DMEK cell count of around 2500 cells/mm^2 seen in the previous DMEK graft eye at 1 month after surgery can be appreciated.

B. Partial and Full Detachments

Similar to DSEK, DMEK grafts may also become partially or completely detached. As stated in the previous section, based on location, extent, and other clinical findings, practitioners may choose to closely observe or intervene appropriately. Several examples of partial DMEK graft detachments are shown in Fig. 15.13; in these cases, there is a prominent area of attachment compared with the area of detachment.

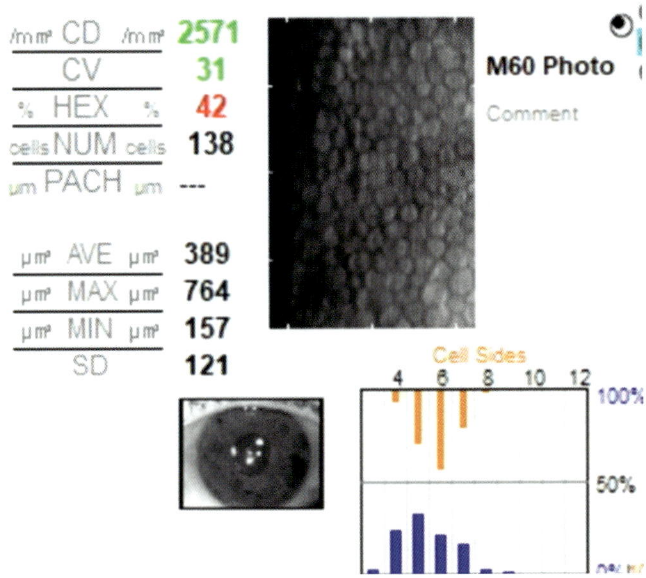

Fig. 15.12 Specular microscopy with a healthy Descemet membrane endothelial keratoplasty (DMEK) cell count at 1 month after surgery of the same eye as Fig. 15.10.

In other instances, complex detachments, wherein there are multiple areas of nonattachment within areas of attachment, also can be visualized by AS-OCT. The DMEK graft may have an undulating or wavelike appearance (Fig. 15.14)

> **CLINICAL PEARL**
>
> DMEK grafts are thinner than DSEK grafts; therefore slit-lamp examination alone may be insufficient to determine apposition and adherence of the graft. In such cases, AS-OCT can be used to visualize questionable areas to ascertain both simple and complex types of detachments.

Similar to DSEK grafts, DMEK grafts are amenable to rebubble procedures. Fig. 15.15 shows an eye that had a fully attached DMEK graft on postoperative day 1, when a large gas bubble was still present, but developed edema 3 weeks after DMEK. AS-OCT performed at 3 weeks after DMEK, on resorption of the gas bubble, showed that the graft was partially detached, and the eye required rebubbling. At 6 weeks after DMEK, the graft was attached, the cornea had cleared, and the patient's vision had improved significantly.

> **CLINICAL PEARL**
>
> Before and after images of rebubbling of DMEK grafts can be very helpful to both the clinician and the patient to demonstrate the success of the intervention.

In some eyes, the DMEK lenticule may fail, either due to poor apposition or endothelial dysfunction. In these eyes, graft failure can also result in edema and bullae (Fig. 15.16). This patient postoperatively developed inferotemporal edema and bullae at postoperative week 1 due to a partially failed graft. The edema decreased over time; however, it did not completely resolve even at 1 year after DMEK. A repeat graft was recommended but was deferred by the patient.

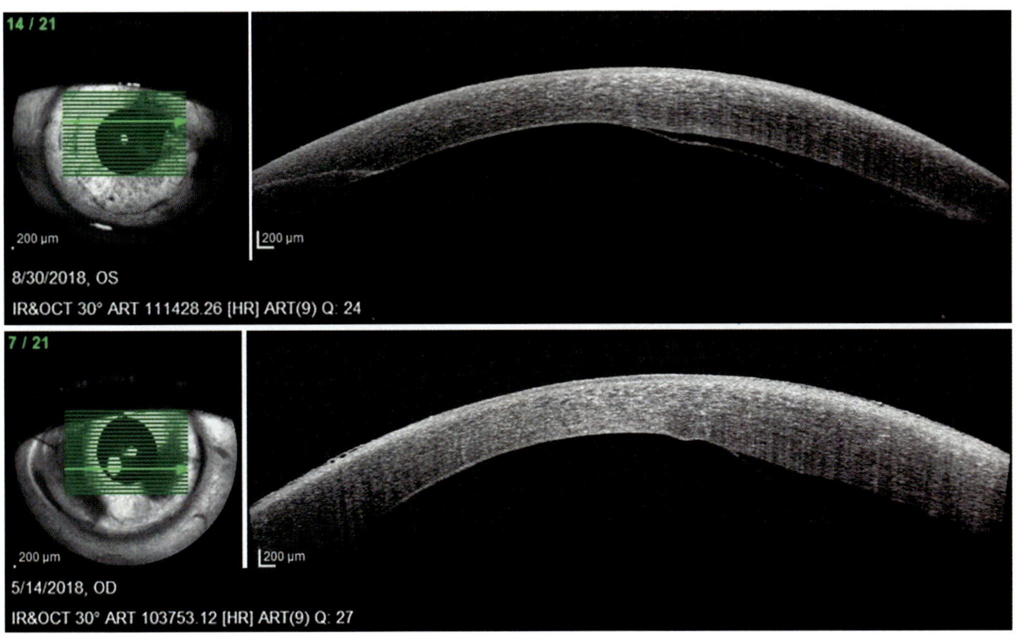

Fig. 15.13 Two examples of partial Descemet membrane endothelial keratoplasty (DMEK) detachment can be readily appreciated with AS-OCT. In both panels, the temporal part of the DMEK graft is attached while the nasal part is not attached. (Courtesy Albert Cheung, MD, Eastern Virginia Medical School, Norfolk, Virginia, United States.)

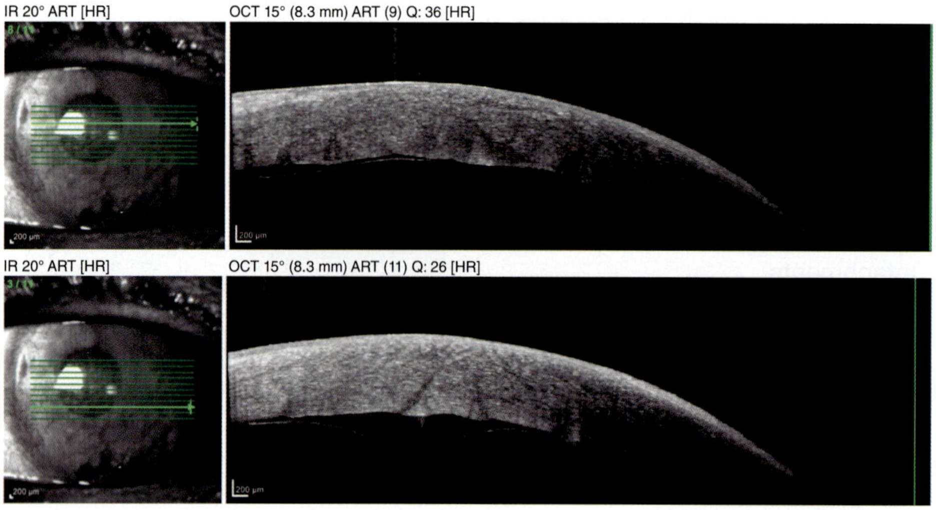

Fig. 15.14 Complex Descemet membrane endothelial keratoplasty (DMEK) detachment. AS-OCT can be used to highlight cases of complex DMEK detachment in which multiple areas of nonattachment are present within areas of attachment. An undulating or wavelike appearance of the DMEK graft is seen. (Courtesy Kamran M. Riaz, MD, Dean McGee Eye Institute, University of Oklahoma, Oklahoma City, Oklahoma, United States.)

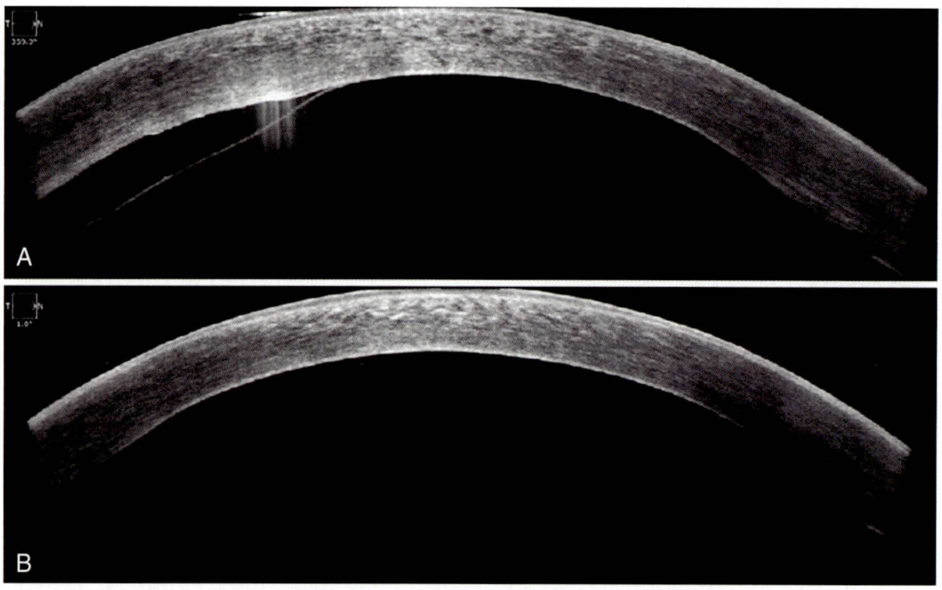

Fig. 15.15 Partially detached Descemet membrane endothelial keratoplasty (DMEK) graft. Partial detachment is seen at 3 weeks (*panel A*) after DMEK, which was successfully rebubbled with a fully attached DMEK graft seen here at 6 weeks (*panel B*) after DMEK.

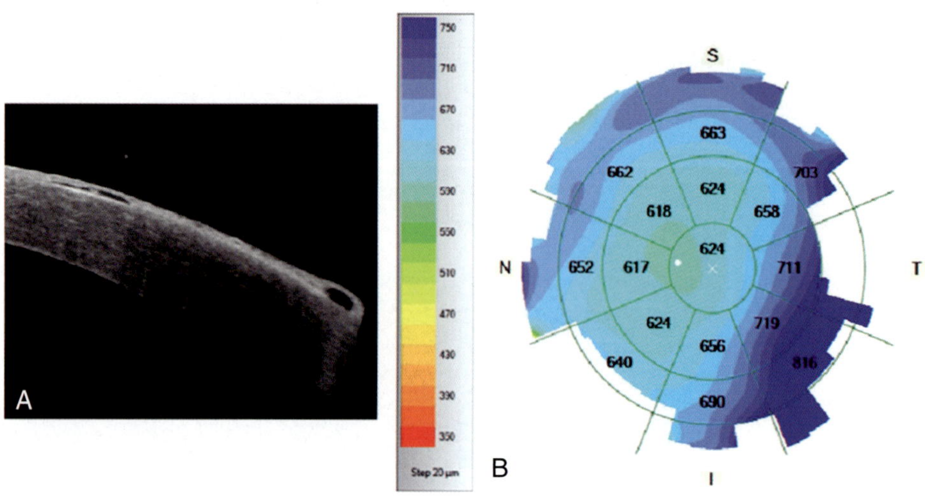

Fig. 15.16 Partial Descemet membrane endothelial keratoplasty (DMEK) graft failure resulting in temporal edema and bullae seen on AS-OCT (*panel A*) and on pachymetry (*panel B*).

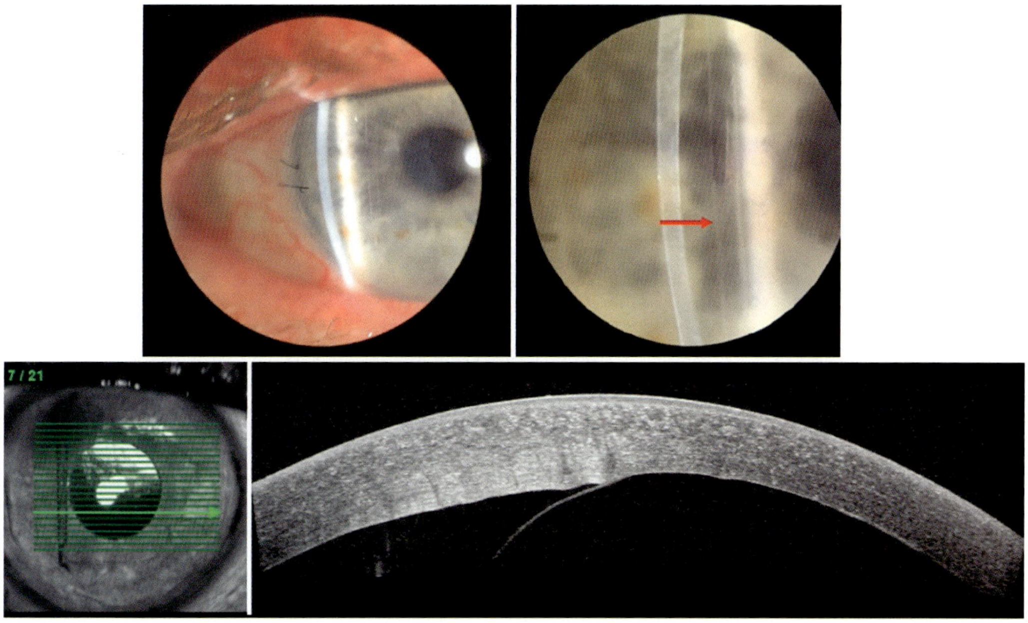

Fig. 15.17 Slit-lamp photographs of a scrolled Descemet membrane endothelial keratoplasty (DMEK) graft, indicated by the *red arrow*. Accompanying AS-OCT image shows the scroll as a prominent area of nonattachment. (Courtesy Dr. Albert Cheung, Eastern Virginia Medical School, Norfolk, Virginia, United States.)

A detached DMEK graft can also become scrolled, as shown in the slit-lamp photographs and AS-OCT images in Fig. 15.17. An eye with a scrolled graft may need to return to the operating room for repositioning and rebubbling. Minor scrolled DMEK grafts or grafts with a small, curled edge may be seen on AS-OCT but may not require further interventions such as repositioning or rebubbling.

Fig. 15.18 shows an eye with a partially detached inferior DMEK graft edge that is slightly curled. The center of the graft remained attached, and there was no obvious edema in the area of the detachment. The eye was able to achieve a best spectacle corrected visual acuity of 20/30 without further intervention.

In other cases, the graft may be attached overall, but central folds may develop within the attached DMEK graft. Fig. 15.19 shows images of a patient with relatively good attachment of the DMEK graft peripherally in the presence of prominent central folds. AS-OCT can be used to further highlight these findings; note the good adherence of the DMEK donor tissue superiorly *(panel A)*, with prominent folds seen on cross-section through the center and inferior views (*panels B and C*, respectively) of the cornea. In this patient, as the corrected visual acuity was 20/30, no additional surgical interventions were pursued.

Thus AS-OCT may reveal subtle interference with EK graft adherence, but not all findings necessarily require intervention if clinical outcomes are satisfactory.

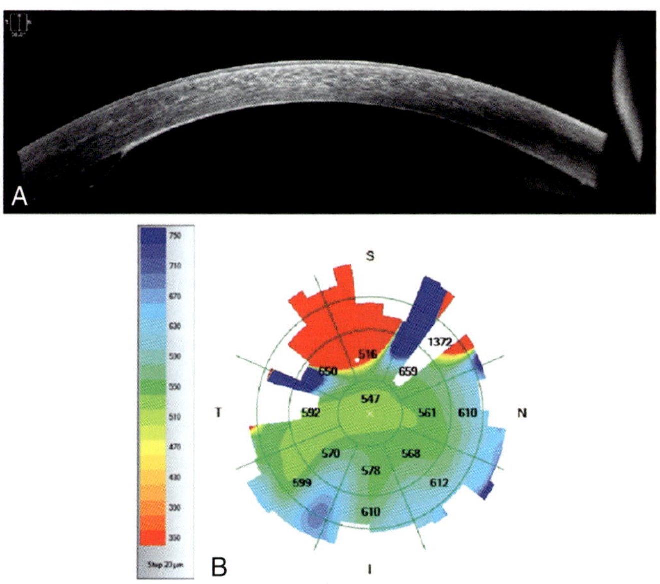

Fig. 15.18 Partially folded Descemet membrane endothelial keratoplasty (DMEK) graft edge. The partially folded graft edge is centrally attached as seen on AS-OCT (*panel A*) and clear with no obvious edema in the area of the detachment based on pachymetry (*panel B*).

CLINICAL PEARL

Despite the presence of folds or focal edema of the DMEK graft on slit-lamp examination or AS-OCT, it is not uncommon for patients to be satisfied with their best corrected visual acuity. In such cases, clinicians should exercise judgment on continued observation versus intervention.

In addition to partial detachments, a DMEK graft also may become completely detached. The DMEK graft in Fig. 15.20 is completely detached from the cornea; significant corneal swelling also can be appreciated on AS-OCT. Complete DMEK detachments require either rebubbling or a repeat DMEK if failure and/or excessive cell loss during the initial surgery is suspected.

IV. OTHER POSTOPERATIVE COMPLICATIONS

Both DSEK and DMEK grafts may have other complications unrelated to detachments and dislocations. For example, there also may be other interface abnormalities with EKs. Epithelial ingrowths may occur between the interface of the graft and cornea. Fig. 15.21 shows slit-lamp photographs *(panel A)* and AS-OCT images (*panel B*) of a post-DMEK eye in which a

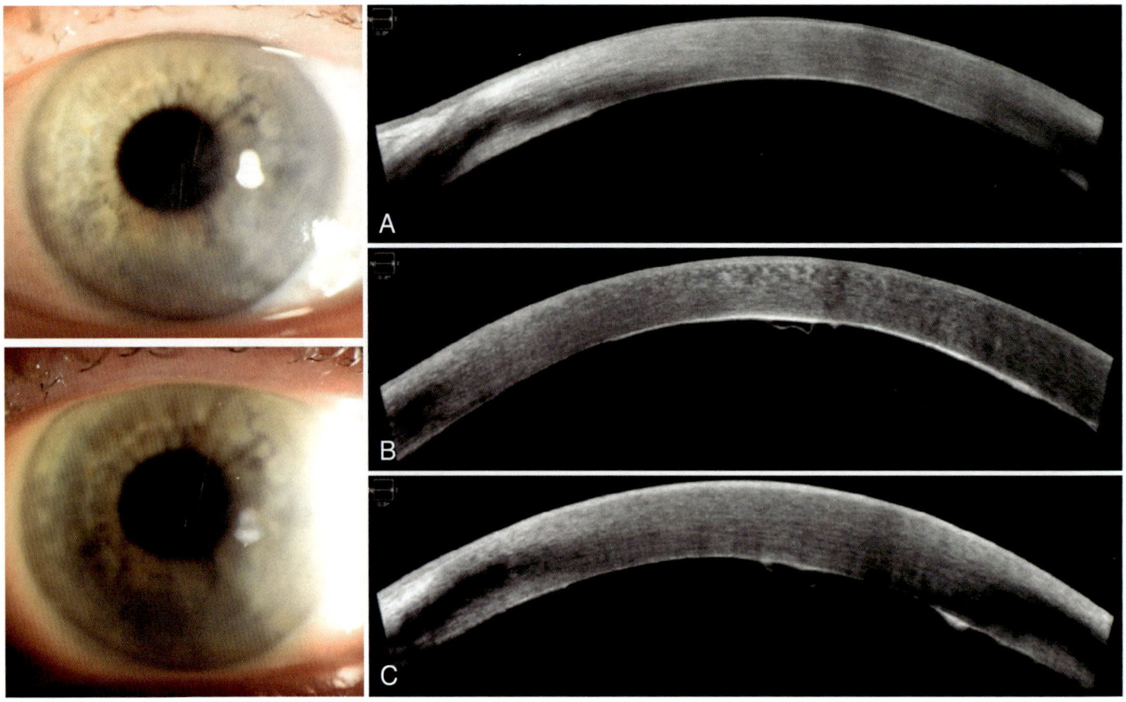

Fig. 15.19 Slit-lamp photographs of a Descemet membrane endothelial keratoplasty (DMEK) graft with good peripheral attachment and the presence of central folds. In the AS-OCT images, the superior aspect of the graft *(panel A)* demonstrates good adherence of the DMEK donor tissue. In *panels B and C,* taken over the central and inferior aspects of the cornea, respectively, the folds are seen in cross-section view. (Courtesy Kamran M. Riaz, MD, Dean McGee Eye Institute, University of Oklahoma, Oklahoma City, Oklahoma, United States.)

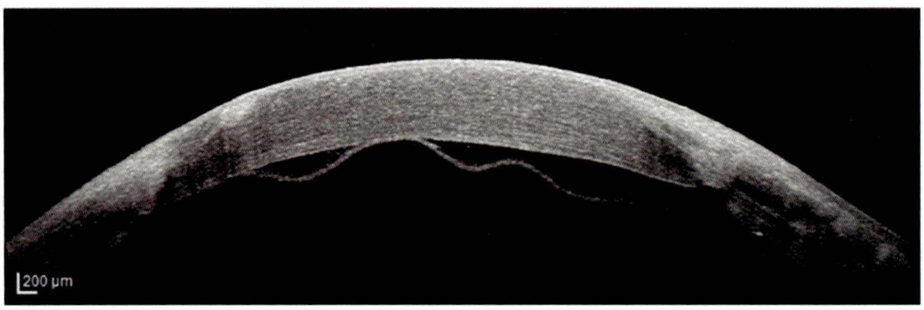

Fig. 15.20 Total Descemet membrane endothelial keratoplasty (DMEK) detachment seen on AS-OCT. (Image Courtesy Dr. Albert Cheung, Eastern Virginia Medical School, Norfolk, Virginia, United States.)

1.1-mm white corneal opacity, identified as an epithelial ingrowth, was seen 6 months after surgery on slit-lamp examination. AS-OCT confirmed that this opacity was located at the interface between the host cornea and the DMEK graft. The epithelial ingrowth was followed serially on AS-OCT and was seen to be enlarging 10 months postoperatively (not shown). Thus 11 months after DMEK, yttrium-aluminum-garnet (YAG) laser was used to treat the opacity. Subsequently, 15 months after DMEK, the opacity resolved and the cornea was clear on slit-lamp examination (Fig. 15.22, *panel A*). AS-OCT images taken 1 month later confirmed resolution of the previously noted opacity (see Fig. 15.22, *panel B*).

Fig. 15.23, *panel A,* shows an eye that originally had a partially detached DMEK graft noted 1 week after surgery that developed edema and bullae. The patient was brought back to the operating room for repositioning and rebubbling. Five weeks after the repositioning, the DMEK graft remained attached to the cornea but had retained DM in the graft interface. The clinical examination and also the AS-OCT in Fig. 15.23, *panel B,* indicate this as a hyperreflective band in the central posterior cornea, as shown by the *red arrow.*

Although rare, postoperative infectious keratitis may develop between the donor lenticule and the host stroma. Fungal keratitis can be especially challenging to treat because of its indolent onset, relatively good vision in early disease states, and subtle examination findings. In such cases, questionable posterior opacities can be better imaged using AS-OCT. Fig. 15.24 shows serial images of a fungal infection that was noted within the interface of a DMEK graft after surgery *(panel A).* Serial intrastromal injections of voriconazole were given, as evidenced by needle tracking *(panel B).* Two years after treatment, a posterior scar remained, and the patient maintained acceptable visual acuity *(panel C).* In other cases, especially in the presence of declining visual acuity, removal of the DMEK graft with intraoperative anterior chamber washout and injection of antifungal agents may be necessary.

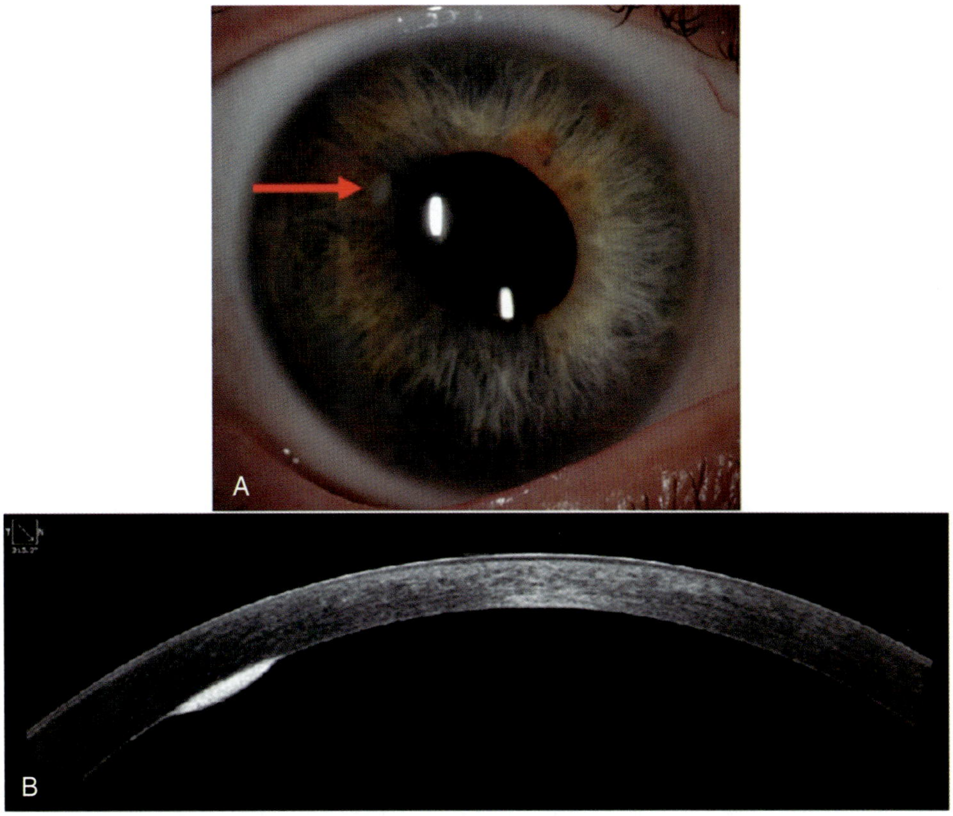

Fig. 15.21 Epithelial ingrowth of a Descemet membrane endothelial keratoplasty (DMEK) shown on slit-lamp photography and on AS-OCT. Six months after DMEK surgery, a 1.1-mm epithelial ingrowth *(red arrow)* was identified on slit-lamp examination *(panel A),* AS-OCT confirmed that the opacity was located at the graft-cornea interface and showed that the opacity increased in size 10 months after DMEK *(panel B).*

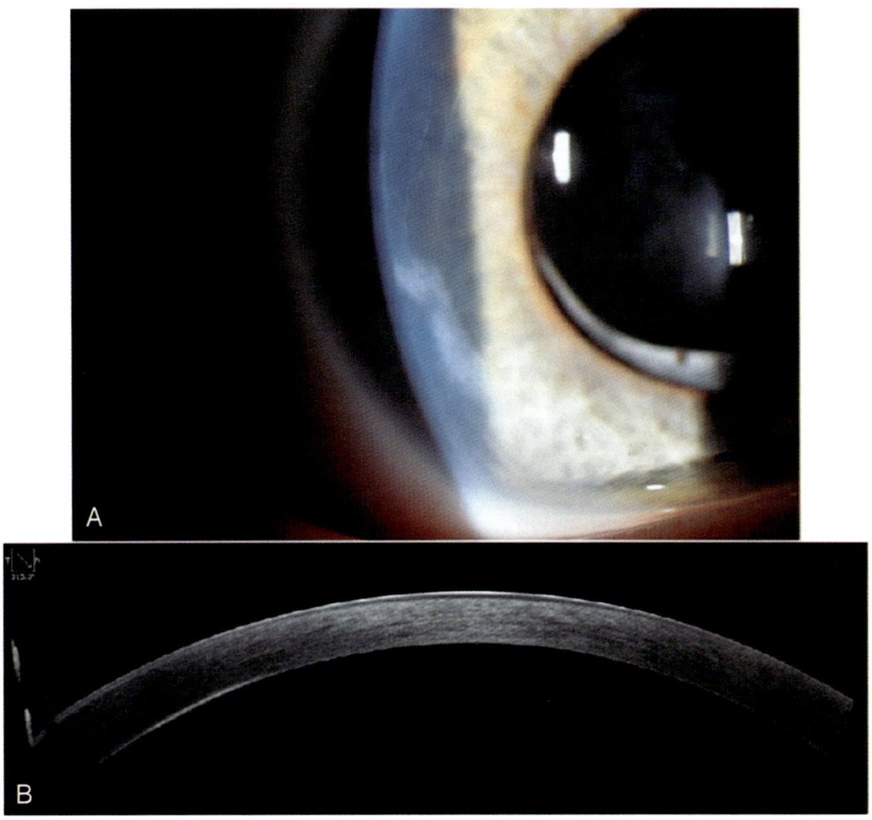

Fig. 15.22 Four months after treatment of epithelial ingrowth of a Descemet membrane endothelial keratoplasty (DMEK) shown on slit-lamp photography and on AS-OCT. Four months after yttrium-aluminum-garnet (YAG) laser treatment and 15 months after the original DMEK surgery, the eye in Fig. 15.21 showed resolution of the previously seen epithelial ingrowth on slit-lamp examination *(panel A).* AS-OCT showed continued resolution of opacity 1 month after YAG laser treatment *(panel B).*

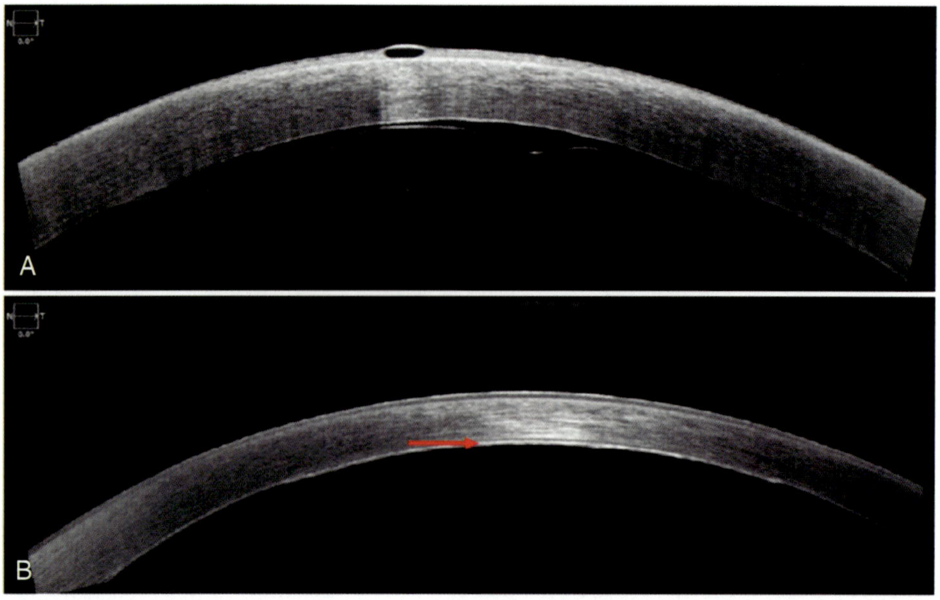

Fig. 15.23 A partially detached Descemet membrane endothelial keratoplasty (DMEK) graft. This partial detachment with corneal edema and bullae was identified 1 week after surgery by AS-OCT (panel A). Five weeks after repositioning the DMEK graft (panel B), the graft remained attached; however, retained Descemet membrane *(red arrow)* can be seen in the graft interface.

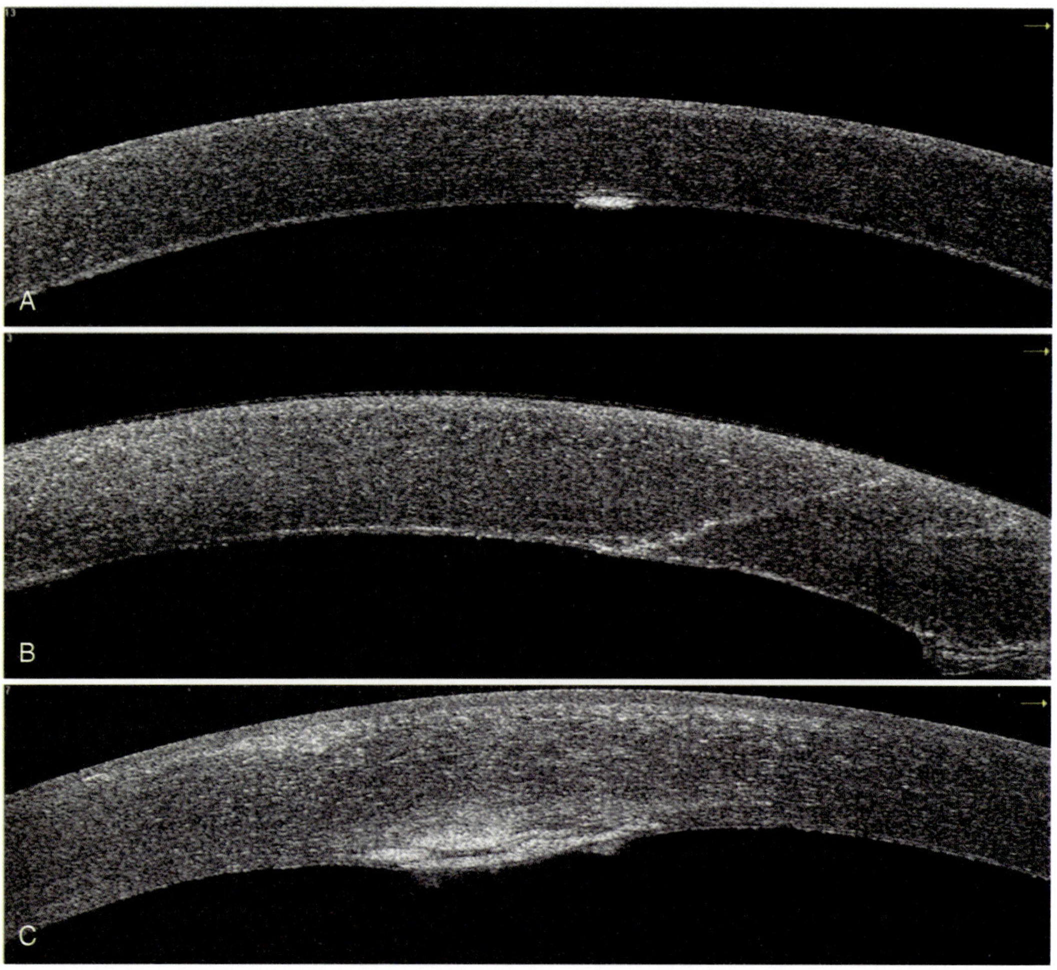

Fig. 15.24 Serial images of fungal infection in a Descemet membrane endothelial keratoplasty (DMEK) graft. *Panel A* shows the initial appearance of the fungal infiltrate as a prominently hyperreflective lesion on the donor endothelium. There is minimal adjacent inflammation. Seral intrastromal injections of voriconazole were given. *Panel B* shows an AS-OCT taken immediately after one of these injections. Two years after treatment *(panel C),* the fungal infiltrate resolved, but a significant posterior stromal scar remains. The patient maintained good visual acuity, and a replacement of the DMEK graft was not required. (Courtesy Parag Majmudar, MD, Rush University, Chicago, Illinois, United States.)

V. FUTURE DIRECTIONS OF ENDOTHELIAL KERATOPLASTY

At the time of this writing, there is significant interest in further developing EK procedures, including surgical techniques to obviate the need for donor endothelium (e.g., Descemet stripping only/Descemets stripping without endothelial keratoplasty). One area of interest is the use of artificial endothelium graft (EndoArt; EyeYon Medical, Ness Ziona, Israel) as a substitute for human donor corneal tissue. The EndoArt implant is an approximately 50 micron-thick, hydrophilic, contact lens–shaped lenticule and resembles an ultrathin DSAEK graft. Fig. 15.25 shows postoperative images taken 1 week after surgery. The donor graft appears as a double-banded hyperreflective lenticule with an optically empty clear space with good adherence to the posterior cornea. There is notable improvement in corneal edema/thickness at the 1-month (Fig. 15.26) and 1-year postoperative time points (Fig. 15.27).

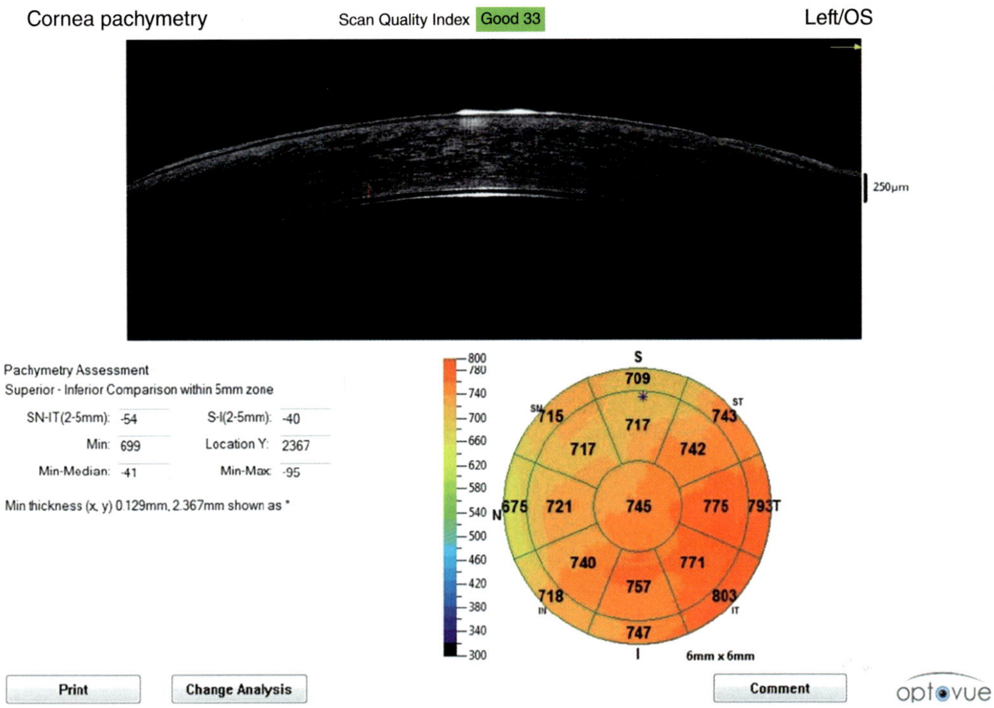

Fig. 15.25 EndoArt (EyeYon Medical, Israel) is an artificial endothelial graft that can be used in lieu of donor corneal tissue for endothelial keratoplasty (EK) surgery. In this postoperative image taken 1 week after surgery, the artificial donor graft can be seen as a prominently hyperreflective double-banded entity with an optically empty space in between them. There is a good apposition between the artificial donor graft and the host cornea. Moderate corneal edema is still present centrally. (Courtesy Michael Mimouni, MD, University of Toronto, Toronto, Canada.)

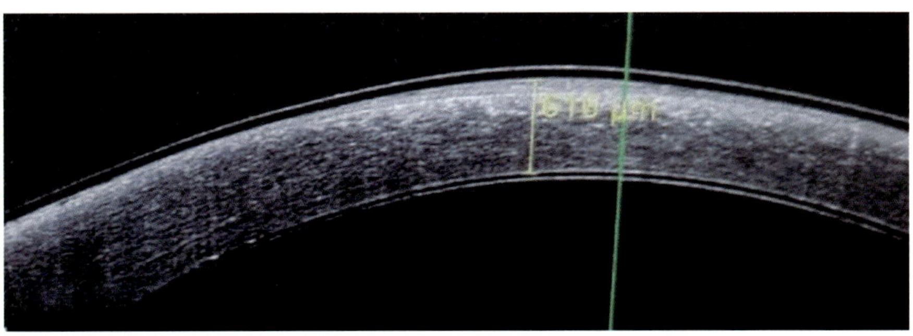

Fig. 15.26 AS-OCT of EndoArt at 1 month shows improvement in corneal edema (610 microns) with good adherence of the artificial donor graft. A bandage contact lens is in place and can be seen as a prominent hyperreflective curved surface overlying the corneal epithelium. Assuming the donor graft is 50 microns, the corneal thickness at this time is approximately 660 microns. (Courtesy Michael Mimouni, MD, University of Toronto, Toronto, Canada.)

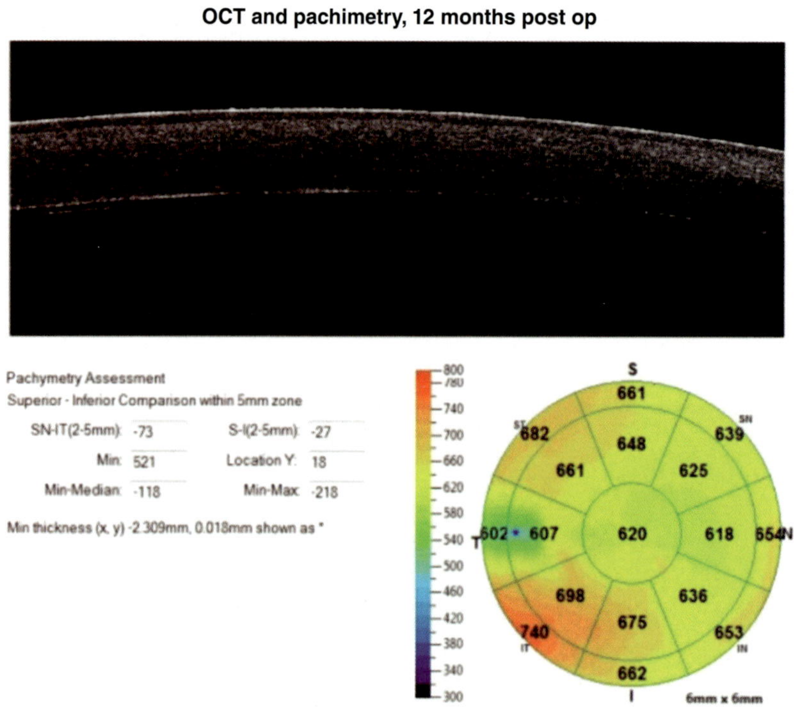

Fig. 15.27 AS-OCT images taken 1 year after EndoArt transplant show an improvement in previously seen corneal thickness. The artificial endothelium remains well attached, and the overlying corneal anatomy appears significantly improved (620 microns) compared with previous measurements in Figs. 15.25 and 15.26. (Courtesy Michael Mimouni, MD, University of Toronto, Toronto, Canada.)

BIBLIOGRAPHY

Allan BDS, Terry MA, Price FW, Price MO, Griffin NB, Claesson M. Corneal transplant rejection rate and severity after endothelial keratoplasty. *Cornea*. 2007;26(9):1039-1042. Available at: https://doi.org/10.1097/ICO.0b013e31812f66e5.

Higashiura R, Maeda N, Nakagawa T, et al. Corneal topographic analysis by 3-dimensional anterior segment optical coherence tomography after endothelial keratoplasty. *Invest Ophthalmol Vis Sci*. 2012;53(7):3286-3295. Available at: https://doi.org/10.1167/iovs.12-9602.

Jenkins SG, Jun AS, Woreta FA, Srikumaran D. YAG laser treatment for epithelial ingrowth in descemet membrane endothelial keratoplasty interface. *Cornea*. 2020;39(11):1439-1441. https://doi.org/10.1097/ico.0000000000002367.

Lee WB, Jacobs DS, Musch DC, Kaufman SC, Reinhart WJ, Shtein RM. Descemet's stripping endothelial keratoplasty: safety and outcomes. a report by the American Academy of Ophthalmology. *Ophthalmology*. 2009;116(9):1818-1830. Available at: https://doi.org/10.1016/j.ophtha.2009.06.021.

Melles GRJ, Ong TS, Ververs B, van der Wees J. Descemet Membrane Endothelial Keratoplasty (DMEK). *Cornea*. 2006;25(8):987-990. Available at: https://doi.org/10.1097/01.ico.0000248385.16896.34.

Mencucci R, Favuzza E, Tartaro R, Busin M, Virgili G. Descemet stripping automated endothelial keratoplasty in Fuchs' corneal endothelial dystrophy: anterior segment optical coherence tomography and in vivo confocal microscopy analysis. *BMC Ophthalmol*. 2015;15(1):99. Available at: https://doi.org/10.1186/s12886-015-0096-x.

Mi H, Tan N, Ang M, Htoon HM, Mehta JS. Comparison of anterior and posterior topographic analysis between 3 imaging systems. *J Cataract Refract Surg*. 2015;41(11):2533-2545. https://doi.org/10.1016/j.jcrs.2015.05.039.

Neff KD, Biber JM, Holland EJ. Comparison of central corneal graft thickness to visual acuity outcomes in endothelial keratoplasty. *Cornea*. 2011;30(4):388-391. Available at: https://doi.org/10.1097/ICO.0b013e3181f236c6.

Price MO, Giebel AW, Fairchild KM, Price FW. Descemet's membrane endothelial keratoplasty. Prospective multicenter study of visual and refractive outcomes and endothelial survival. *Ophthalmology*. 2009;116(12):2361-2368. Available at: https://doi.org/10.1016/j.ophtha.2009.07.010.

Tarnawska D, Wylegala E. Monitoring cornea and graft morphometric dynamics after descemet stripping and endothelial keratoplasty with anterior segment optical coherence tomography. *Cornea*. 2010;29(3):272-277. Available at: https://doi.org/10.1097/ICO.0b013e3181b61496.

van Rij G, Bartels M. Descemet's stripping with endothelial keratoplasty in 50 eyes: a refractive neutral corneal transplant. *J Refract Surg*. 2006;22(6):529-530.

Yeh RY, Quilendrino R, Musa FU, Liarakos VS, Dapena I, Melles GR. Predictive value of optical coherence tomography in graft attachment after Descemet's membrane endothelial keratoplasty. *Ophthalmology*. 2013;120(2):240-245. doi:10.1016/j.ophtha.2012.08.011.

SECTION 6

Pediatrics, Trauma, Contact Lenses and Other Pathologies

16 Pediatric Cornea and Anterior Segment Imaging

Angela Zhu Y. | Asim Ali

I. INTRODUCTION

Anterior segment optical coherence tomography (AS-OCT) imaging can be invaluable in pediatric ophthalmology. As a noncontact imaging modality, it can aid in visualization of anterior segment abnormalities associated with congenital corneal opacities that may not be directly visible on clinical examination. Particularly for inattentive or photophobic children who may be uncooperative with slit-lamp examination, the near-infrared light used by OCT is generally well tolerated by even the most photosensitive of children. The rapid image acquisition time is also advantageous for imaging active children with short attention spans. AS-OCT images can be more reliable than a limited clinical examination in these patients, even obviating the need for examination under anesthesia in some cases (Mireskandari K, Tehrani NN, Vandenhoven C, 2011).

Different AS-OCT technologies have a variety of uses in pediatric cornea and anterior segment pathologic conditions. With time-domain systems such as the standalone Visante AS-OCT (Carl Zeiss Meditec, Dublin, California, United States), a long-wavelength (1310 nm) light source is used that can image the entire anterior segment from limbus-to-limbus and take high-resolution corneal images for patients who can sit upright. This allows for delineation of corneal and ocular surface pathologic conditions, preoperative planning for anterior segment reconstruction and refractive procedures, postoperative visualization of intraocular lens (IOL) and glaucoma drainage device placement, and evaluation of angle and lenticular anomalies. For higher resolution corneal imaging, a spectral domain system such as the upright Cirrus OCT (Carl Zeiss Meditec) or handheld Bioptigen OCT (Bioptigen, Inc., Morrisville, North Carolina, United States) can be configured to image the anterior segment. These systems use an 840-nm wavelength and are most useful for detailed imaging of corneal pathologic findings and structures, such as measuring depth of a lesion for preoperative planning or demarcating Descemet membrane (DM)/endothelial abnormalities (Mireskandari K, Tehrani NN, Vandenhoven C, 2011; Rodrigues EB, Johanson M, Penha FM, 2012).

Here, we illustrate some examples where AS-OCT imaging proves highly useful in the diagnosis and/or management of pediatric patients. Tomographic correlation with clinical and/or structural abnormalities is emphasized in these pathologic conditions.

II. CORNEA AND EXTERNAL DISEASE PATHOLOGIC CONDITIONS

A. Corneolimbal Dermoid

Corneolimbal dermoids are choristomas, commonly located in the limbal epibulbar area but may also extend into the visual axis (Fig. 16.1, *panel A*). In some cases, these lesions can be quite extensive and even invade the anterior chamber (Nischal KK, 2015). Although they are generally benign with good prognosis, the more extensive lesions can be associated with significant amblyopia, anterior segment dysgenesis, and rarely secondary glaucoma, especially in auriculo-oculo-vertebral (Goldenhar) syndrome.

Management can include observation (if small and not visually significant) or surgical excision, which may require lamellar or even penetrating keratoplasty (PKP) depending on depth and extent of the lesion. AS-OCT can be useful in these cases to delineate the depth of the epibulbar lesion for preoperative planning purposes, especially if lamellar or PKP tissue may be necessary for reconstruction (see Fig. 16.1, *panel B*). However, because of the dense homogeneity of these lesions, there may be difficulty visualizing the posterior aspect of lesions of interest; some AS-OCT systems may be unable to penetrate deep into the underlying tissue; in these cases, other imaging modalities such as high-resolution ultrasound biomicroscopy (UBM) may be more useful (Mireskandari K, Tehrani NN, Vandenhoven C, 2011).

B. Blepharokeratoconjunctivitis

Blepharokeratoconjunctivitis (BKC) is a chronic inflammatory disorder of childhood in which pediatric lid margin disease (blepharitis) is accompanied by episodes of conjunctivitis and keratopathy. Although the prevalence depends on racial demographics, the

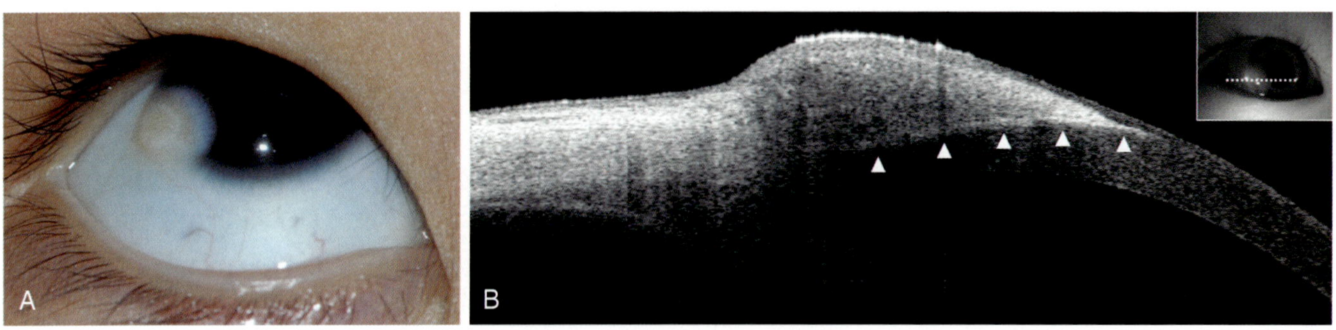

Fig. 16.1 Limbal dermoid. A, Slit-lamp photograph of the right eye of a 5-year-old boy with a raised, inferotemporal epibulbar lesion at the inferotemporal limbus. B, AS-OCT image slice through the corneolimbal area reveals an epithelialized, homogeneous, hyperreflective lesion extending from perilimbal sclera to corneal stroma. The base of the lesion is clearly demarcated *(arrowheads),* with normal-appearing stromal tissue deep to the lesion suggesting no intraocular extension.

mean age of onset has been reported as 3 to 7 years in most populations (Hammersmith KM, 2015). Moderate to severe corneal involvement associated with BKC has been reported in up to 40% of some cohorts, ranging in severity from acute marginal infiltrates/phlyctenules, to chronic central or paracentral scars with or without neovascularization, to even thinning and perforation in severe cases (Fig. 16.2, *panel A*) (Jones SM, Weinstein JM, Cumberland P, 2007). For this reason, BKC can lead to significant visual morbidity, with up to 10% requiring surgical intervention and 60% of patients developing associated amblyopia (Hammersmith KM, 2015).

Given the degree of ocular surface inflammation generally present in the acute phase, these patients tend to be highly photosensitive so detailed corneal examination can be difficult. However, the low-intensity light used by the AS-OCT often can be tolerated enough by these patients to better depict the degree of corneal involvement, from evaluating presence of any corneal ulceration or thinning to delineating extent of a chronic scar for preoperative planning after medical management of the underlying BKC (see Fig. 16.2, *panel B*).

C. Vernal Keratoconjunctivitis

Vernal keratoconjunctivitis (VKC) is a chronic, allergy-associated inflammatory condition of the ocular surface predominantly affecting children. Although the clinical features can vary depending on ethnic and geographic distribution, the hallmark manifestations of limbal, tarsal, or mixed giant papillae differentiate this entity from other forms of allergic conjunctivitis (Pattnaik L, Acharya L, 2015). Severe cases can lead to corneal neovascularization, microepithelial or macroepithelial erosions, and shield ulcers (Fig. 16.3, *panel A*). These are often prominent in the superior half of the cornea, where repetitive mechanical trauma from upper eyelid tarsal conjunctival giant papillae can perpetuate corneal ulceration and underlying stromal haze formation.

Even after the atopic pathophysiology has been medically treated, persistent epithelial defects and shield ulcers may require surgical debridement or excimer laser phototherapeutic keratectomy to promote reepithelialization (Pattnaik L, Acharya L, 2015). Symptomatic patients also tend to be extremely photophobic, so AS-OCT can greatly aid in identifying any corneal involvement and help distinguish eosinophilic inflammatory material plaques from underlying anterior stromal haze/scar formation associated with shield ulcers (see Fig. 16.3, *panel B*).

CLINICAL PEARL

When deciding whether corneal surgery is indicated, AS-OCT imaging can provide quantitative assessment of lesion or scar depth for preoperative planning. For example, corneal dermoids that extend into deeper intrastromal planes may require lamellar keratoplasty for reconstruction; other superficial lesions may only necessitate keratectomy to debulk the irregular superficial aspect (e.g., Fig. 16.1). Some lesions also may be more apparent on AS-OCT than on clinical examination, such as quiescent BKC scars that may no longer appear dense clinically but can have significant anterior stromal and epithelial irregularity seen on high-resolution corneal imaging that can be extremely visually significant. Similarly, shield ulcers associated with VKC can have epithelial defects with underlying stromal opacity and superficial plaque deposition; the difference between these can be distinguished on AS-OCT to determine whether superficial keratectomy, deeper phototherapeutic keratectomy, or anterior lamellar keratoplasty may be the optimal procedure for visual rehabilitation.

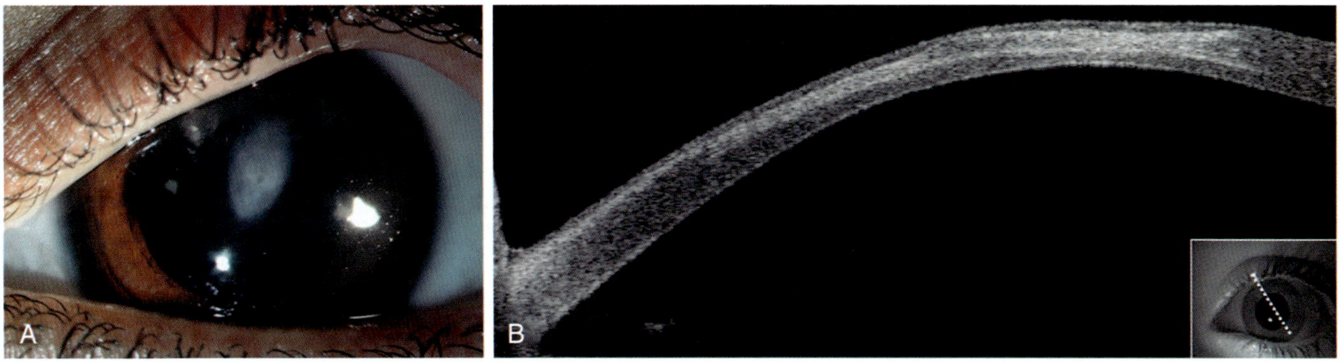

Fig. 16.2 Central corneal scar secondary to blepharokeratoconjunctivitis (BKC). A, Slit-lamp photograph of the left eye of a 4-year-old girl with central quiescent, anterior to midstromal opacity after treatment of chronic BKC. No significant neovascularization is present. B, AS-OCT high-resolution corneal image shows a hyperreflective stromal scar extending past 50% depth centrally with overlying surface irregularity.

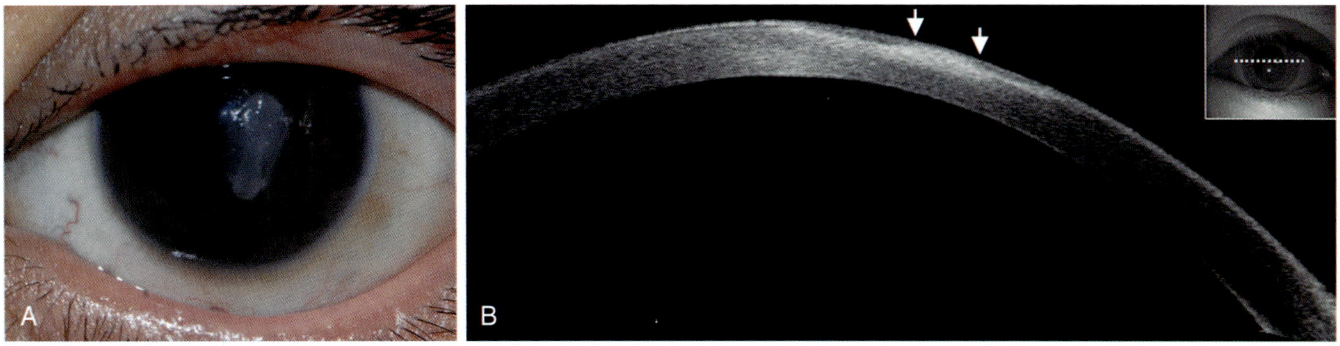

Fig. 16.3 Shield ulcer with central plaque. A, Slit-lamp photograph of the left eye of a 10-year-old girl with vernal keratoconjunctivitis and giant upper tarsal conjunctival papillae presenting with a persistent, superior paracentral corneal epithelial defect with central plaque consistent with shield ulcer. B, AS-OCT high-resolution corneal image shows hyperreflective material within epithelial defect (edges denoted by *arrows*), consistent with inflammatory plaque. Mild underlying anterior stromal hyperreflectivity is also present, corresponding to anterior stromal haze seen underlying the base of the shield ulcer.

D. Aniridia-Associated Keratopathy

Congenital aniridia caused by a mutation in *PAX6* can be associated with other anterior segment abnormalities, including central corneal opacities, iridotrabecular dysgenesis and glaucoma, keratolenticular adhesions, and cataracts (often anterior polar or pyramidal) (Nischal KK, 2015). *PAX6* mutations can also involve limbal stem cells to varying degrees, resulting in a progressive aniridic keratopathy affecting about 20% of these patients (Lee H, Khan R, O'Keefe M, 2008). In the early stages, minimal limbal stem cell dysfunction causing metastatic epithelial changes can exist, evolving to peripheral pannus formation and ultimately complete conjunctivalization of the cornea (Fig. 16.4, *panel A*). On AS-OCT, even subtle epithelial changes associated with limbal stem cell dysfunction can be visible, as conjunctival epithelium is generally more hyperreflective (opaque), irregular, and thinner than normal corneal epithelium (see Fig. 16.4, *panel B*).

E. Endothelial Dystrophies

I. CONGENITAL HEREDITARY ENDOTHELIAL DYSTROPHY

Congenital hereditary endothelial dystrophy (CHED) is a congenital, autosomal recessive (*SLC4A11* mutation) disease. Patients generally present within the neonatal period with bilateral, symmetric, diffuse corneal edema (Fig. 16.5, *panel A*). Histologic features characteristic of CHED include diffuse epithelial and stromal edema, Bowman membrane abnormalities, thickening of DM, and a paucity of normal endothelial cells (Nischal KK, 2015). These structural changes are clearly visible on AS-OCT high-resolution corneal imaging, which can be used to visualize the DM appearance despite significant epithelial and stromal edema (see Fig. 16.5, *panel B*).

II. POSTERIOR POLYMORPHOUS CORNEAL DYSTROPHY

Posterior polymorphous corneal dystrophy (PPCD) comprises a more heterogeneous spectrum of clinical presentations associated with multiple genetic variants, generally inherited in an autosomal dominant manner (Nischal KK, 2015). It rarely manifests at birth but is characterized by polymorphous posterior stromal or endothelial opacities, blister-like vesicles, and/or band-like "snail track" lesions (Fig. 16.6, *panel A*). It may be bilaterally asymmetric and associated with a variable degree of stromal edema. The typical histologic appearance involves multilayering of endothelial cells with an irregular, jagged "saw-toothed" thickening pattern of the DM. These posterior stromal and DM changes are fairly pathognomonic on AS-OCT imaging (see Fig. 16.6, *panel B*).

CLINICAL PEARL

Even in the presence of significant corneal edema, AS-OCT imaging can provide a clear outline of the DM structure and morphology. This can help differentiate between various causes of corneal edema in pediatric patients, from congenital causes (CHED, PPCD) to secondary causes (congenital glaucoma, bullous keratopathy). Particularly in CHED or bullous keratopathy, some patients have minimal DM, which may be difficult to remove during endothelial keratoplasty (EK), so some surgeons have demonstrated that it may not be necessary to strip the DM in these cases. The authors have found AS-OCT imaging to be a helpful guide for this type of preoperative planning, as a distinct hyperreflective layer of DM on AS-OCT generally reflects a membrane that can be stripped, whereas other patients may have a less-defined layer that does not require stripping during EK. Furthermore, slit-lamp evaluation of infants and young children is often difficult and limited, so AS-OCT imaging can be essential in the postoperative period for confirming EK graft attachment and identifying early signs of graft rejection or failure (e.g., preclinical corneal edema).

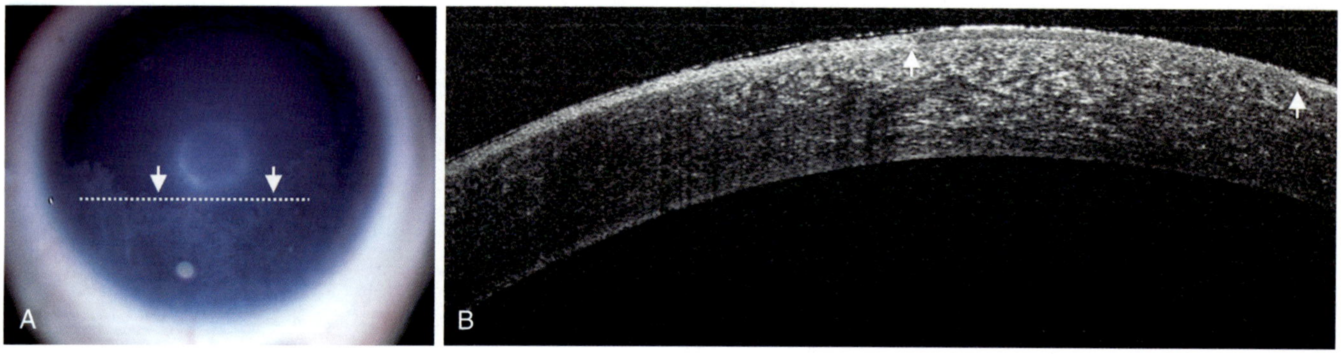

Fig. 16.4 Metastatic corneal epithelium associated with aniridia. A, External RetCam (Clarity Medical Systems, Pleasanton, California, United States) photograph of left eye of 7-year-old boy with bilateral congenital aniridia (*PAX6* mutation), showing early peripheral corneal epithelial metastatic changes associated with limbal stem cell deficiency (edges denoted by *arrows*). B, AS-OCT high-resolution corneal image shows hyperreflective peripheral epithelial keratinization with abrupt transition to residual central normal epithelium *(arrows)*.

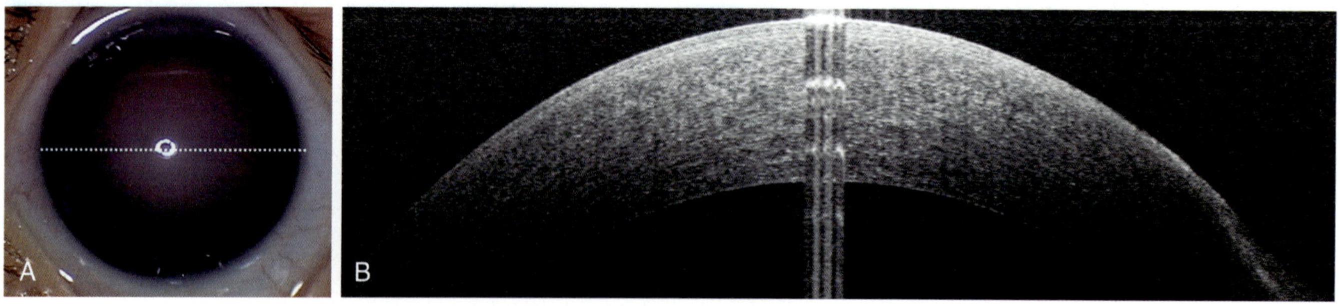

Fig. 16.5 Congenital hereditary endothelial dystrophy (CHED). A, External RetCam (Clarity Medical Systems) photograph of right eye of 6-month-old boy with bilateral congenital corneal clouding showing moderate diffuse corneal haze and edema. B, AS-OCT high-resolution corneal image shows significant diffuse corneal stromal edema (central pachymetry 1104 μm) with associated epithelial edema and thickening/irregularity of the Bowman layer. A pronounced Descemet membrane appears present without significant irregularity.

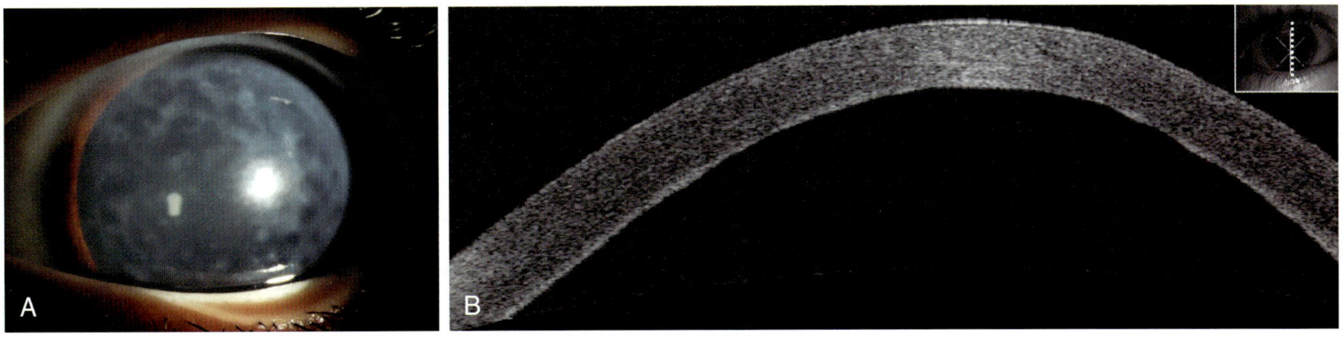

Fig. 16.6 Posterior polymorphous corneal dystrophy (PPCD). A, Slit-lamp photograph of right eye of 6-year-old boy with bilateral, polymorphous posterior stromal opacities with focal scattered vesicles. B, AS-OCT high-resolution corneal image shows hyperreflective and thickened Descemet membrane with irregular jagged areas.

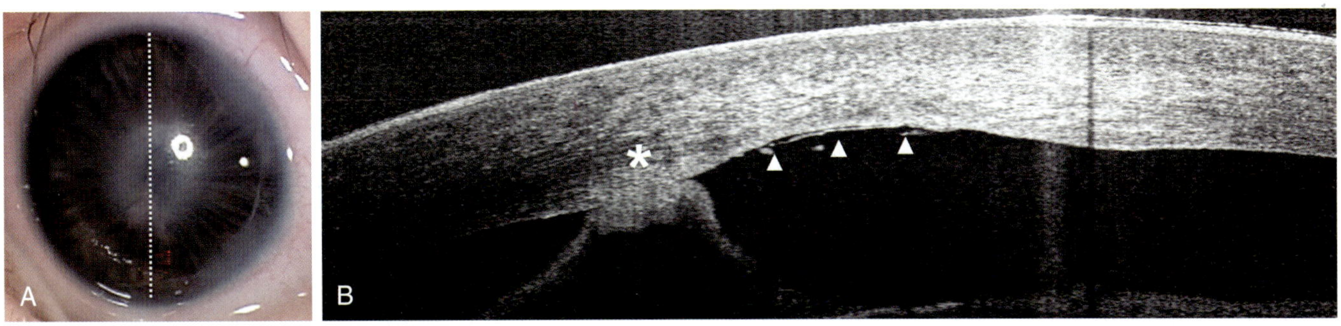

Fig. 16.7 Peters anomaly type 1. A, External RetCam (Clarity Medical Systems) photograph of left eye of 1-year-old boy with unilateral congenital central corneal opacity. Peripheral hypoplastic iris with inferior iridocorneal adhesion is apparent. B, AS-OCT image shows focal iridocorneal adhesion *(asterisk)* with adjacent posterior corneal defect (*arrowheads* marking posterior stromal invagination) corresponding with central corneal leukoma.

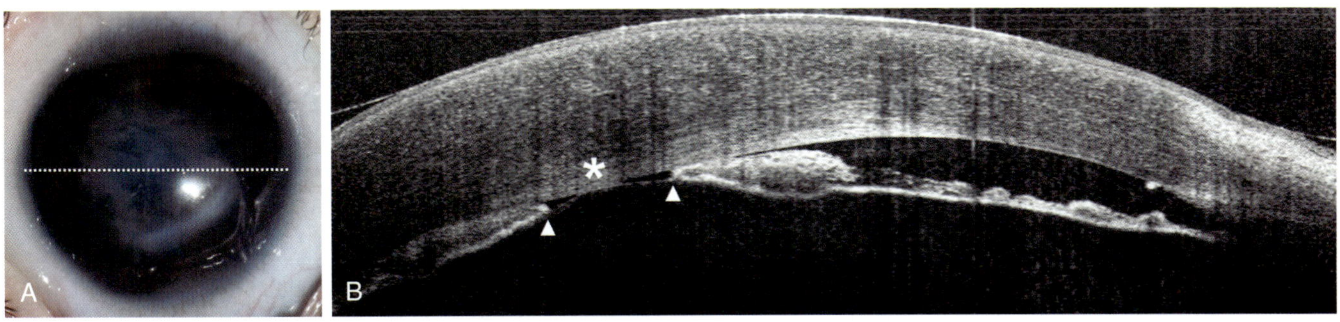

Fig. 16.8 Peters anomaly type 2. A, External RetCam (Clarity Medical Systems) photograph of right eye of 3-month-old boy with bilateral congenital central corneal opacities. Peripheral hypoplastic iris with multiple iridocorneal adhesions are apparent. B, Bioptigen (Bioptigen, Inc.) AS-OCT image reveals diffuse posterior corneal defect with multiple iridocorneal adhesions (edges denoted by *arrowheads*) and focal area of corneolenticular adhesion *(asterisk).*

F. Other Posterior Corneal Defects

I. PETERS ANOMALY TYPE 1

Peters anomaly describes a collection of anterior segment developmental abnormalities associated with a congenital corneal opacity. It can be seen in a variety of genetic mutations (e.g., *PITX2, FOXC1, CYP1B1,* and *PAX6*) and can also have systemic associations (Nischal KK, 2015). Peters anomaly type 1 generally refers to the less severe phenotype in which a central or total corneal opacity secondary to a focal absence of DM and endothelium is associated with iridocorneal adhesions, with a normal lens (Fig. 16.7, *panel A*). These adhesions and posterior corneal defects may be difficult to visualize clinically because of the corneal opacity, but they are easily visible on AS-OCT imaging (Fig. 16.7, *panel B*).

II. PETERS ANOMALY TYPE 2

In the more severe type 2 phenotype, there is lens involvement, either in the form of an associated cataract or keratolenticular adhesion. These adhesions are the result of a developmental failure of separation of the invaginating lens vesicle from the overlying surface ectoderm (Nischal KK, 2015). Clinically, the central or total corneal opacity is often vascularized and a cataractous lens may be seen (Fig. 16.8, *panel A*). It is important to note that these are not distinct genotypic diagnoses, as Peters anomaly type 1 (solely iridocorneal adhesions) may be seen in one eye and Peters anomaly type 2 (kerato-irido-lenticular adhesions) may be present in the other eye of a patient with a single known genetic mutation. High-resolution anterior segment imaging is critical in visualizing these keratolenticular adhesions, as the anterior lens capsule may be difficult to discern clinically (see Fig. 16.8, *panel B*).

III. ANTERIOR STAPHYLOMA

Congenital anterior (corneal) staphyloma is a total corneal opacification and ectactic protrusion distinguished by the presence of uveal tissue lining the inner surface. It generally has a nonspecific and sporadic inheritance, affects one or both eyes, and can be associated with other ocular developmental anomalies (Fig. 16.9, *panel A*). Histopathologically, it shares some similarities to Peters anomaly in that there is a total absence of DM and endothelium, but congenital anterior staphyloma is more extreme with concomitant corneal ectasia and thinning reflecting severe mesenchymal dysgenesis (Salour H, Owji N, Sadeghipour A, 2009). The corneal epithelium is generally intact but may be keratinized secondary to exposure; the Bowman membrane can be fragmented and atrophic; and the stroma is often hypercellular and disorganized. Although the clinical presentation is often dramatic with significant thinning and protrusion of an opaque, vascularized cornea, the pathologic diagnosis can be confirmed on AS-OCT imaging via presence of a hyperreflective uveal layer (atrophic iris) lining the posterior aspect of the ectactic, irregular stroma (see Fig. 16.9, *panel B*).

CLINICAL PEARL

When presented with a congenital corneal opacity, evaluation with AS-OCT can provide invaluable insight into the posterior corneal and anterior segment structure. This can be critical for determining the underlying cause and guiding further diagnostic testing (e.g., genetic screening), management, and prognosis. For example, the difference between Peters anomaly types 1 and 2 may not be obvious on clinical examination if there is only a focal area of keratolenticular adhesion, but the prognosis for penetrating keratoplasty is more guarded in Peters anomaly type 2 (Elbaz U, Strungaru H, Mireskandari K, 2020). A good preoperative assessment with AS-OCT can be helpful to demonstrate the pathologic features and direct management decision-making during discussions with the patient's family.

IV. DM RUPTURE SECONDARY TO BIRTH FORCEPS TRAUMA

Trauma from birth forceps at the time of delivery can cause DM rupture and secondary corneal edema. Changes are usually unilateral and typically seen in the left eye (Figs. 16.10 and 16.11) Because of refractive errors secondary to corneal scarring, patients may develop anisometropic amblyopia. Of note, DM ruptures secondary to birth forceps have a vertical or oblique orientation, although horizontal changes may occur as well. Horizontal breaks are classically associated with congenital glaucoma (Haab striae).

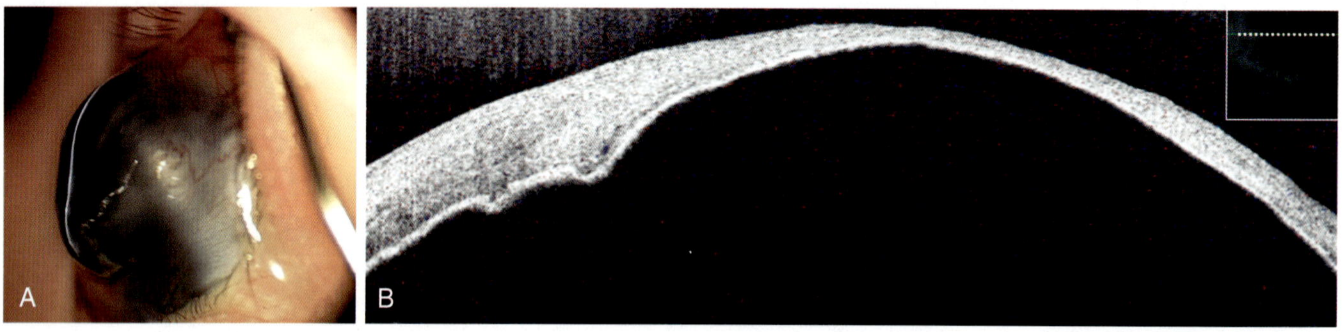

Fig. 16.9 Anterior staphyloma. A, RetCam (Clarity Medical Systems) external slit-beam photograph of left eye of 2-month-old girl with bilateral congenital diffuse corneal opacity, thinning, and ectasia. B, AS-OCT image confirms pronounced corneal thinning and ectasia with diffuse, hyperreflective uveal lining of entire posterior cornea, consistent with anterior staphyloma.

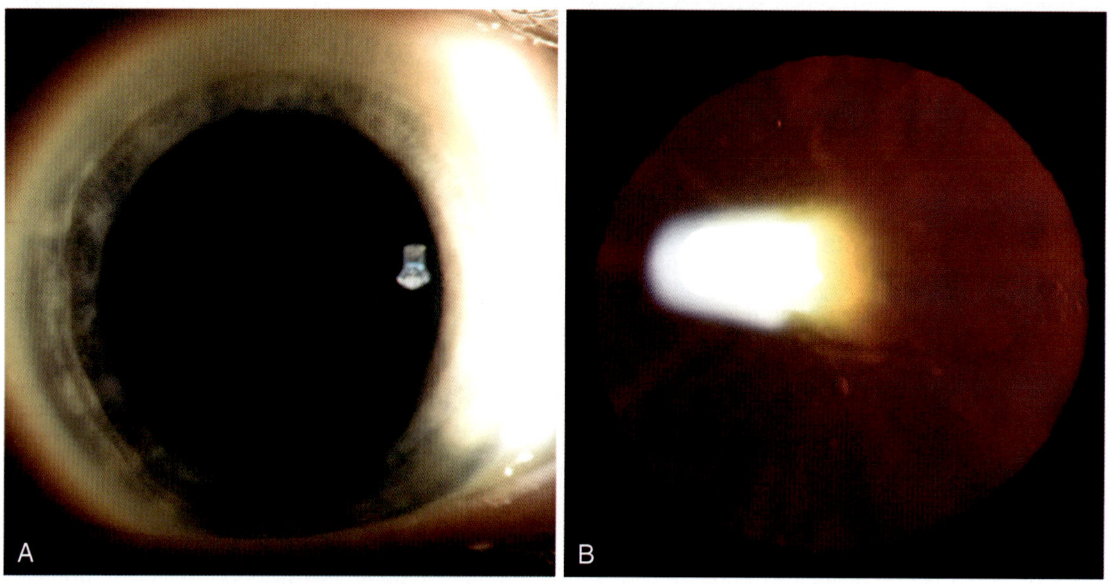

Fig. 16.10 Descemet membrane rupture secondary to birth forceps trauma. Slit-lamp photos demonstrate linear, horizontal breaks best appreciated in retro-illumination views. These ruptures should be distinguished from horizontal ruptures classically seen in congenital glaucoma (Haab striae).

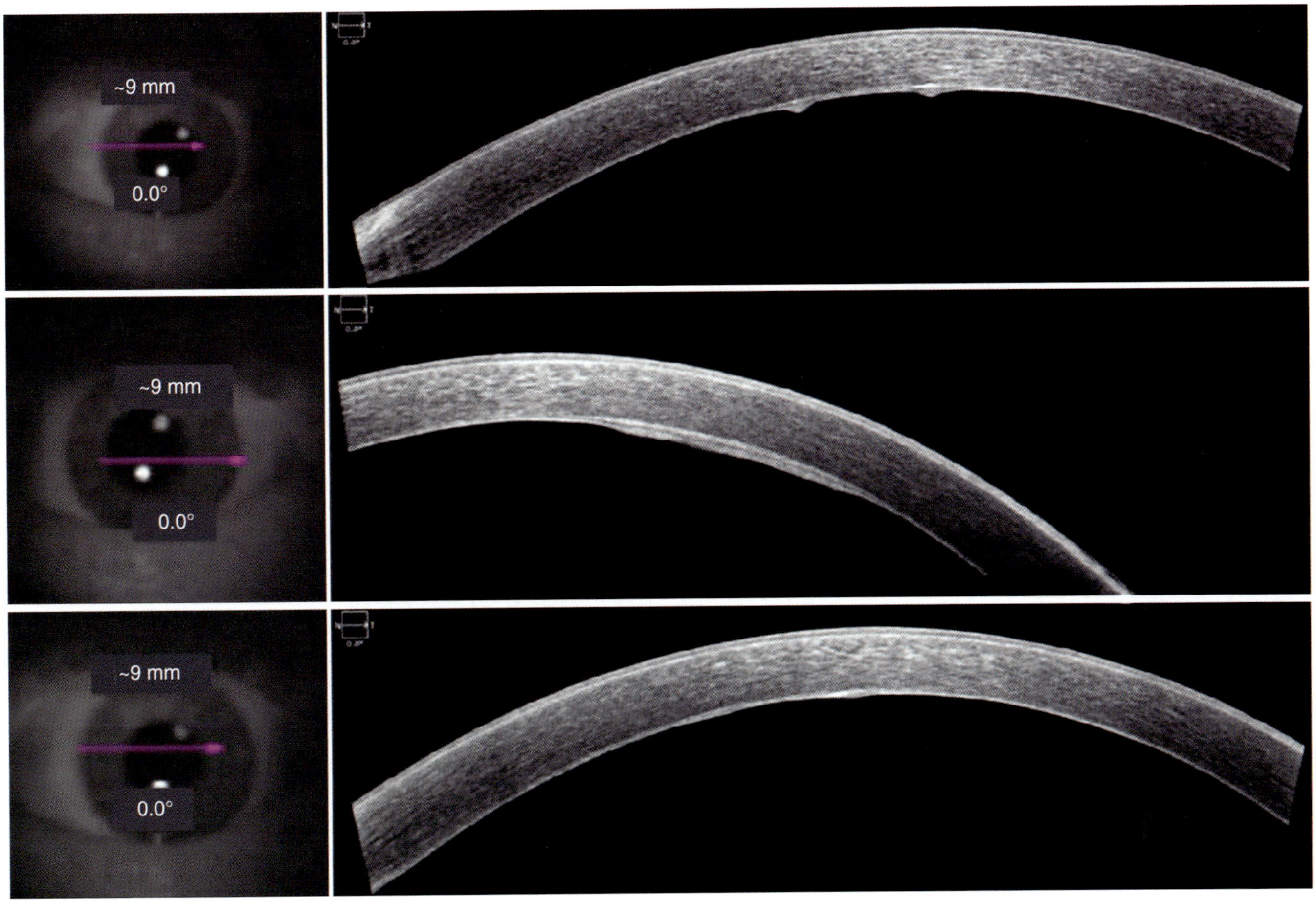

Fig. 16.11 AS-OCT images through the Descemet membrane rupture secondary to birth forceps trauma. Posterior scarring is seen as areas of increased hyperreflectivity in horizontal slice views through the scars seen on slit-lamp photographs.

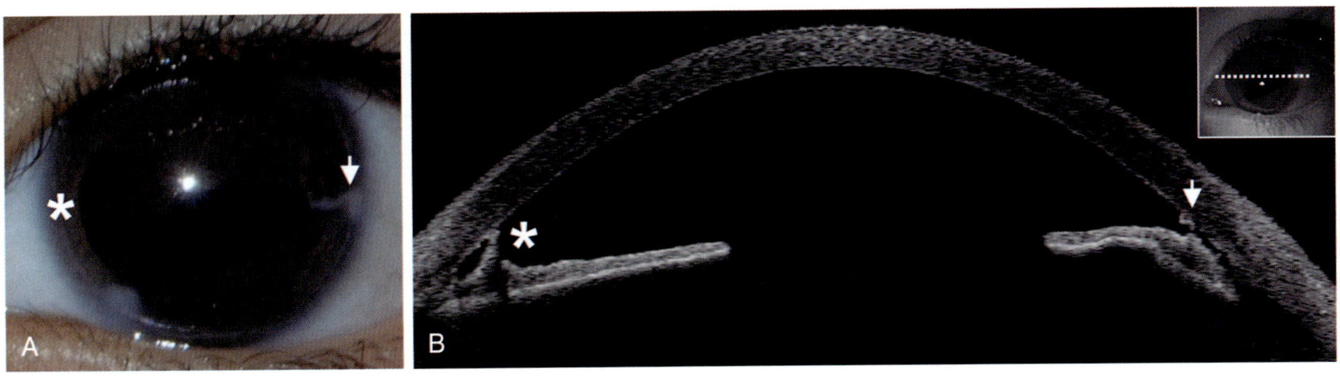

Fig. 16.12 Corectopia and posterior embryotoxon associated with Axenfeld-Rieger syndrome. A, Slit-lamp photograph of the left eye of 7-year-old girl with bilateral congenital iris hypoplasia, corectopia with peripheral iridocorneal adhesions *(asterisk)*, posterior embryotoxon *(arrow)*, and glaucoma secondary to Axenfeld-Rieger syndrome (*FOXC1* mutation). B, AS-OCT image of entire limbus-to-limbus anterior segment showing peripheral anterior synechiae *(asterisk)* and prominent anterior Schwalbe line *(arrow)*.

III. ANTERIOR SEGMENT AND LENS PATHOLOGIC CONDITIONS

A. Axenfeld-Rieger Syndrome

Axenfeld-Rieger syndrome involves a primary iridotrabecular dysgenesis, most commonly caused by pathogenic mutations in the *PITX2* or *FOXC1* genes (Nischal KK, 2015). Although the syndrome includes multiple systemic findings (i.e., maxillofacial, dental, cardiac, umbilical, and neurodevelopmental abnormalities), the characteristic anterior segment manifestations are posterior embryotoxon with adherent iris strands (Axenfeld anomaly) and congenital iris hypoplasia, corectopia, and/or polycoria (Rieger anomaly). The clinical presentation can vary in this bilateral, heterogeneous condition, but corneal opacities and elevated intraocular pressure are often associated with the structural anomalies (Fig. 16.12, *panel A*). AS-OCT imaging of the iris and angle structures can demonstrate the posterior embryotoxon and iridocorneal adhesions to the anteriorly displaced Schwalbe line (see Fig. 16.12, *panel B*).

B. Primary Congenital Glaucoma

I. BUPHTHALMOS

Primary congenital glaucoma (PCG) implies developmental anomalies in the trabecular meshwork and anterior chamber angle and can be associated with mutations in *CYP1B1* or *LTBP2* (Nischal KK, 2015). It generally presents in the first few months of life with the classic "triad" of symptoms (photophobia, epiphora, and blepharospasm) secondary to elevated intraocular pressure causing buphthalmos. Definitive treatment of glaucoma can reverse the corneal edema associated with PCG. However, permanent stromal scarring and corneal opacification can also occur with formation of Haab striae, which are horizontal or oblique breaks in DM secondary to rapid corneal enlargement (Fig. 16.13, *panel A*). Evidence of these DM breaks on high-resolution AS-OCT corneal imaging can corroborate a suspected diagnosis of PCG in the setting of corneal edema (see Fig. 16.13, *panel B*).

II. POSTOPERATIVE USE AFTER GLAUCOMA DRAINAGE DEVICE PLACEMENT

In many cases of congenital glaucoma either secondary to primary iridotrabecular dysgenesis (PCG) or other anterior segment structural abnormalities (e.g., Axenfeld-Rieger syndrome, Peters anomaly, sclerocornea), associated dense corneal opacification can obscure the view of the anterior chamber. However, precise placement of the tube portion of glaucoma drainage devices in a specific location (anterior chamber vs. sulcus vs. pars plana) may be critical for ensuring long-term function and preventing associated complications, such as corneal decompensation. In these cases, AS-OCT imaging can be invaluable both intraoperatively and postoperatively for visualizing the exact location of a glaucoma drainage tube that may not be clinically evident (Fig. 16.14). Particularly in pediatric patients in whom a glaucoma drainage device placed at a young age may retract over time as a result of growth of the patient's eye and orbit, AS-OCT imaging may be used to confirm location and patency of the tube opening.

C. Microspherophakia

Microspherophakia is a condition in which the crystalline lens has a smaller horizontal diameter with increased anterior-posterior diameter, rendering it more spherical than normal (Fig. 16.15, *panel A*). It can be associated with genetic mutations in *LTBP2* and *ADAMTS17,* as well as various systemic syndromes (Senthil S, Rao HL, Hoang NT, 2014). Clinical manifestations can include zonular instability, lens subluxation, high myopia, accommodative insufficiency, and progressive glaucoma in over 50% of patients as a result of secondary angle closure (Senthil S, Rao HL, Hoang NT, 2014). As the early clinical signs may be subtle and challenging to diagnose, anterior segment imaging can be a useful adjunct to elucidate lens morphology and position in relation to angle architecture (see Fig. 16.15, *panel B*). In cases in which a progressive anterior lens subluxation causes worsening pupillary block, peripheral iridotomy and/or lensectomy may be indicated to prevent irreversible synechial angle closure glaucoma.

D. Posterior Lenticonus

Posterior lenticonus is another structural congenital anomaly of the crystalline lens in which a cone-shaped herniation of the

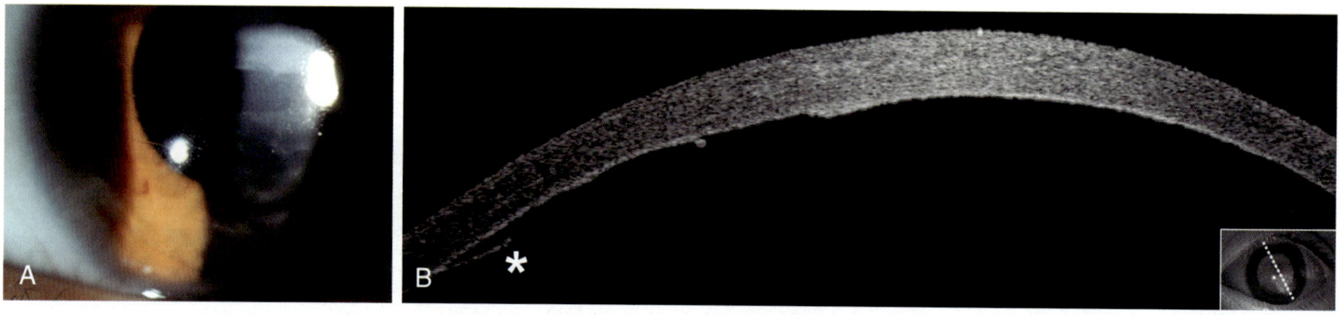

Fig. 16.13 Haab striae secondary to primary congenital glaucoma. A, High-magnification slit-lamp photograph of the left eye of 7-year-old boy with unilateral buphthalmos, Haab striae, and corneal clouding secondary to primary congenital glaucoma. B, AS-OCT high-resolution corneal image shows diffuse central stromal hyperreflectivity (haze/scarring) with associated Descemet membrane break *(asterisk).*

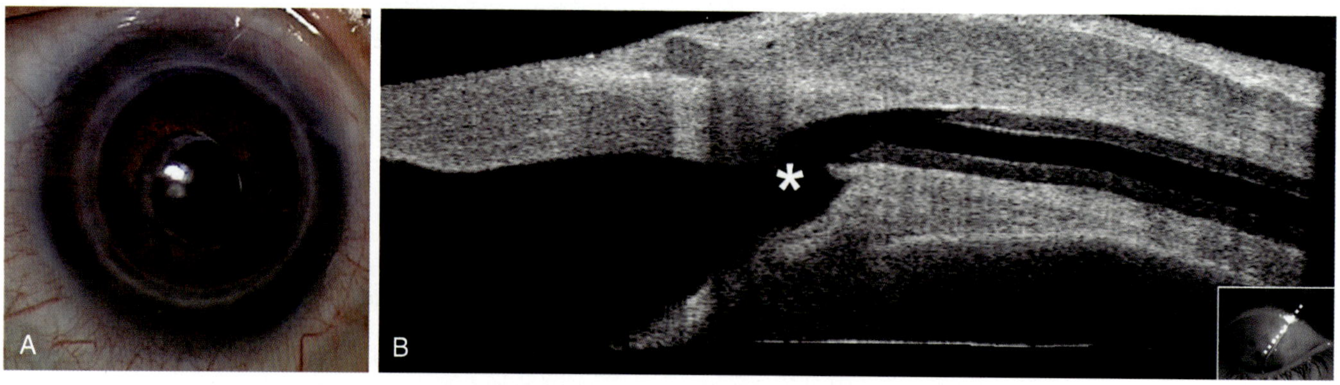

Fig. 16.14 Intrascleral position of glaucoma drainage tube. A, Slit-lamp photograph of the left eye of 14-year-old girl with history of bilateral penetrating keratoplasty (PKP) for congenital corneal opacities and subsequent glaucoma, status post–Ahmed glaucoma valve implants in both eyes. Although the PKP graft appears clear centrally, anterior chamber position of the superotemporal glaucoma tube is unable to be visualized at slit-lamp because of peripheral corneal opacity. B, AS-OCT image slice through superotemporal limbus confirms posterior migration of the tube from the anterior chamber, with stable overlying patch graft and patent opening into the anterior chamber *(asterisk).*

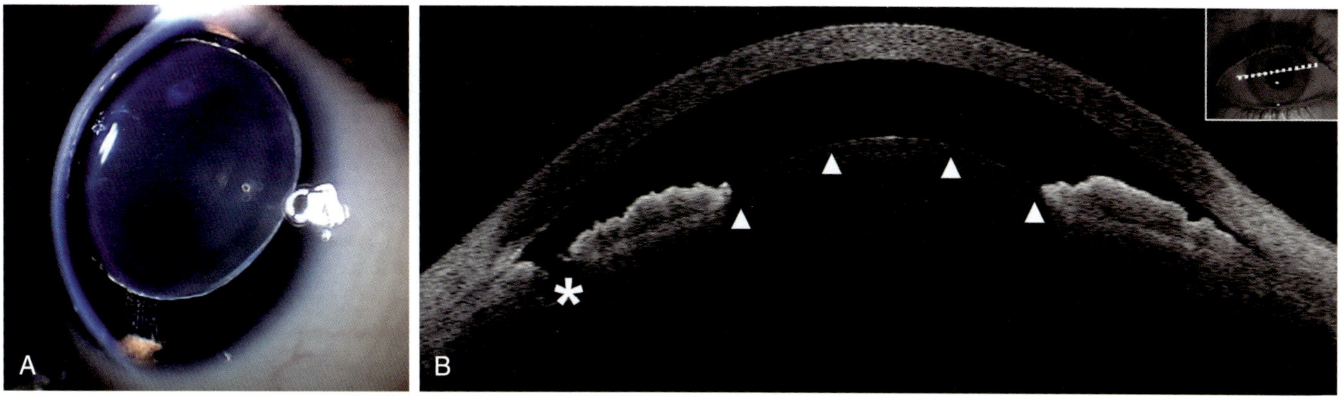

Fig. 16.15 Microspherophakia with anterior lens subluxation. A, Slit-lamp photograph of the right eye of 11-year-old boy with bilateral microspherophakia and narrow angles with progressive anterior lens subluxation. With the pupil pharmacologically dilated, significant anterior chamber shallowing and zonular stretching from the microspherophakic crystalline lens is visible on slit beam. B, AS-OCT image shows protrusion of anterior lens capsule through pupil *(arrowheads)* causing peripheral narrow angles. A patent peripheral iridotomy is visible temporally *(asterisk)* with the angle appearing slightly more open in that area.

posterior lens capsule and cortex extends posteriorly (Fig. 16.16, *panel A*). It is typically unilateral and axial in location but can occur bilaterally, peripherally, or eccentrically in any direction (Agarwal R, Jain V, Kaur M, 2021). This condition generally worsens throughout childhood causing progressive myopia and irregular astigmatism, as well as posterior cortical opacification that can become more visually significant. These lenticular changes can be severely amblyogenic, so early lens extraction is often indicated for visual rehabilitation. Especially early in unilateral cases without associated cataractous changes, this anomaly can be difficult to detect on limited clinical examination, but AS-OCT imaging of the lenticular plane can clearly delineate the posterior capsular morphology (see Fig. 16.16, *panel B*).

E. Lens Material Proliferation

Despite advances in surgical techniques and technology for lens extraction with IOL implantation, visual axis opacification remains the most common complication after pediatric cataract surgery (Kletke SN, Mireskandari K, Ali A, 2018). Use of hydrophobic acrylic IOL materials, square-edge IOL designs, and in-the-bag IOL implantation all help delay retro-IOL lens material proliferation. Whereas most surgeons will perform primary posterior capsulotomy with anterior vitrectomy in younger patients to prevent visual axis opacification, many may defer this extra step in patients who are old enough to tolerate neodymium-doped yttrium aluminum garnet (Nd:YAG) laser capsulotomy in clinic or are at higher risk for complications (e.g., history of uveitis or retinal detachment).

Posterior capsule opacification can become visually significant at some point in nearly 100% of pediatric eyes after cataract extraction (Kletke SN, Mireskandari K, Ali A, 2018). In many cases, bubble-like clusters of proliferated lens epithelial cells can accumulate on the posterior capsule, seen clinically as Elschnig pearls (Fig. 16.17, *panel A*). These can be imaged by AS-OCT and appear as vacuoles among a thickened posterior lens capsule, posterior to a clear IOL plane (see Fig. 16.17, *panel B*). Given its more scattered and less dense appearance, this type of posterior capsule opacification is often amenable to Nd:YAG laser capsulotomy for clearing the visual axis, but recurrent proliferation may still occur over the intact hyaloid face in the Berger space (Kletke SN, Mireskandari K, Ali A, 2018).

In other cases, significantly denser retro-IOL lens material proliferation can occur, such as in uveitic patients (Fig. 16.18, *panel A*). AS-OCT imaging can demonstrate different densities and reflectivities within a thick band of regenerated lens material posterior to a clear IOL plane (see Fig. 16.18, *panel B*). Higher reflectivity on AS-OCT imaging is associated with increased opacity and thus greater effect on visual acuity. Based on its cross-sectional appearance, surgical membranectomy with anterior vitrectomy is often the procedure of choice to manage these thicker, denser bands of visual axis opacification.

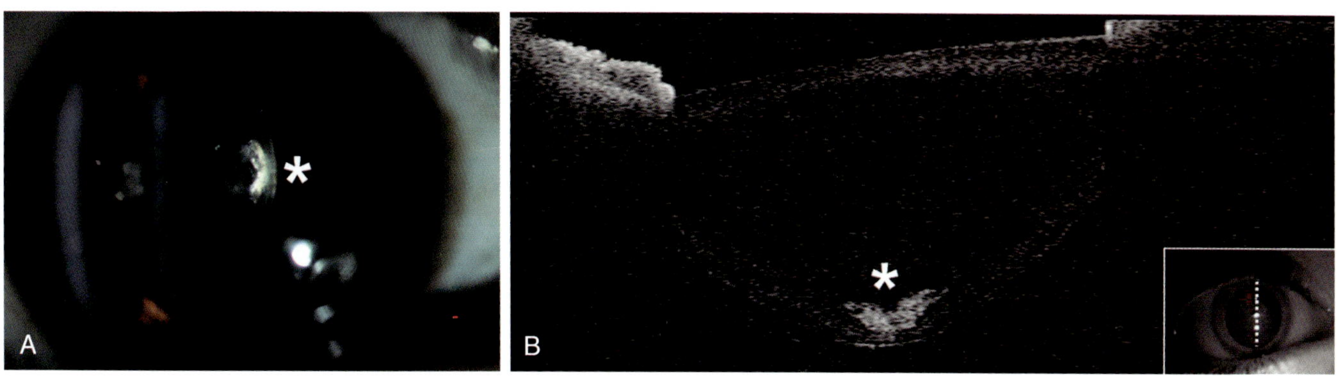

Fig. 16.16 Posterior lenticonus. A, Slit-lamp photograph of the right eye of 10-year-old girl with unilateral congenital cataract. Significant posterior lenticonus can be appreciated on slit beam with focal posterior polar cataract *(asterisk)*. B, AS-OCT deep anterior segment image through lenticular plane delineates posterior lenticonus appearance of lens capsule, with focal posterior subcapsular hyperreflective opacity at base *(asterisk)*.

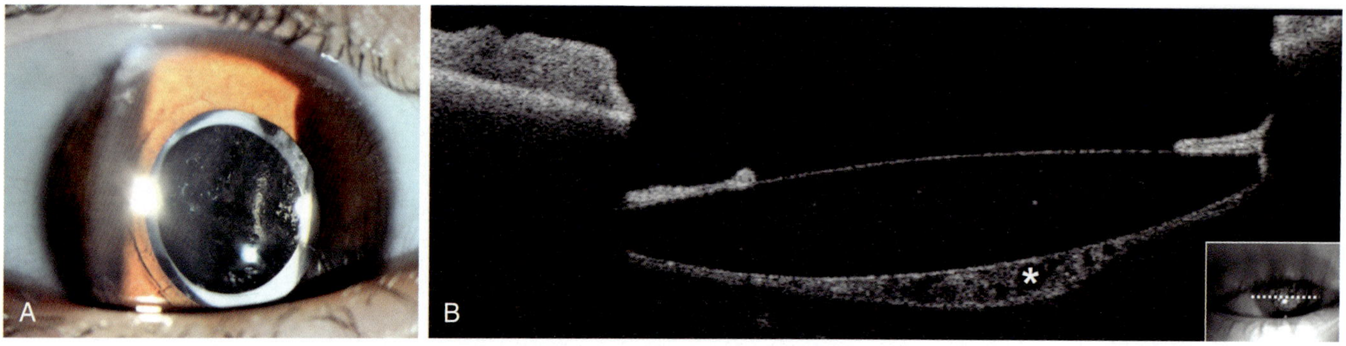

Fig. 16.17 Elschnig pearls. A, Slit-lamp photograph of the right eye of 7-year-old girl with history of unilateral congenital cataract status post-cataract extraction with intraocular lens (IOL) implantation 2 years prior. Diffuse posterior capsular opacification is noted posterior to IOL. B, AS-OCT deep anterior segment image through lenticular plane shows retro-IOL capsular thickening with scattered vacuolar spaces *(asterisk),* consistent with Elschnig pearls.

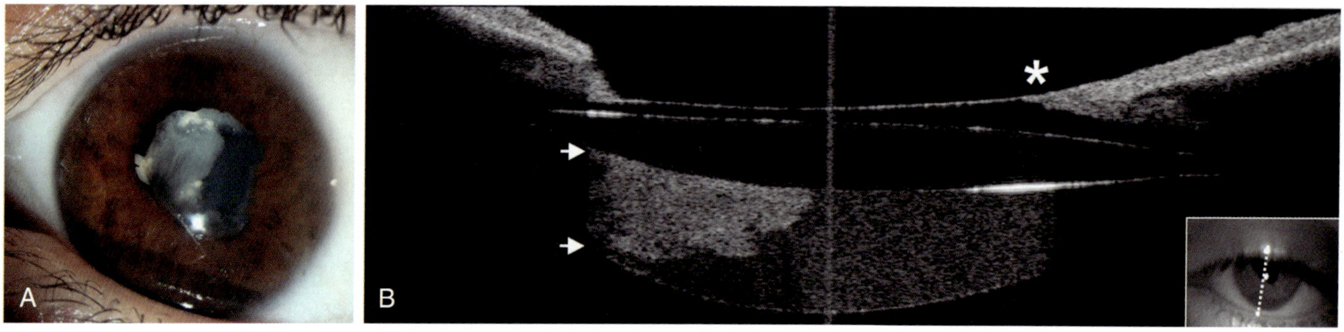

Fig. 16.18 Retro-intraocular lens (IOL) material proliferation. A, Slit-lamp photograph of the left eye of 10-year-old boy with history of uveitic cataract status post–cataract extraction with IOL implantation 2 years previously. Diffuse lens material proliferation with posterior capsular opacification is noted posterior to IOL. B, AS-OCT deep anterior segment image through lenticular plane reveals significant thickness and density of hyperreflective lens material proliferation posterior to IOL within capsular bag (thickness denoted by *arrows*). The AS-OCT image also shows a thin, mildly hyperreflective pupillary membrane anterior to the IOL *(asterisk),* which is transparent on slit-lamp examination.

CLINICAL PEARL

Congenital lenticular anomalies often can be subtle initially if there are no associated cataractous changes, and detailed examination of the lens configuration can be challenging in awake children. Anterior segment imaging of the lenticular plane by AS-OCT or UBM can clearly illustrate any abnormalities of the lens shape and the thickness and extent of any pathologic findings, because lens opacities appear distinctly hyperreflective on AS-OCT. For example, it can help distinguish whether a posterior polar cataract involves the lens capsule, or whether an apparent posterior subcapsular cataract is actually retrocapsular and may instead be focal/peripheral anterior persistent fetal vasculature, or whether retro-IOL lens material proliferation may be too thick for Nd:YAG laser capsulotomy. These subtle differences are vital for preoperative planning, prognostication, and postoperative visual rehabilitation.

BIBLIOGRAPHY

Agarwal R, Jain V, Kaur M, et al. Atypical presentation of peripheral posterior lenticonus and role of multi-modal ocular imaging in its diagnosis and management. *BMJ Case Rep*. 2021;14(2):e238801.

Elbaz U, Strungaru H, Mireskandari K, et al. Long-term visual outcomes and clinical course of patients with Peters anomaly. *Cornea*. 2021;40(7):822-830.

Hammersmith KM. Blepharokeratoconjunctivitis in children. *Curr Opin Ophthalmol*. 2015;26(4):301-305.

Jones SM, Weinstein JM, Cumberland P, et al. Visual outcome and corneal changes in children with chronic blepharokeratoconjunctivitis. *Ophthalmology*. 2007;114(12):2271-2280.

Kletke SN, Mireskandari K, Ali A. Update on pediatric cataract surgery and the Delphi panel paper. *Curr Ophthalmol Rep*. 2018;6:207-216.

Lee H, Khan R, O'Keefe M. Aniridia: current pathology and management. *Acta Ophthalmol*. 2008;86(7):708-715.

Mireskandari K, Tehrani NN, Vandenhoven C, et al. Anterior segment imaging in pediatric ophthalmology. *J Cataract Refract Surg*. 2011;37(12):2201-2210.

Nischal KK. Genetics of congenital corneal opacification: impact on diagnosis and treatment. *Cornea*. 2015;34(suppl 10):S24-S34.

Pattnaik L, Acharya L. A comprehensive review on vernal keratoconjunctivitis with emphasis on proteomics. *Life Sci*. 2015;128:47-54.

Rodrigues EB, Johanson M, Penha FM. Anterior segment tomography with the cirrus optical coherence tomography. *J Ophthalmol*. 2012;2012:806989.

Salour H, Owji N, Sadeghipour A. Congenital corneal staphyloma. *J Ophthalmic Vis Res*. 2009;4(3):182-184.

Senthil S, Rao HL, Hoang NT, et al. Glaucoma in microspherophakia: presenting features and treatment outcomes. *J Glaucoma*. 2014;23(4):262-267.

Trauma

Hursuong Vongsachang | Kamran Riaz | Fasika Woreta

17

I. INTRODUCTION

Eye injuries pose a significant public health burden with major social and economic consequences. As the external aspect of the eye, the anterior chamber and cornea are frequent locations of ocular trauma, and foreign bodies, blunt force and contrecoup, penetrating injuries, chemical insults, and burns, amongst others. Anterior segment optical coherence tomography (AS-OCT) is a useful tool and adjunct imaging modality in the diagnosis, evaluation, management, and monitoring of ocular trauma. AS-OCT provides a noninvasive, rapaid, and high-resolution cross-sectional imaging modlity, especially in eyes in which prolonged clinical examination may be difficult.

This chapter will present examples of frequently encountered traumatic ocular injuries in which AS-OCT imaging can be applied. Posterior segment injuries, which are difficult to visualize with AS-OCT, are better evaluated with other modalities, such as B-scan, ultrasound, computed tomography, or magnetic resonance imaging.

II. CORNEAL INJURIES

A. Corneal Abrasion

Corneal abrasions refer to the traumatic loss of the corneal epithelium and are some of the most common forms of anterior segment injury seen by clinicians. Multiple types of contact with the epithlium can causse corneal abrasions including digital trauma including fingernails and traumatic contact lens removal, foreign object touching the ocular surface, including, makeup brushs, and sports injuries. Patients often present with severe pain, tearing, foreign body sensation, blurry vision, and photophobia. AS-OCT will demonstrate loss of the epithelial layer and help assess the depth of involvement in cases of trauma. (Fig. 17.1).

B. Corneal Foreign Bodies

Corneal foreign bodies can be organic, inorganic or a combintion of both and are one of the most common types of ocular trauma seen in the emergency setting and the clinic. While some foreign bodies can be comprised on inert matter and can be present for days or weeks, others can cause an inflammatory reaction with hypermeia and pain. When a corneal foreign body is suspected and the depth is unclear based on slit-lamp examination alone, AS-OCT can help in determining the shape, size, and depth of the foreign body in the cornea. AS-OCT imaging can help guide clinical decision-making, including in-office and preoperative surgical planning. In addition, AS-OCT may be helpful in determining the composition of the foreign body based on its unique appearance on AS-OCT (Figs. 17.2 to 17.4).

CLINICAL PEARL

In situations in which visualization of the foreign body is difficult, different characteristics seen on AS-OCT may give clues to the material of the foreign body and provide further guidance on the need for urgent removal. Most materials will have a hyperreflective anterior border on AS-OCT. Opaque materials, such as pencil graphite and wood, may also have posterior shadowing or appear as a hyperreflective mass. Metals have additionally been associated with the presence of a chain of inverted signals posteriorly on AS-OCT. Conversely, transparent materials, such as glass and plastic, are hyporeflective in the corneal stroma but have a sharp, hyperreflective border when extruding into the air or intruding into the anterior chamber.

C. LASIK Flap Trauma

Laser in-situ keratomileusis (LASIK) is the most common refractive surgical procedure using the excimer laser to alter the

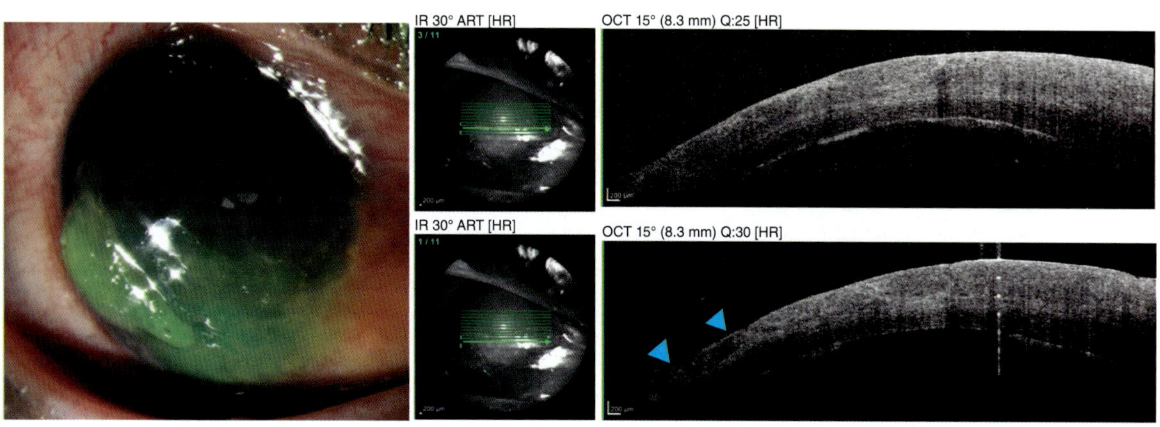

Fig. 17.1 Corneal abrasion. This 33-year-old patient received a grazing bullet injury to the the cornea. The shearing force resulted in a corneal abrasion. Amazingly, the Seidel test was negative, and there was no signs of an open globe. AS-OCT demonstrates areas of epithelial disruption as evidenced by loss of the hyperreflectivity *(arrowheads)* of the epithelium. There is associated epithelial and stromal edema, and areas of increased stromal hyperreflectivity. (Courtesy Kamran M. Riaz, MD, Dean McGee Eye Institute, University of Oklahoma, Oklahoma City, Oklahoma, United States.)

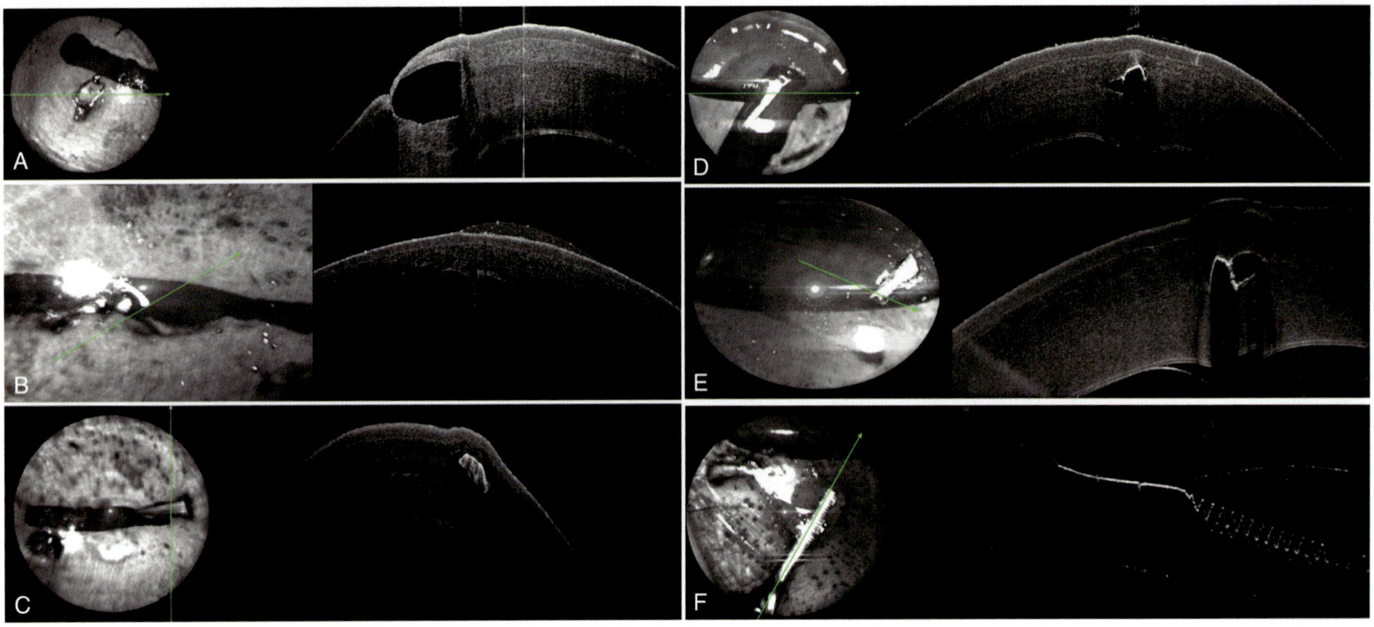

Fig. 17.2 Common corneal foreign bodies. Features of commonly seen corneal foreign bodies pictured here in the stroma of calf corneas include (A) glass, (B) plastic, (C) wood, (D) iron, (E) pencil graphite, and (F) gold. (Courtesy Michael Mimouni, MD, University of Toronto, Toronto, Ontario, Canada.)

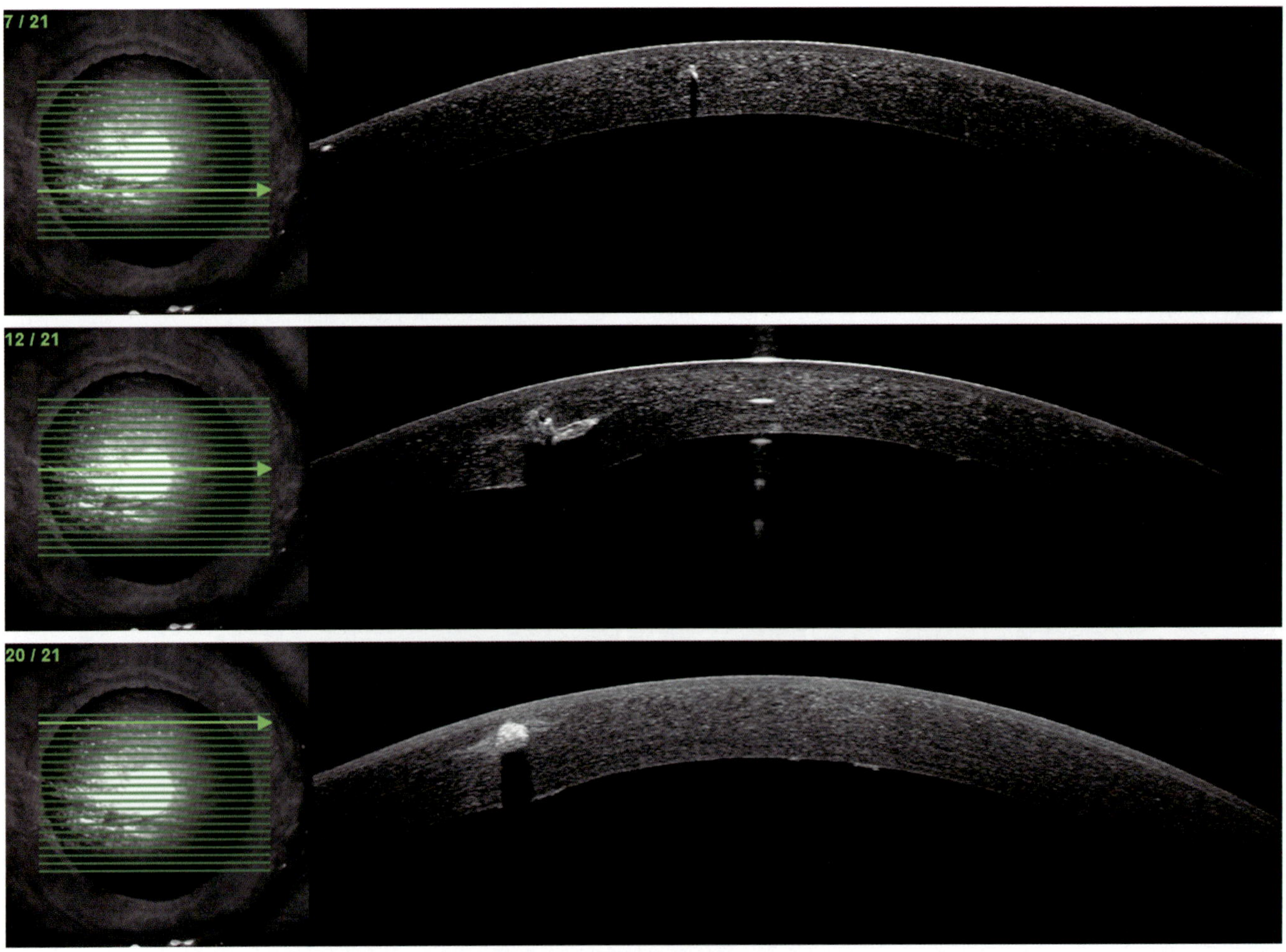

Fig. 17.3 Superficial corneal foreign body. AS-OCT demonstrates the extent of the injury caused by the corneal foreign body. This visualization is helpful for guiding management and treatment and for monitoring outcomes postoperatively. In this case the foreign body appears hyperreflective with posterior shadowing and is limited to the anterior and midstromal layers. There is no sign of pentration through the cornea into the anterior chamber.

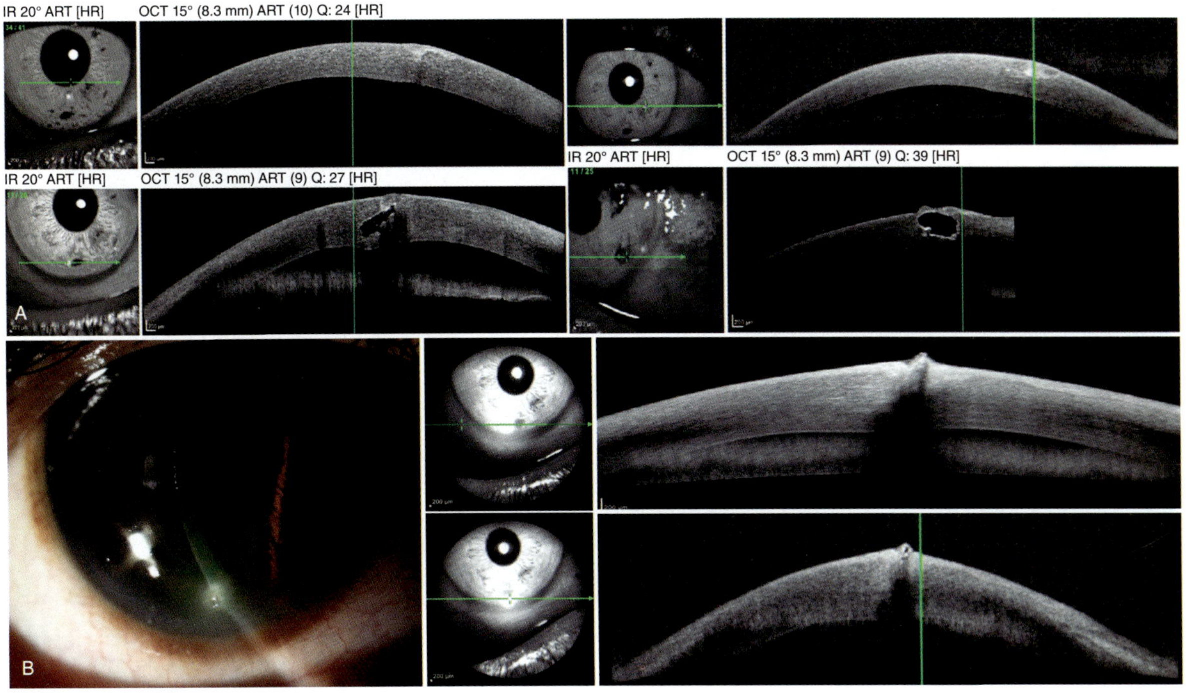

Fig. 17.4 Corneal foreign body (glass). A 34-year-old patient presented after a gunshot wound with multiple glass debris in corneal stroma bilaterally. A, After initial removal of multiple glass shards on slit-lamp examination, AS-OCT helped visualize the remaining glass shards and confirmed no full-thickness penetration. The decision was made to follow closely and remove residual shards as they progressed forward. B, Follow-up one year later demonstrating that the foreign body seen in the inferior cornea had risen to a more superficial position. (Courtesy Kamran M. Riaz, MD, Dean McGee Eye Institute, University of Oklahoma, Oklahoma City, Oklahoma, United States.)

corneal shape, and involves the creation of a corneal flap, using either a microkeratome or a femptosecond laser. Traumatic flap dislocations, detachment, and tears of the flap are rare but can still occur years after surgery. In these instances, AS-OCT can evaluate the extent of flap trauma, identify the presence of epithelial ingrowth, and guide management strategies, including observation versus surgical interventions (Fig. 17.5).

CLINICAL PEARL

When surgical interventions for flap repositioning are performed, especially in the presence of epithelial ingrowth, AS-OCT can be extremely useful to assess the efficacy of the surgical intervention. Residual epithelial ingrowth may be difficult to visualize on clinical examination, but may be better visualized on AS-OCT as epithelial hyperreflectivity contrasts with the hyporeflectivity of the stroma.

Traumatic LASIK flap injuries also can be associated with retained or embedded foreign bodies. Figs. 17.6 to Fig. 17.10 show images from a patient with traumatic corneal injury in the context of previous LASIK. Fig. 17.6 shows slit-lamp photographs and AS-OCT image at the time of presentation. Notably, there is a triangular flap tear with retained vegetative foreign body material. The foreign body is seen as a hyperreflective area at the flap interface. Intraoperative images (Figs. 17.7 and 17.8) demonstrate the use of AS-OCT to favorably visualize and remove the foreign body material and perform flap repair. Fig. 17.9 shows serial slit-lamp and tomography images of this patient over the course of approximately nine months until excellent final visual acuity. Notably, this patient had AS-OCT imaging with two different devices as shown in Fig. 17.10. Compared with the preoperative AS-OCT image, the image taken nine months later demonstrates minimal scarring with good preservation of the flap and overlying corneal contour.

D. Corneal Perforation

Corneal perforations from trauma are true ocular emergencies. and a high level clincial suspicion is required—urgent exploration and repair of the injury in the operating room is often required. The presentation of corneal perforation is protean and can be quite subtle, with a mild change in the shape of the iris and a slight shallowing of the anterior chamber with minimal if any leakage, to a flat chamber with uveal prolapse and egress of aquous fluid onto the ocular surface. A flat chamber is a particaully concerning sign and in this case, the Seidel test may be "negative" as there is not enough remaining anterior chamber fluid to "leak out". Decreased vision, conjunctival hyperemia, pain, and "tearing" from flow of anterior chamber fluid are all possible clinical findings. In addition to a careful slit-lamp examination and Seidel testing, AS-OCT can noninvasively show the corneal wound shape, depth, and corneal thickness, identify the presence of intracorneal foreign bodies, and guide and monitor treatment (Figs. 17.11 and 17.12).

E. Corneal Scarring

Trauma to the cornea and the ensuing healing process often results in corneal scarring and sometimes neovascularization. as well. Stromal scarring can lead to decreased visual acuity, from irregular astigmatism, and patients often complain of glare, halos and ghosting of images—RGP, scleral or hybrid contact lenses are sometimes needed to restore high acuity vision. AS-OCT can be used to monitor corneal remodeling after trauma and the epithelial hypertrophy that occurs in areas of stromal loss. Corneal scars manifest as hyperreflective lines on AS-OCT. AS-OCT also can serve as a pachymetry tool to measure scar thickness. Serial AS-OCT can be used to evaluate and monitor corneal scars before and after treatment and assist with surgical planning (Figs. 17.13 and 17.14).

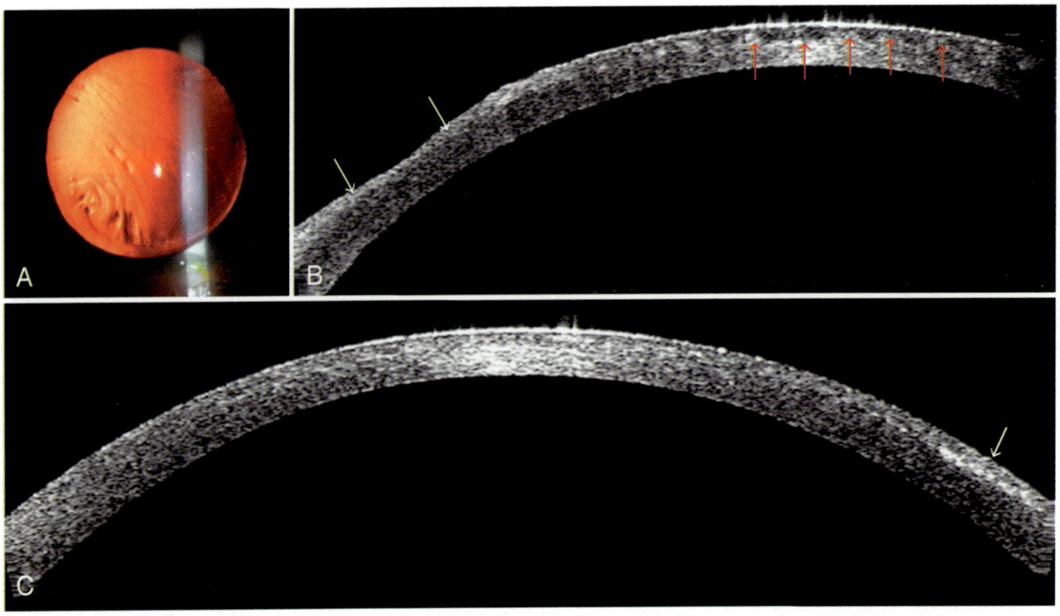

Fig. 17.5 LASIK flap dislocation. A 58-year-old man presented with left eye traumatic LASIK flap dislocation several months after a motor vehicle collision. A, Red reflex photograph shows macrostriae and epithelial ingrowth. B, On AS-OCT, the *red arrows* point to drape-like folds in the flap representing macrostriae. *White arrows* show the area where the dislocated flap has retracted to uncover the underlying stroma (except for the epithelium that filled in the exposed gap). C, After flap repositioning and removal of epithelial ingrowth, postoperative AS-OCT demonstrates resolution of macrostriae, but a small area of epithelial ingrowth remains at the flap edge *(white arrow)*. (Courtesy Kraig Bower, MD, Wilmer Eye Institute/Johns Hopkins University, Baltimore, Maryland, United States.)

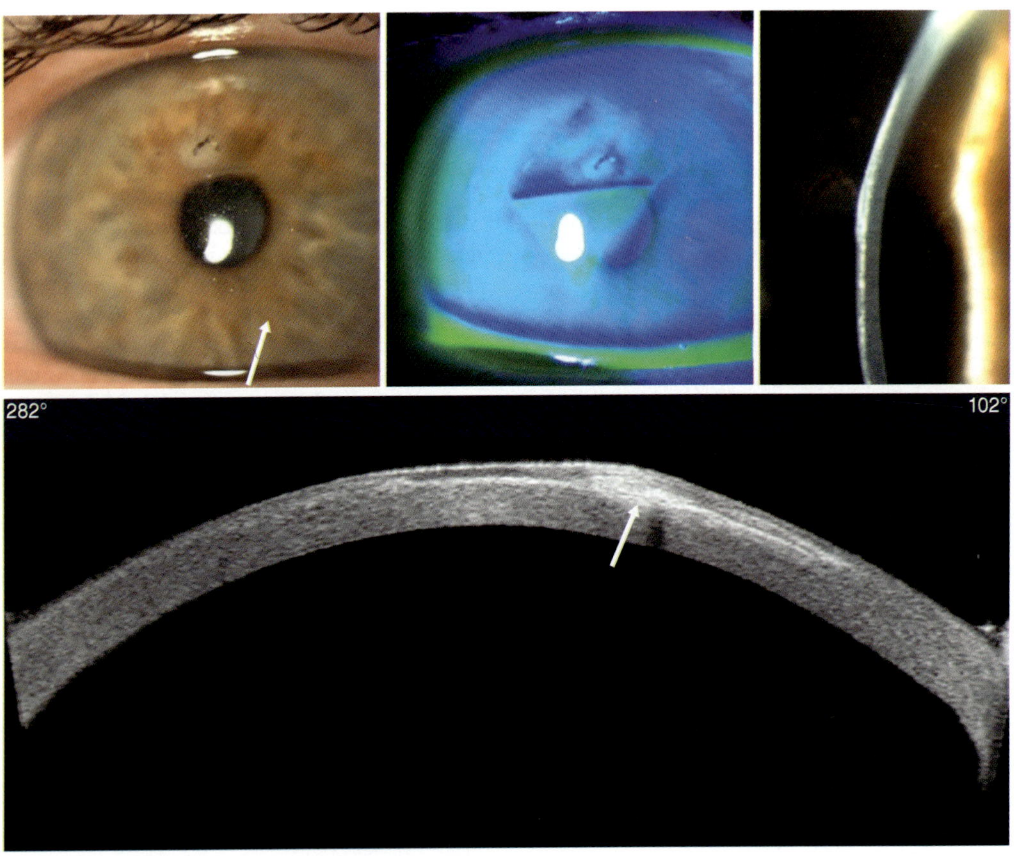

Fig. 17.6 Triangular LASIK flap tear with retained vegetative foreign body material. Slit-lamp photographs *(top panels)* show a triangular flap tear within the previous LASIK flap. A foreign body is present. AS-OCT shows the foreign body material as a hyperreflective area at the flap interface *(lower panel, arrow)*. (Courtesy Kraig Scot Bower, MD, Wilmer Eye Institute, Johns Hopkins University, Baltimore, Maryland, United States.)

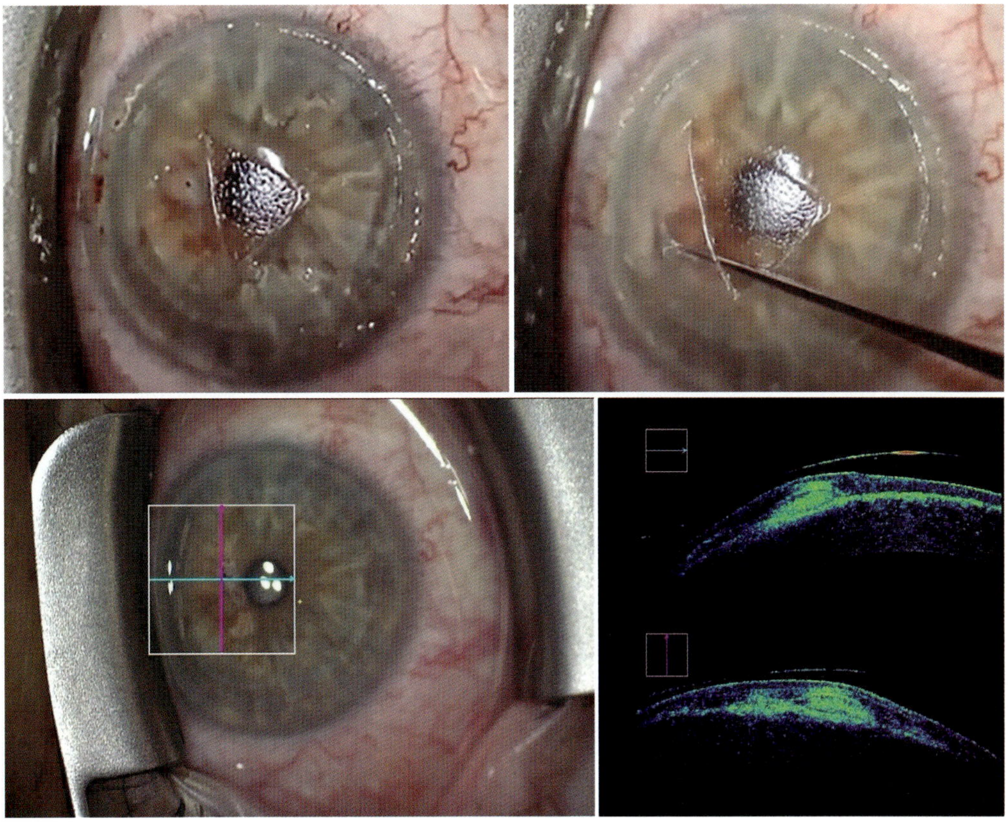

Fig. 17.7 Intraoperative images and intraoperative AS-OCT taken before foreign body removal and flap repair. (Courtesy Kraig Scot Bower, MD, Wilmer Eye Institute, Johns Hopkins University, Baltimore, Maryland, United States.)

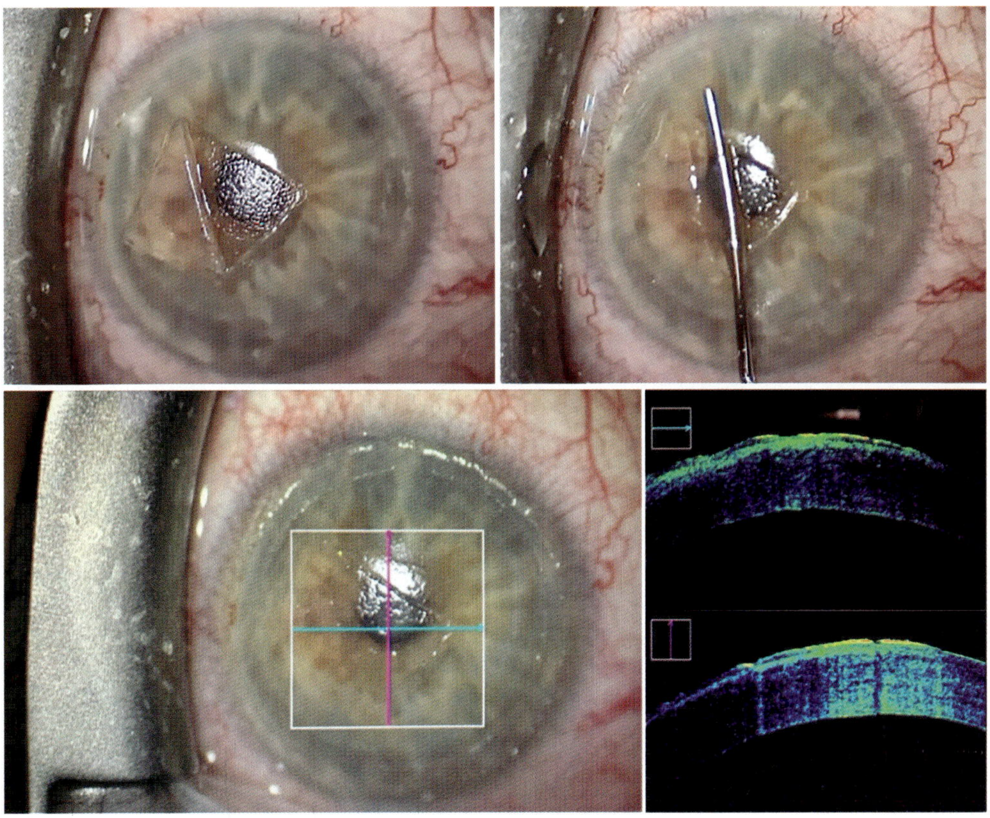

Fig. 17.8 Intraoperative images and intraoperative AS-OCT taken immediately after foreign body removal and flap repair. (Image Courtesy Kraig Scot Bower, MD, Wilmer Eye Institute, Johns Hopkins University, Baltimore, Maryland, United States.)

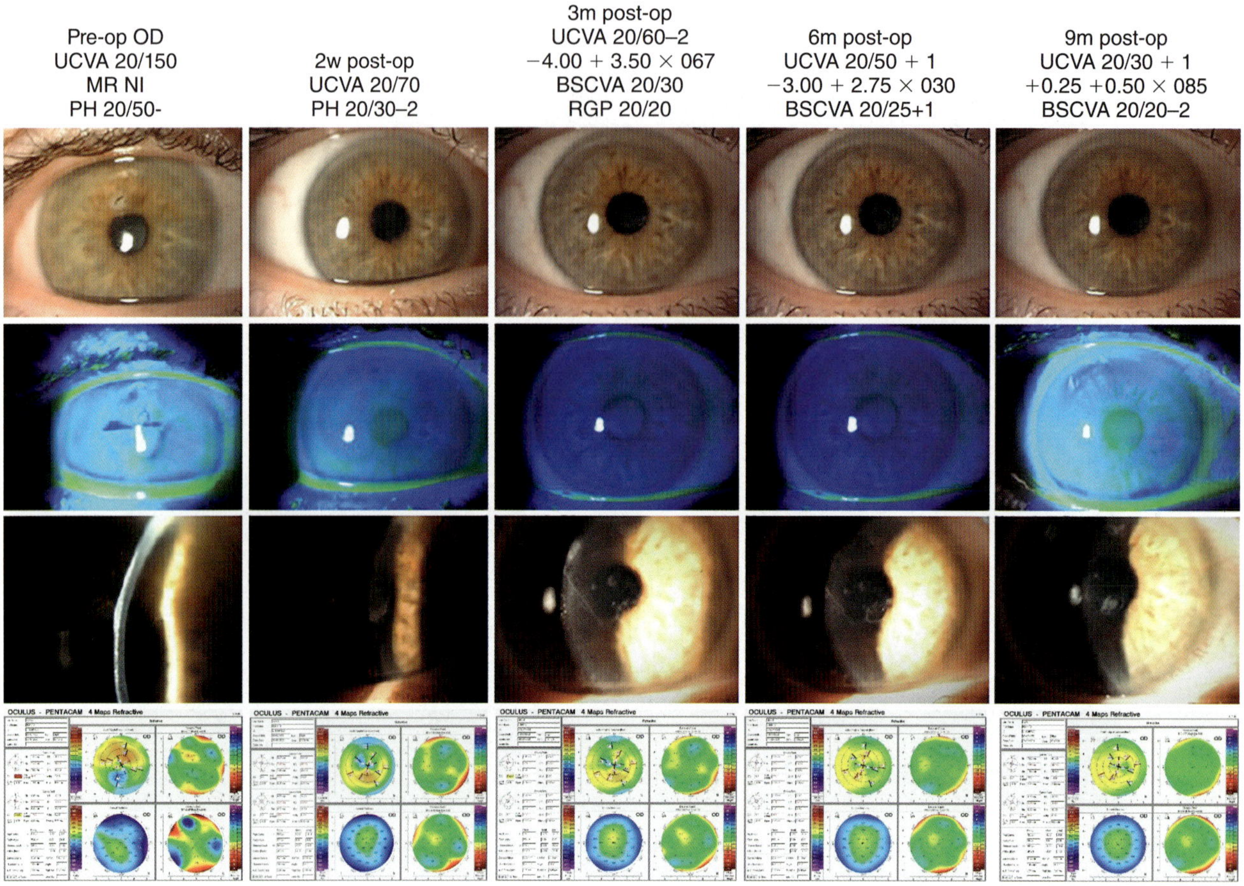

Fig. 17.9 Serial slit-lamp photographs and tomography images over nine months of the patient seen in Figs. 17.6 to 17.8. There is notable improvement in corneal irregularity with excellent final visual acuity. (Courtesy Kraig Scot Bower, MD, Wilmer Eye Institute, Johns Hopkins University, Baltimore, Maryland, United States.)

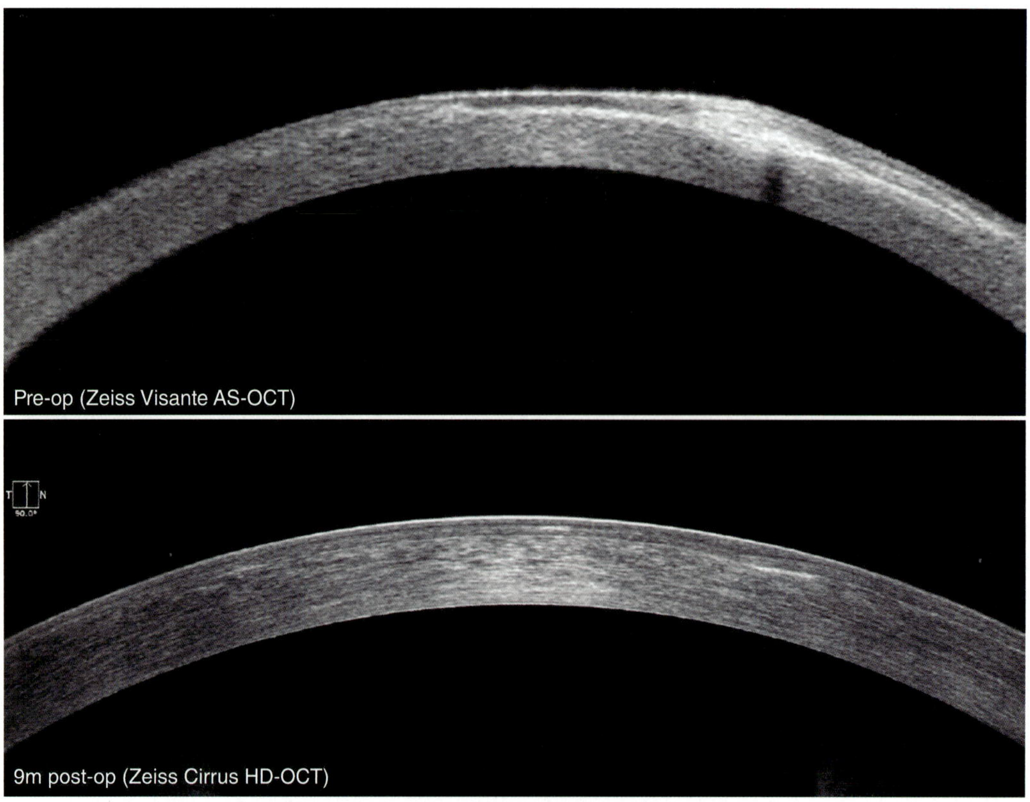

Fig. 17.10 Preoperative AS-OCT image with Zeiss Visante AS-OCT device compared with postoperative (nine months later) taken with Zeiss Cirrus AS-OCT device. (Courtesy Kraig Scot Bower, MD, Wilmer Eye Institute, Johns Hopkins University, Baltimore, Maryland, United States.)

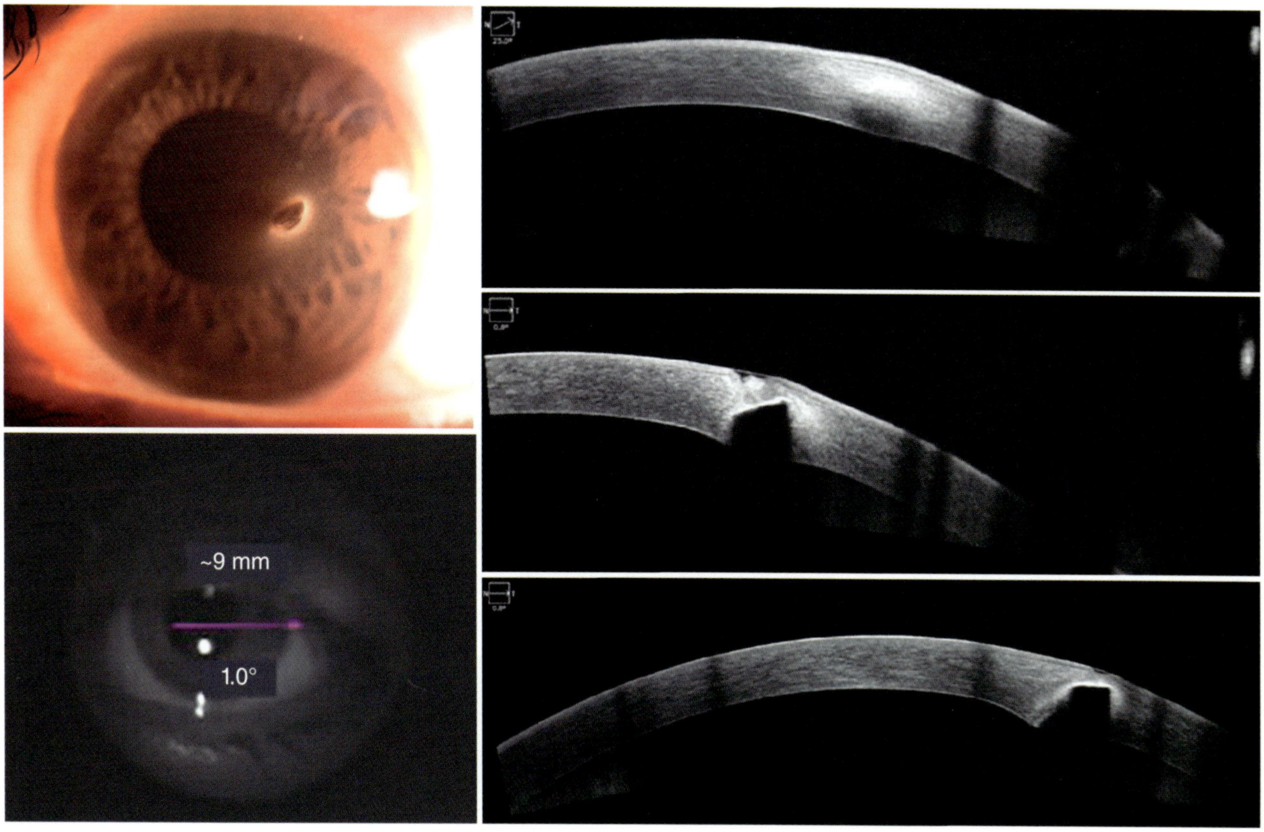

Fig. 17.11 Case of corneal perforation resulting from full-thickness corneal foreign body. AS-OCT shows perforation at the cornea through the Descemet membrane. The foreign body was surgically removed. (Courtesy Kamran M. Riaz, MD, Dean McGee Eye Institute, University of Oklahoma, Oklahoma City, Oklahoma, United States.)

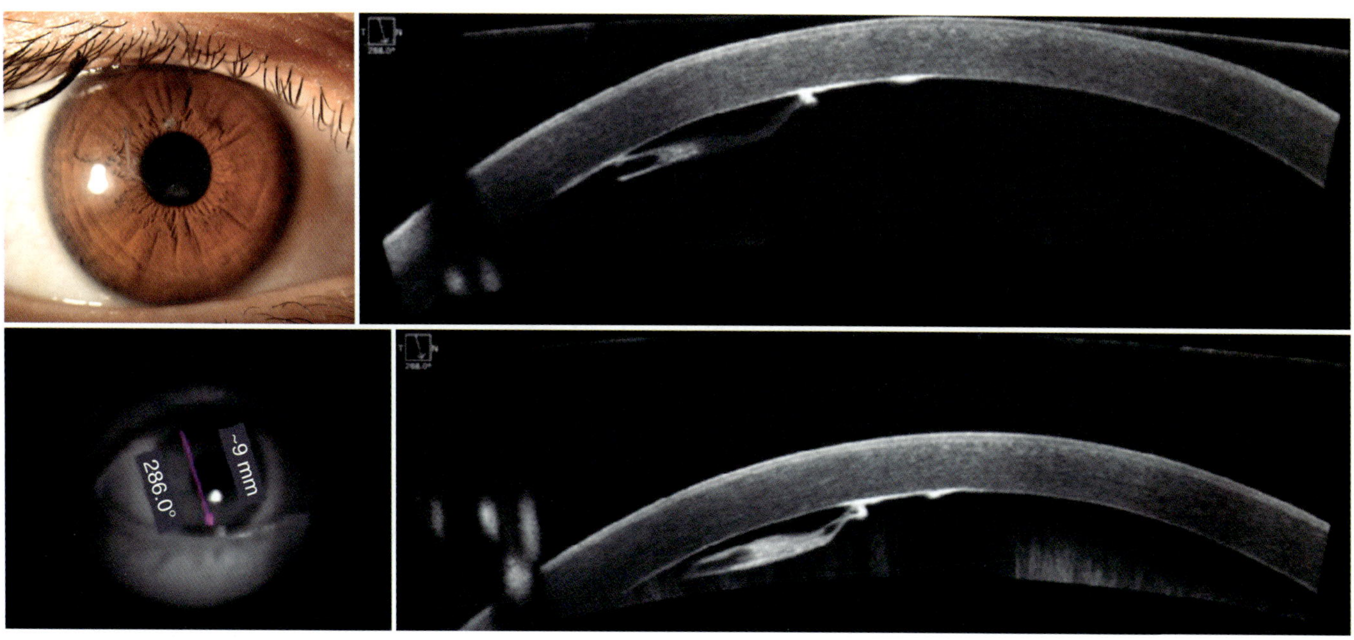

Fig. 17.12 Full-thickness corneal laceration. A 27-year-old man with history of penetrating trauma was referred after removal of a metallic foreign body causing a full-thickness corneal laceration in the right eye. Notably, detachment of the Descemet membrane and scrolling can be seen on AS-OCT. (Courtesy Kamran M. Riaz, MD, Dean McGee Eye Institute, University of Oklahoma, Oklahoma City, Oklahoma, United States.)

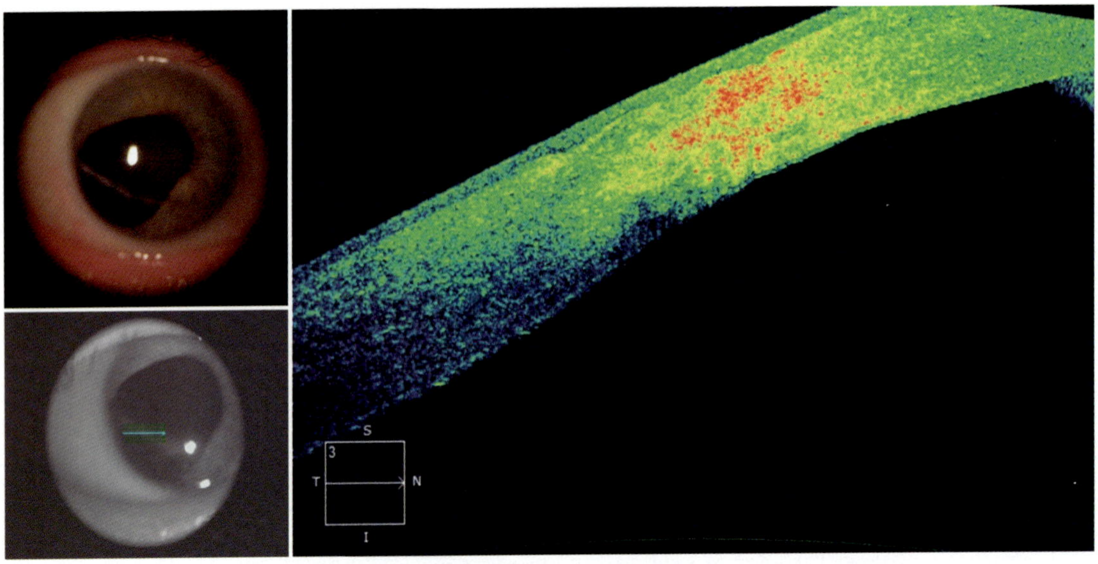

Fig. 17.13 Corneal scarring. Slit-lamp photographs and AS-OCT images of a 77-year-old patient with an old corneal scar and prominent iris defect from prior trauma. AS-OCT through the scar demonstrates prominent hyperreflectivity of the scar tissue within the corneal stroma.

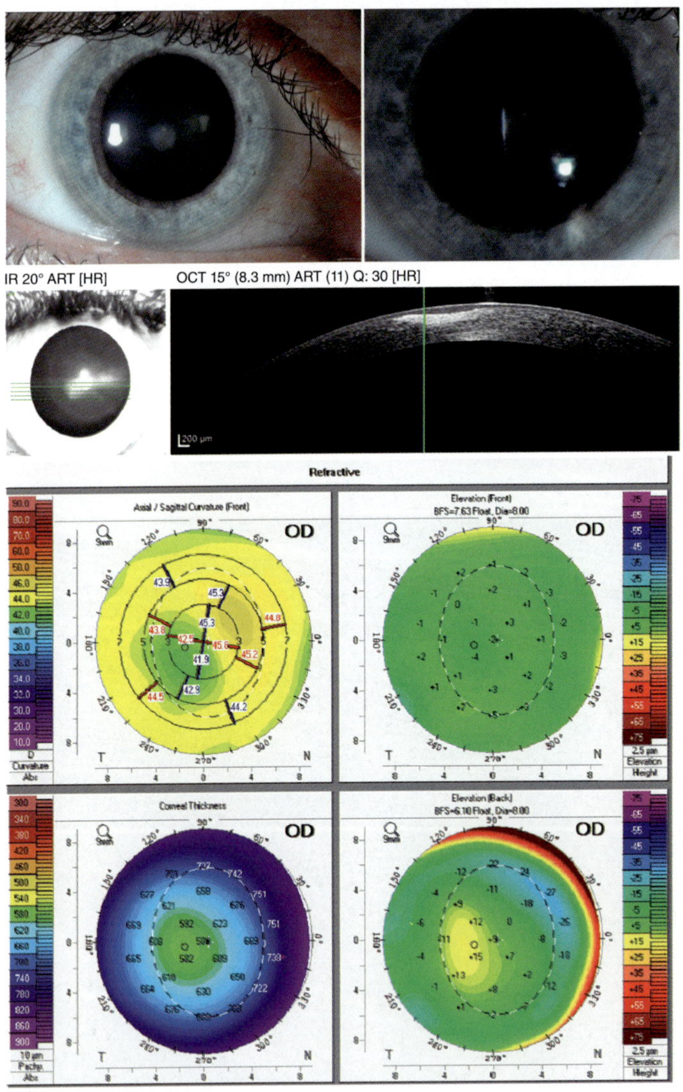

Fig. 17.14 Corneal scarring. Slit-lamp photographs, tomography, and AS-OCT images of a 48-year-old patient after right eye metallic foreign body removal resulting in central corneal scar. Patient presented with poor vision, light sensitivity, and inability to tolerate any activity with right eye open. Corneal scarring is appreciated as a crescentic area of hyperreflectivity on AS-OCT. Epithelial hypertrophy is also noted in the area of stromal thinning, helping to restore the normal refractive surface of the cornea. (Courtesy Kamran M. Riaz, MD, Dean McGee Eye Institute, University of Oklahoma, Oklahoma City, Oklahoma, United States.)

III. ANTERIOR CHAMBER AND IRIS

A. Hyphema

While a hyphema, the presence of blood in the anterior chamber can sometimes occur spontaneously from intra-pcular pathology, it is much more commonly linked with trauma, eother blunt force or due to a pentrating injury. Intra-ocular surgery and occasionally intra-ocular lenses can lead to anterior chamber bleeding as well. Although hyphema may be directly visualized at the slit-lamp, ultrasonography may be needed to assess for additional injuries. Because hyphema can be accompanied by damage to angle structures and elevated intraocular pressure, AS-OCT can provide a noncontact method to assess the angle and help assess the rik for increased intra-ocular pressure or hypotony from angle trauma (Fig. 17.15). AS-OCT can show the hyperreflective migration of red blood cells into the stroma in resultant corneal blood staining, which can be an indication for surgical evacuation.

B. Iridodialysis

Iridodialysis refers to the separation of the iris from the ciliary body and may arise from blunt trauma. AS-OCT can serve as a noncontact, fast, and high-resolution tool to visualize the anterior segment angle structures and document outcomes after repair (Fig. 17.16).

CLINICAL PEARL

When iris trauma can be readily identified at the slit-lamp, the extent of the trauma, including damage to the anterior chamber angle structures, may be difficult, especially in cases in which gonioscopy cannot be performed or corneal edema obscures the examiner's view. AS-OCT can be used to characterize the locations and extent of iris-angle trauma and help surgical planning for iris repair procedures.

C. Iris Cyst

Iris cysts can arise secondary to trauma and subsequent epithelial implantation. Treatment of the cyst may be needed depending on symptoms and complications secondary to the cyst. In addition to ultrasound biomicroscopy, AS-OCT can be used to make the diagnosis of iris cysts (Fig. 17.17).

D. Traumatic Iritis

Any type of trauma can cause anterior segment inflammation and iritis. Careful anterior segment examination is needed during the evaluation of traumatic iritis, in which AS-OCT can be helpful. Common findings include cell and flare and keratic precipitates (Fig. 17.18).

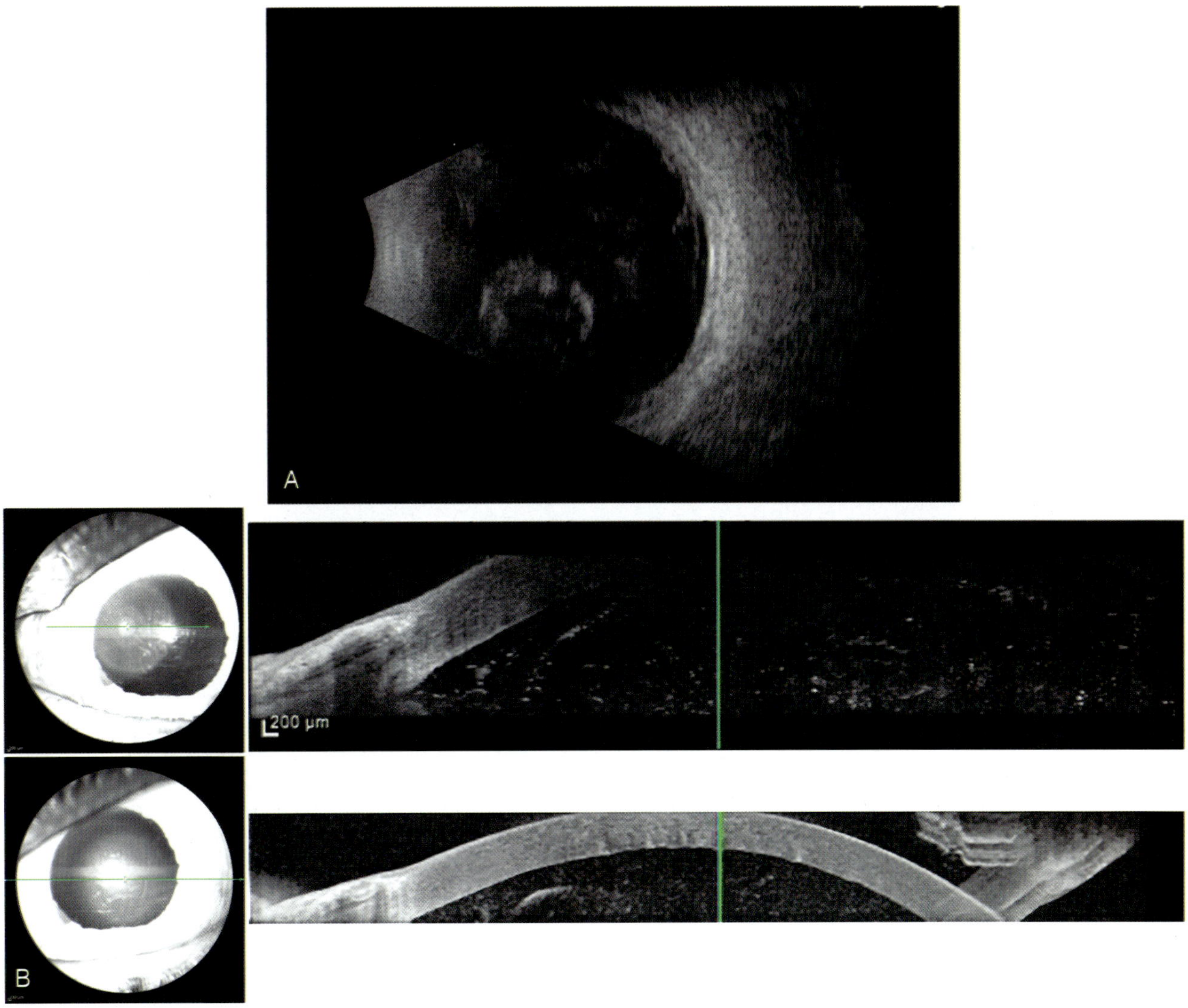

Fig. 17.15 Traumatic hyphema. A 56-year-old patient presented with left eye traumatic hyphema with zonular instability. A, B-scan demonstrating posterior dislocation of lens. B, Hyphema appears as accumulations of hyporeflective (darker) areas on AS-OCT. (Courtesy Kamran M. Riaz, MD, Dean McGee Eye Institute, University of Oklahoma, Oklahoma City, Oklahoma, United States.)

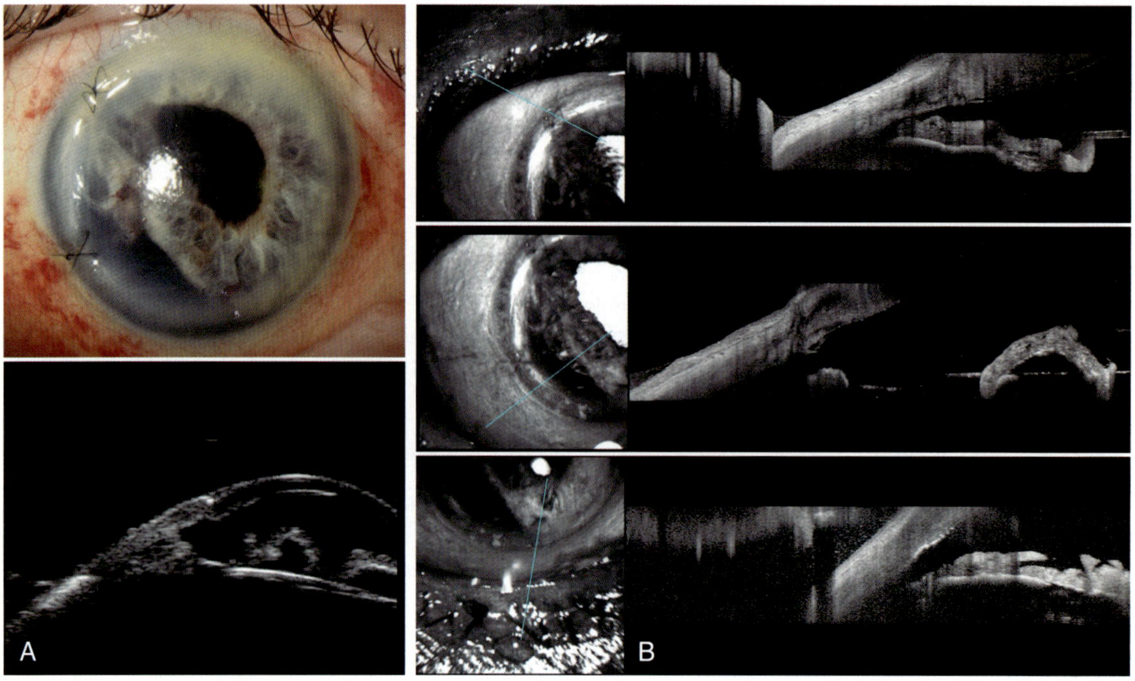

Fig. 17.16 Iridodialysis. Appearance of iridodialysis and zonular instability on (A) ultrasound biomicroscopy and (B) AS-OCT. AS-OCT is helpful to visualize areas of attachment compared with areas of profound detachment. Surgeons can use this information to appropriately plan for surgical repair of such cases if the clinical course warrants. (Courtesy Kamran M. Riaz, MD, Dean McGee Eye Institute, University of Oklahoma, Oklahoma City, Oklahoma, United States.)

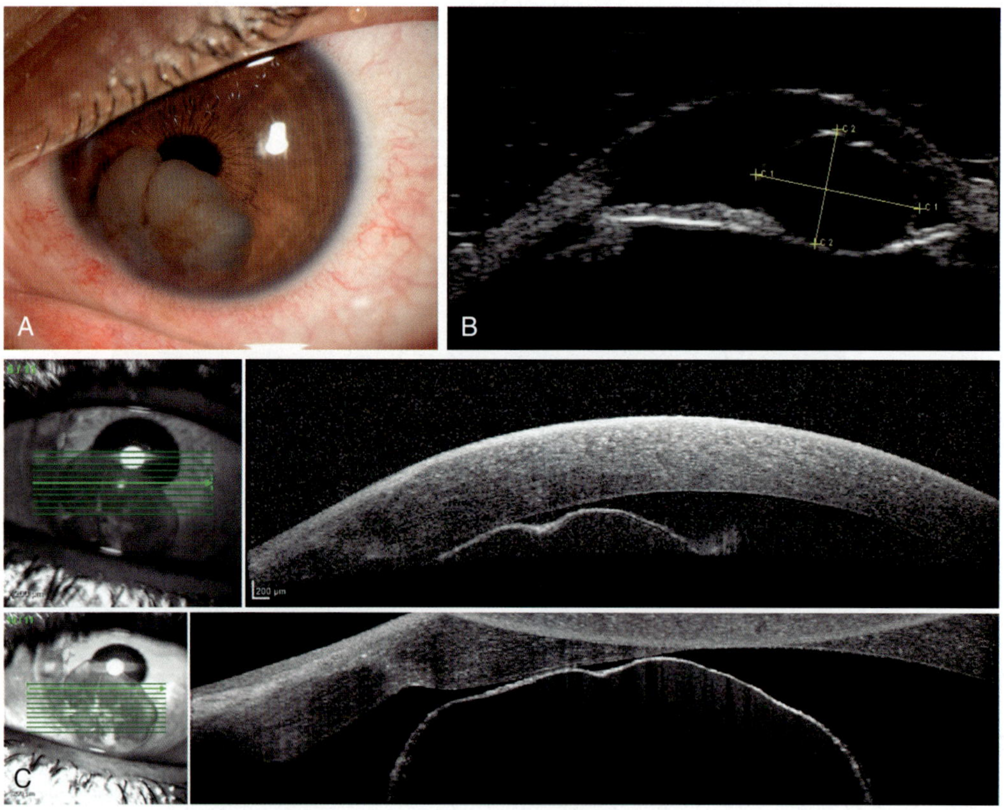

Fig. 17.17 Iris cyst secondary to trauma. A 22-year-old patient presented with stromal iris cyst secondary to penetrating trauma during childhood which appeared to the patient to be getting larger over time As the cyst was blocking part of the visual axis, the patient had decreased vision, most likely due to deprevation ambylopia. Slit-lamp image *(panel A)* demonstrates the size and location of the iris cyst, including extent of pupil obscuration. Ultrasound biomicroscopy (UBM; *panel B*) can be used to further visualize the lesion, including confirmation of its cystic nature as evidenced by hyporeflectivity within the lesion. The lesion also can be measured for documentation purposes. AS-OCT *(panel C)* further highlights features of the cyst, including a hyporeflective center and hyperreflective outer wall. Of note, there is significant corneal touch seen on AS-OCT views that is not readily evident on UBM. The corneal endothelium is seen to be intact. (Courtesy Kamran M. Riaz, MD, Dean McGee Eye Institute, University of Oklahoma, Oklahoma City, Oklahoma, United States.)

IV. LENS

Capsule Violation and Traumatic Cataract

Ocular trauma can lead to traumatic cataracts shortly after the injury, or years later. With penetrating injuries, there may be violation of the anterior or posterior capsule. Rupture of the lens capsule can lead to leakage of lens material into the anterior chamber with resultant inflammation and sometimes increased intraocular pressure. Significant blunt trauma can lead to stellate or rosette cataracts and zonular instability. AS-OCT can assess the integrity of the lens capsule and help determine the treatment approach (Fig. 17.19). Various appearances of traumatic cataracts are further discussed in Chapter 11.

Inadvertent trauma to the endothelium during cataract surgery is an occasionally seen iatrogenic trauma and can be imaged on AS-OCT (Fig. 17.20).

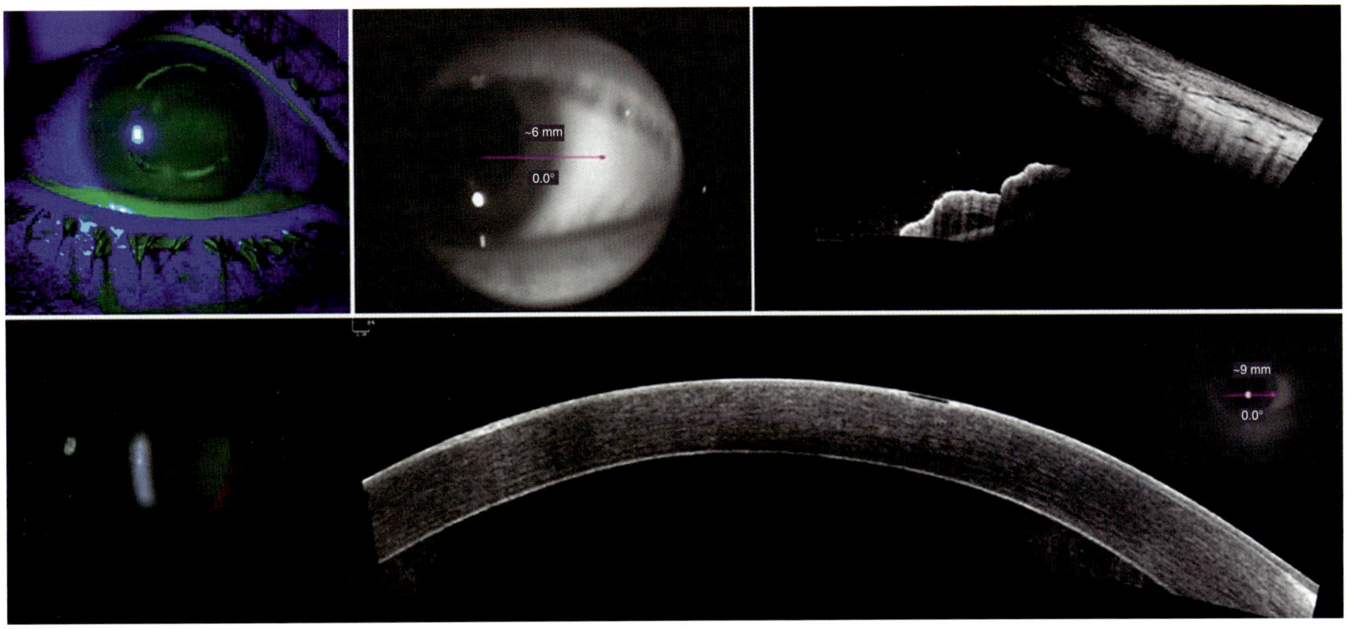

Fig. 17.18 Traumatic iris sustained from a tennis ball. On AS-OCT, 3+ to 4+ cell can be seen in the anterior chamber. Hyphema is not present.

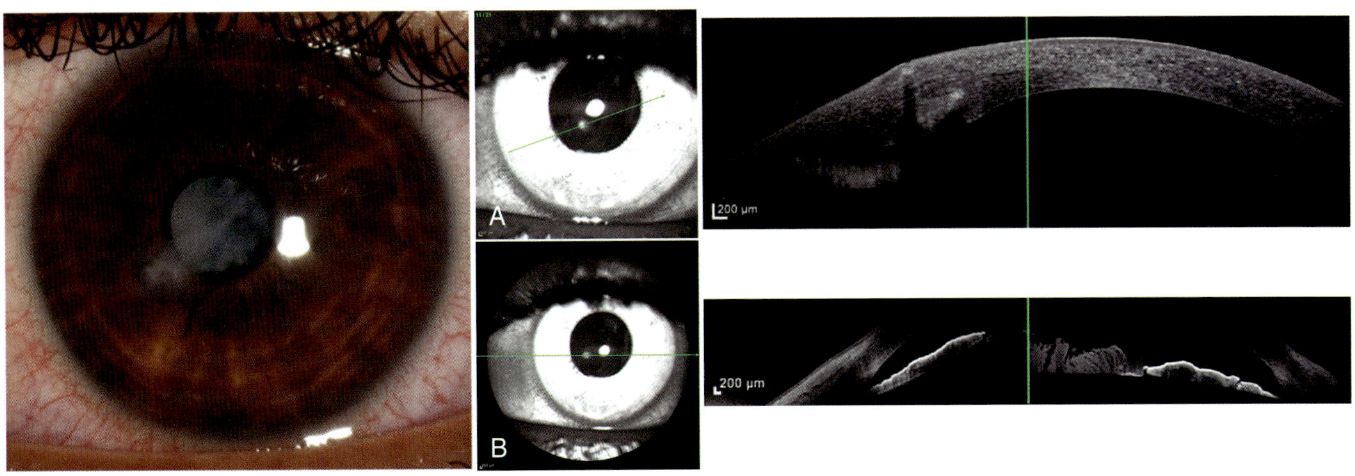

Fig. 17.19 Anterior capsule violation in the context of full-thickness corneal laceration. AS-OCT images of a 16-year-old patient after penetrating ocular trauma reveal (A) full-thickness corneal laceration and (B) anterior capsule violation. (Courtesy Kamran M. Riaz, MD, Dean McGee Eye Institute, University of Oklahoma, Oklahoma City, Oklahoma, United States.)

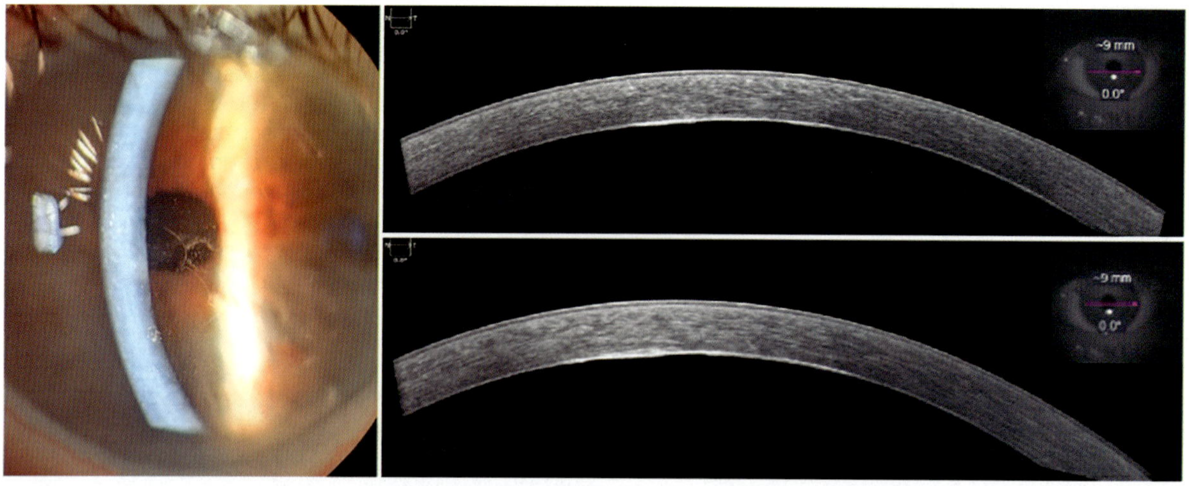

Fig. 17.20 Iatrogenic endothelial scarring from trauma during cataract surgery. The patient presented with visual acuity of 20/50. AS-OCT shows a hyperreflective area of scarring on the endothelium. The corneal thickness is within normal limits. Neither guttae nor excrescences are present. (Courtesy Kamran M. Riaz, MD, Dean McGee Eye Institute, University of Oklahoma, Oklahoma City, Oklahoma, United States.)

BIBLIOGRAPHY

Ang M, Baskaran M, Werkmeister RM, et al. Anterior segment optical coherence tomography. *Prog Retin Eye Res*. 2018;66:132-156. Available at: https://doi.org/10.1016/j.preteyeres.2018.04.002.

Armarnik S, Mimouni M, Goldenberg D, et al. Characterization of deeply embedded corneal foreign bodies with anterior segment optical coherence tomography. *Graefes Arch Clin Exp Ophthalmol*. 2019;257(6):1247-1252. Available at: https://doi.org/10.1007/s00417-019-04309-y.

Han SB, Liu YC, Noriega KM, Mehta JS. Applications of anterior segment optical coherence tomography in cornea and ocular surface diseases. *J Ophthalmol*. 2016;2016:4971572. Available at: https://doi.org/10.1155/2016/4971572.

Jancevski M, Foster CS. Anterior segment optical coherence tomography. *Semin Ophthalmol*. 2010;25(5-6):317-323. Available at: https://doi.org/10.3109/08820538.2010.518473.

Ryan DS, Sia RK, Colyer M, et al. Anterior segment imaging in combat ocular trauma. *J Ophthalmol*. 2013;2013:308259. Available at: https://doi.org/10.1155/2013/308259.

Venkateswaran N, Galor A, Wang J, Karp CL. Optical coherence tomography for ocular surface and corneal diseases: a review. *Eye Vis (Lond)*. 2018;5:13. Available at: https://doi.org/10.1186/s40662-018-0107-0.

Wylegala E, Dobrowolski D, Nowińska A, et al. Anterior segment optical coherence tomography in eye injuries. *Graefes Arch Clin Exp Ophthalmol*. 2009;247:451-455. Available at: https://doi.org/10.1007/s00417-008-0937-x.

18 Applications in Contact Lens Fitting

Amanda Crum | Laura Di Meglio

I. INTRODUCTION

There is no singular, defined, or standardized approach adapted by all practitioners when fitting contact lenses. At a minimum, an eye care provider is likely to include subjective observation using a slit-lamp biomicroscope and vital dyes. However, many providers will collect corneal measurements and images via keratometry, corneal topography, and anterior segment optical coherence tomography (AS-OCT). These technologies are not only useful in establishing a baseline and tracking disease progression but also can assist contact lens specialists in fitting and troubleshooting a contact lens fit and to detect and document adverse events.

Although the original purpose of AS-OCT might not have been intended for contact lenses, it has been useful in expanding our understanding of corneal and scleral shape and the physical interaction of a contact lens with the eye. A report by Kojima and colleagues outlines the various uses for AS-OCT in patients who wear contact lenses. These include sagittal depth measurements to assist in lens fitting, corneal thicknesses before and after lens wear to screen for corneal edema, and troubleshooting peripheral landing zones to minimize lens awareness or mechanical irritation. This technology has become a valuable tool for fitters by reducing uncertainties in the fitting relationships between the back surface of the lens and the corneal, limbal, or conjunctival epithelium.

II. SOFT CONTACT LENSES

Subclinical morphologic changes have been documented on AS-OCT, specifically at the level of the corneoscleral junction after silicone hydrogel contact lens wear. Additionally, there may be some value in using AS-OCT to assess reepithelialization of the epithelium after refractive surgery, corneal abrasions, or recurrent corneal erosions without removing the therapeutic bandage contact lens.

III. RIGID GAS-PERMEABLE

Rigid gas-permeable (RGP) lenses are typically evaluated at the slit-lamp, using fluorescein dye to assess the fitting relationship: corneal alignment, clearance, or touch. Based on the degree of hyperfluorescence, the relationship between the posterior surface of the lens and the corneal epithelium is qualified. AS-OCT can be used to quantify the amount of clearance or the extent of touch. It is particularly useful for examining edge profiles on the cornea and may simplify the troubleshooting process when a patient is struggling to adapt to RGP lenses. Clinically, the aim of RGP lenses is to distribute weight across multiple points with faint contact with the corneal epithelium. Tear exchange must be optimal to maintain corneal health.

IV. HYBRID

Hybrid lenses have evolved since their introduction into the market; newer gas-permeable and soft skirt materials have led to improved breathability and tear exchange, reducing the risk of hypoxia. Radial AS-OCT segmentation allows a provider to screen for areas of touch, impingement, or vault. In Fig. 18.1, the lacrimal lens and fitting relationship can be observed. More specifically, calipers are used to quantify the lacrimal lens in Fig. 18.2. The lacrimal lens is identified as the space between the posterior lens surface and anterior cornea. Quantification of this space is useful when determining whether the lens falls within the manufacturers' intended fitting guidelines. AS-OCT can also help identify poor fit patterns, as seen in Fig. 18.3.

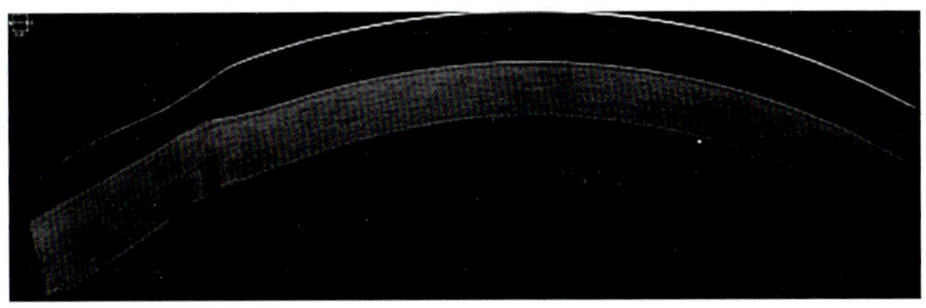

Fig. 18.1 AS-OCT cross-section of hybrid contact lens. Note the transition between the central rigid gas-permeable and peripheral soft skirt. Tracing the hyperreflective posterior surface of the lens relative to the shape of the corneal epithelium assists in identifying ideal versus ill-fitting lenses. (Courtesy Brett Levinson.)

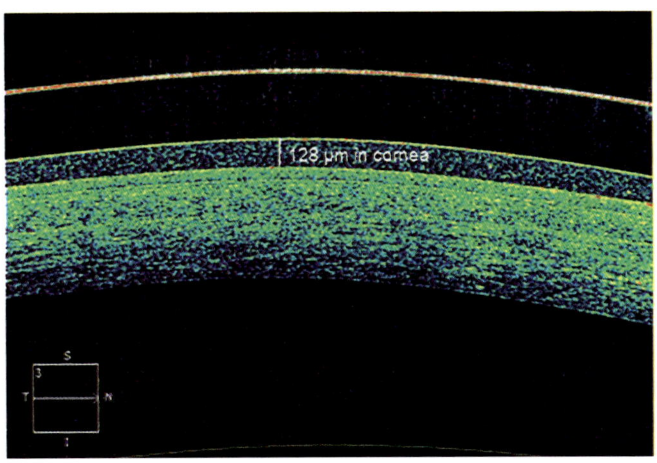

Fig. 18.2 AS-OCT calipers measure the lacrimal lens in this temporal-to-nasal corneal cross-section. In this cut, 128 microns of central corneal clearance at the apex of the cornea is quantified with a hybrid contact lens on the eye. (Courtesy Brett Levinson.)

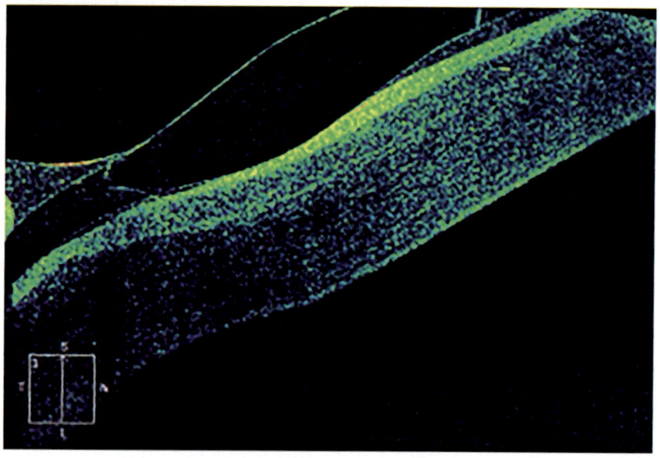

Fig. 18.3 Inferior to superior cross-section of mid-peripheral hybrid contact lens. Image highlights the steep approach at the rigid gas-permeable and soft contact lens junction with notable compression of the anterior corneal surface. (Courtesy Brett Levinson.)

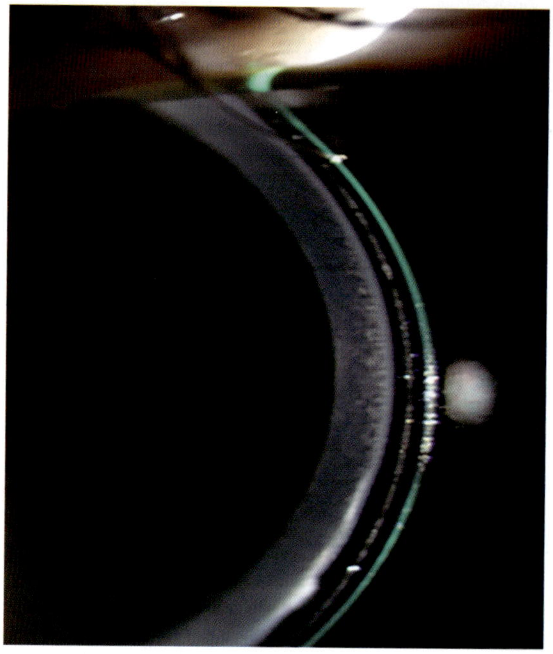

Fig. 18.4 Slit-lamp image of a scleral contact lens on a cornea. The structures (right to left) are the front surface of the contact lens (highlighted with fluorescein), the reflective back surface of the contact lens, the corneal epithelium, and the corneal endothelium. The lacrimal lens is the space between posterior lens and anterior cornea and is quantified by comparing the contact lens thickness or the corneal thickness to the lacrimal lens. (Courtesy Tom Arnold.)

V. SCLERAL CONTACT LENSES

The use of AS-OCT has broadened our understanding of the scleral profile, by demonstrating a correlation between corneal and scleral shape. Notably, the scleral shape is not spherical and is affected by extraocular muscle insertion. This has removed some of the mystery of fitting large-diameter lenses, particularly scleral contact lens designs.

Traditionally, multiple diagnostic lenses are placed on the eye until an ideal fit is achieved. Careful scrutiny of the post-lens tear film, or lacrimal lens, at the slit-lamp is critical to balance clearance over corneal structures while optimizing oxygen permeability. AS-OCT assessment of the lacrimal lens may usurp slit-lamp assessment. A study by Yeung and Sorbara found that providers tend to overestimate the clearance by about 103 microns at the slit-lamp biomicroscope. Use of AS-OCT technology may help practitioners identify ill-fit patterns, which is useful in patients with fragile corneal transplants or low endothelial cell counts.

A scleral lens comprises corneal, limbal, and peripheral zones. The aim of a scleral lens is to vault the corneal apex and clear the limbal stem cells, while aligning and distributing weight equally across the conjunctival/scleral tissue. Fig. 18.4 shows an image of an optic cross-section taken at a biomicroscope of a scleral lens on the eye. The lacrimal lens can be estimated by comparing the scleral lens thickness or corneal thickness to the lacrimal lens. Instead of estimating, Figs. 18.5 and 18.6 show how AS-OCT can be used to quantify the lacrimal lens at the corneal apex and limbus of the same scleral lens. The ideal apical corneal clearance is 150 to 250 microns, which tapers to 50 to 100 microns at the limbus. The weight of the lens should be distributed evenly across the landing and peripheral curves, avoiding any blanching and edge liftoff.

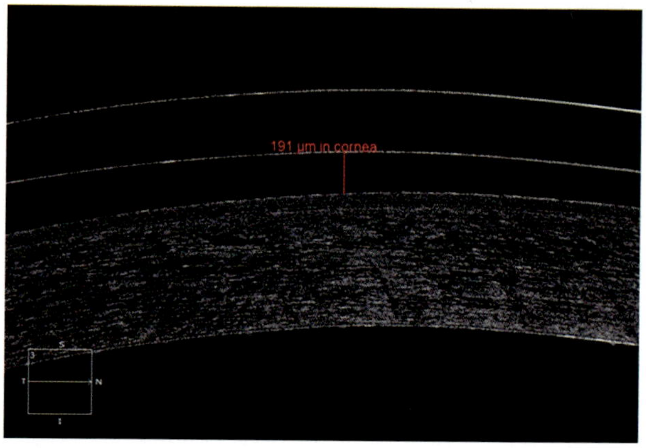

Fig. 18.5 Using AS-OCT to quantify the corneal clearance, 191 microns measured at the apex. (Courtesy Tom Arnold.)

A. Central Clearance

Figs. 18.7 and 18.8 demonstrate two examples of scleral lenses with an adequate amount of corneal clearance. Notably, the lens fitting relationship on application usually changes over several hours as the lens settles on the eye. Figs. 18.9 and 18.10 show the change in corneal clearance of the same lens after a few hours of wear. The risk with settling is inadequate clearance and corneal touch, as seen in Fig. 18.11. Conversely, excessive corneal vault increases the risk of reduced oxygen availability, vascularization, and post-lens tear debris. Anything over 250

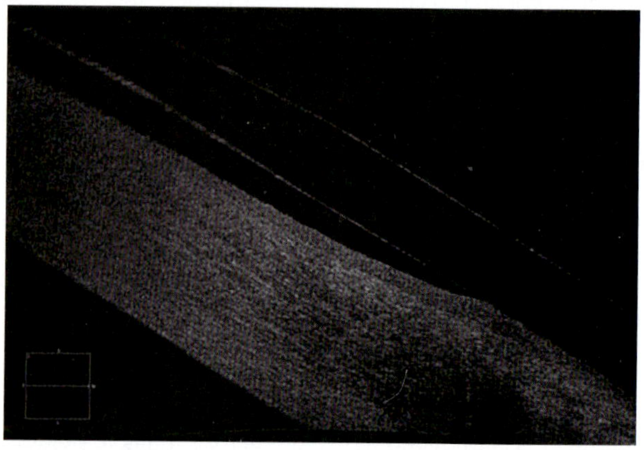

Fig. 18.6 Mid-peripheral image showing a tapered lacrimal lens peripherally, nearing the limbal stem cells. (Courtesy Tom Arnold.)

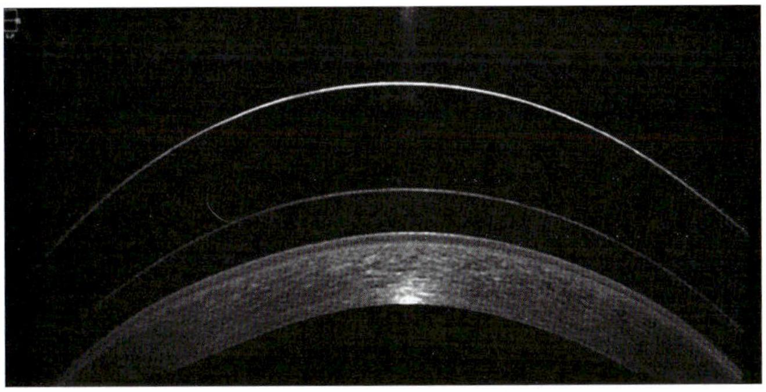

Fig. 18.7 If the corneal thickness or lens thickness is known, the post-lens reservoir can be estimated at the slit lamp, otherwise AS-OCT can assist in these measurements. (Courtesy Tom Arnold.)

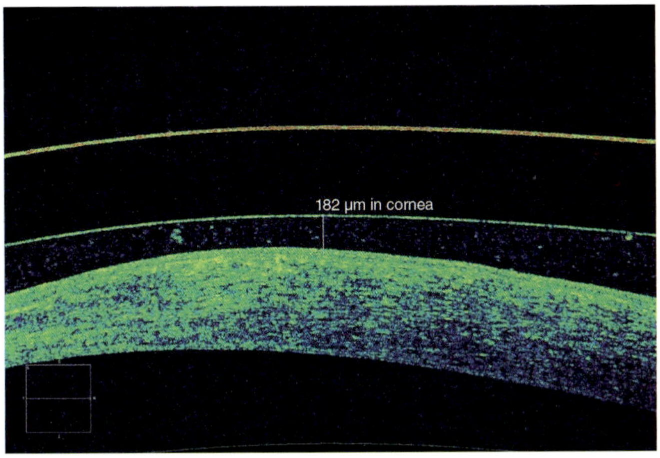

Fig. 18.8 Using AS-OCT to quantify the post-lens reservoir. The AS-OCT caliper measures 182 microns of clearance over the apex of the cornea. (Courtesy Tom Arnold.)

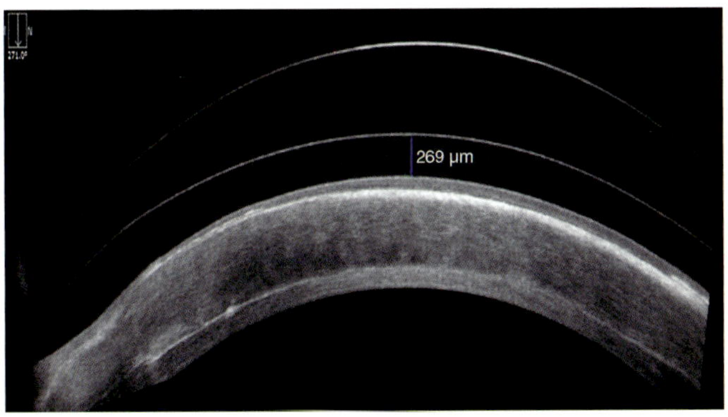

Fig. 18.9 Central clearance of 269 microns upon application. (Courtesy Clarke Newman.)

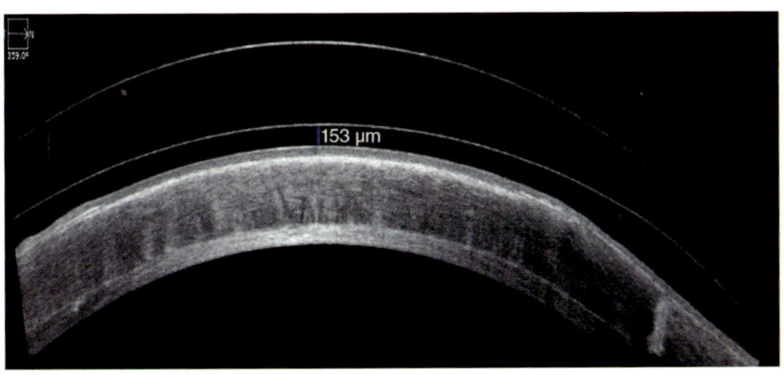

Fig. 18.10 Scleral lens after settling with reduced central clearance of 153 microns. (Courtesy Clarke Newman.)

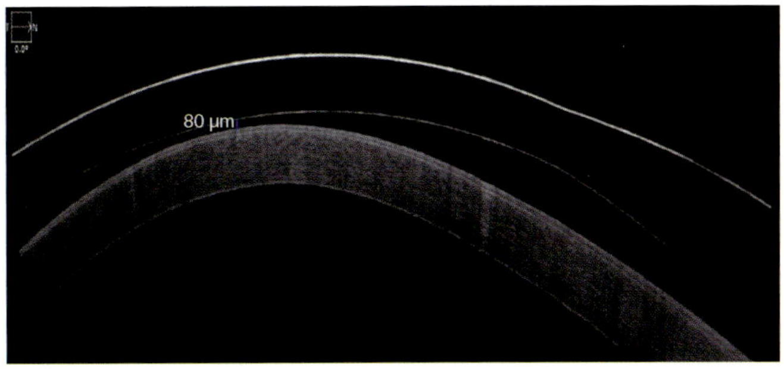

Fig. 18.11 Minimal apical clearance exhibited over an eye with keratoconus. (Courtesy Clarke Newman.)

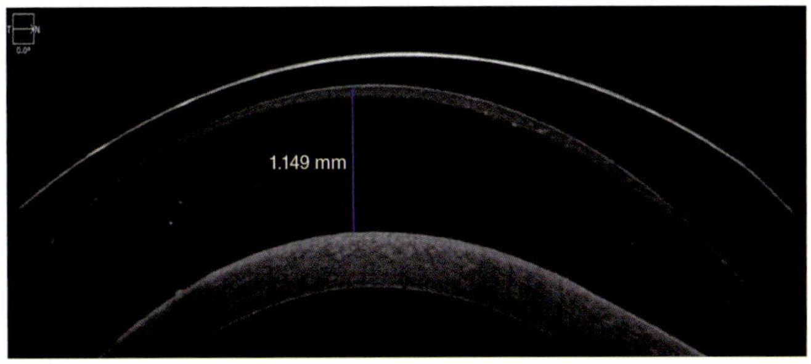

Fig. 18.12 Excessive apical clearance quantified as 1149 microns of clearance. (Courtesy Clarke Newman.)

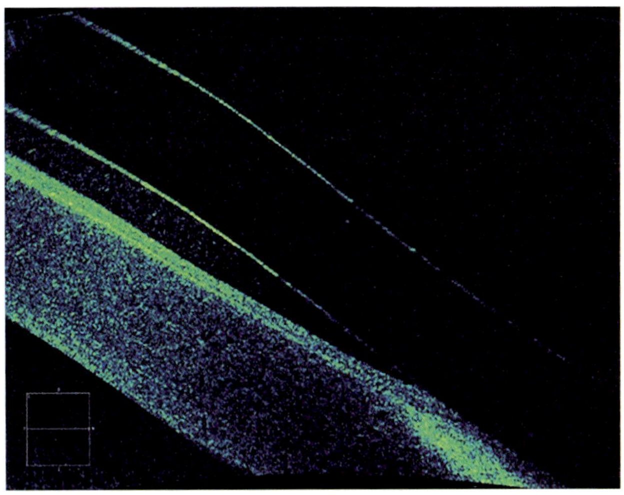

Fig. 18.13 Tapering of the post-lens reservoir nearing the limbal stem cells relative to the midperipheral corneal tissue. (Courtesy Tom Arnold.)

microns would be defined as excessive clearance, as demonstrated in Fig. 18.12.

B. Limbal Clearance

By gross examination, the limbus is identified as a thin blue-gray ring between the corneal and scleral tissues. Given the high-resolution capabilities of AS-OCT, direct visualization of the anatomic boundaries of the limbus is attainable. As limbal clearance tapers, it can be difficult to visualize the limbal structures using slit-lamp biomicroscope and to quantify the amount of space between the posterior lens and limbal stem cells. AS-OCT technology is a useful tool in ensuring adequate fitting relationships, which is particularly useful in patients with compromised limbal stem cell health. Fig. 18.13 demonstrates the ideal taper seen in AS-OCT at the limbal stem cells.

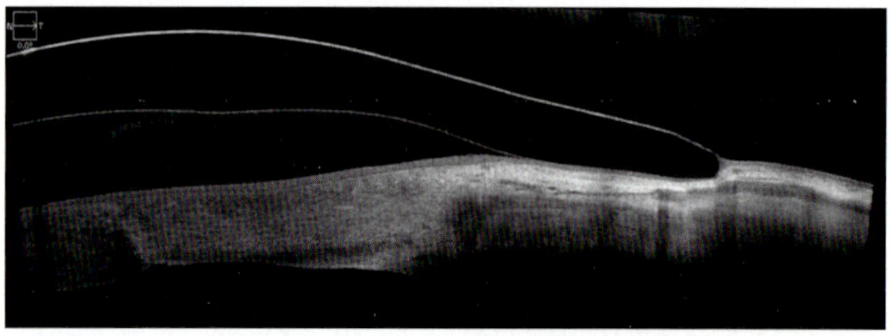

Fig. 18.14 Peripheral scan of scleral lens demonstrating more significant corneal and limbal vault with haptic alignment with the scleral tissue. (Courtesy Clarke Newman.)

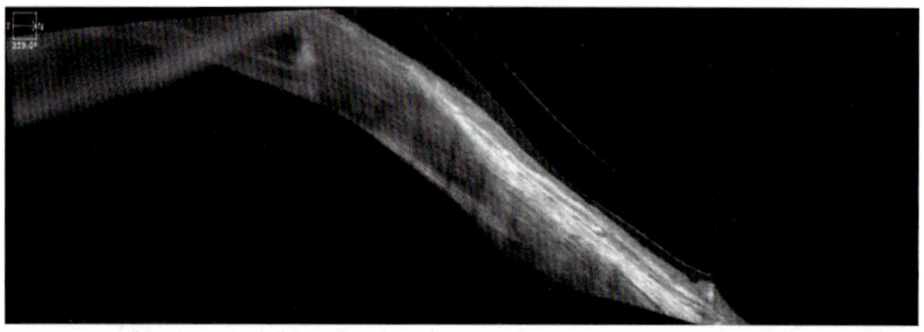

Fig. 18.15 Scan demonstrating peripheral edge liftoff with unequal weight distribution at the landing curve. (Courtesy Clarke Newman.)

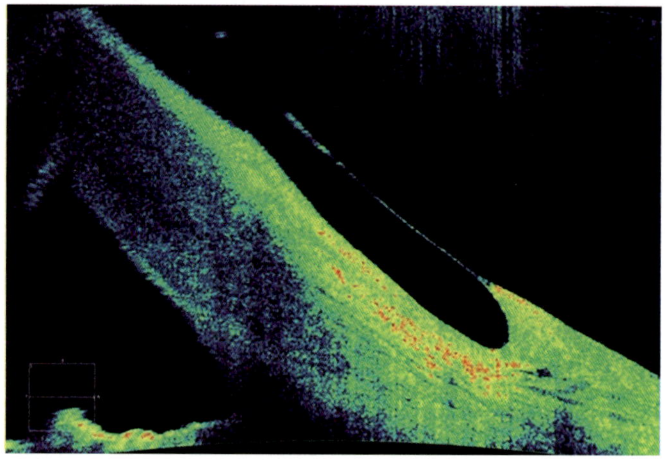

Fig. 18.16 Peripheral impingement of the haptic. This clinical presentation is generally paired with impingement of conjunctival vasculature. (Courtesy Tom Arnold.)

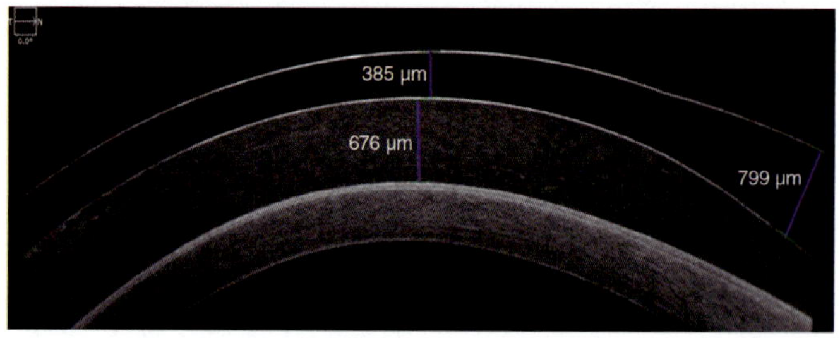

Fig. 18.17 Scleral lens with excessive corneal vault with a cloudy post-lens tear reservoir. (Courtesy Clarke Newman.)

C. Landing and Peripheral Alignment

Weight distribution across the landing and peripheral curves is critical for an ideal fit. A steep approach can result in a tight fit and blanching of the underlying vasculature and compression of the conjunctival and scleral tissue. A loose or flat approach may result in excessive movement, lens awareness, and increased midday fogging. Figs. 18.14 through 18.16 demonstrate the range of peripheral fitting patterns. Given the scleral asymmetry noted in previous AS-OCT studies, toric haptics are often used and have been shown to improve centration and enhance vision, comfort, and general wearability.

D. Complications

Various case series have been published documenting contact lens fit–related complications using AS-OCT technology. Figs. 18.17 to 18.19 demonstrate images of scleral lens-related complications documented by AS-OCT.

VI. CONTACT LENSES AND OCULAR PATHOLOGY

AS-OCT technology is not required to successfully fit contact lenses but is rather a useful tool in a prescriber's armamentarium for troubleshooting contact lens fits over normal and diseased corneas. Additionally, as discussed in earlier chapters, this technology provides another mechanism for monitoring disease progression. The remaining images, Figs. 18.20 to 18.29, demonstrate various lens fits over pathologic, postsurgical, and posttransplanted corneas. Combining data collected from various equipment, including AS-OCT, may enhance our understanding of lens patterns on the eye and the eye's response to the lens.

ACKNOWLEDGMENT

The authors gratefully acknowledge the contribution of Dr. Rachel Caywood.

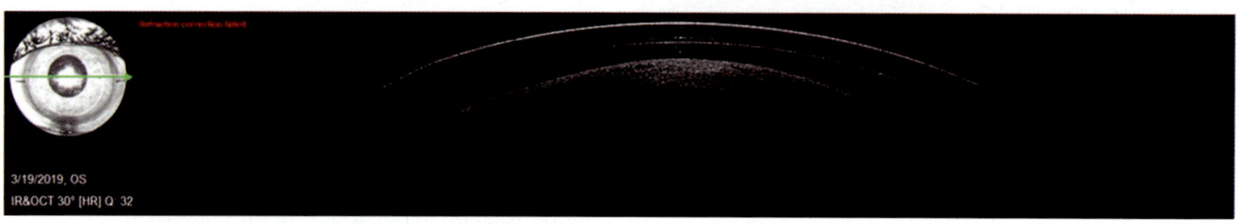

Fig. 18.18 Scleral lens with poor wettability seen on the anterior lens surface. (Courtesy Brian Silverman.)

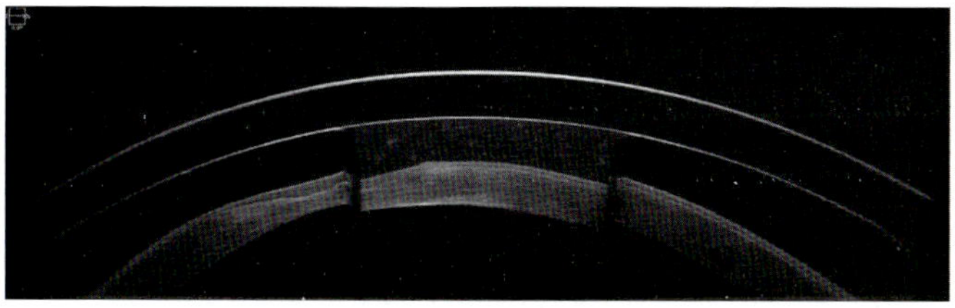

Fig. 18.19 Cross-section of scleral lens with an air bubble trapped between lens and corneal surfaces. (Courtesy Tom Arnold.)

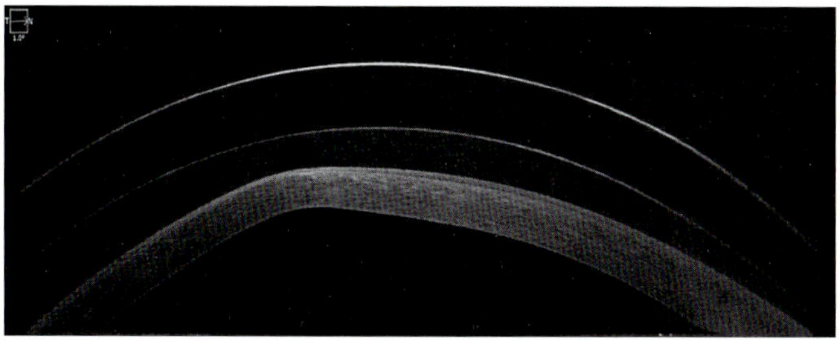

Fig. 18.20 A scan of scleral lens over a cornea with keratoconus. It is important to assess the post-lens tear reservoir at the apex of the cornea. (Courtesy Tom Arnold.)

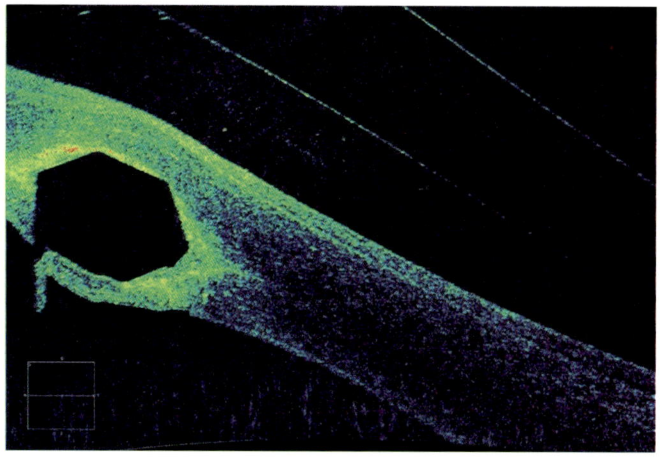

Fig. 18.21 Cross-sectional scan of a scleral lens over a cornea with intrastromal rings. (Courtesy Tom Arnold.)

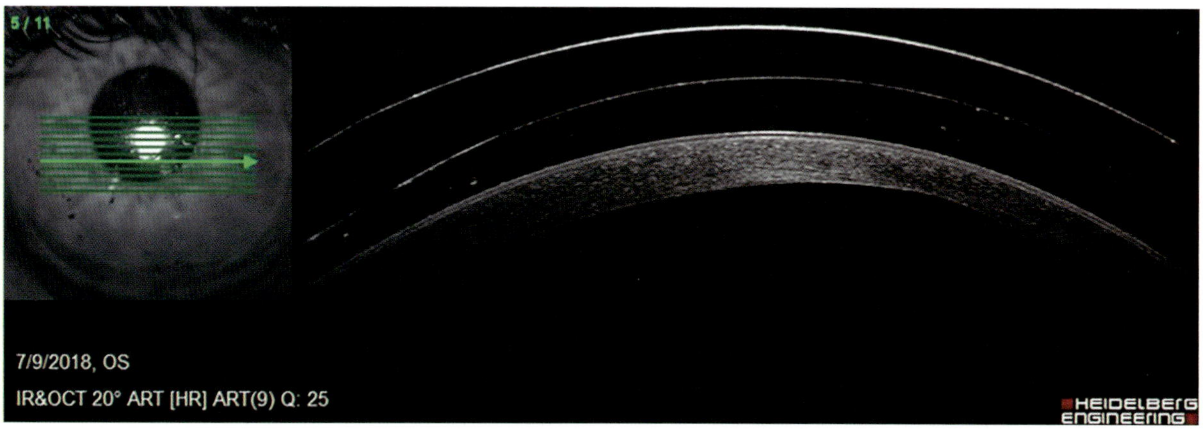

Fig. 18.22 Scleral lens with adequate to excessive vault over a cornea with keratoglobus and history of hydrops. (Courtesy Brian Silverman.)

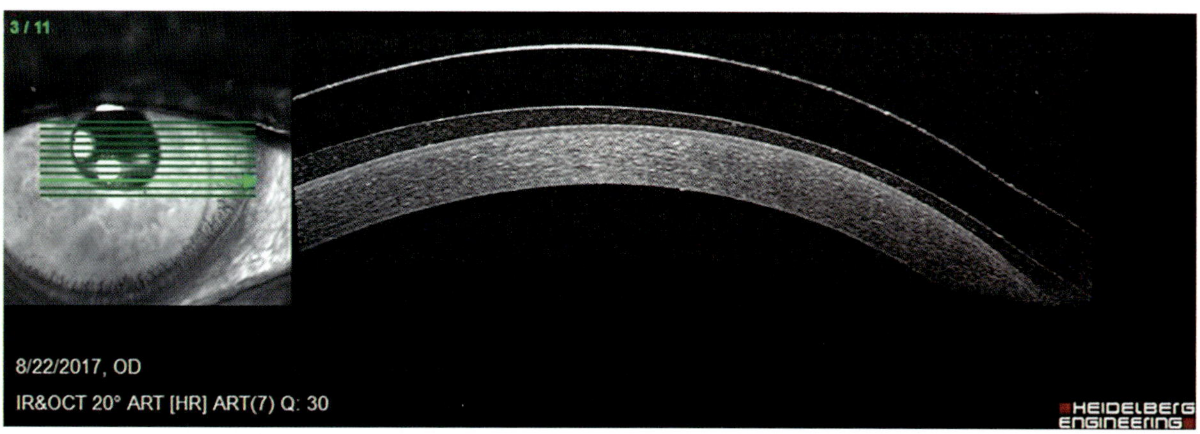

Fig. 18.23 Scleral lens over a cornea with history of advanced pellucid marginal degeneration. (Courtesy Brian Silverman.)

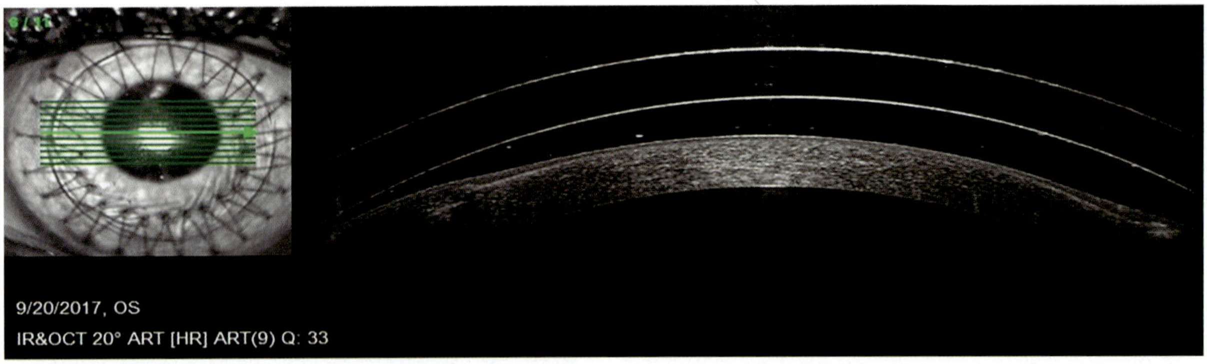

Fig. 18.24 Heidelberg AS-OCT image of scleral lens over post-penetrating keratoplasty with running sutures intact. The image illustrates an adequate amount of central clearance which tapers near the graft-host junction. (Courtesy Brian Silverman.)

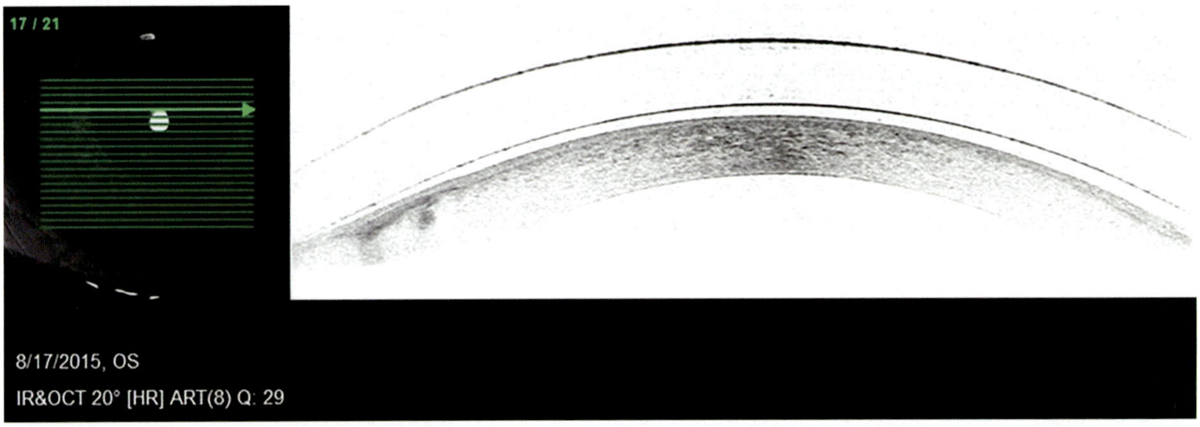

Fig. 18.25 Central scan illustrating a minimal amount of corneal vault over a full-thickness corneal graft. (Courtesy Brian Silverman.)

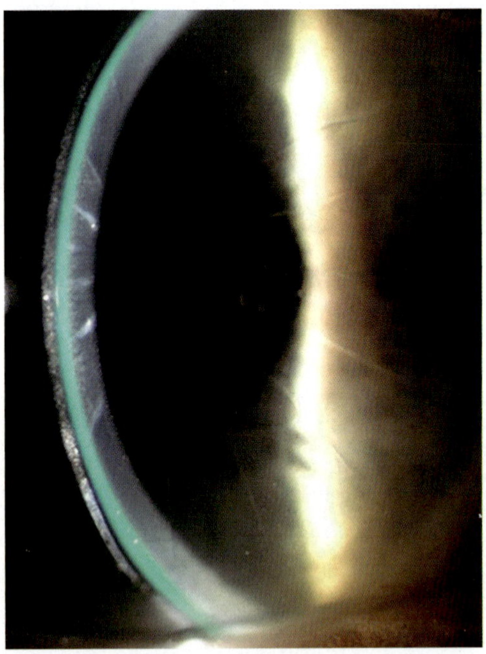

Fig. 18.26 Slit-lamp image of a scleral lens on an eye previously treated with radial keratectomy (RK). The lacrimal lens is highlighted with fluorescein dye. This image illustrates a scleral lens vaulting a cornea with the radial scars following RK. (Courtesy Tom Arnold.)

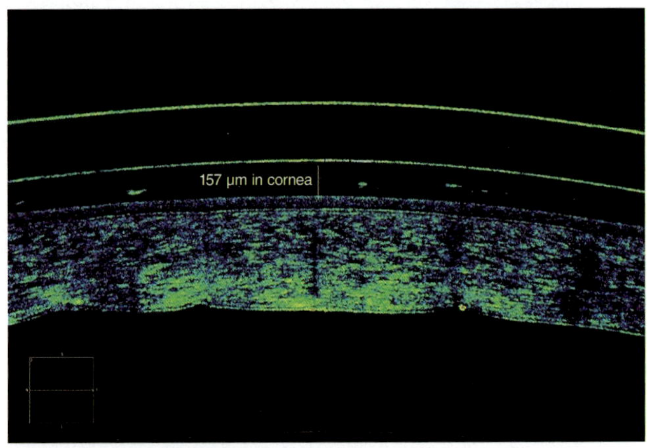

Fig. 18.27 AS-OCT image of a scleral lens over a cornea after RK. (Courtesy Tom Arnold.)

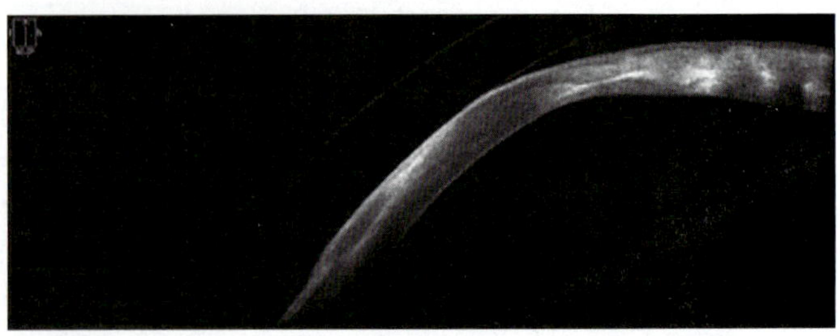

Fig. 18.28 Impression-based lens system on a patient with ectasia following RK and laser-assisted in-situ keratomileusis (LASIK). (Courtesy Buddy Russell.)

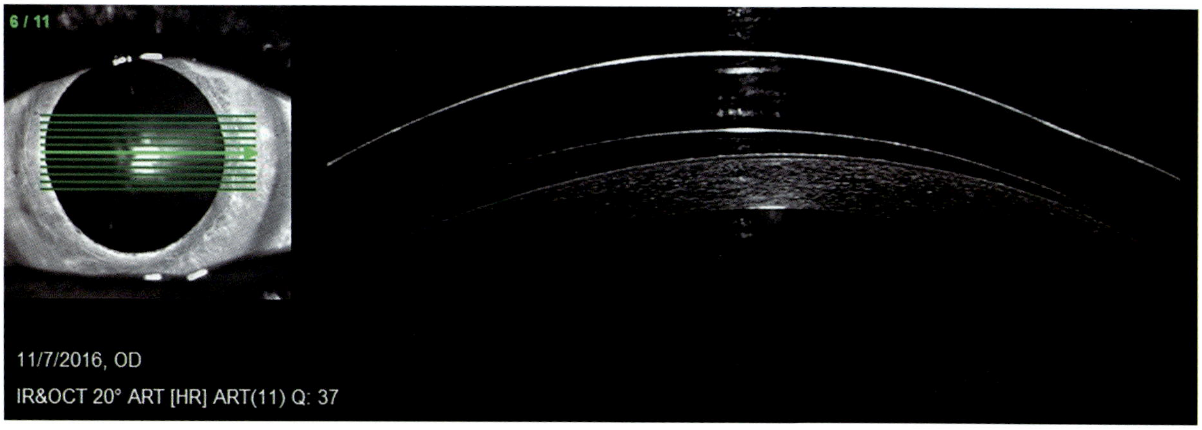

Fig. 18.29 Scleral lens image on a patient with history of graft-versus-host disease (GVHD). (Courtesy Brian Silverman.)

BIBLIOGRAPHY

Alonso-Caneiro D, Shaw AJ, Collins MJ. Using optical coherence tomography to assess corneoscleral morphology after soft contact lens wear. *Optom Vis Sci*. 2012;89(11):1619-1626.

Elbendary A, Abou Samra W. Evaluation of rigid gas permeable lens fitting in keratoconic patients with optical coherence tomography. *Graefes Arch Clin Exp Ophthalmol*. 2013;251(6):1565-1570.

Eliaçık M, Erdur SK, Gülkılık G, Özsütçü M, Karabela Y. Compare the effects of two silicone-hydrogel bandage contact lenses on epithelial healing after photorefractive keratectomy with anterior segment optical coherence tomography. *Cont Lens Anterior Eye*. 2015;38(3):215-219.

Isozaki VL, Chiu GB. Transient corneal epithelial bullae associated with large diameter scleral lens wear: A case series. *Cont Lens Anterior Eye*. 2018;41(5):463-468.

Kojima R, Caroline P, Walker M, Kinoshita B, André M, Lampa M. Benefits of OCT when fitting specialty lenses. *Cont Lens Spectrum*. 2014;29:46, 48-51, 63.

Le Q, Cordova D, Xu J, Deng SX. In vivo evaluation of the limbus using anterior segment optical coherence tomography. *Trans Vis Sci Tech*. 2018;7:12. Available at: http://doi.org/10.1167/tvst.7.4.12.

Nguyen L, Yang D, Vien L. Case series: corneal epithelial macrocysts in scleral contact lenses post–penetrating keratoplasty. *Optom Vis Sci*. 2018;95(7):616-620.

Nixon AD, Barr JT, VanNasdale DA. Corneal epithelial bullae after short-term wear of small diameter scleral lenses. *Cont Lens Anterior Eye*. 2017;40(2):116-126.

Piotrowiak I, Kaluzny B, Danek B, Chwiedacz A, Sikorski B, Malukiewicz G. Spectral optical coherence tomography vs. fluorescein pattern for rigid gas-permeable lens fit. *Med Sci Monit*. 2014;20:1137-1141. Available at: http://doi.org/10.12659/MSM.890269.

van der Worp E. Beyond the cornea part I. *Global CONTACT*. 2009:42-45.

Xu M, Randleman JB, Chiu GB. Long-term descemetocele management with prosthetic replacement of the ocular surface ecosystem (PROSE) treatment. *Eye Contact Lens*. 2020;46(2):e7-e10.

Yeung D, Sorbara L. Scleral lens clearance assessment with biomicroscopy and anterior segment optical coherence tomography. *Optom Vis Sci*. 2018;95(1):13-20.

19 Corneal Infections

Paula A. Sepulveda-Beltran | Diego S. Altamirano | Guillermo Amescua

I. INTRODUCTION

Although diagnosis and management of routine ocular infections, especially infectious keratitis, may be accomplished with clinical examination, anterior segment optical coherence tomography (AS-OCT) may be a useful adjunct imaging modality because of its ability to provide high-resolution images through noncontact means. AS-OCT images can therefore play an important role in the clinical evaluation, diagnosis, surgical planning, and monitoring of therapeutic interventions in patients with ocular infections. In addition, the anatomic illustration that it provides may enhance patients' understanding of disease diagnosis and treatment progress, thus improving compliance. Patients and practitioners benefit from the detailed findings of this imaging device, which may continue to yield a greater extent of applications.

This chapter will primarily focus on the applicability of AS-OCT for corneal infections, though it also may be used for conjunctival and scleral infection. Images from commonly encountered infections are presented with salient features on AS-OCT highlighted.

II. BACTERIAL INFECTIONS

A. Contact Lens–Related Bacterial Keratitis

Contact lens use, particularly in the setting of extended lens wear, overnight use of soft contact lenses, unhygienic contact lens practices, and/or exposure to water, significantly increases the risk for microbial keratitis, which includes bacterial, fungal, and acanthamoeba keratitis. Although the use of daily disposable lenses and use of hydrogen peroxide cleaning solutions have decreased incidence, contact lens–related keratitis (CLRK) is frequently seen by eye care practitioners.

CLRK itself may range from mild pathologic findings with minimal impact on vision to severe pathologic conditions with vision-threatening implications. Patients with mild cases of CLRK may present with nonspecific symptoms such as mild decrease in visual acuity, pain, redness, epiphora, and photophobia. The practitioner may need to elicit important details regarding contact lens use, including but not limited to contact lens type, material, brand; overnight wear; exposure to fresh water/swimming pools; and previous history of corneal infections.

CLRK can be readily detected at the slit-lamp, especially in conjunction with fluorescein staining. Corneal cultures may be taken depending on the severity, location, and clinical experience of the practitioner. In these cases, AS-OCT can be used to identify the location of the infiltrate, assess its depth, and determine the presence of other lesions that may not readily be seen on examination. Fig. 19.1 shows AS-OCT images of a patient with mild CLRK. This patient was successfully treated with a two-week course of topical antibiotics and discontinuation of contact lens wear.

CLINICAL PEARL

Although contact lens–related keratitis can be readily seen at the slit-lamp, AS-OCT can be used to determine the presence or absence of other infiltrates that may be missed on clinical examination. Detecting multiple infiltrates may guide the clinician toward management options, such as whether to obtain corneal cultures and choice of topical antibiotics (i.e., nonfortified vs. fortified antibiotics). AS-OCT also can be used at follow-up examinations to assess response to treatment and guide the clinician toward the need for additional or alternative therapeutic interventions.

B. Bacterial Keratitis

Bacterial keratitis may occur outside of contact lens wear, usually in the setting of trauma or other mechanical injury to the eye that allows for opportunistic infections to occur. Ocular adnexa and eyelid flora, such as *Staphylococcus* and *Cutibacterium acnes,* are common infectious organisms.

Although AS-OCT is often not required for initial diagnosis, a scar frequently remains after successful treatment of the corneal infection. Clinicians may then be faced with options for visual rehabilitation, ranging from conservative measures (e.g., glasses or specialty contact lenses) to surgical interventions. In these cases, AS-OCT is extremely helpful to measure the vertical depth and horizontal extent of the scar. In Fig. 19.2,

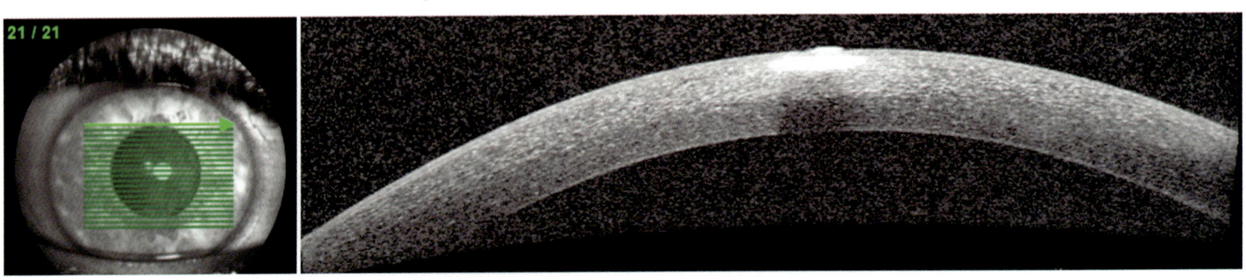

Fig. 19.1 Contact lens–related keratitis (CLRK). Although a variety of microbial agents (including fungal and acanthamoeba) may be implicated, bacterial CLRK remains most common. AS-OCT can be used to identify the location and depth of the infiltrate. In this image, the infiltrate is seen as a hyperreflective lesion limited to the subepithelial-anterior stromal space with overlying epithelial disruption. No additional lesions are seen. (Courtesy Albert Cheung, MD, Eastern Virginia Medical School, Norfolk, Virginia, United States.)

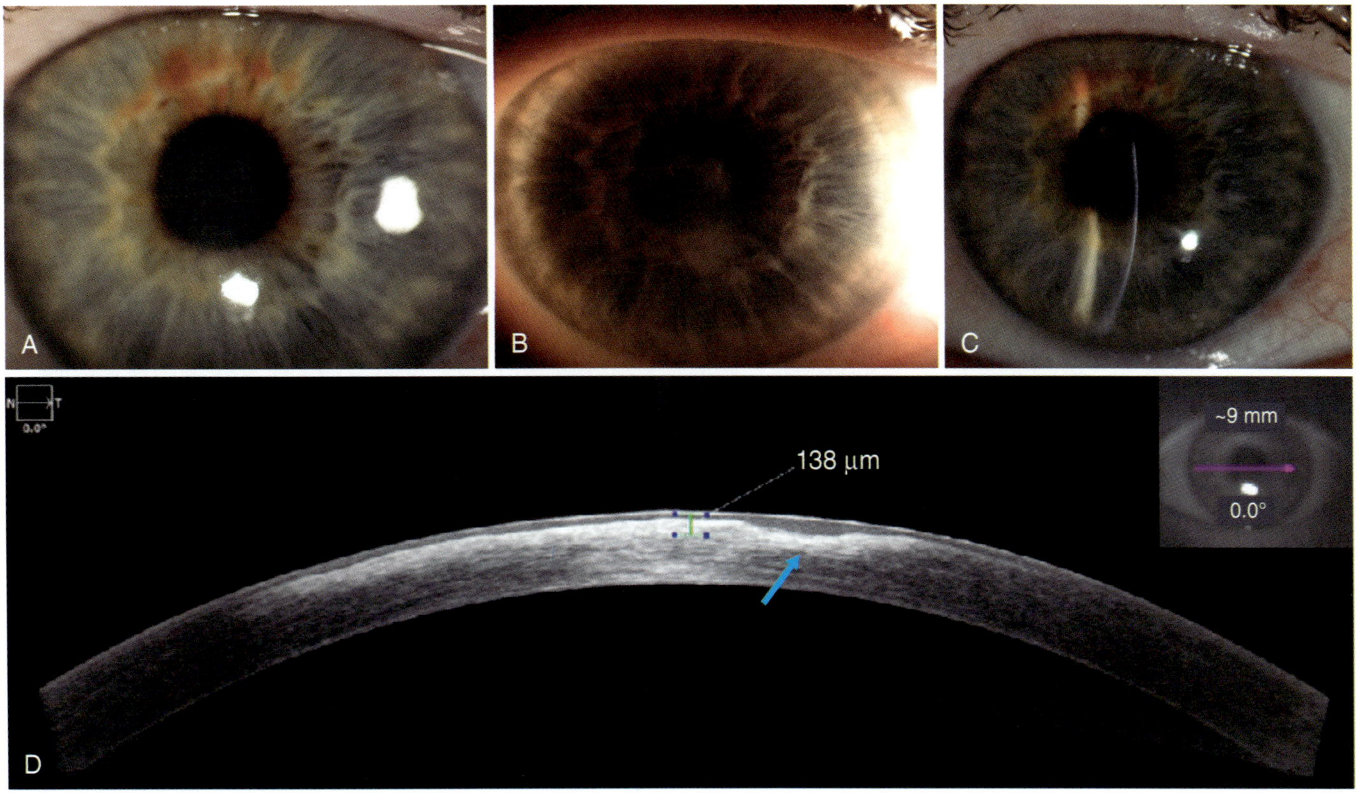

Fig. 19.2 Corneal scarring after treatment of bacterial corneal ulcer. Slit-lamp photograph in direct illumination *(panel A),* sclerotic scatter *(panel B)*, and thin slit-beam cross-section *(panel C)* show various features of the scar, including its partial light-blocking composition, nonhomogeneity, and limitation to the anterior cornea. AS-OCT through the visual axis shows the scarring as a band of hyperreflectivity limited to the anterior 140 to 150 microns of the cornea. Additionally, there is an area of deeper extension *(blue arrow)* with corresponding hypertrophy of the overlying epithelium to maintain a smooth outer corneal surface *(panel D)*.

a 63-year-old female patient was referred after successful treatment of a corneal ulcer with culture-positive *Staphylococcus epidermidis.* Visual acuity at the time of presentation was 20/500, and a 1+ to 2+ nuclear sclerotic cataract was also present. The patient was presented with several options, including scleral contact lens assessment, phototherapeutic keratectomy (PTK) to debulk the scarring followed by scleral contact lens assessment, and cataract extraction followed by scleral contact lens assessment. AS-OCT was helpful in this scenario because it showed that the scarring was limited to the anterior 140 to 150 microns of the cornea. The patient was successfully fitted with a scleral contact lens and achieved 20/40 vision; any further surgery was delayed indefinitely.

C. Pseudomonas Keratitis

The previous section discussed bacterial keratitis; however, pseudomonas keratitis merits additional discussion because of its frequent finding in a variety of settings, though it is more frequent in contact lens wearers with poor hygiene, overnight use, and exposure to water. Pseudomonas corneal infections may be particularly virulent because the bacteria are known to secrete proteases that can cause rapid necrosis of the cornea, leading to corneal thinning and perforation.

In addition to the previously discussed signs and symptoms of CLRK, patients usually present with significant mucopurulent discharge and profound vision loss. Slit-lamp examination findings include rapidly progressive ulceration with associated stromal inflammation, stromal thinning, and corneal edema. A central location is common, but peripheral locations also may be found. The tear film is usually filled with green-yellow exudates. A significant anterior chamber reaction, including hypopyon formation, may be present.

Treatment usually requires diagnostic cultures of the cornea (and contact lenses/cases if available); intense topical antibiotics, including fortified antibiotics, for centrally located and vision-threatening ulcers; and anticollagenase therapy (e.g., systemic doxycycline). The use of steroids is extremely controversial, and they should be used only once identification of the organism and clinical improvement have been confirmed. Severe cases may require therapeutic keratoplasty, especially if the infiltrate borders encroach on the limbus or sclera.

Fig. 19.3 shows images from a patient with a rapidly progressive, centrally located pseudomonas ulcer. Slit-lamp photography demonstrates significant thinning centrally with a peripheral ring of suppuration and profound corneal edema. AS-OCT images show significant corneal edema, loss of corneal architecture, and multiple areas of epithelial disruption. Despite treatment with fortified antibiotics, significant thinning was present and the decision was made to place amniotic membrane (AM). Fig. 19.4 shows slit-lamp photographs taken immediately after AM placement *(panels A and B);* AS-OCT taken two days later and one month later (*panels C and D,* respectively) show incorporation of the AM into the cornea with eventual remodeling during healing. One month later, the AM has melted and a significant scar remains.

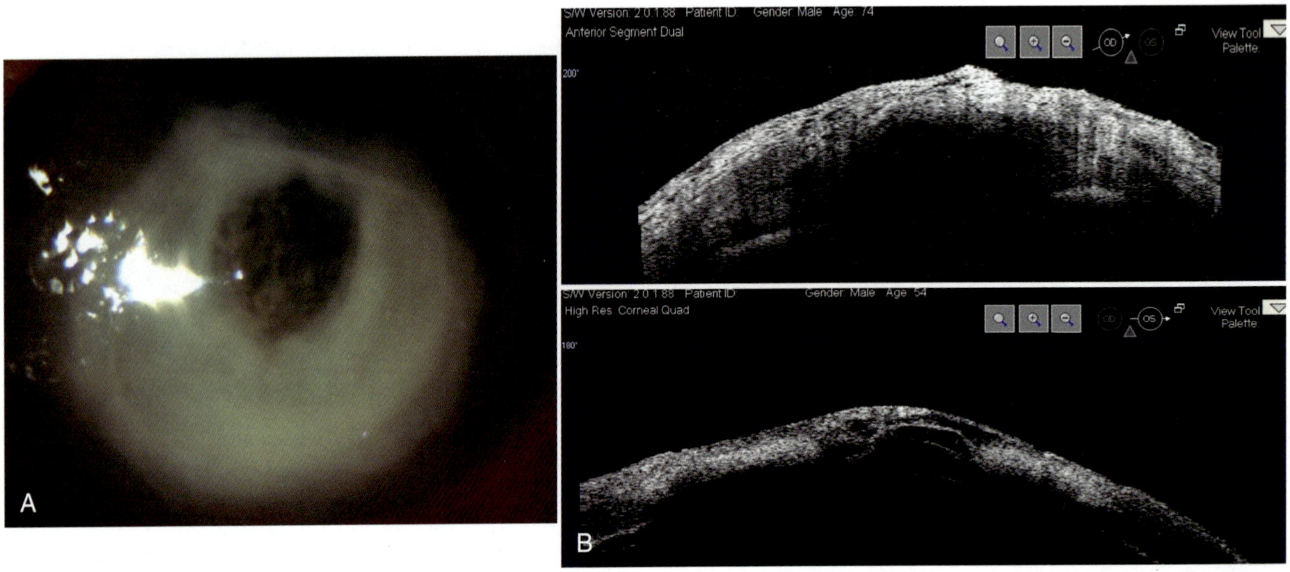

Fig. 19.3 Pseudomonas keratitis. Slit-lamp photograph displays a rapidly progressive pseudomonas ulcer with significant central thinning surrounded by a ring of suppurative inflammation and necrosis. AS-OCT images highlight the extent of stromal inflammation, corneal edema, loss of corneal architecture, and multiple areas of epithelial disruption.

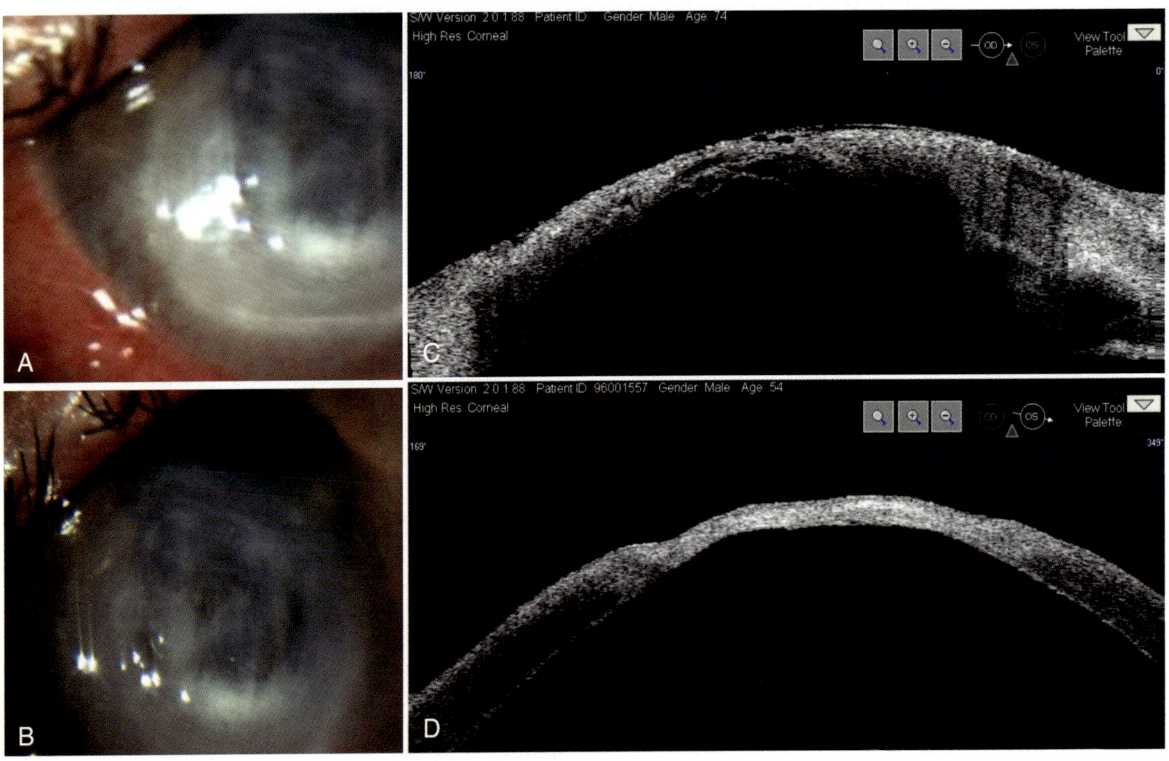

Fig. 19.4 For progression of the pseudomonas ulcer (shown in Fig. 19.2), amniotic membrane was placed *(panels A and B).* AS-OCT taken two days later *(panel C)* shows incorporation of the amniotic membrane (AM) into the cornea with improved epithelialization. After several weeks *(panel D),* the AM has melted and a corneal scar remains. Note the overall thinning and stromal compaction compared with the previous images. Full epithelialization is present, though the corneal surface remains significantly irregular.

> **CLINICAL PEARL**
>
> In cases of rapidly progressive ulcers, clinical examination may be limited because of patient cooperation or significant corneal inflammation/edema. In these instances, slit-lamp examination may be insufficient to determine the presence of severe, rapidly progressive corneal thinning and/or descemetocele. AS-OCT can be used to quickly determine the rate of stromal thinning. This may guide the clinician toward interventions such as tarsorrhaphy and amniotic membrane placement.

Fig. 19.5 shows images of another patient with progressively worse infection in which AM was placed because of severe stromal thinning with near descemetocele. Figs. 19.6 and 19.7 show AS-OCT raster images after AM placement that highlight the healing process as corneal edema and inflammation subside and scarring occurs. There is notable thinning after several months of healing. Fig. 19.8 shows serial AS-OCT images that demonstrate improvement of the suppurative process after AM

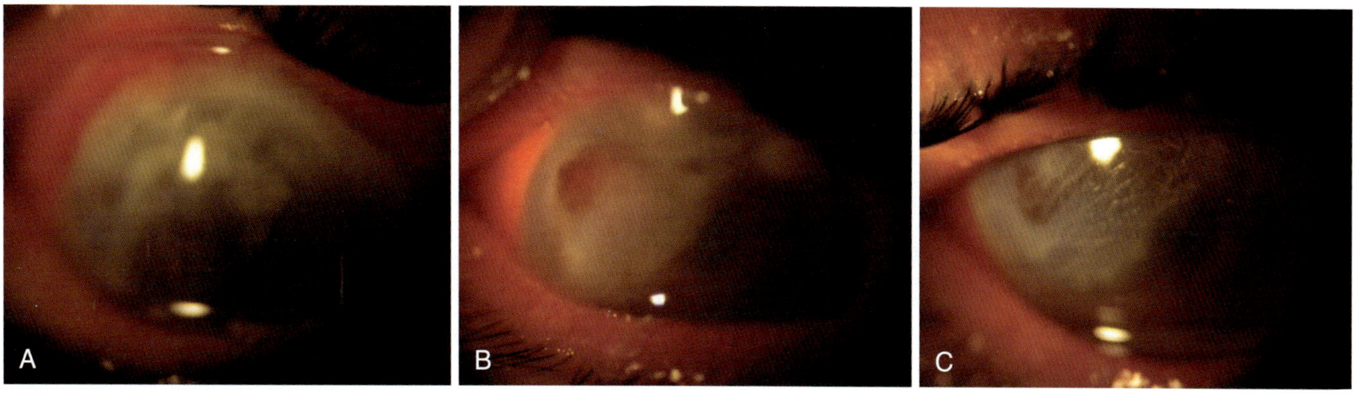

Fig. 19.5 Pseudomonas ulcer of the right eye in a patient who wears contact lenses. *Panel A* shows images taken at the time of referral after unsuccessful treatment by a primary eye care provider. Significant suppurative inflammation is present. Despite prompt initiation of fortified antibiotics (tobramycin), two days later, notable stromal thinning with borderline descemetocele was observed in the superotemporal cornea *(panel B)*. Amniotic membrane was placed to promote epithelialization and prevent further stromal ulceration *(panel C)*.

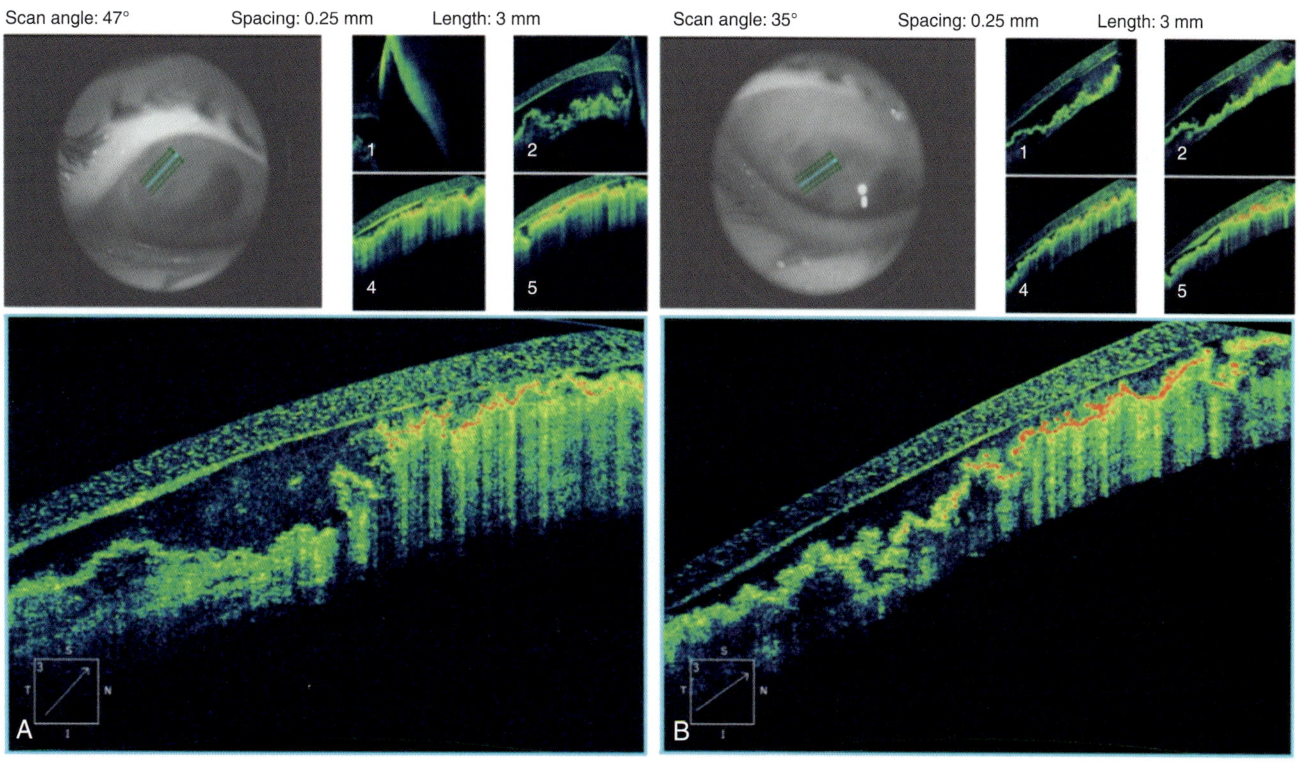

Fig. 19.6 Anterior segment raster images taken immediately after amniotic membrane transplant placement *(panel A)*. One week later, repeat raster image *(panel B)* shows interval improvement of the previously noted inflammation and thinning.

placement with stromal scarring initially; however, there is continued thinning and a descemetocele has formed nearly six months later. Fig. 19.9 shows preoperative and postoperative images of this patient who then underwent an eccentric penetrating keratoplasty (PKP) and cataract removal; three months later, there is significant improvement in corneal clarity. AS-OCT taken at this time (Fig. 19.10) shows restoration of corneal thickness though considerable central stromal scarring remains.

Fig. 19.11 shows serial images of another patient with pseudomonas keratitis who was successfully managed with medical therapy alone. AS-OCT images taken one month after presentation (Fig. 19.12) highlight areas of subepithelial/anterior stromal scarring with overlying epithelial irregularity. A partial light-blocking scar remains. Visual acuity was subsequently improved with scleral contact lenses several months later.

In other cases, despite successful therapy with topical antibiotics, stromal scarring with prominent extent and depth may be present. Fig. 19.13 shows AS-OCT images of a patient with deep stromal scarring after pseudomonal infection. Given the depth of scarring, it was determined that PTK would be insufficient to remove scarring. The patient was then referred for contact lens fitting but was unsuccessful and ultimately underwent PKP for visual rehabilitation.

D. Marginal Keratitis

Marginal keratitis is an inflammatory disease of the peripheral cornea that occurs as a result of epithelial breakdown and ulceration caused by eyelid and skin flora. Ocular surface disease, especially the presence of rosacea, meibomian gland dysfunction, and blepharitis, is strongly associated with this classically

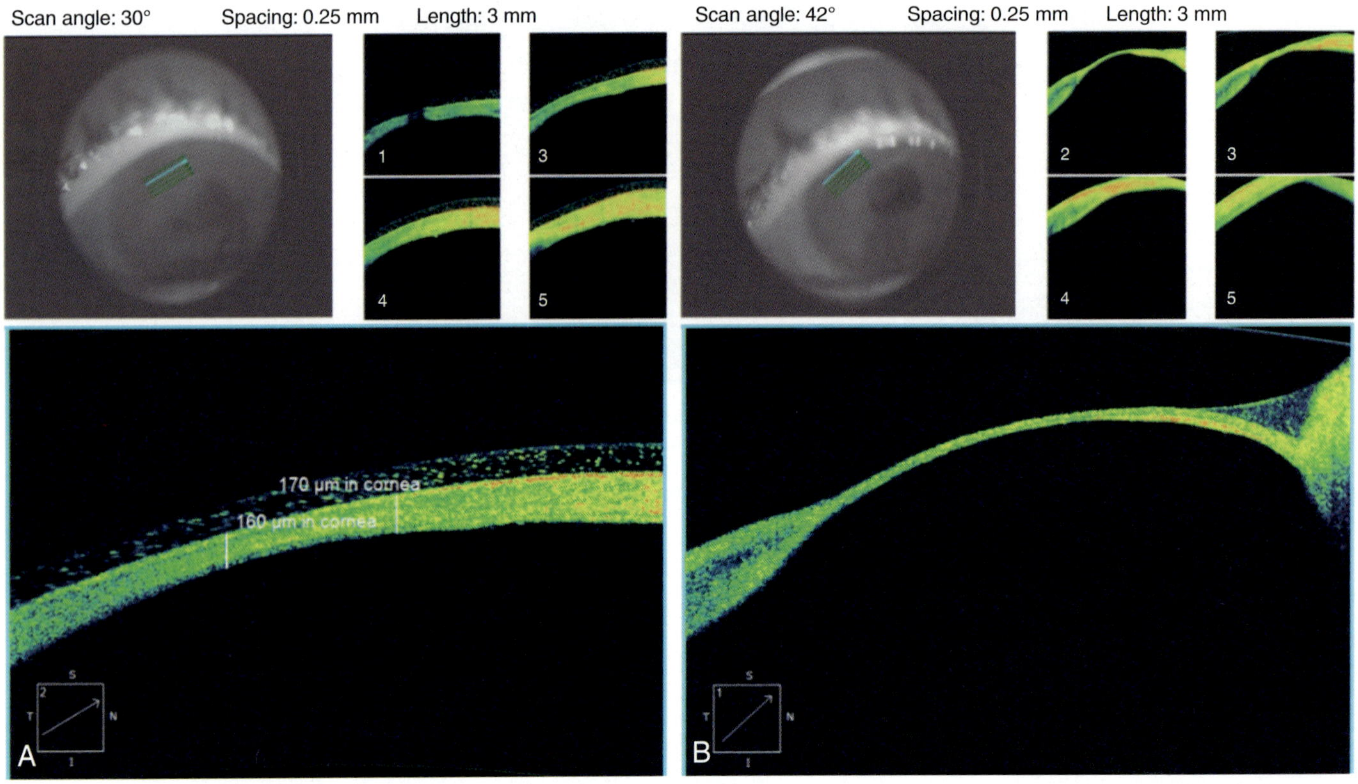

Fig. 19.7 Follow-up images taken at one month *(panel A)* and three months *(panel B).* There is considerable resolution of previously seen corneal edema and inflammation, though a markedly thinner cornea remains after scarring has completed.

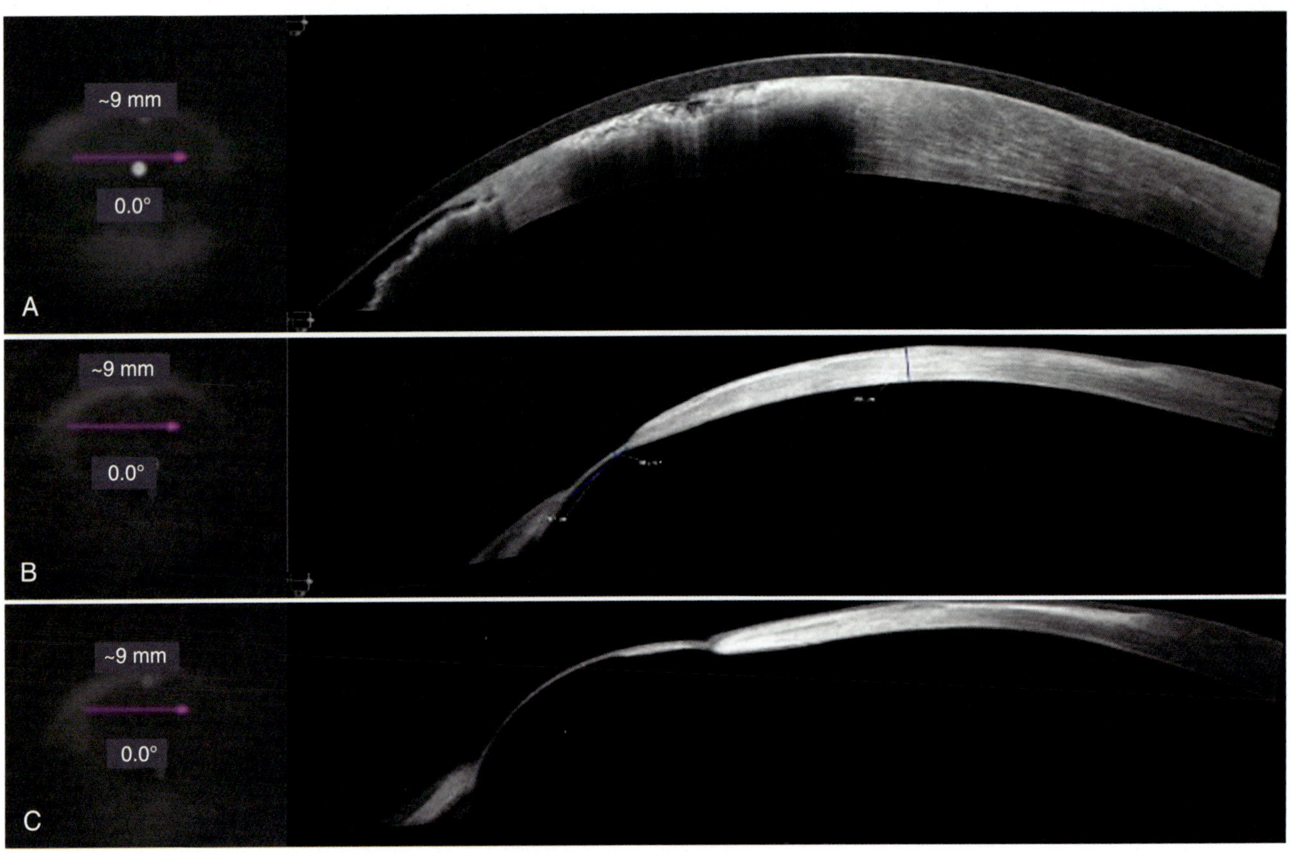

Fig. 19.8 Serial AS-OCT images of the patient from Fig. 19.4 at one week *(panel A),* one month *(panel B),* and six months *(panel C)* after amniotic membrane placement. Note the progressive improvement in corneal edema between one week and one month. However, there is continued thinning, and at six months after the infection, a descemetocele has formed. The overlying cornea remains extremely thin.

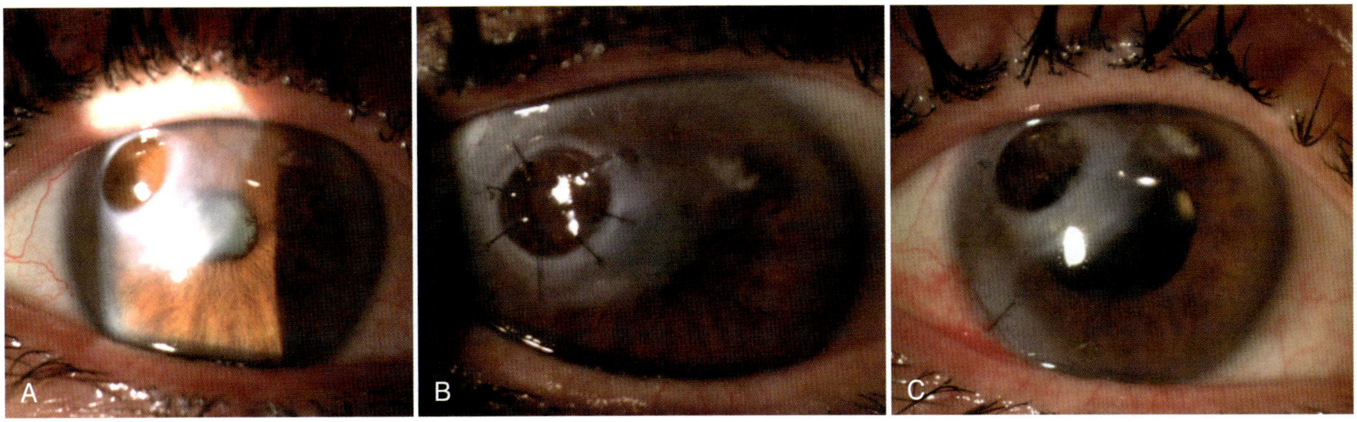

Fig. 19.9 Although the infectious process has nearly resolved, a descemetocele remains and the cornea was at risk for perforation *(panel A).* The patient underwent an eccentric penetrating keratoplasty combined with cataract extraction and intraocular lens placement. Immediate postoperative images are shown in *panel B.* Three months later *(panel C),* sutures were removed. There is notable and marked appearance in corneal clarity and visual acuity.

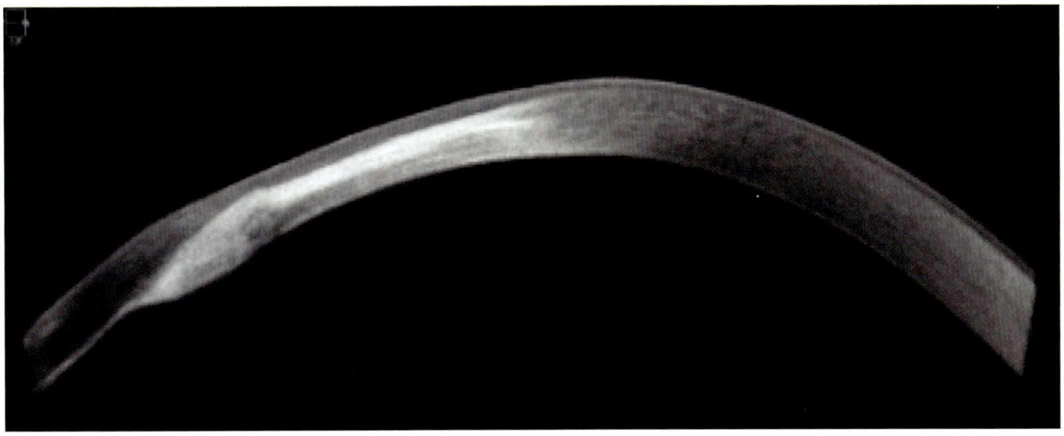

Fig. 19.10 AS-OCT taken three months after combined penetrating keratoplasty and cataract surgery. Restoration of corneal thickness is readily apparent though considerable stromal scarring remains.

peripheral keratitis. Bacterial antigens, especially those produced by *Staphylococcus aureus,* trigger a type III hypersensitivity reaction that causes lesions (immunocomplexes) to be deposited in the peripheral corneal stroma. Notably, there is an intervening "clear space" between the lesions and limbus.

Clinical examination is usually sufficient to identify stromal infiltrates in the peripheral cornea, classically located at the points of intersection between the eyelid margins and limbus (10-, 2-, 4-, and 8-o'clock positions). Treatment usually consists of typical management strategies for blepharitis and topical antibiotics and steroids with close observation.

Fig. 19.14 shows slit-lamp images of a patient with staphylococcal marginal keratitis *(panels A and B).* AS-OCT images highlight the multiple, discrete, focal lesions limited to the subepithelial and anterior stromal spaces. Notably, there is no ulceration of the overlying epithelium, though there is some focal elevation of the epithelium overlying several lesions.

E. Infectious Crystalline Keratopathy

Infectious crystalline keratopathy (ICK) is a slowly progressing keratitis characterized by needle-like branching opacities and an absence of corneal or anterior segment inflammation. ICK occurs more commonly in corneal grafts or otherwise immunocompromised corneas. Infective microorganisms enter the corneal stroma through an epithelial defect and proliferate. In ICK, the usual immune response is blunted by localized immunosuppression, allowing microorganisms to become sessile pathogens surrounded by biofilm, which results in a discrete keratitis with limited inflammation in the surrounding tissues. Although ICK is mostly associated with *Streptococcus* spp. (α-hemolytic *Streptococcus* is the most common cause).

Initial treatment consists of prolonged use of topical antibiotics along with tapering and/or cessation of topical steroid use. Many cases may require a repeat PKP or lamellar keratectomy despite appropriate antimicrobial therapy.

Fig. 19.15 shows the slit-lamp and AS-OCT images of a patient with ICK. AS-OCT can be used to assess the depth and location of ICK lesions. Notably, lesions are seen in the subepithelial and anterior stromal layers as focal areas of hyperreflectivity. The overlying epithelium may or may not be intact.

F. Nontuberculous Mycobacteria Keratitis

Nontuberculous mycobacteria (NTM) have become increasingly recognized as important causes of infectious keratitis. NTM

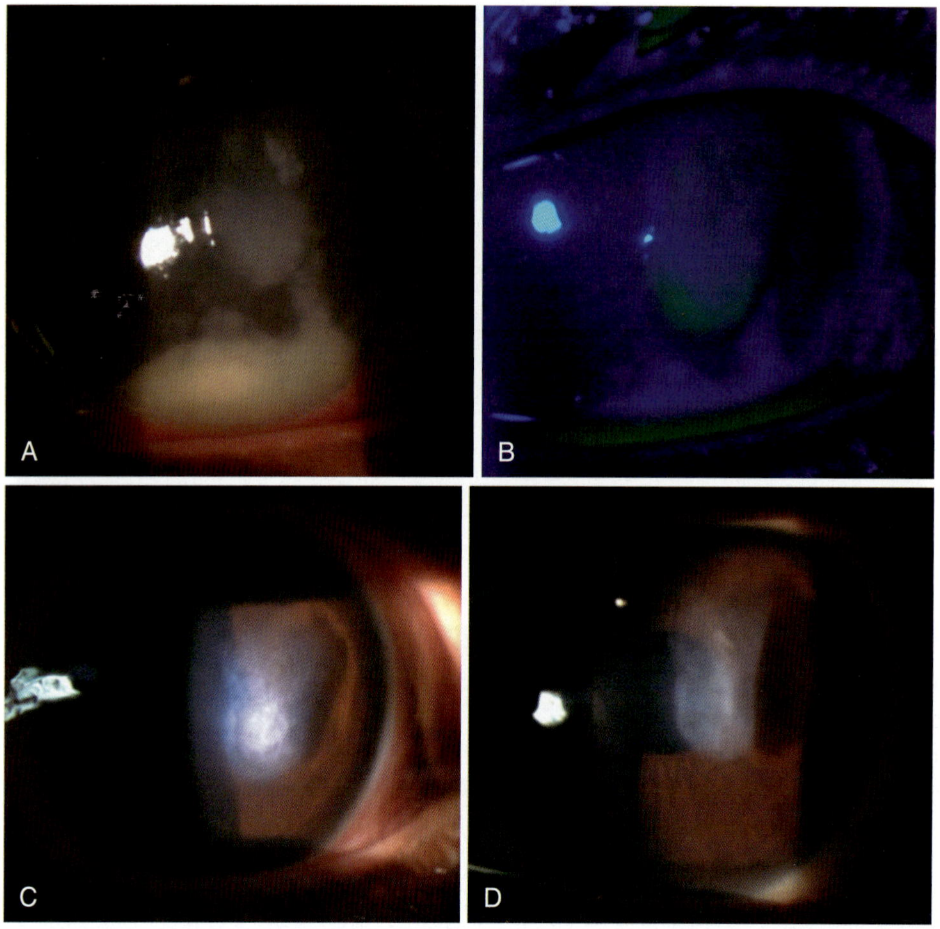

Fig. 19.11 Central pseudomonas ulcer with hypopyon. *Panels A and B* show images of the left eye of a patient who presented with corneal infiltrate with cultures positive for pseudomonas. The patient was promptly started on fortified antibiotics, including fortified tobramycin. Two weeks later *(panel C)*, there is notable improvement in the previously seen infiltrate. One month later *(panel D)*, the infiltrate has resolved and a partial light-blocking scar remains.

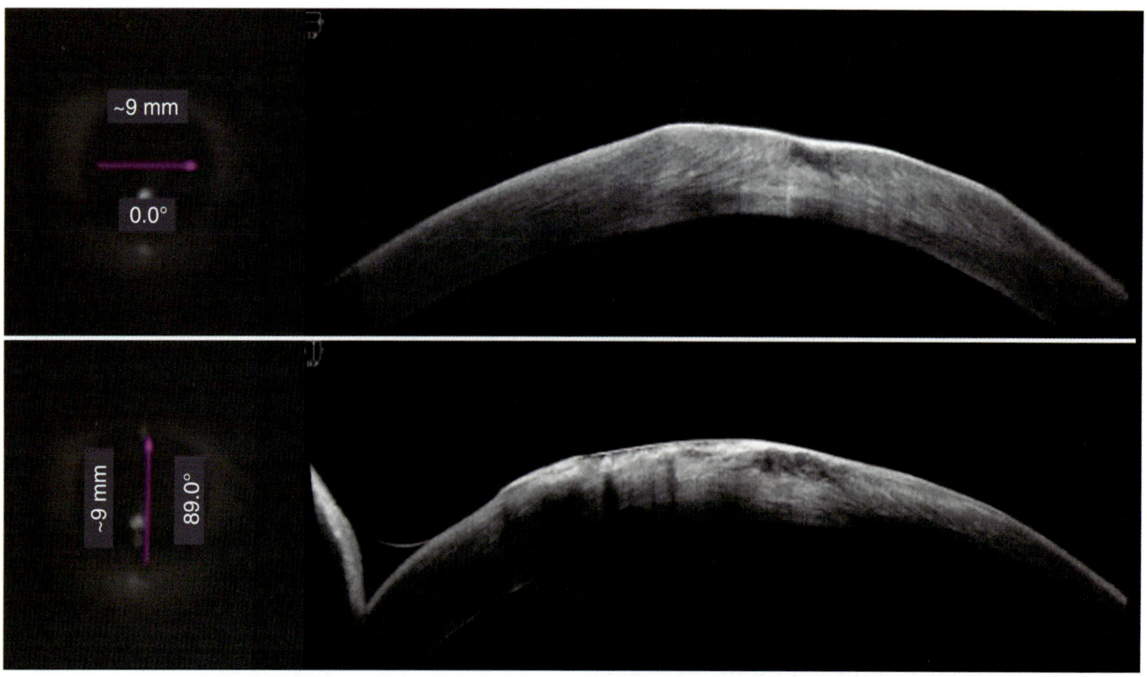

Fig. 19.12 AS-OCT images taken of the patient from Fig. 19.10 at one month after treatment initiation demonstrates epithelial irregularity with subepithelial and anterior stromal scarring.

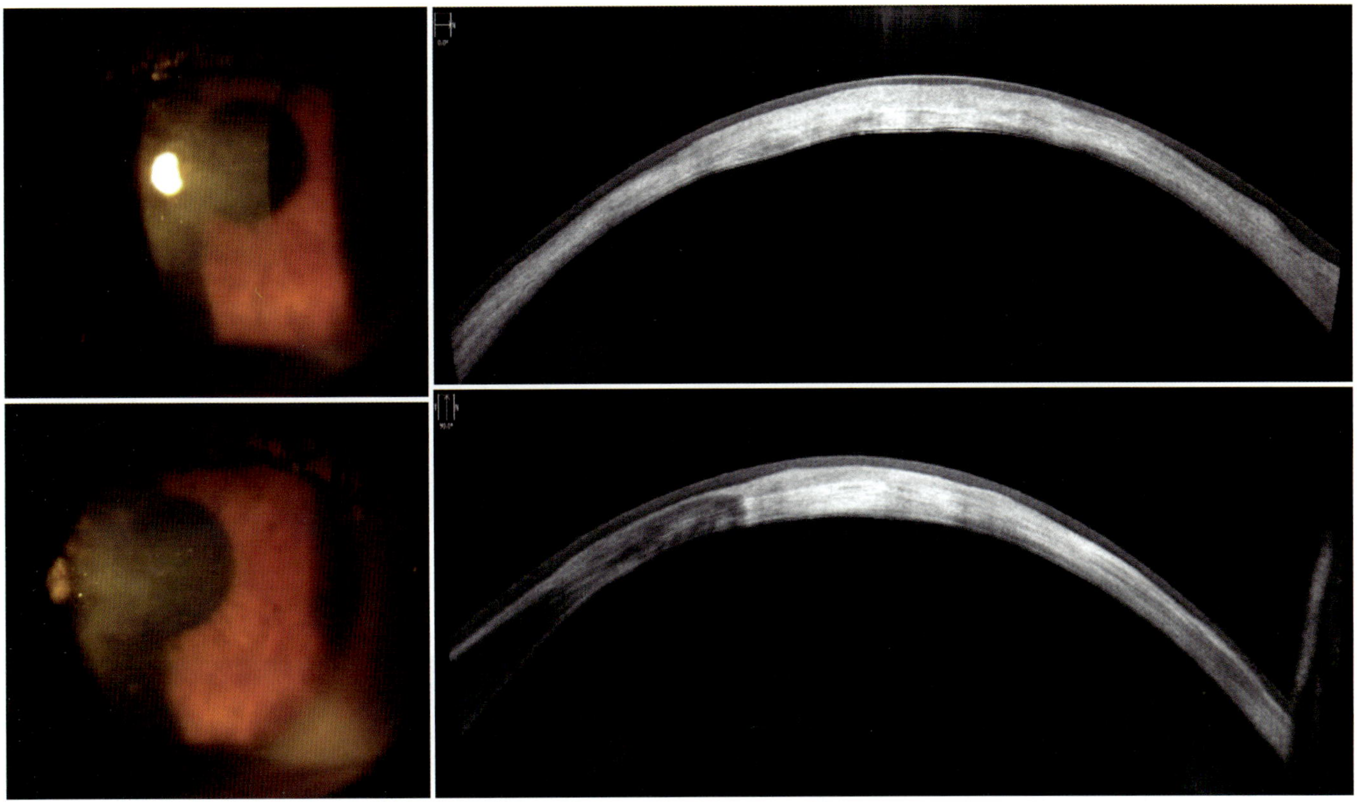

Fig. 19.13 AS-OCT of deep stromal scarring after medical treatment of pseudomonas keratitis. There is notable extension of the scarring into the deeper stromal layers. Contact lens fitting was unsuccessful, and the patient ultimately required penetrating keratoplasty.

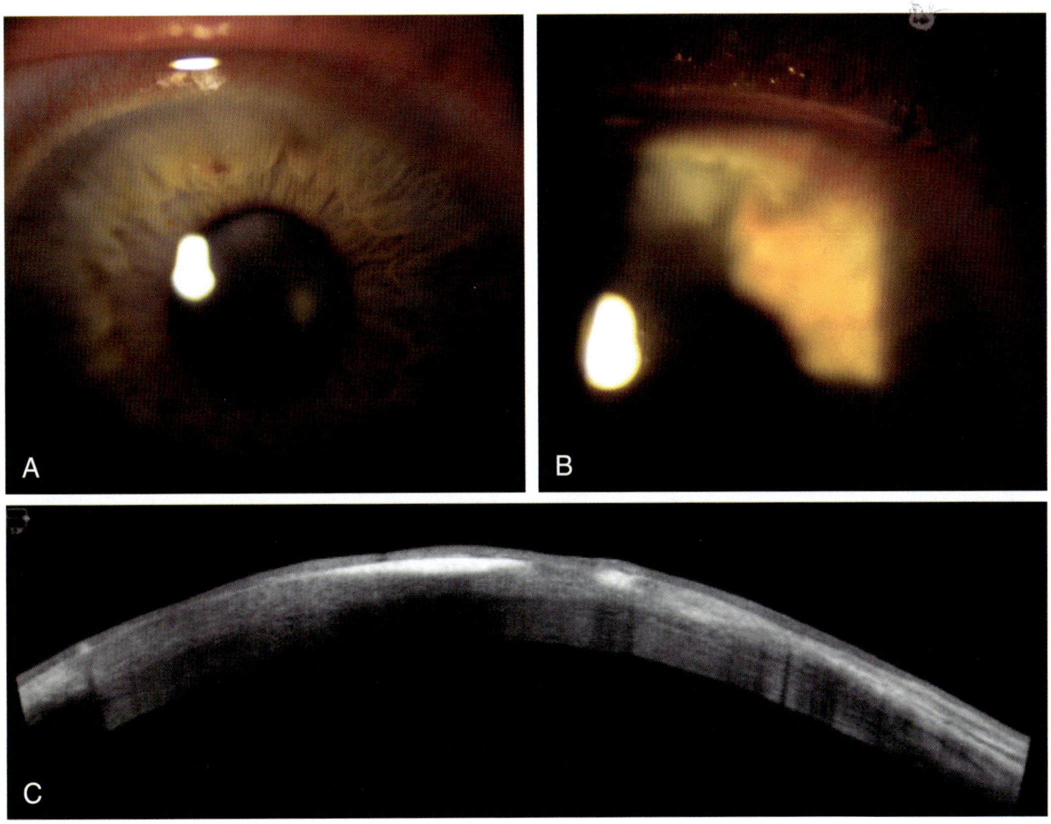

Fig. 19.14 Staphylococcal marginal keratitis. Slit-lamp images *(panels A and B)* show the appearance of peripheral corneal infiltrates without epithelial defect. AS-OCT images *(panels C–E)* demonstrate focal, discrete, hyperreflective lesions limited to the subepithelial and anterior stromal spaces. Notably, there is some elevation of the overlying epithelium over some of the lesions.

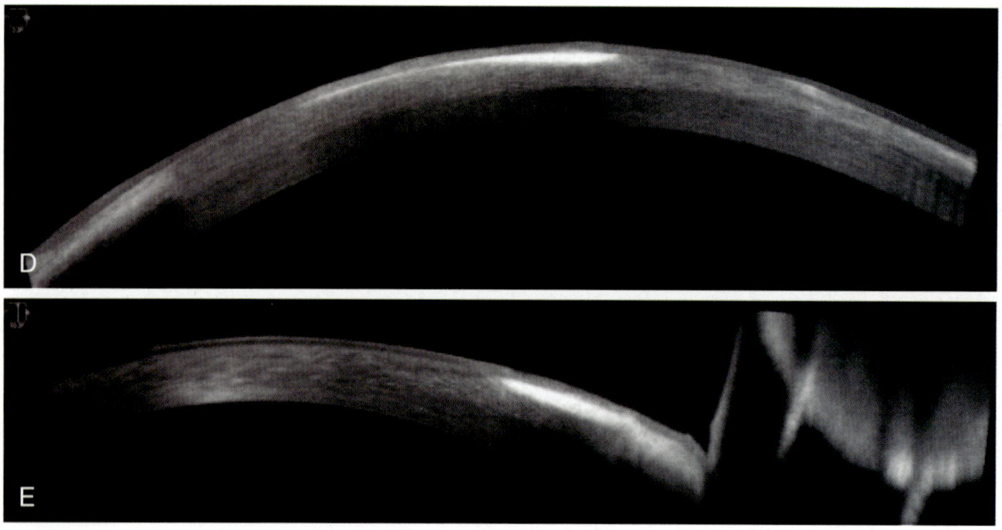

Fig. 19.14, cont'd

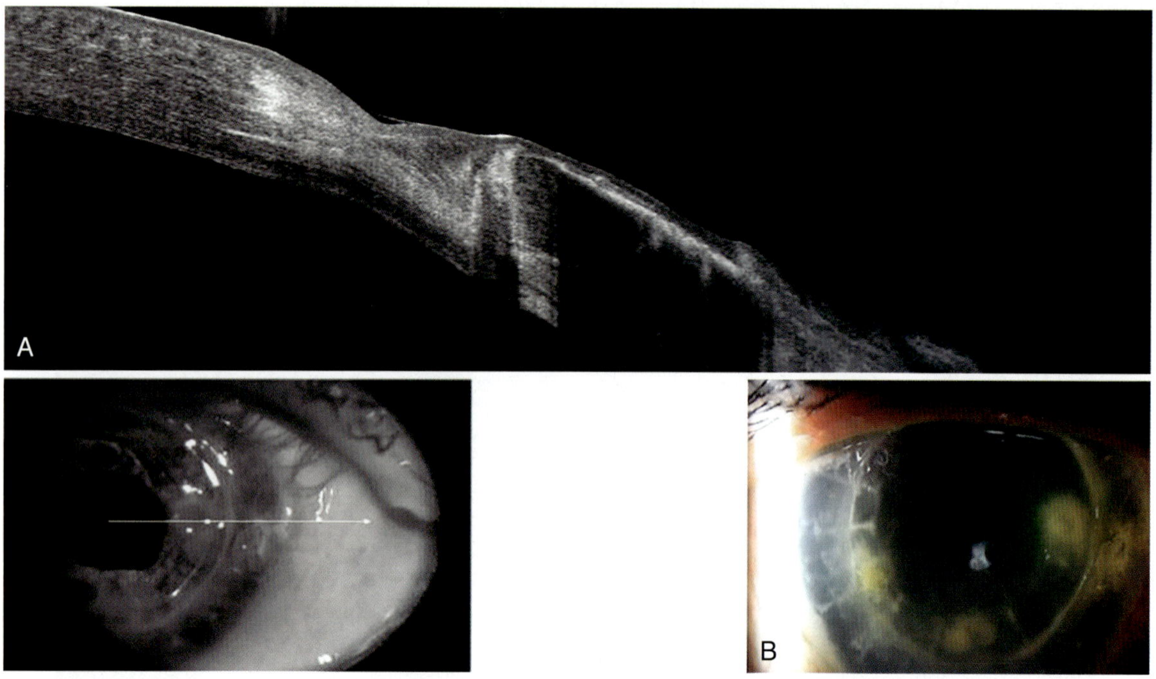

Fig. 19.15 Infectious crystalline keratopathy (ICK) secondary to infection with *Streptococcus viridans* in a patient with prior penetrating keratoplasty. *Panel A* shows appearance of ICK lesion at three-o'clock location on the cornea. The lesion appears as a prominently hyperreflective area within the anterior stroma. This corresponds to the slit-lamp image shown in *panel B,* which shows multiple infiltrates at three-, six-, and eight-o'clock locations. The white, arborizing, crystalline infiltrates are present in the anterior third of the corneal stromal underneath the epithelial defects.

keratitis is largely caused (83.5%) by two subgroups: *Mycobacterium fortuitum* and *Mycobacterium chelonae–abscessus.* NTM are present in natural waters and soils worldwide.

Similar to ICK, an important pathogenic property of NTM is in their ability to develop biofilm that protects bacteria from disinfectants and facilitates their attachment to the surface interface. As a result, they can survive in artificial environments, such as daily water distribution systems in operating theaters and swimming pools.

Patients with NTM keratitis often have a history of trauma with corneal foreign bodies or ocular surgery. The cases can be divided into two main groups, post-LASIK and non–LASIK-related groups.[1] The simultaneous use of multiple culture media, including Löwenstein–Jensen medium, blood agar, MacConkey agar, and Middlebrook media, aids in the identification of specific NTM, particularly the slow growers.

NTM infections are very difficult to eradicate, have poor response to treatment, and require long-term treatment with a combination of two or more drugs. Triple therapy with amikacin, topical clarithromycin, and fourth-generation fluoroquinolones is suggested for treatment. Systemic antibiotics, such as clarithromycin and doxycycline, also may be used for recalcitrant cases. Topical steroids should be avoided as much as possible.

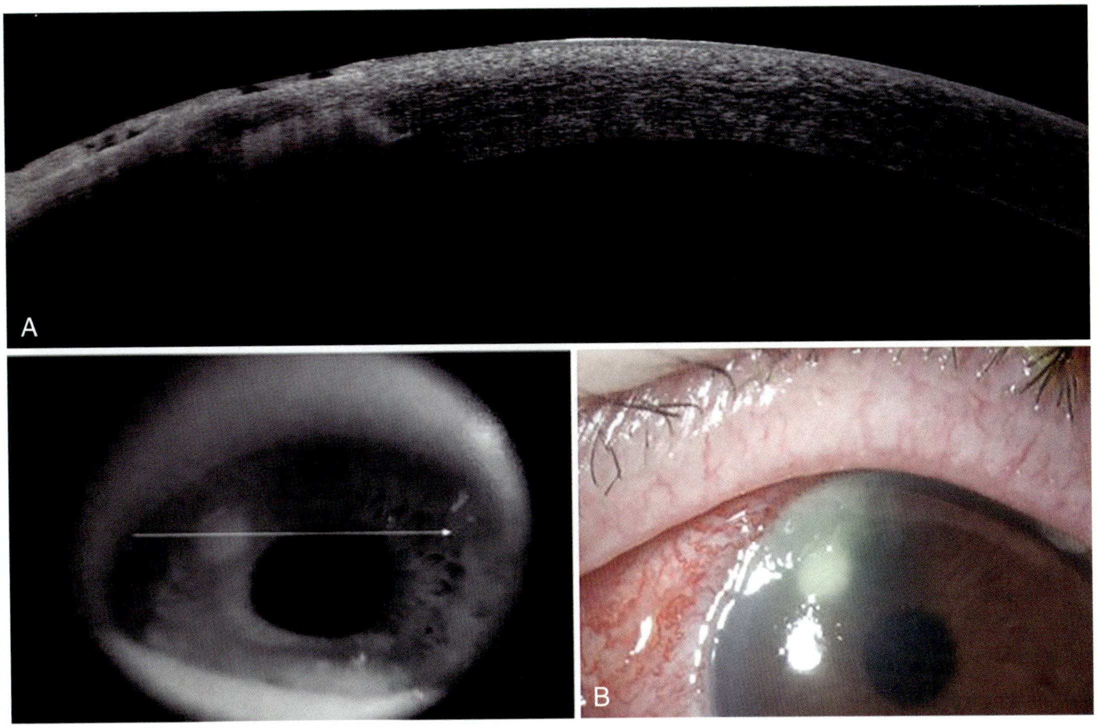

Fig. 19.16 Nontuberculous mycobacteria (NTM) keratitis. *Panel A* shows AS-OCT images of a patient with NTM keratitis. Notably, there is a stromal infiltrate with considerable surrounding stromal inflammation. The overlying epithelium is disrupted. Accompanying slit-lamp photograph *(panel B)* shows the clinical appearance of the stromal infiltrate near the superior limbus with overlying epithelial defect and prominent conjunctival injection.

Fig. 19.16 displays images of a patient with NTM keratitis. The AS-OCT image *(panel A)* highlights the stromal infiltrate with surrounding inflammation and overlying epithelial defect that correspond to the stromal infiltrate seen on slit-lamp images *(panel B)*.

III. VIRAL INFECTIONS

A. Herpes Simplex

Herpes simplex virus type 1 (HSV-1) is the leading cause of infectious blindness in the developed world. It is estimated that 50% of adults are seropositive for the HSV antigen in the United States with approximately 500,000 cases of active ocular HSV infections seen annually. The mechanism of infection may be primary or secondary. Primary infection occurs by way of direct contact between mucous membranes, and secondary infection (which accounts for most cases) occurs as a result of reactivation of a latent HSV infection that is usually triggered by environmental factors or immunosuppressed states. It can involve any part of the eye but predominantly affects the cornea, particularly the epithelium (60%) and the stroma (20%–48%). It has a relapsing and remitting course that renders the greatest morbidity through corneal scarring and neovascularization.

I. EPITHELIAL AND STROMAL KERATITIS

Epithelial keratitis begins as a punctate defect that evolves into a branching lesion with terminal bulbs (dendritic ulcer) that may coalesce to form a geographic ulcer (Fig. 19.17).

Nummular keratitis can occur as a feature of any viral keratoconjunctivitis, including herpetic infections. Nummular lesions appear as coin-shaped anterior stromal infiltrates that appear as granular deposits surrounded by stromal haze. There is likely considerable overlap in disease pathophysiology between nummular keratitis–like clinical presentation from HSV compared with stromal (interstitial) keratitis discussed later. Fig. 19.18 displays images of a patient with HSV-associated nummular keratitis with associated corneal neovascularization. Coin-shaped stromal opacities are seen in the superior corneas of both eyes with temporal stromal neovascularization on slit-lamp examination. AS-OCT demonstrates subepithelial opacity as areas of increased hyperreflectivity. Treatment with systemic valacyclovir and topical prednisolone acetate was sufficient for resolution of symptoms and return of 20/20 visual acuity.

Stromal keratitis can be necrotizing or nonnecrotizing and may occur without a history of epithelial keratitis, thus manifesting with an intact epithelium. Stromal inflammation may be focal, multifocal, or diffuse and may be associated with anterior uveitis. The inflammation may lead to stromal scarring, thinning, neovascularization, and lipid deposition. Stromal neovascularization may be sectorial or diffuse and affect several layers of the cornea. Fig. 19.19 shows slit-lamp and AS-OCT raster images of a patient with mild stromal keratitis. Notably, there is an intact epithelium with a minimal, focal subepithelial infiltrate that presents with increased hyperreflectivity in the AS-OCT image. This is contrasted with Fig. 19.20, which presents images from a more severe presentation of stromal keratitis. AS-OCT images *(panel A)* show significant stromal thinning from necrotic, melting processes with intact overlying epithelium that can be readily seen on slit-lamp examination *(panel B)*. Notably, there is significant sectoral neovascularization with corneal edema extending toward and involving the central visual axis.

Patients with HSV stromal keratitis can often present with repeated episodes of reactivation, corneal inflammation, and lipid keratopathy. In Figs. 19.21 to 19.23, serial images of a patient with HSV lipid keratopathy are shown. In Fig. 19.21

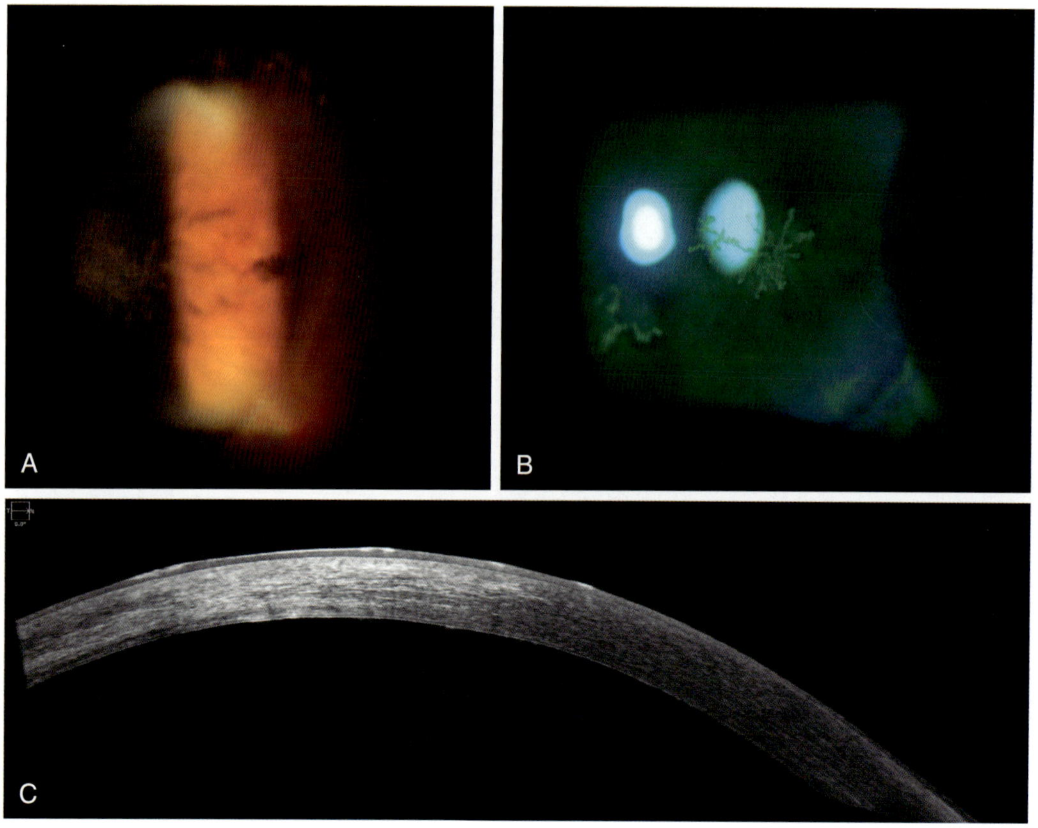

Fig. 19.17 Slit-lamp photographs of dendrites seen in herpes simplex virus epithelial keratitis (Panels A and B). AS-OCT (Panel C) image demonstrates areas of focal hyperreflectivity in the epithelium.

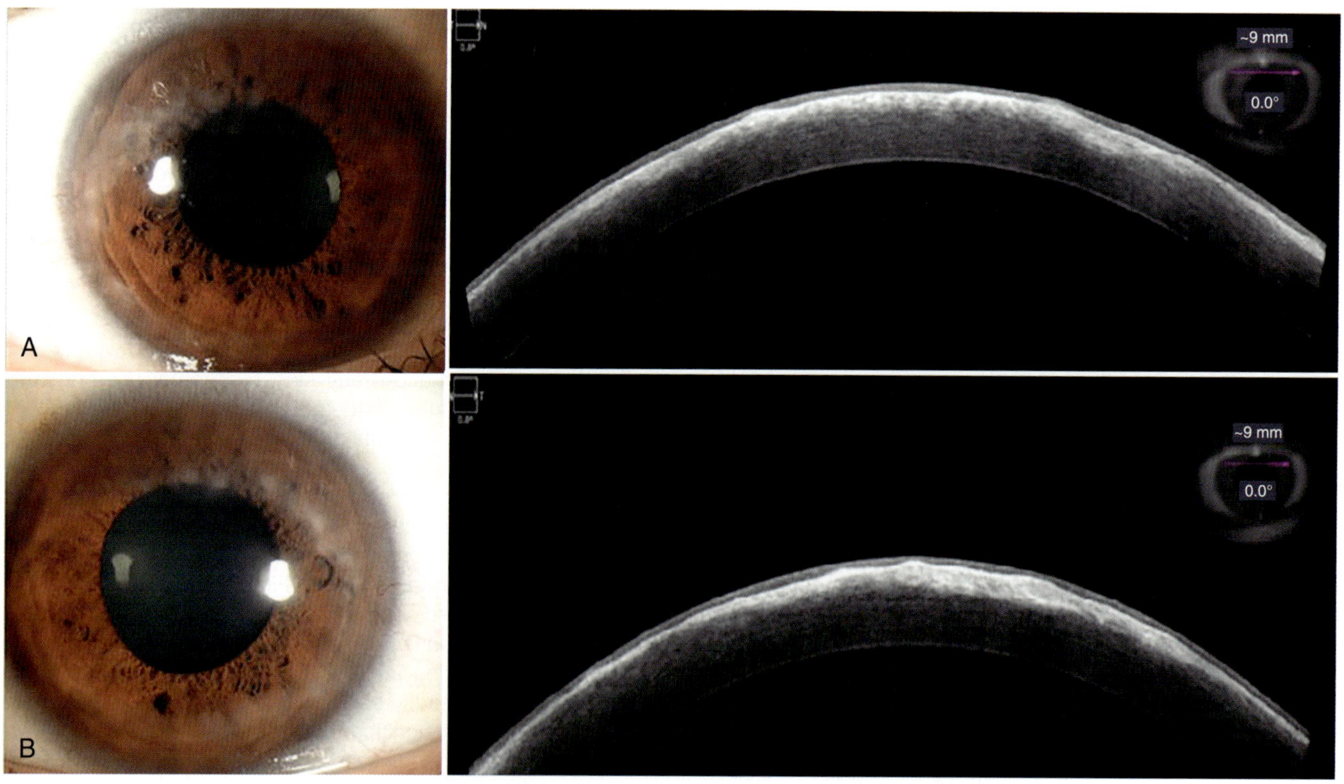

Fig. 19.18 Herpes simplex virus–associated nummular keratitis. Slit-lamp image of the right eye *(panel A)* demonstrates an area of sectoral neovascularization temporally with associated nummular lesions with haze. There are some interval areas of clear space seen. Accompanying AS-OCT through the area of interest shows the stromal opacities as a prominent area of hyperreflectivity with focal disruptions of the Bowman layer. There is some extension into the middle stromal layers. Notably, the overlying epithelium is intact. Similar features are seen in the left eye *(panel B)* slit-lamp and AS-OCT images.

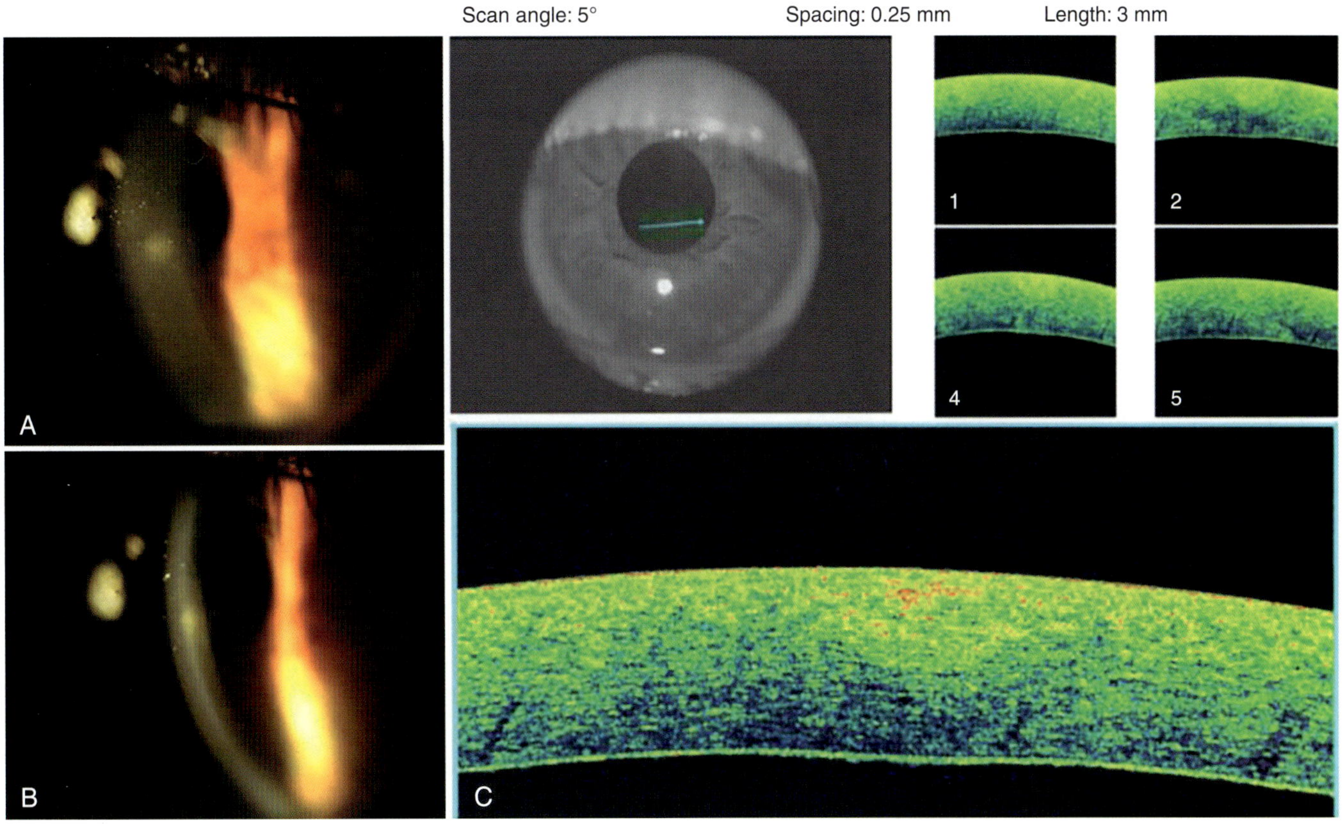

Fig. 19.19 Slit-lamp photographs *(panels A and B)* of a patient with mild HSV-related stromal keratitis. The overlying epithelium is intact, and a focal, minimally light-blocking infiltrate is present. On AS-OCT raster images *(panel C),* the observed lesion is seen as a focal, intense area of increased hyperreflectivity.

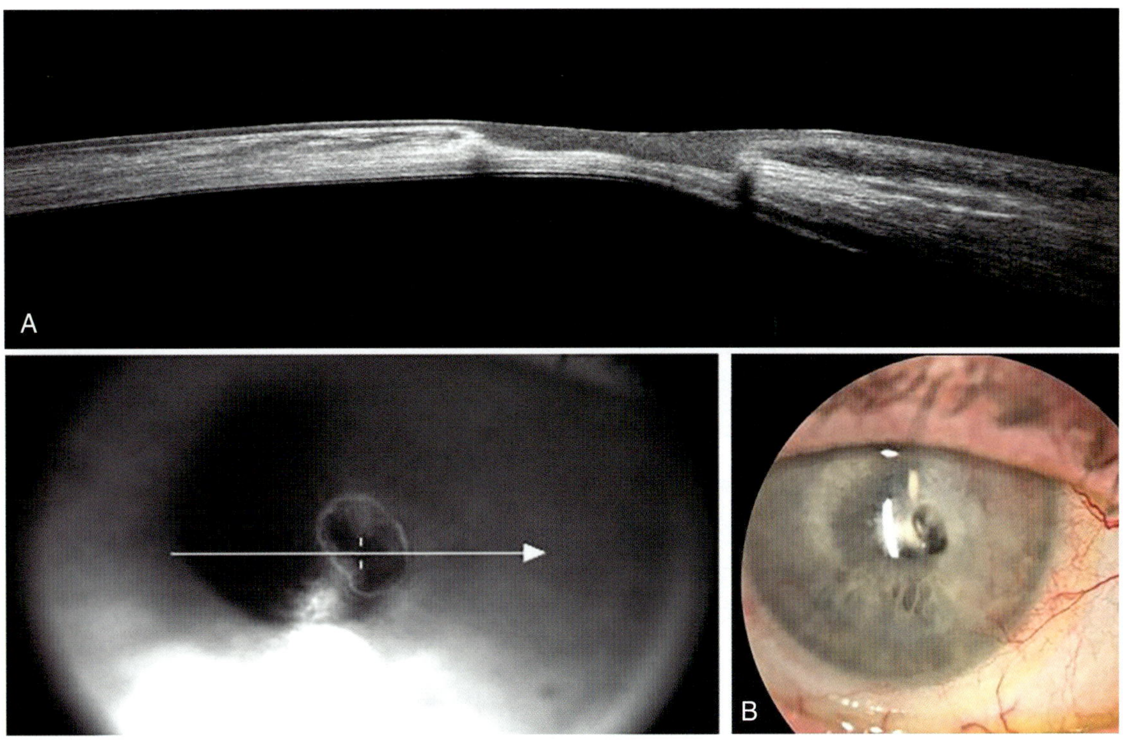

Fig. 19.20 Severe case of herpes simplex virus stromal keratitis with stromal thinning and melting. AS-OCT image *(panel A)* highlights the extent of stromal thinning with an intact overlying epithelium. There is increased edema (hyporeflectivity) temporally. These findings correspond with the clinical features seen on slit-lamp examination *(panel B),* which additionally shows areas of sectoral corneal neovascularization, thinning, and associated edema.

OD

OS

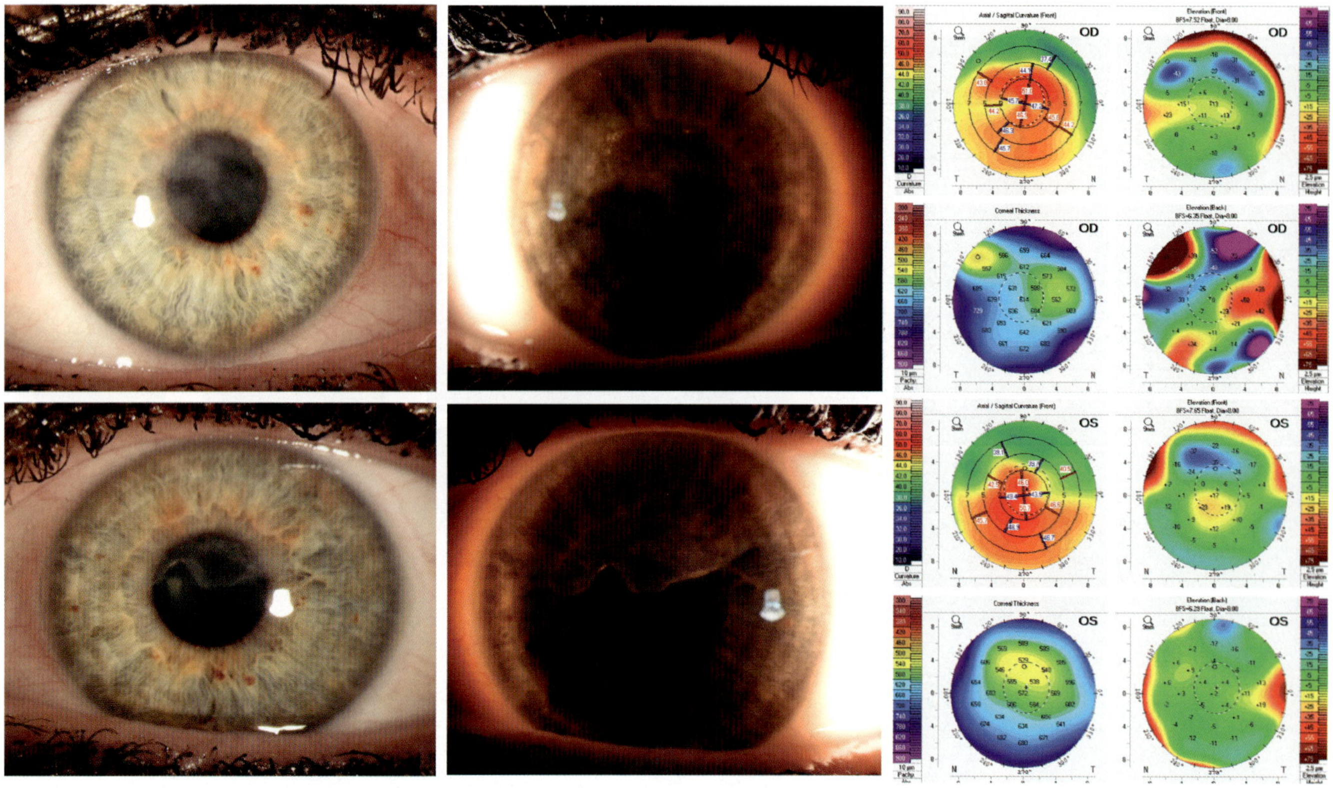

Fig. 19.21 Herpes simplex virus stromal keratitis with lipid keratopathy. Slit-lamp photographs of both eyes demonstrate involvement of the superior stroma with a wavelike region of superior anterior stromal opacification with partial light-blocking effect. There are prominent areas of thicker lipid deposition within the superior opacity and a leading edge of finer, thinner lipid deposits extending into the visual axis. Tomography images of both eyes reveal the presence of significant irregular astigmatism and front surface changes.

OD, IR 20° ART + OCT 15° Q: 30 [HR]

OS, IR 20° ART + OCT 15° Q: 28 [HR]

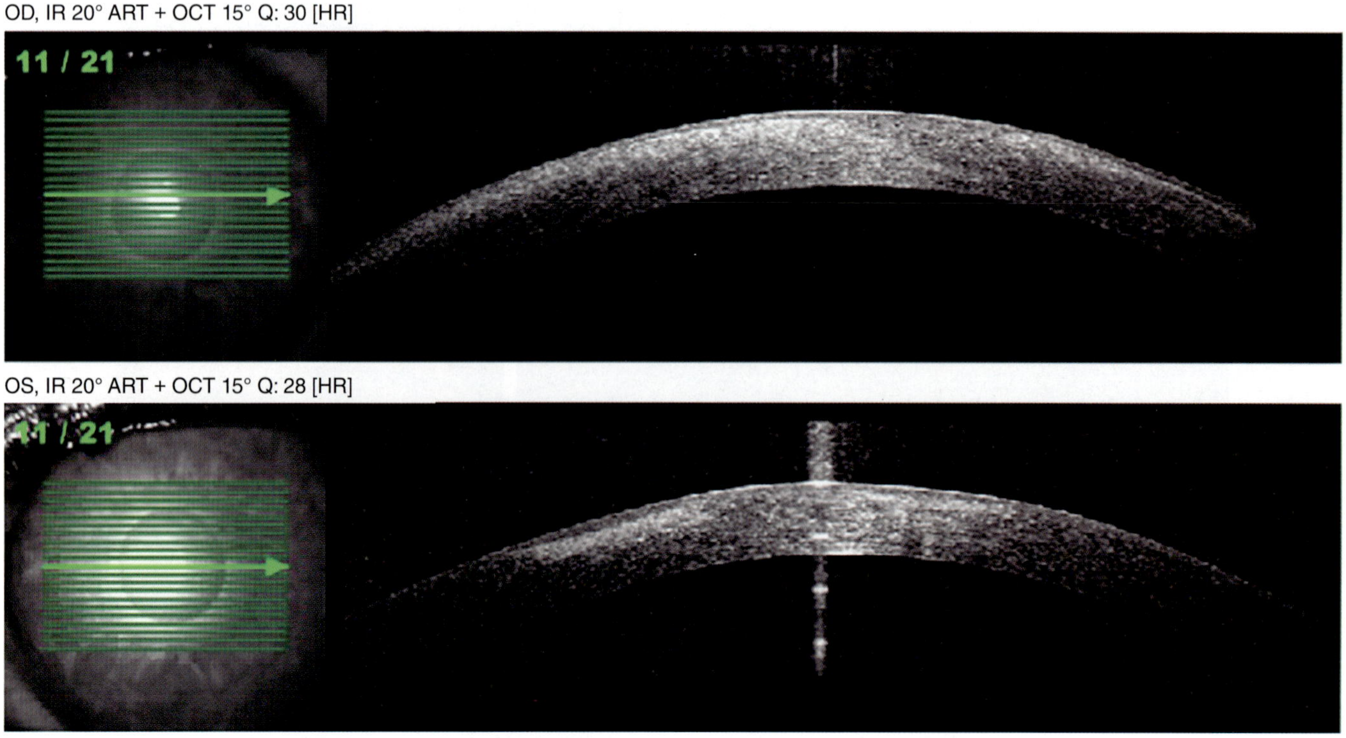

Fig. 19.22 AS-OCT images of the patient shown in Fig. 19.21. Stromal opacity corresponds to increased areas of hyperreflectivity.

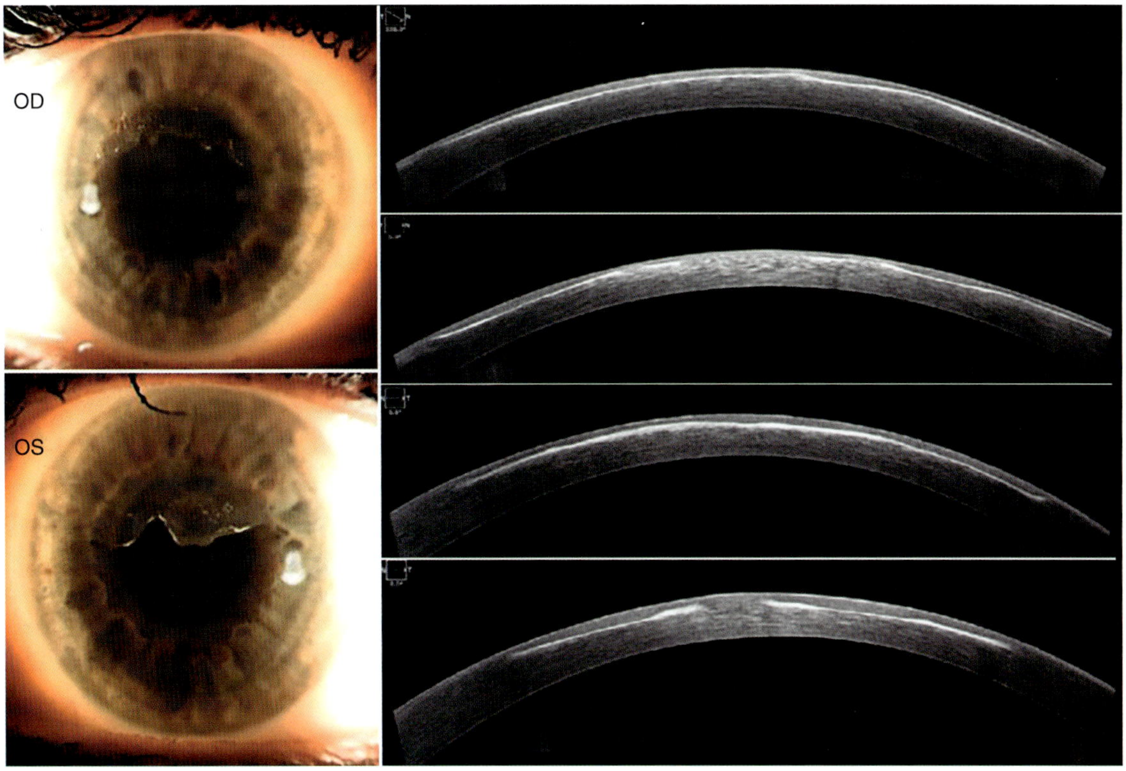

Fig. 19.23 Herpes simplex virus stromal keratitis with lipid keratopathy after treatment with systemic antivirals and topical steroids. Slit-lamp photographs of the right and left eye demonstrate interval resolution and improvement of previously seen stromal opacity with near-resolution of denser lipid deposits. The thin and fine lipid deposits at the leading edge remain essentially similar. AS-OCT images through the areas of interest show stromal compaction and scarring evidenced by areas of hyperreflectivity primarily located in the anterior stroma. The overlying epithelium is normal.

taken at the time of presentation, there is a significant area of sectoral stromal inflammation with leading edge of lipid deposition superiorly in both eyes. Corresponding tomography images are also shown. Fig. 19.22 shows AS-OCT images taken at the time of presentation highlighting multiple areas of stromal hyperreflectivity corresponding to the changes seen on clinical examination. After treatment with systemic antivirals and topical steroids, repeat images taken three months later (Fig. 19.23) show improvement of lipid deposition on clinical examination. AS-OCT is notable for consolidation and increased hyperreflectivity corresponding to the areas of inactive subepithelial fibrosis and scarring that primarily involve the anterior stroma. The overlying epithelium is thickened, but intact images of a patient with repeated stromal keratitis are shown.

CLINICAL PEARL

For patients with HSV-related scarring limited to the subepithelium/anterior stroma, AS-OCT can be used to measure the depth of lesions. After a period of quiescence, PTK may be cautiously performed with appropriate antiviral prophylaxis and/or treatment, to decrease corneal scarring and facilitate visual rehabilitation with glasses and/or contact lenses.

II. ENDOTHELIITIS

There is often considerable overlap between stromal keratitis and endotheliitis because HSV can have protean manifestations in the cornea and anterior segment. Often, stromal opacity and inflammation occur with both stromal keratitis and endotheliitis, and thus the two entities may be difficult to separate clinically.

Endotheliitis from HSV infection may occur either as a result of direct infection of endothelial cells or secondary to inflammation caused by the virus. Fig. 19.24 shows slit-lamp photographs and AS-OCT images of a patient with HSV endotheliitis. Although there is some stromal edema and folds, there is a notable lack of prominent infiltrate as seen in the previous images of stromal keratitis. Focal areas of endothelial disease are subtle on slit-lamp images *(panels A and B).* AS-OCT *(panels C–E)* can be used to further identify areas of focal endothelial disease and assess response to antiviral and antiinflammatory treatment. Fig. 19.25 shows an AS-OCT image of a different patient with endotheliitis. Multiple hyperreflective lesions with focal outpouching can be seen on this image.

III. SCARRING

Stromal scarring can occur despite adequate treatment, especially in recurrent cases. Corneal neovascularization may additionally accompany scarring, and these vessels may leak proteins and exudates in and around the scar. Fig. 19.26 shows images of a patient with marked subepithelial and anterior stromal scarring, neovascularization, and pigmentary epithelial changes as a response to chronic and recurrent HSV stromal keratitis. AS-OCT images highlight both local and global changes of the scarring. In this patient, the scarring extended to approximately two-thirds of the cornea.

Stromal scarring can additionally be challenging, as the depth and extent of lesions may be difficult to assess on clinical examination alone. In these cases, AS-OCT can be used to provide both “global” (high-definition [HD]-OCT) and “regional” (raster) views of the area(s) of interest that may help

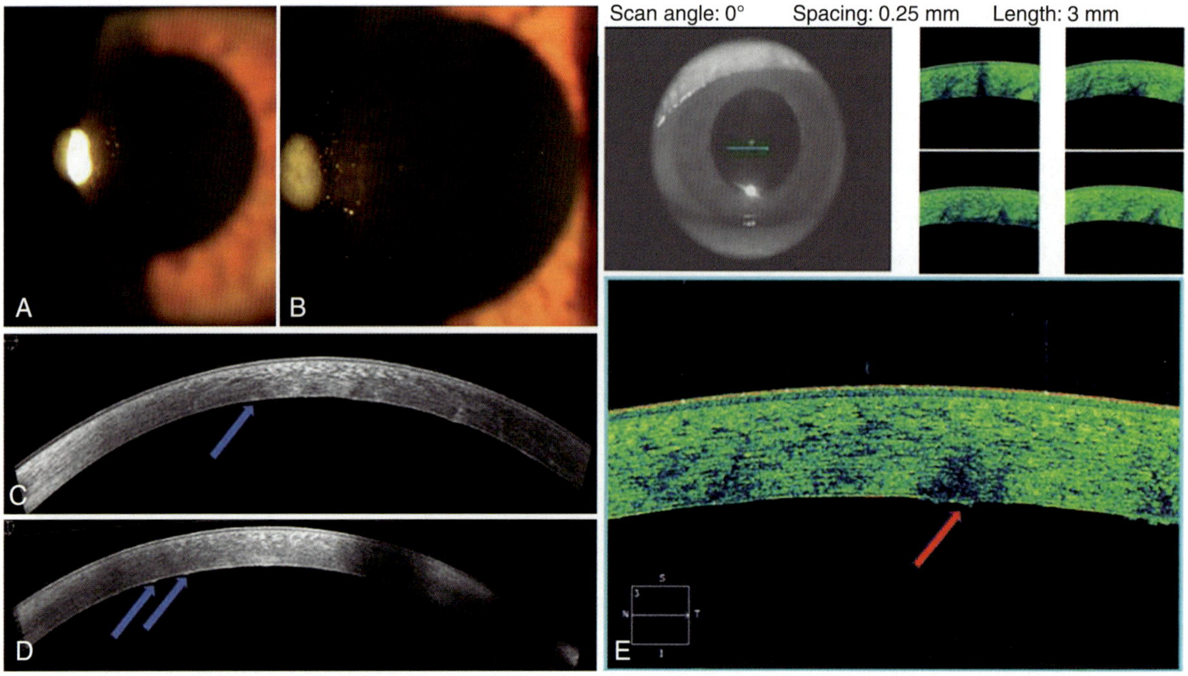

Fig. 19.24 Herpes simplex virus (HSV) endotheliitis. Slit-lamp findings in HSV endotheliitis *(panels A and B)* may be subtle and include corneal edema and focal endothelial opacities. In such cases, AS-OCT *(panels C and D)* can highlight areas of focal endothelial disease that are fleck-like areas of hyperreflectivity *(blue arrows)* in the endothelium. AS-OCT raster images *(panel E)* can show an outpouching of the endothelium *(red arrow).*

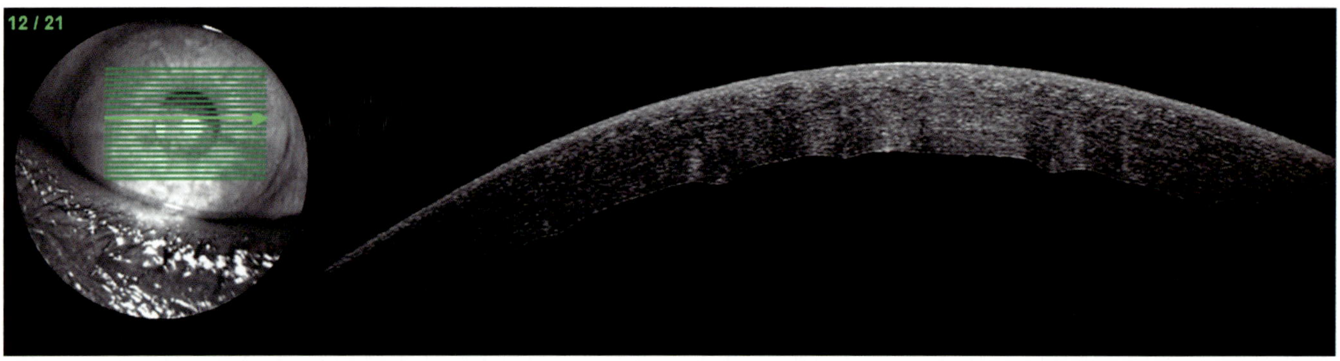

Fig. 19.25 Herpes simplex virus endotheliitis. Multiple, hyperreflective lesions with focal outpouching can be observed on AS-OCT.

guide decision-making. Figs. 19.27 to 19.30 show an example of a patient with stromal scarring. Slit-lamp images show different levels and extent of scarring depending on the lighting technique used. Similarly, the AS-OCT images show varying levels of scarring that depend on the technique and image used. Such information can help guide the clinician toward recommending further management options, such as contact lens rehabilitation versus surgical interventions.

B. Herpes Zoster

Varicella-zoster virus (VZV) is prevalent worldwide, with lifetime risk for development of 30%, and causes two distinct disease entities. The first is a primary infection known as *varicella*, or more commonly, *chickenpox*. It is spread by respiratory droplets and is easily contracted by susceptible individuals.

After a primary infection, the virus migrates to the sensory spinal or cerebral ganglia, where it remains dormant. Reactivation of this latent virus results in the second clinical manifestation of VZV known as *herpes zoster* or *shingles*. Herpes zoster presents acutely with pain and vesicular lesions of the skin in a single dermatomal distribution. Herpes zoster ophthalmicus specifically affects the V1 distribution. Patients tend to present with unilaterally marked swelling and vesicles of the forehead, scalp, and eyelids that may be preceded by fever, malaise, and headaches. These lesions may continue to develop over the course of a week and may take several weeks before resolving completely. Keratitis (76%) is the most common associated complication followed by uveitis/iritis (46.6%), conjunctivitis (35.4%), severe eye pain (14%), increased intraocular pressure (13.2%), scleritis/episcleritis (10.6%), and corneal scarring (10%). Other manifestations occur in less than 10% of the population.

Similar to HSV, VZV can infect and cause inflammatory reactions in all layers of the cornea. Fig. 19.31 shows external photographs, slit-lamp images, and AS-OCT images of a patient with VZV stromal keratitis. AS-OCT again can be used to

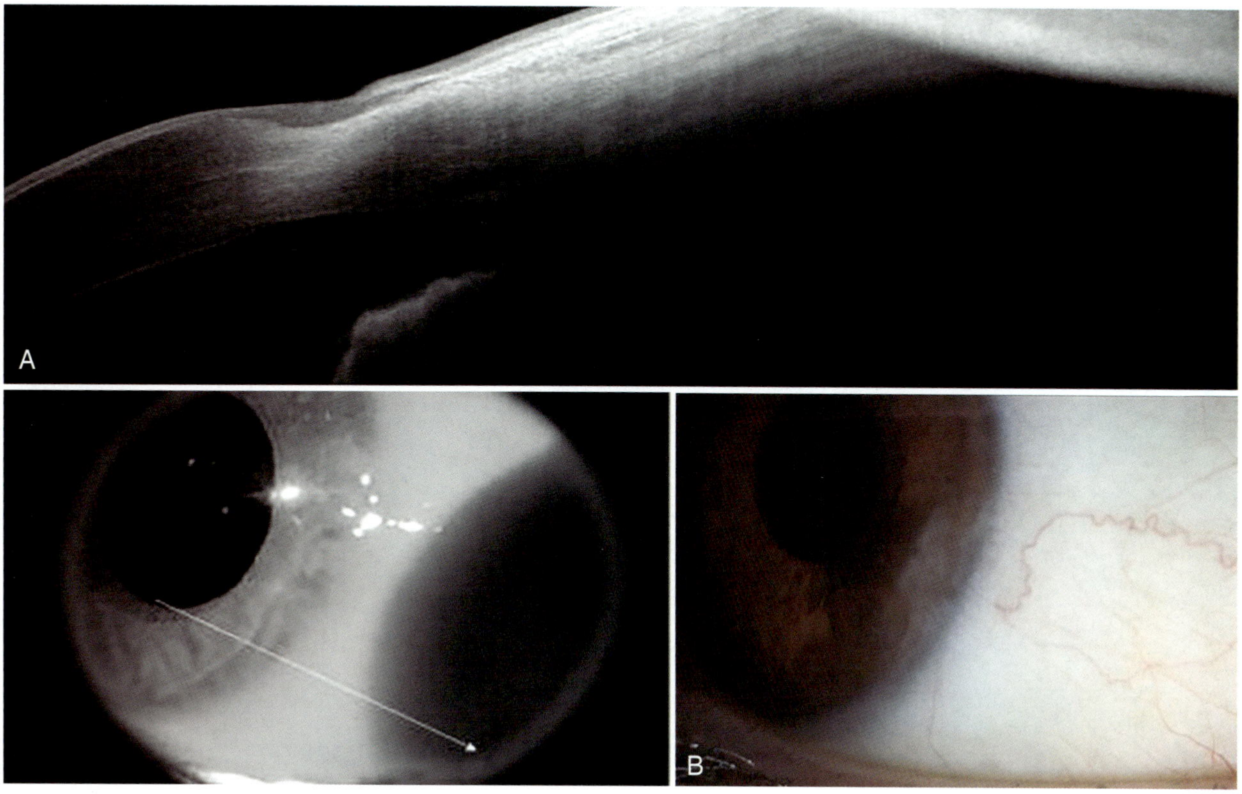

Fig. 19.26 Recurrent herpes simplex virus (HSV) stromal keratitis. The images displayed are representative of a patient who presented with recurrent episodes of inflammation in the right eye. AS-OCT image *(panel A)* shows a thicker epithelium overlying the stromal thinning, with a subepithelial hyperreflective fibrous layer. This corresponds to the slit-lamp finding seen in *panel B.* There is peripheral thinning of the cornea without epithelial defects and presence of fibrovascular tissue overlying the area of corneal thinning. The patient was treated empirically with antivirals for possible HSV with a good clinical response.

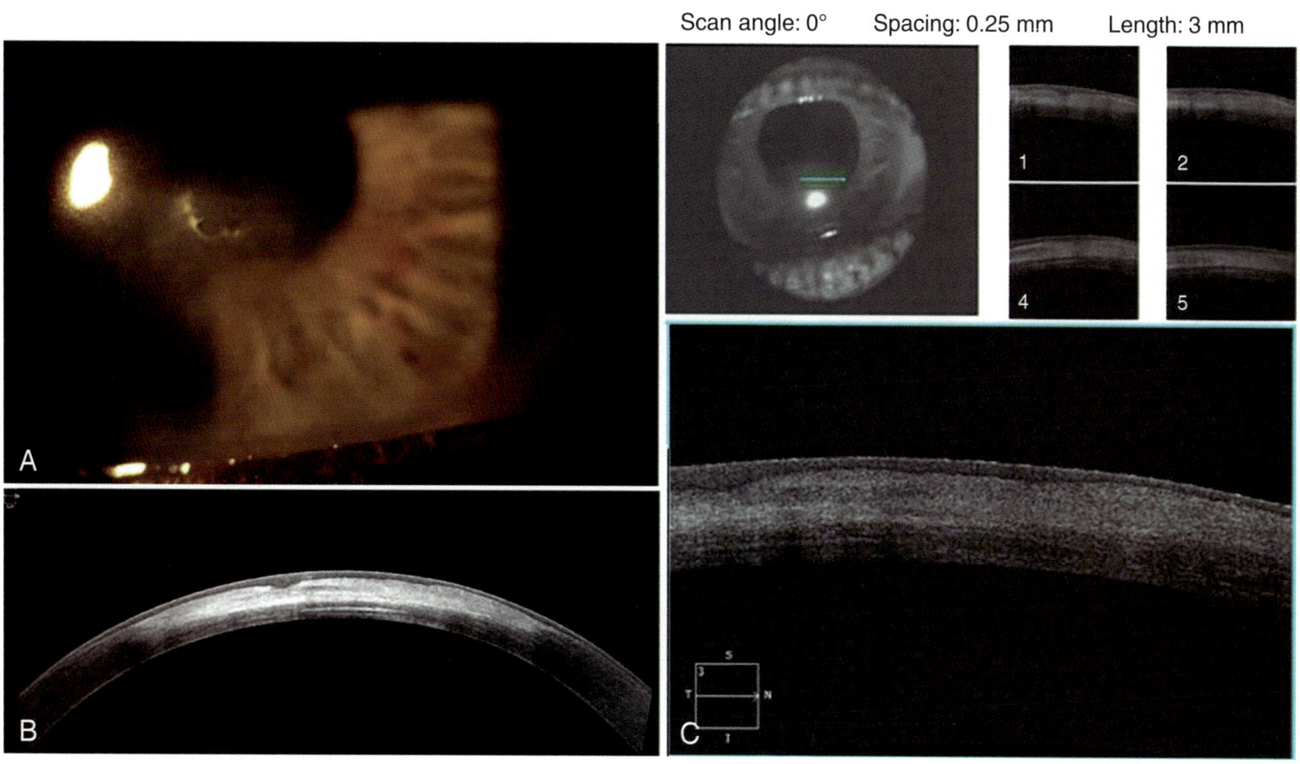

Fig. 19.27 Stromal scarring from recurrent herpes simplex virus keratitis. Slit-lamp photograph *(panel A)* shows a centrally located area of corneal scarring with associated corneal neovascularization inferiorly. There is additional subepithelial linear scarring and overlying pigmentary changes in the epithelium. AS-OCT of the scar *(panel B)* further highlights the extent and depth of the stromal scarring. Notably, the scarring involves approximately two-thirds of the cornea. Raster images *(panel C)* further show local changes underlying the stromal scarring.

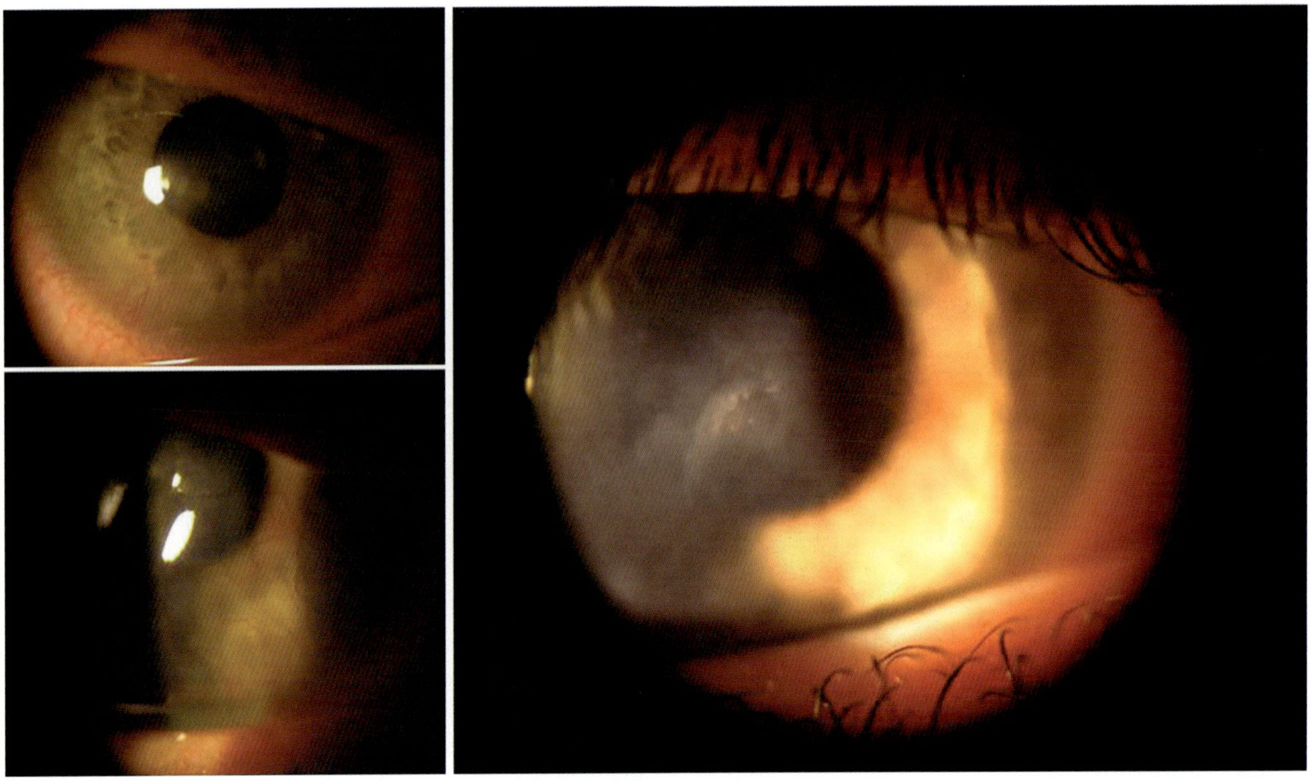

Fig. 19.28 Slit-lamp photographs of a patient with stromal scarring secondary to herpes simplex virus infection. Note the variable appearance of the stromal scarring, subepithelial haze, and corneal neovascularization involving the inferior half of the cornea depending on the lighting technique.

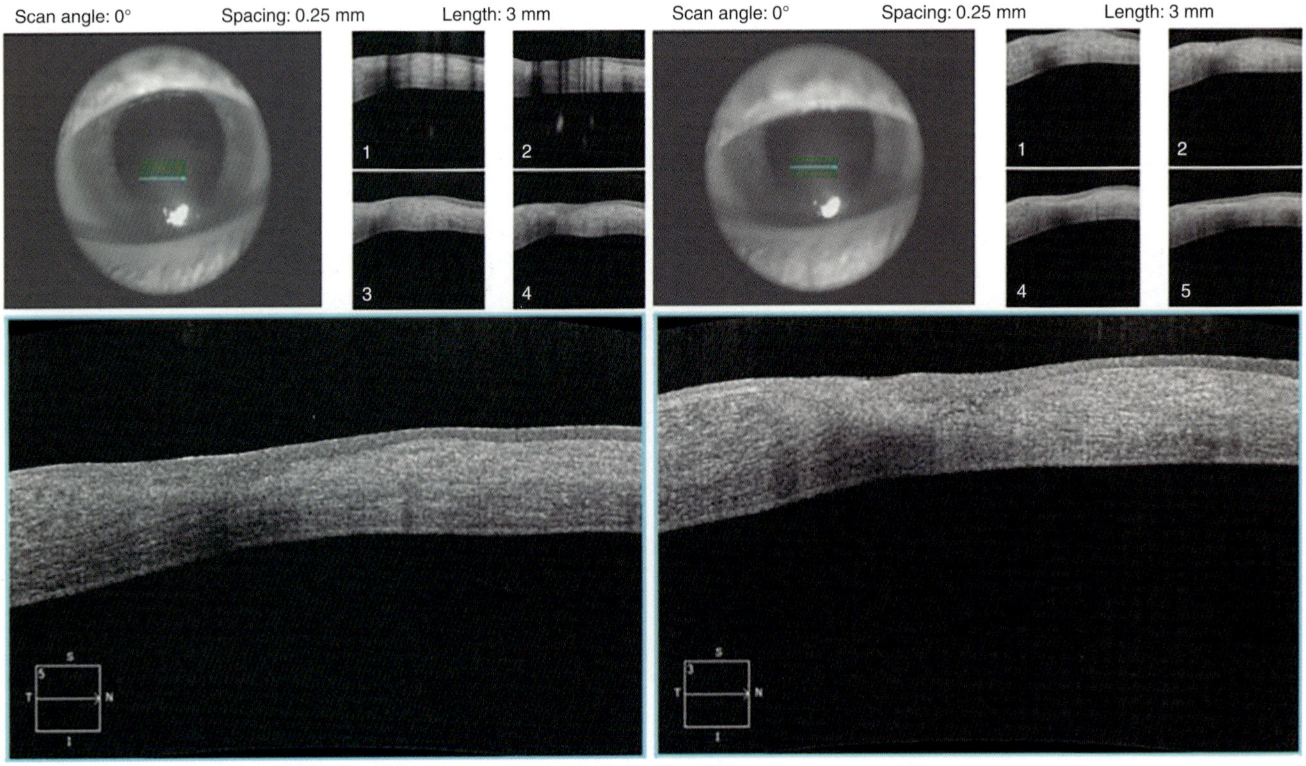

Fig. 19.29 AS-OCT raster images of the previous patient. Stromal thinning with epithelial remodeling is evident.

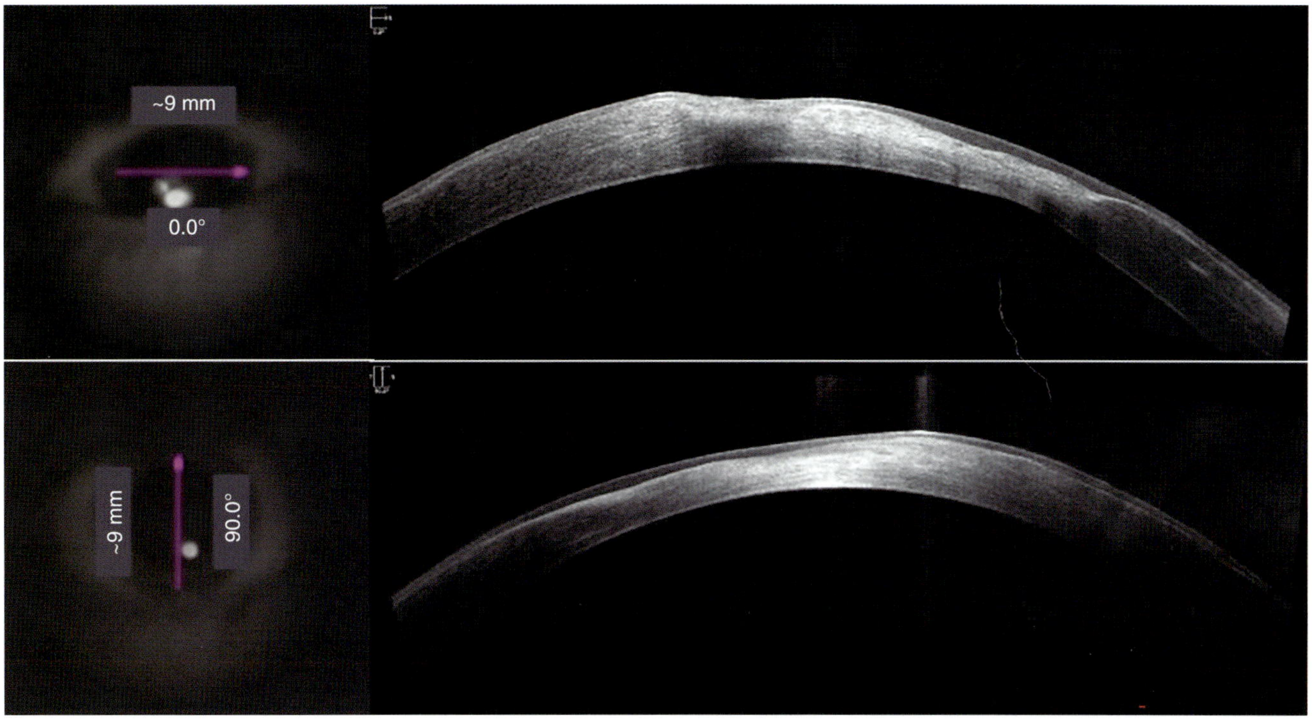

Fig. 19.30 AS-OCT high-definition cornea views (horizontal and vertical slices) of the patient from Fig. 19.23. This "global" view provides the clinician with information regarding the depth and extent of the stromal scarring changes.

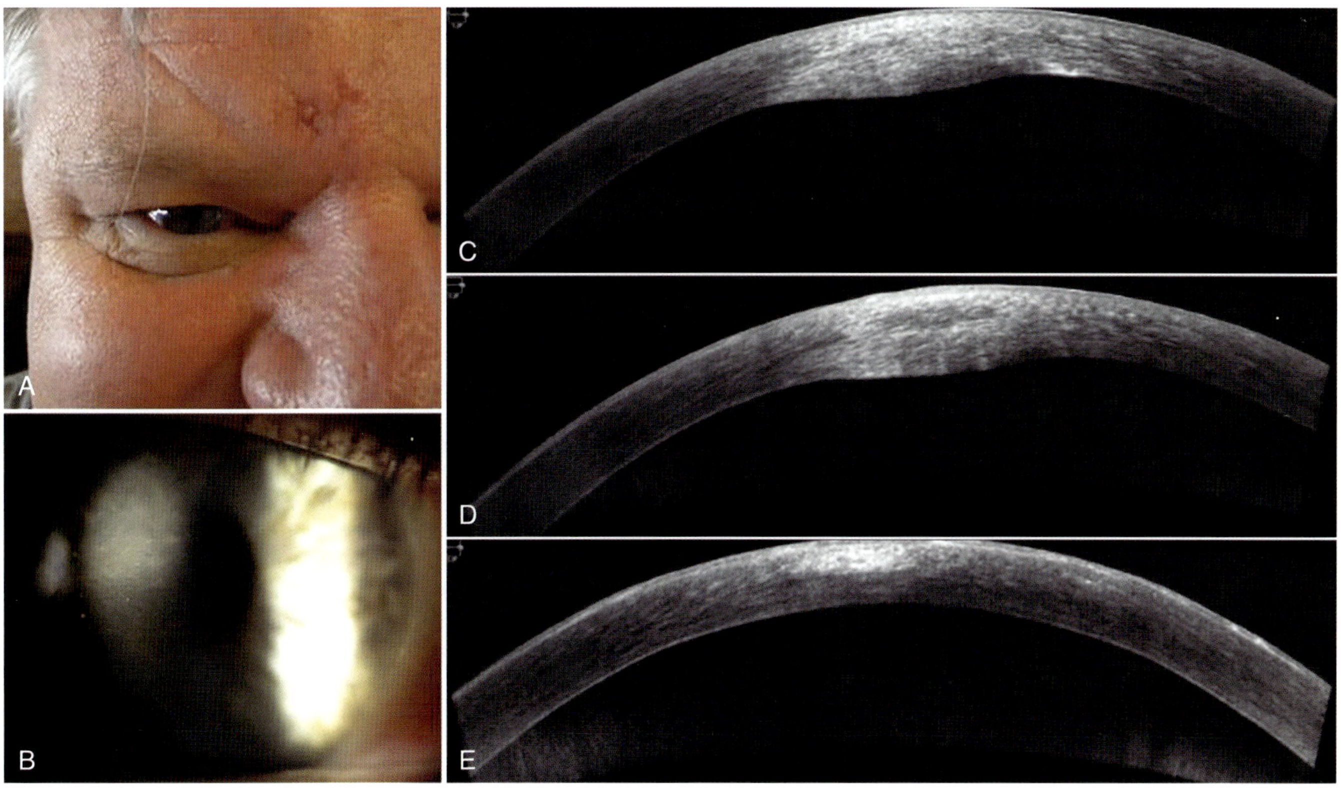

Fig. 19.31 Stromal keratitis secondary to varicella-zoster virus infection. *Panel A* shows external photographs of a patient with vesicular skin lesions in the V1 distribution. *Panel B* shows slit-lamp image of stromal keratitis with prominent central corneal edema. Notably, there is a lack of corneal neovascularization in this patient. *Panels C to E* display various AS-OCT images through the area of stromal keratitis. The stromal keratitis appears as an area of increased hyperreflectivity primarily involving the anterior half of the stroma. There is increased corneal edema seen in *panels C and D.*

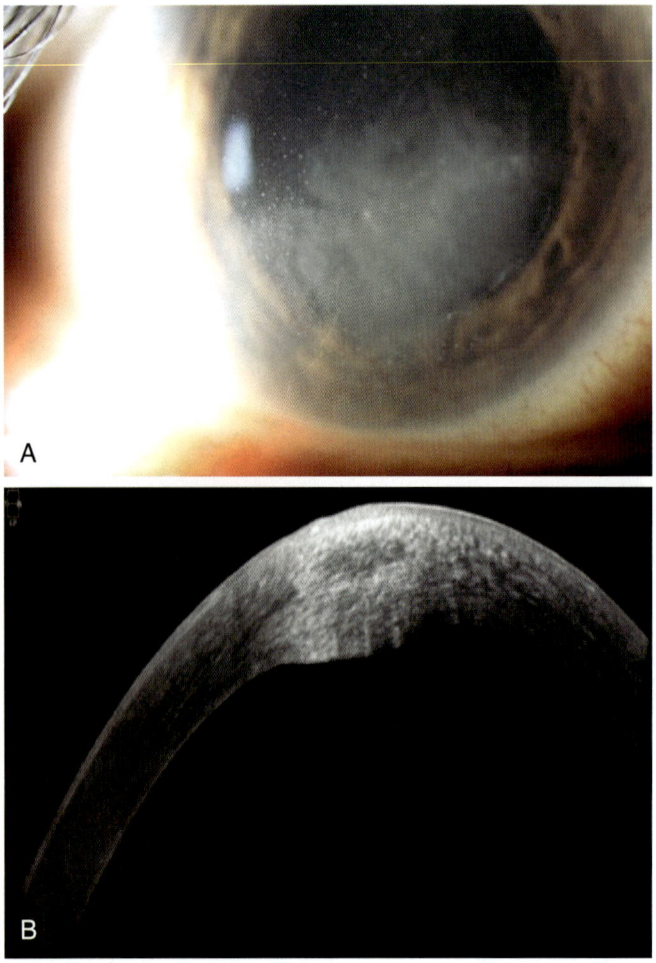

Fig. 19.32 Stromal keratitis secondary to varicella-zoster virus infection. Slit-lamp photograph *(panel A)* shows stromal opacification and edema with fine keratic precipitates and an intact epithelium. AS-OCT image *(panel B)* displays findings compatible with stromal edema and inflammation with an intact epithelium.

highlight the extent of stromal keratitis. Fig. 19.32 shows images from a different patient with recurrent VZV infection that manifested with stromal edema, stromal opacification, and fine keratic precipitates.

Figs. 19.33 to 19.36 display images from a patient with severe stromal keratitis with advanced stromal melting and descemetocele for which AM placement was performed.

C. Adenovirus Subepithelial Infiltrates

Adenoviral keratoconjunctivitis (AK) is a highly contagious infection that mainly affects the surface of the eye. It accounts for up to 75% of conjunctivitis cases and is caused by adenoviruses, which belong to the *Adenoviridae* family, comprising more than 130 different serotypes. Serotypes 8, 11, 19, and 37 are known to cause keratoconjunctivitis, with serotypes 8 and 19 being particularly responsible for epidemic outbreaks. The corneal disease usually manifests after a period of incubation that takes about 2 to 14 days in the form of diffuse epithelial keratitis, focal epithelial punctate keratitis, and subepithelial corneal infiltrates (SEIs).

The pathogenesis of SEIs involves persisting viral replication in keratocytes, which triggers an immunologic host reaction. Histopathologic investigation reveals lymphocytes, histiocytes, and fibroblasts that are accompanied by disruption of the collagen fibers of the Bowman layer. SEIs are usually bilateral and asymmetric. They are small, round, grayish lesions that are composed of residues of antigen and lymphocyte accumulations adhered to surface stromal cells and have the potential to cause significant ocular morbidity, reduced vision, photophobia, glare, halos, and foreign body sensation that can persist for months or years after the initial infection.

Long-term topical steroid use is usually effective in the treatment of SEIs; however, it is associated with important side effects such as cataract, glaucoma, and prolonged viral seeding. These side effects after long-term treatments with topical steroids prompted the search for alternative treatments such as cyclosporine and tacrolimus, which have been shown to be safe and effective for the treatment of SEIs in different studies.

Figs. 19.37 and 19.38 show images of a typical patient with SEIs secondary to AK. Slit-lamp findings are notable for subepithelial infiltrates without overlying epithelial defect. AS-OCT can be used to highlight the focal, diffuse nature of SEIs. In some patients, AS-OCT may further reveal SEIs that may have been missed on clinical examination.

CLINICAL PEARL

Patients with adenovirus can be extremely photophobic and averse to prolonged examination at the slit-lamp. As a result of its noncontact nature and rapid acquisition time, AS-OCT can be used to assess the number and location of SEIs. Follow-up AS-OCT images also can be used to assess the effectiveness of treatment with antiinflammatory medications and to show patients' interval improvement. Because symptoms of AK and SEIs can take a significant amount of time to heal, interval images also may be helpful for clinicians to show patients that progress is occurring and persistent treatment and patience are often required.

A particularly useful role of AS-OCT in these patients is to help distinguish between active SEIs and inactive scarring from previous SEIs. Anatomically, the SEI scarring involves disruption of the Bowman layer and extends into the anterior stroma. Clinically, this may be difficult to appreciate on slit-lamp examination alone. In such cases, AS-OCT can highlight differences between active SEIs and inactive scarring from old SEIs. Fig. 19.39 shows slit-lamp photographs and AS-OCT images comparing and contrasting features of active SEIs and inactive scarring from previous SEIs.

D. Epstein-Barr Virus

Epstein-Barr virus (EBV) is a DNA virus that is a well-known causative agent of infectious mononucleosis but has a wide range of anterior segment manifestations, including follicular conjunctivitis, keratitis, and uveitis. In the cornea, EBV can have protean manifestations similar to previously mentioned viruses, including a nummular, anterior stromal keratitis that occurs as a secondary result of subclinical and/or prolonged infection. Superficial and SEIs similar to Thygeon superficial keratitis and multifocal keratitis with neovascularization also have been described. Treatment strategies for all three types of EBV-associated keratitis involve a combination of topical/systemic antiinflammatory medications, with or without systemic antiviral treatment, because there is no clear consensus regarding preferred practice patterns.

Figs. 19.40 to 19.47 show serial images from a 15-year-old female patient who developed EBV-associated nummular keratitis. Figs. 19.40 and 19.41 show slit-lamp, tomography, and AS-OCT images of the right eye and left eye, respectively, at the time of presentation. Of note, the lesions are limited to mid and

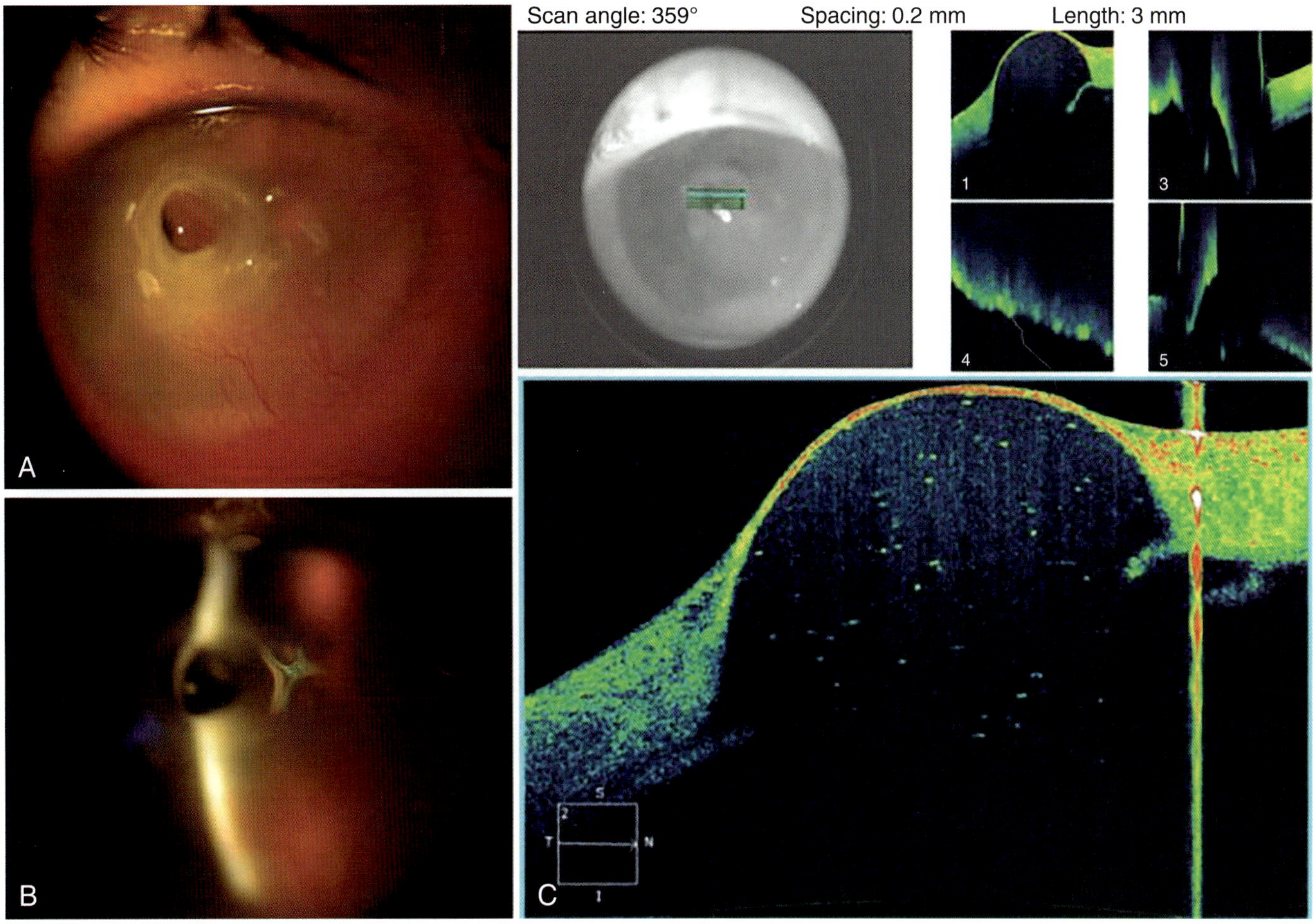

Fig. 19.33 Severe case of stromal keratitis secondary to varicella-zoster virus. Slit-lamp photographs *(panels A and B)* display marked thinning, surrounding necrosis, and prominent peripheral corneal neovascularization. A hypopyon is present. Notably, there is a descemetocele within the area of thinning. AS-OCT raster images *(panel C)* further highlight the extent of the descemetocele.

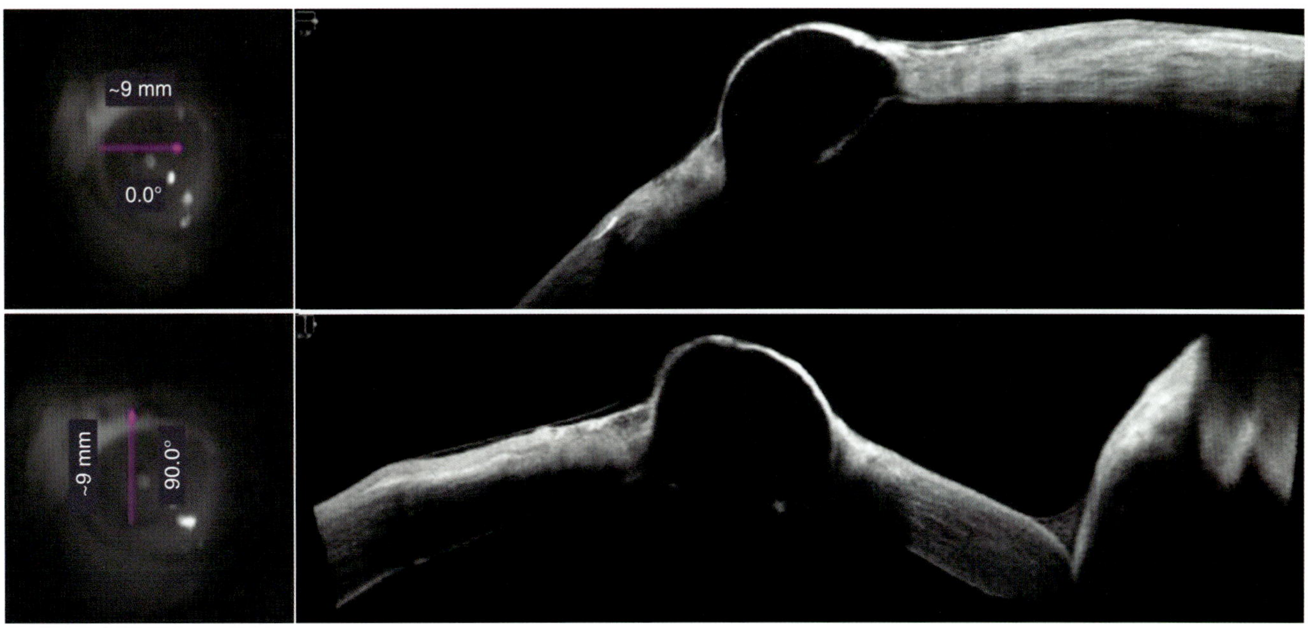

Fig. 19.34 AS-OCT high-definition images from the patient shown in Fig. 19.27. Horizontal and vertical slices (*top and bottom panels,* respectively) show the architecture of the descemetocele. There is marked inflammation surrounding the descemetocele as evidenced by marked hyperreflectivity in the anterior stroma.

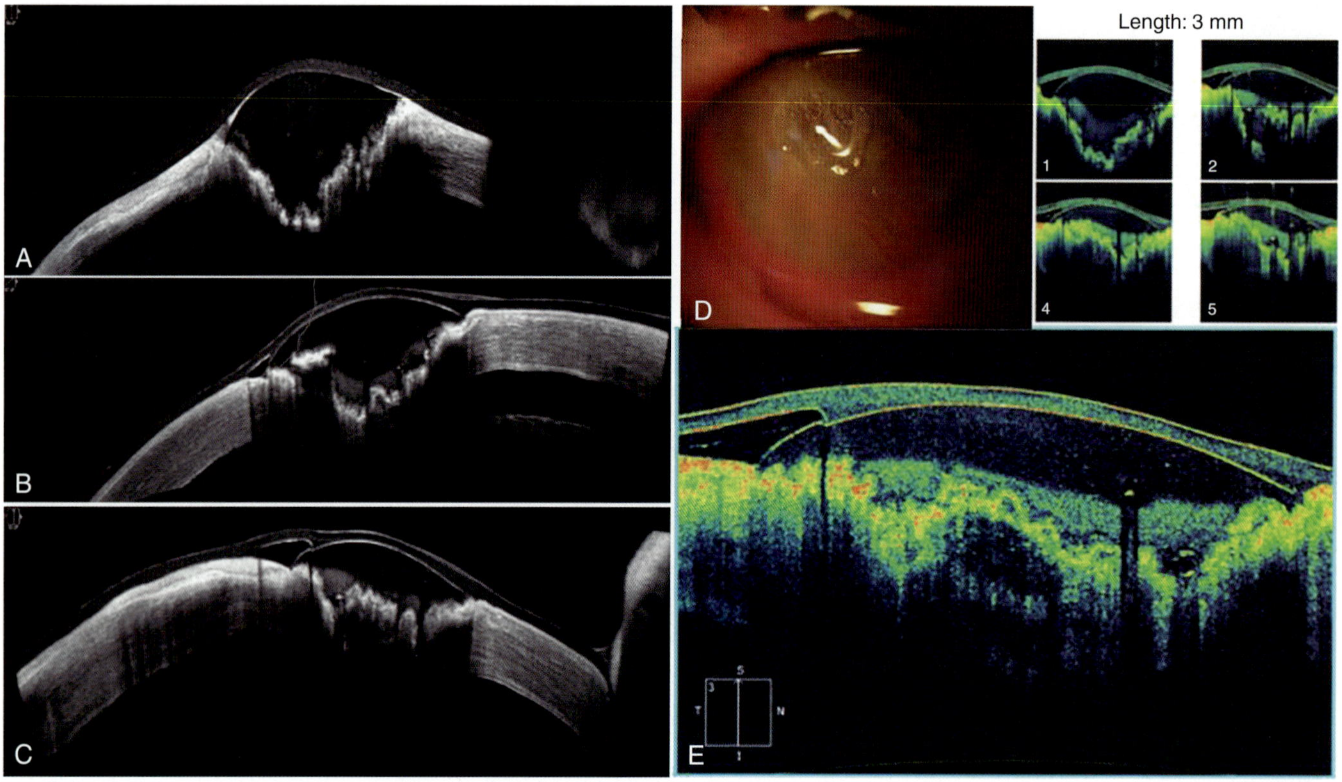

Fig. 19.35 Because of concerns for impending perforation secondary to descemetocele, an amniotic membrane (AM) was placed. AS-OCT high-definition images show the appearance of the descemetocele immediately after AM placement. Slit-lamp photograph *(panel D)* taken immediately after AM placement confirms good coverage of the area of severely thinned cornea. AS-OCT raster images *(panel E)* similarly confirm AM placement.

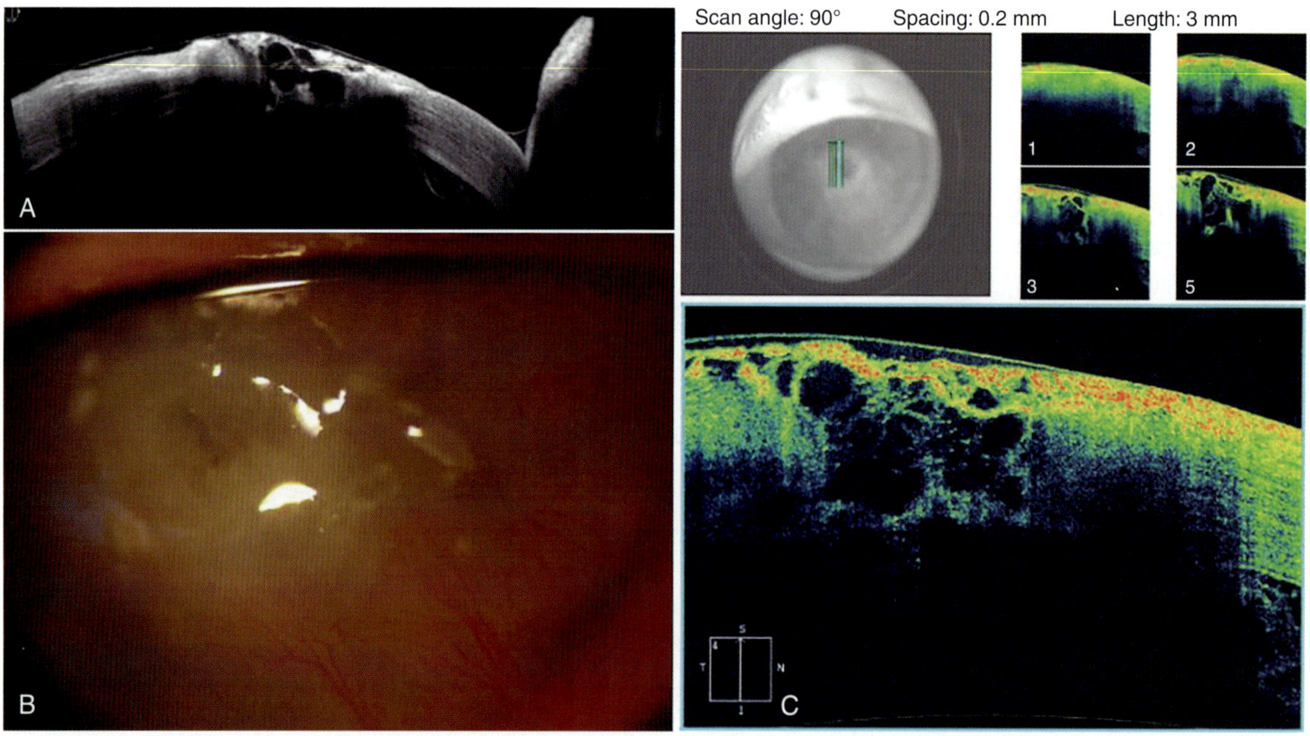

Fig. 19.36 One week after amniotic membrane (AM) placement, repeat AS-OCT *(panel A)* shows improvement of the descemetocele as the AM has become incorporated into the corneal stroma. Slit-lamp photograph *(panel B)* shows markedly persistent inflammation and corneal neovascularization with notable improvement of previously seen central corneal thinning. AS-OCT raster images *(panel C)* similarly shows improvement of the descemetocele with secondary healing changes within the corneal stroma.

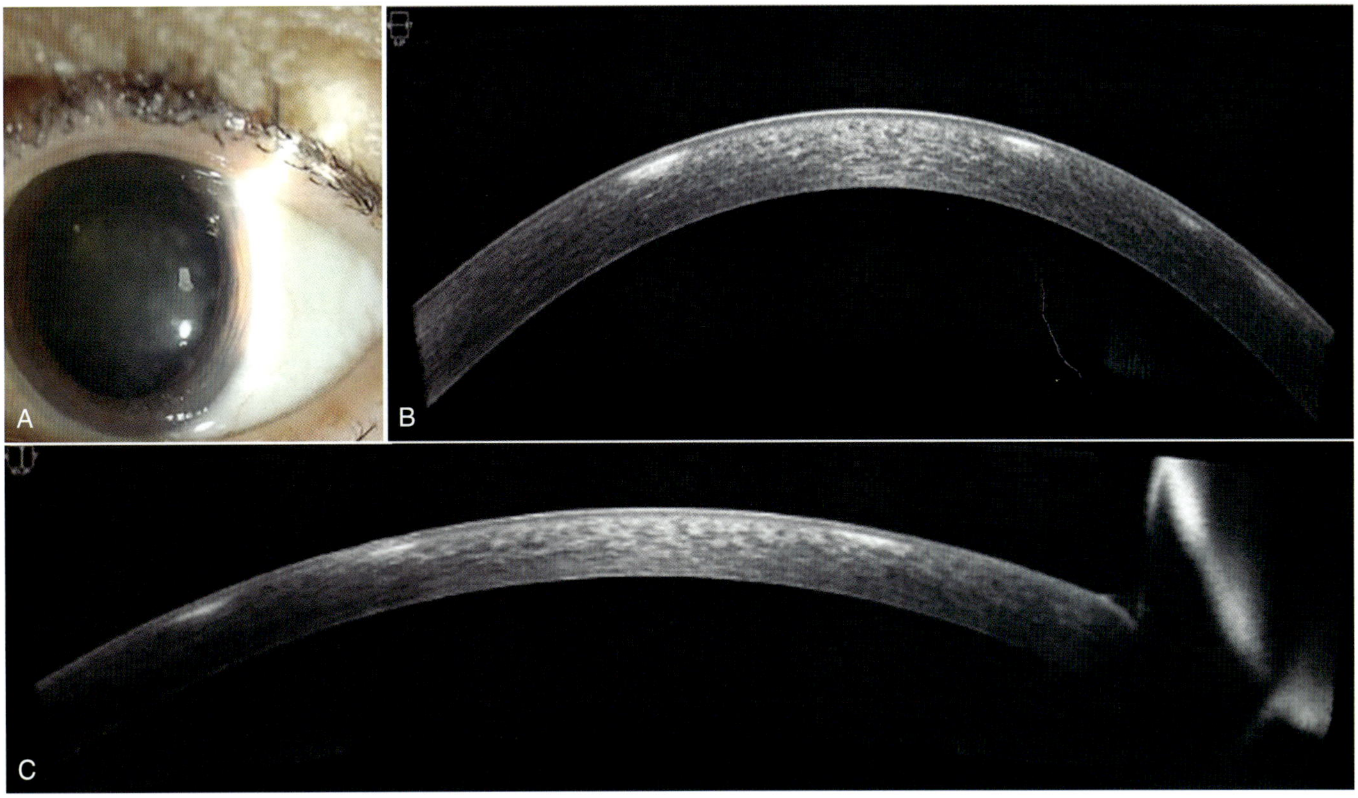

Fig. 19.37 Subepithelial infiltrates (SEIs) secondary to adenovirus keratoconjunctivitis. Images are representative of a patient with a history of pink eye who presented to the clinic complaining of foreign body sensation. Slit-lamp photograph *(panel A)* show subepithelial opacities that compromise almost the entirety of the cornea secondarily to adenoviral conjunctivitis. AS-OCT images *(panels B and C)* highlight the SEIs as focal, discrete hyperreflective lesions limited to the subepithelial space without involvement of the middle and posterior stroma. AS-OCT can be used to highlight SEIs that may be difficult to appreciate on clinical examination.

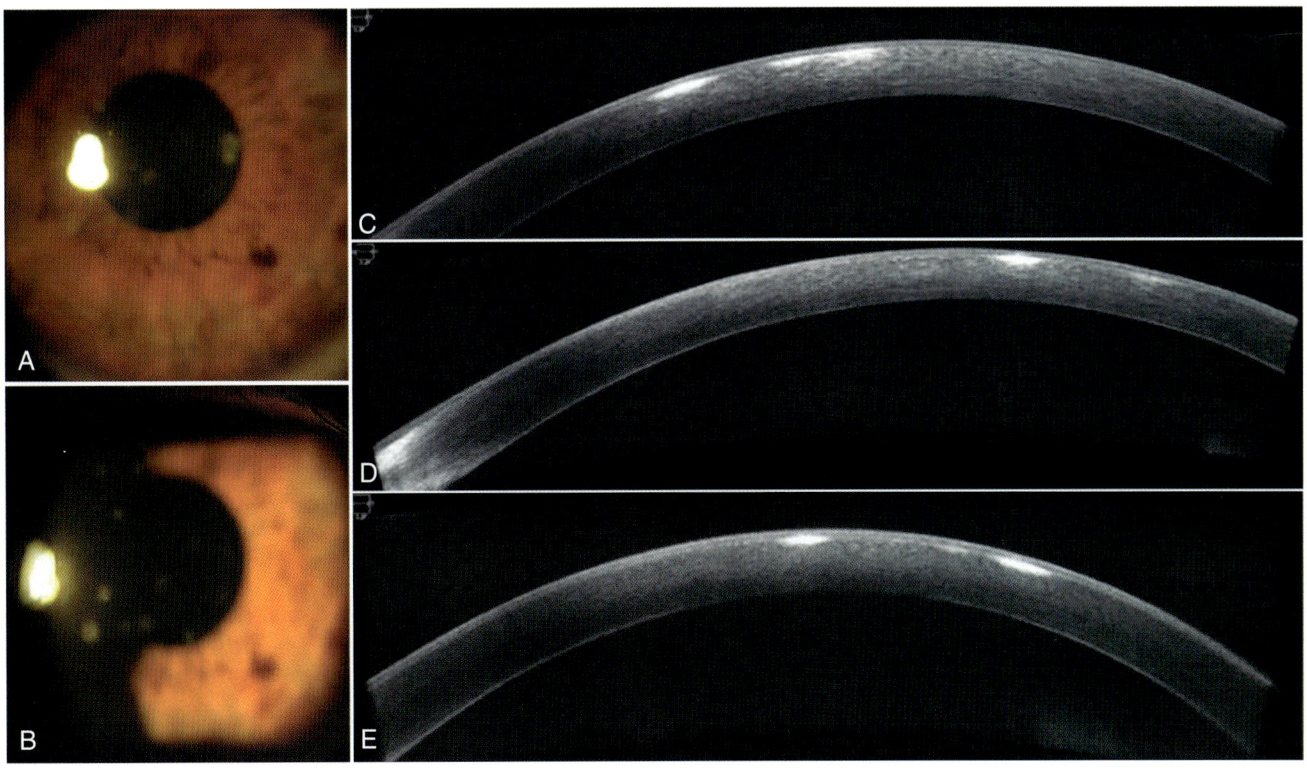

Fig. 19.38 Subepithelial infiltrates (SEIs) secondary to adenovirus keratoconjunctivitis in another patient. Slit-lamp photographs *(panels A and B)* show subepithelial opacities that compromise almost the entirety of the cornea. AS-OCT images *(panels C–E)* again highlight the SEIs as focal, discrete hyperreflective lesions limited to the subepithelial space without involvement of the middle and posterior stroma. AS-OCT can be used to highlight SEIs that may be difficult to appreciate on clinical examination.

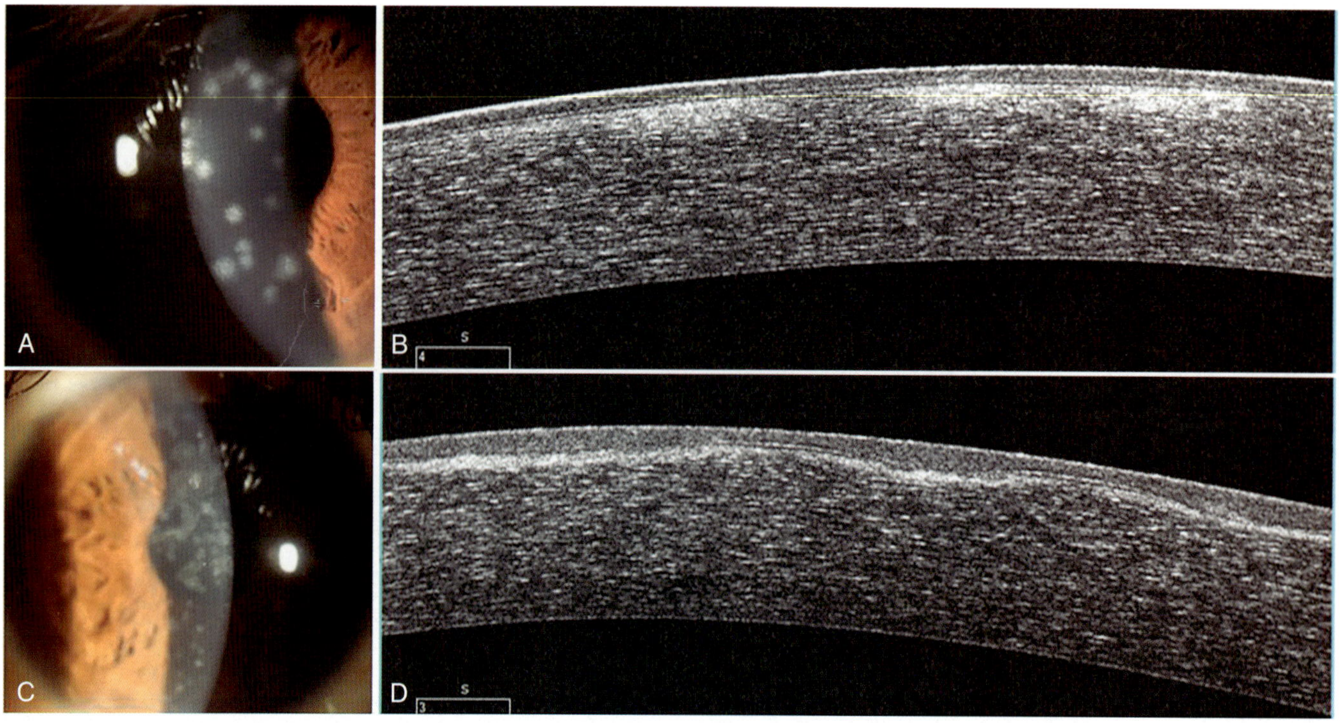

Fig. 19.39 Subepithelial infiltrates and scarring due to adenovirus infection. In the *top panel,* slit-lamp photograph *(panel A)* and AS-OCT image *(panel B)* of active subepithelial infiltrates are shown. These findings are similar to features seen in previous images. Notably, the Bowman layer is intact. The slit-lamp photograph *(panel C)* and AS-OCT image *(panel D)* of scarring after adenovirus infection are shown. In *panel C,* the lesions are smaller, have coalesced, and lack the intervening clear spaces as seen in *panel A.* In *panel D,* AS-OCT highlights multiple areas of disruption of the Bowman layer, which can be contrasted with *panel B.* (Courtesy Nikhil Gokhale, MD, Gokhale Eye Center, Mumbai, India.)

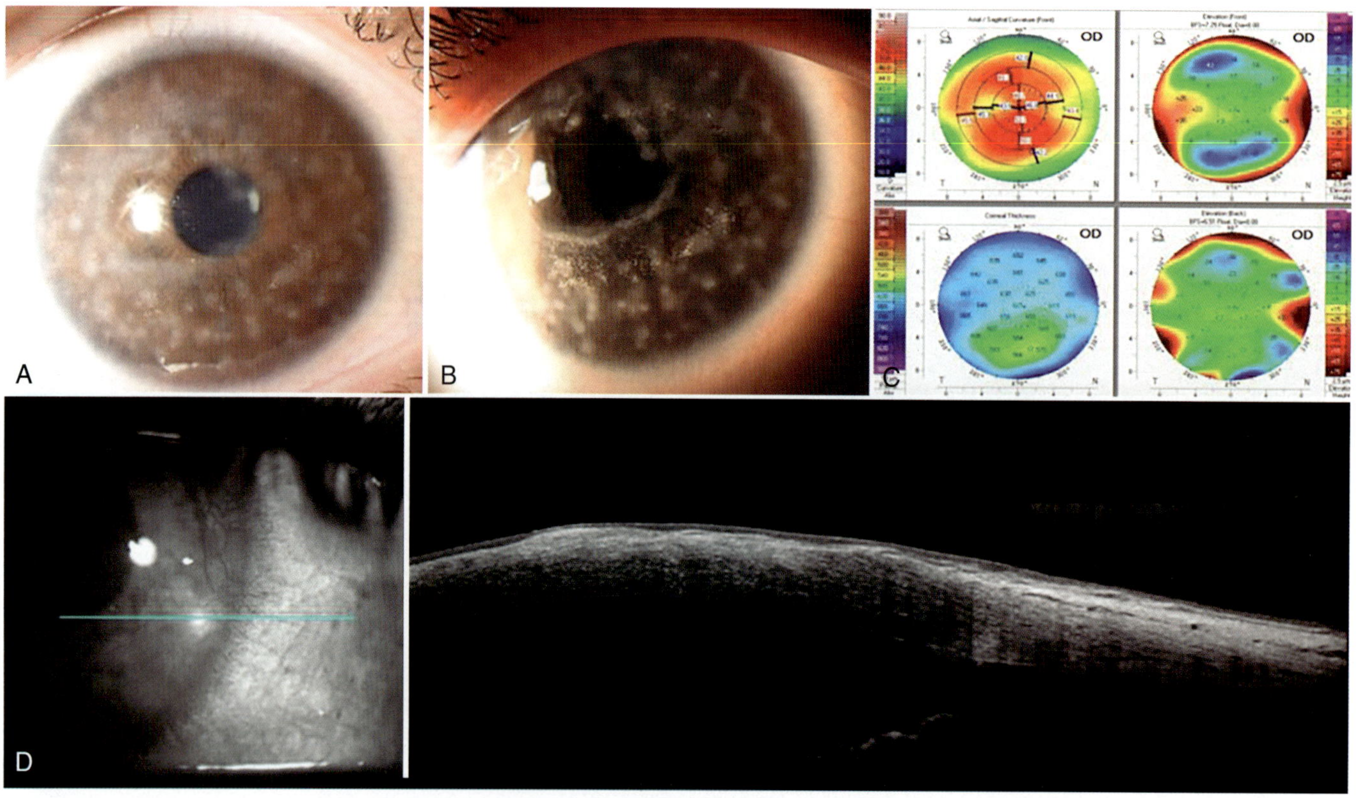

Fig. 19.40 Epstein-Barr virus–associated nummular keratitis. Slit-lamp photographs, tomography, and AS-OCT images taken at the time of presentation of the right eye. Slit-lamp photographs *(panels A and B)* demonstrate nummular appearance of multiple lesions involving the mid and far periphery with a relatively clear central cornea. Tomography images *(panel C)* show irregular astigmatism without significant anterior or posterior elevation changes. On AS-OCT *(panel D),* there is prominent hyperreflectivity within the subepithelial and anterior stromal layers without intervening clear spaces as seen in previous images.

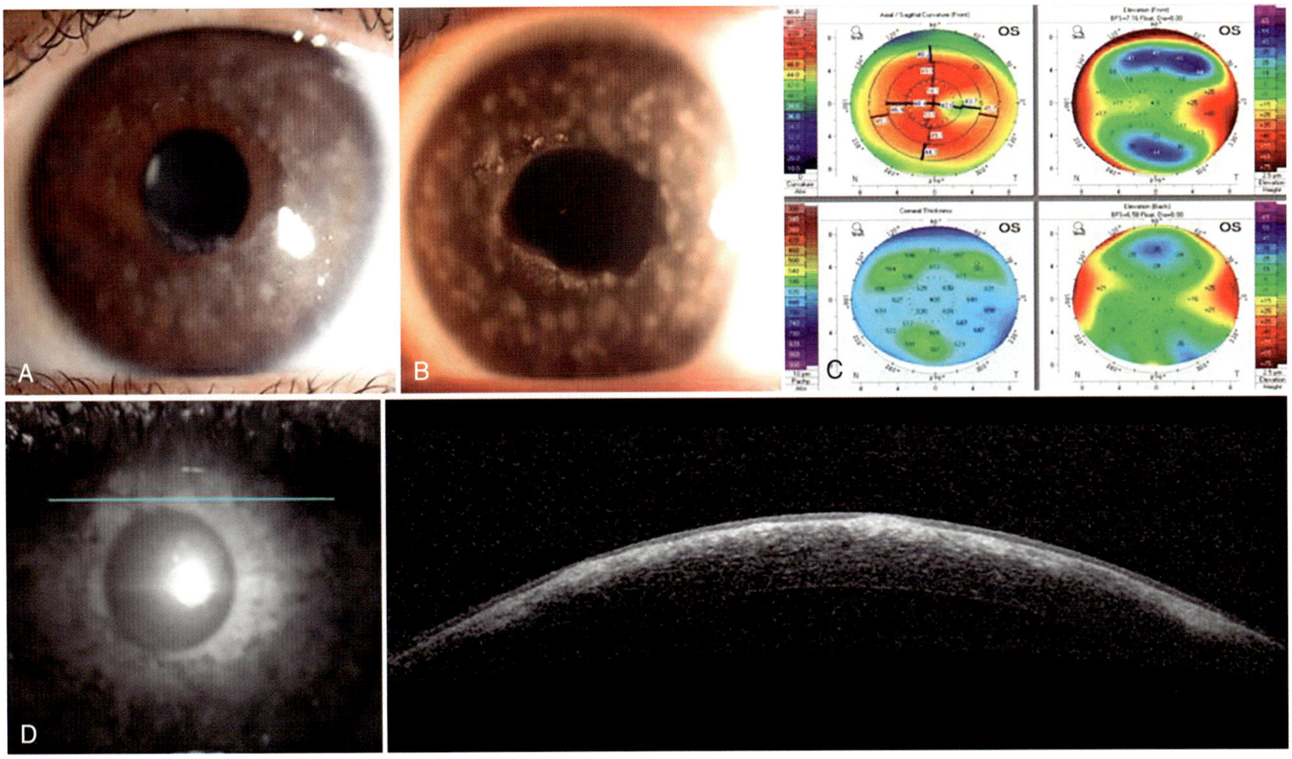

Fig. 19.41 Epstein-Barr virus–associated nummular keratitis. Slit-lamp photographs, tomography, and AS-OCT images taken at the time of presentation of the left eye. Slit-lamp photographs *(panels A and B)* demonstrate nummular appearance of multiple lesions involving the mid and far periphery with a relatively clear central cornea. Tomography images *(panel C)* show irregular astigmatism without significant anterior or posterior elevation changes. On AS-OCT *(panel D),* there is prominent hyperreflectivity within the subepithelial and anterior stromal layers without intervening clear spaces as seen in previous images.

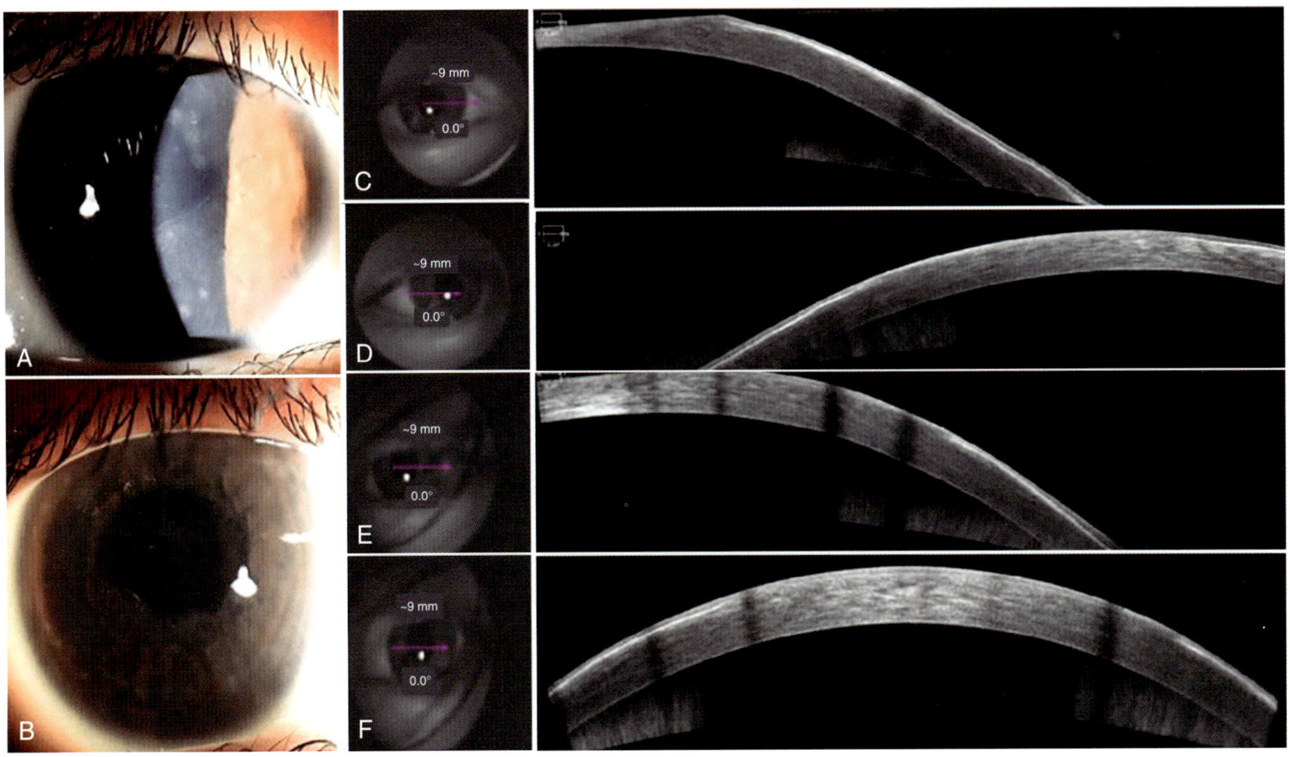

Fig. 19.42 Epstein-Barr virus–associated nummular keratitis. The patient was started on systemic antiviral medication and topical steroids after confirmatory laboratory workup. Follow-up images taken at three months of the right eye and left eye (*panel A and B,* respectively) show interval improvement. AS-OCT images (*panels C and D,* right eye; *panels E and F,* left eye) show consolidation of the previously seen subepithelial lesions into areas of uniform subepithelial scarring that appears as prominent areas of hyperreflectivity. The central cornea remains unaffected.

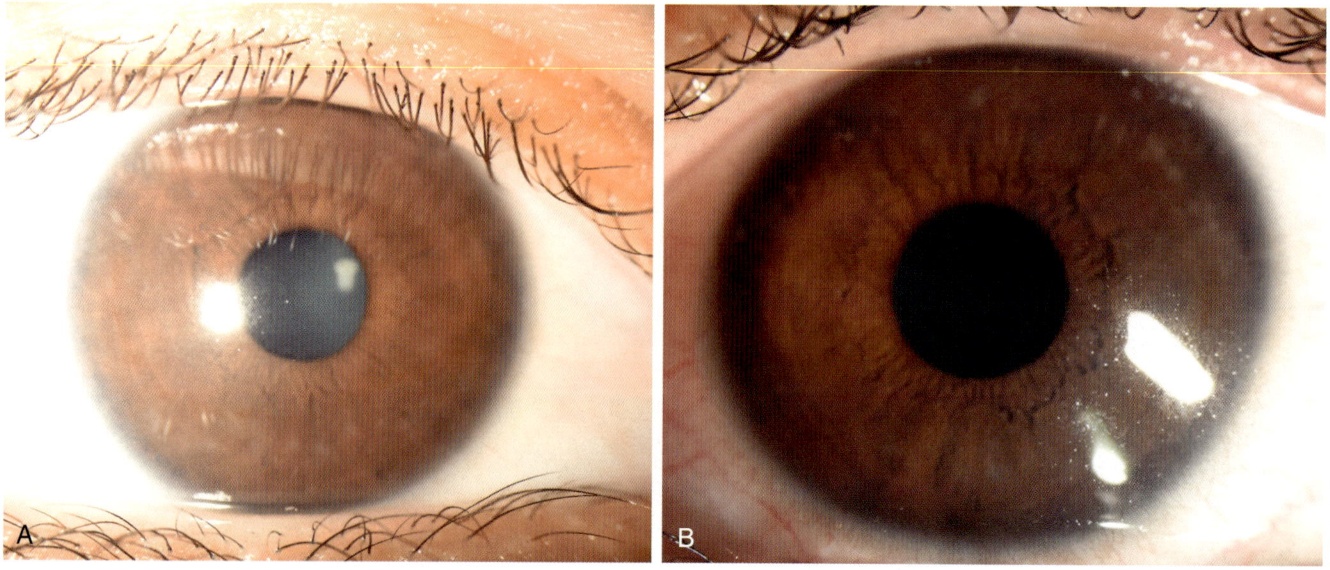

Fig. 19.43 Epstein-Barr virus–associated nummular keratitis. One-year follow-up slit-lamp photographs of the right eye *(panel A)* and left eye *(panel B)* show significant improvement of nummular keratitis lesions seen at the time of presentation (see Figs. 19.35 and 19.36).

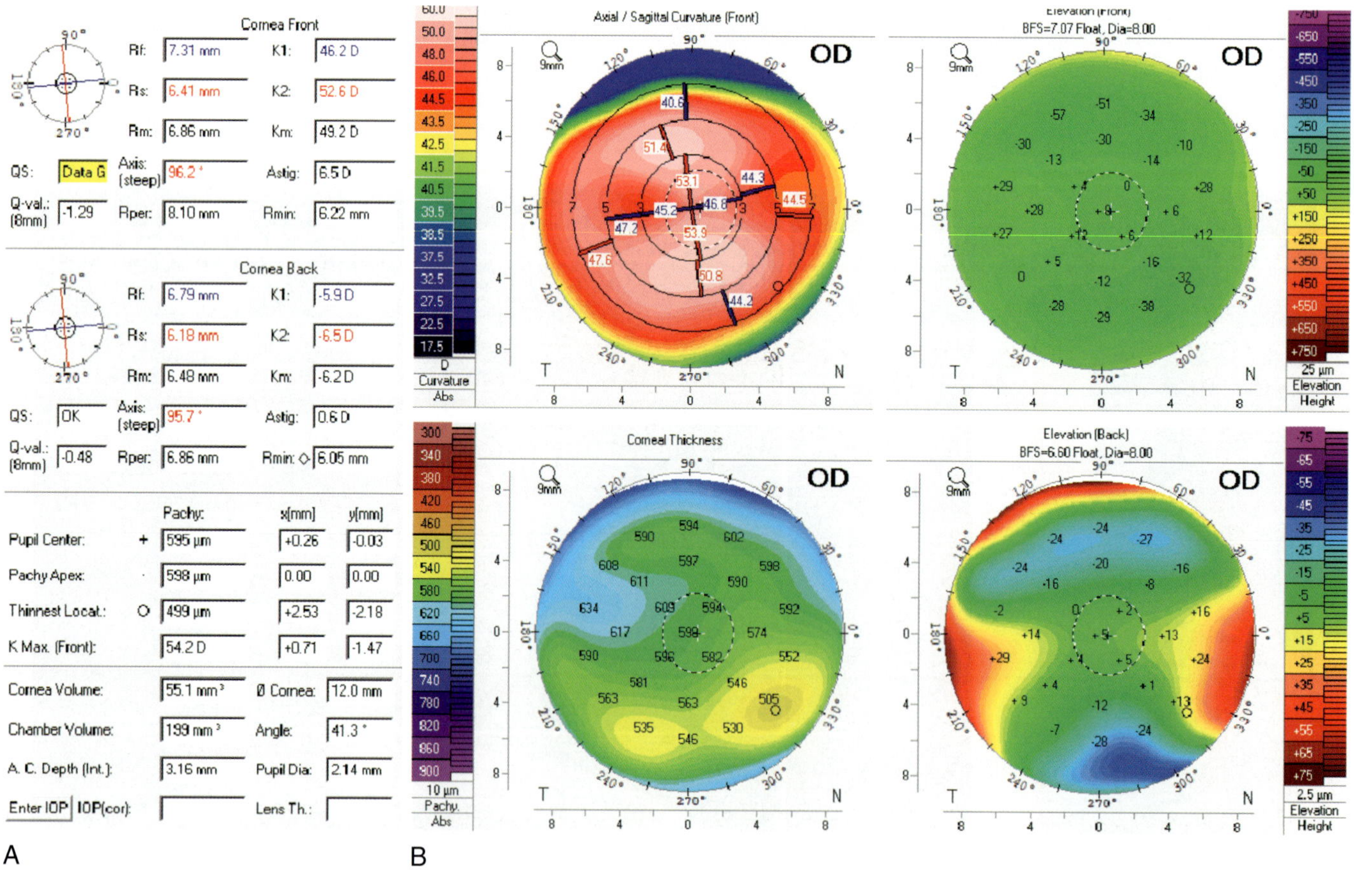

Fig. 19.44 Epstein-Bar virus–associated nummular keratitis. Tomography images of the right eye at one year show a dramatic increase in astigmatism compared with images taken at the time of presentation in Fig. 19.35.

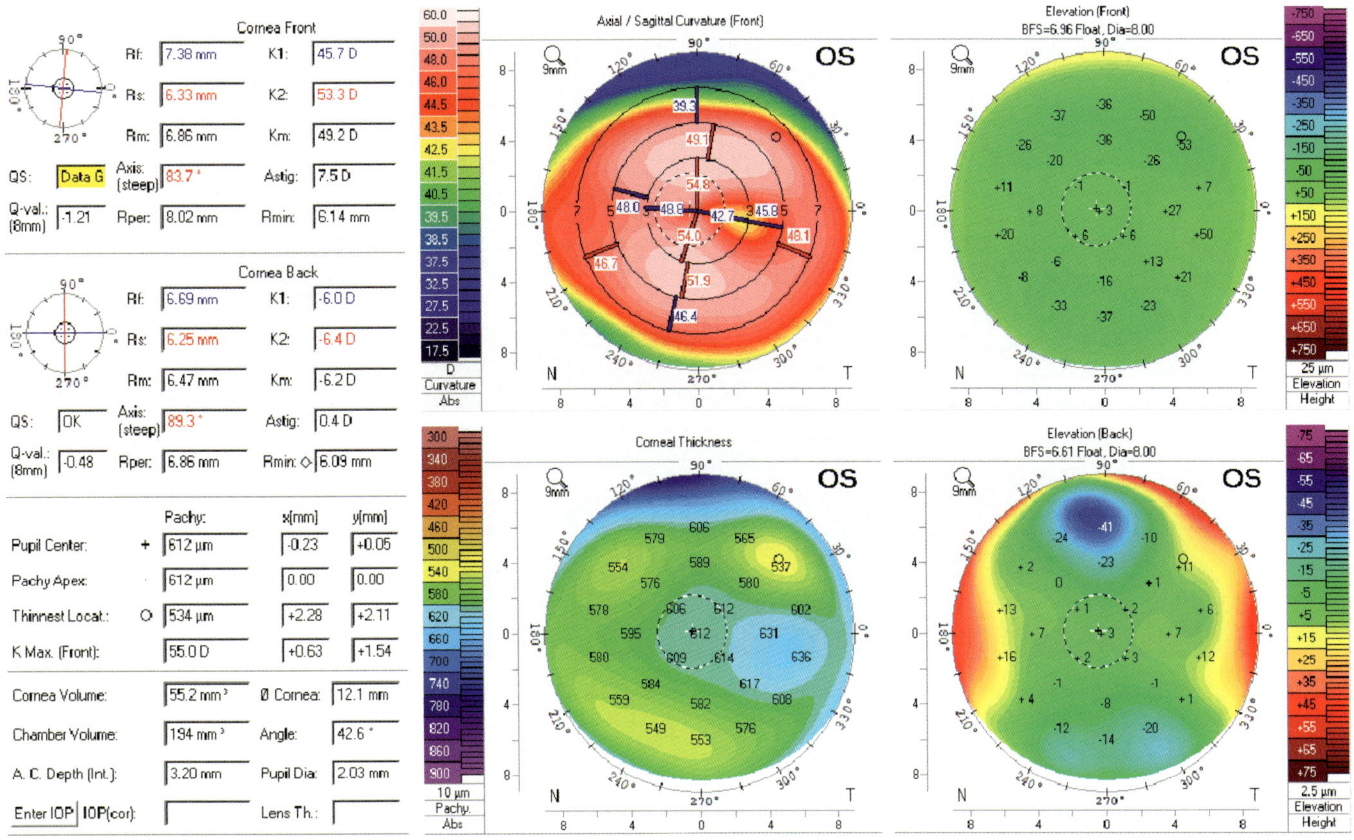

A B

Fig. 19.45 Epstein-Barr virus–associated nummular keratitis. Tomography images of the left eye at one year show a dramatic increase in astigmatism compared with images taken at the time of presentation in Fig. 19.36.

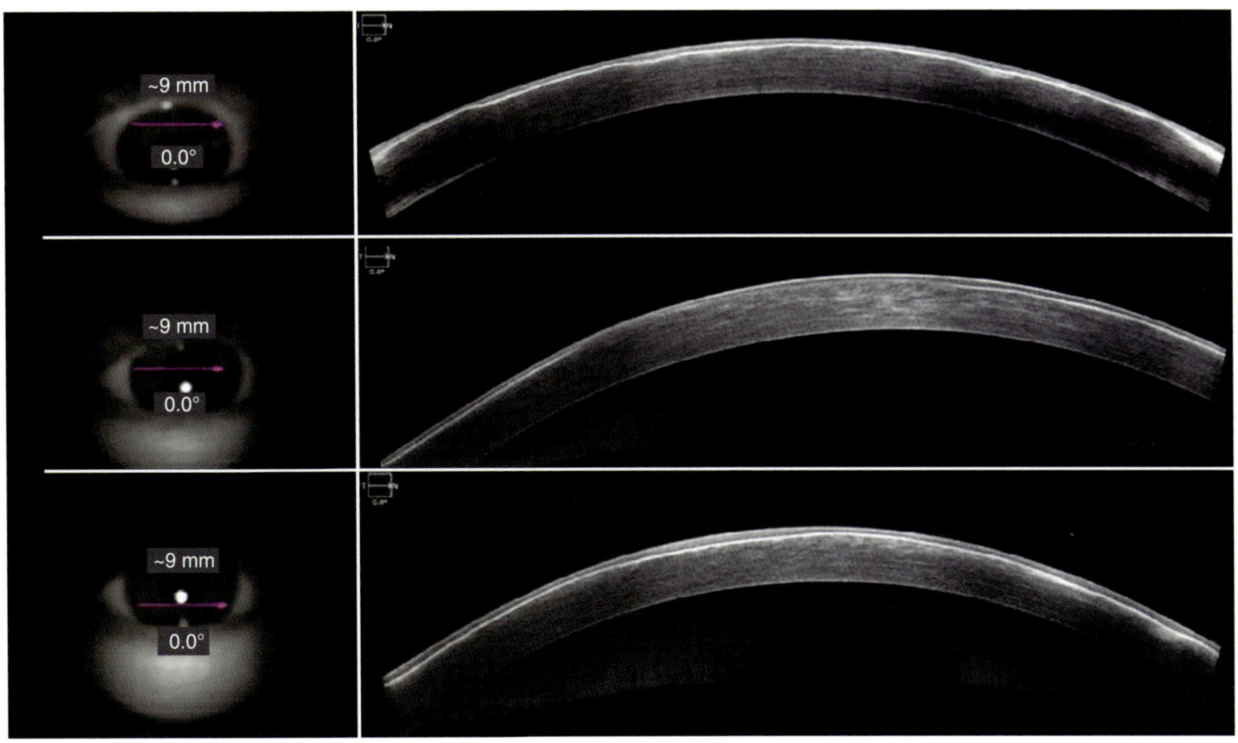

Fig. 19.46 Epstein-Barr virus–associated nummular keratitis. AS-OCT images of the right eye taken at one year after presentation show further improvement of previously seen subepithelial nummular lesions and consolidation of subepithelial scarring. The central cornea remains unaffected.

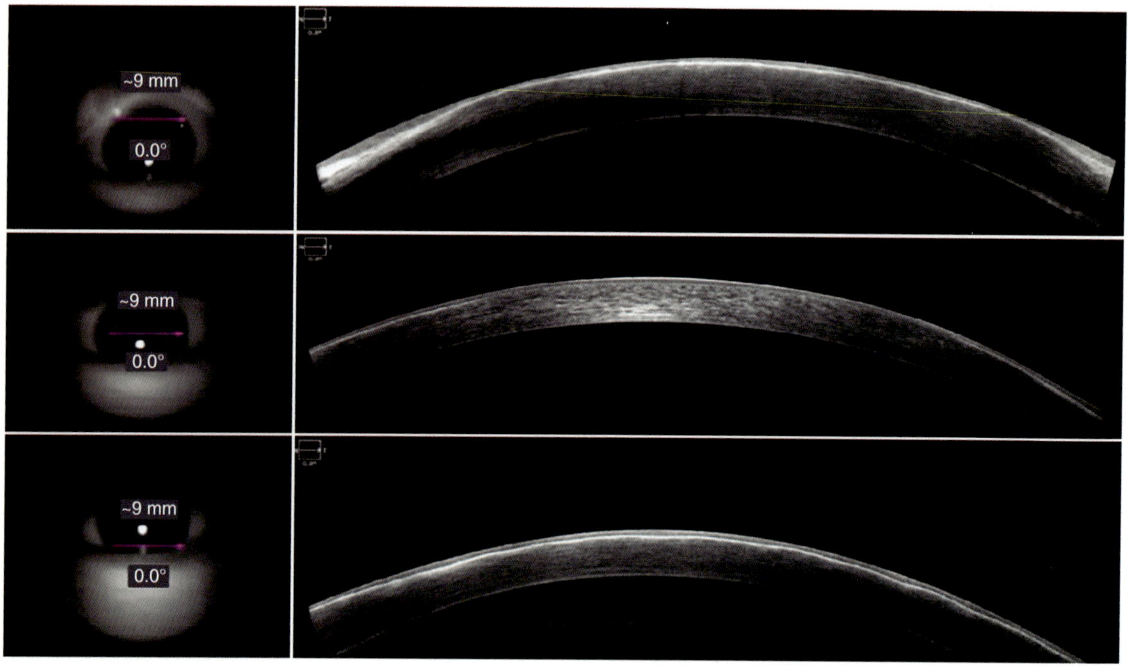

Fig. 19.47 Epstein-Barr virus–associated nummular keratitis. AS-OCT images of the left eye taken at one year after presentation show further improvement of previously seen subepithelial nummular lesions and consolidation of subepithelial scarring. The central cornea remains unaffected.

distal periphery of the cornea, with a central clear space. AS-OCT again demonstrates multiple areas of hyperreflectivity in the subepithelial/anterior stromal spaces. However, compared with previously seen SEIs that had a focal, discrete nature, there are not readily appreciable clear spaces because the lesions have considerable intervening haze. After confirmatory laboratory workup, the patient was started on systemic antiviral therapy and topical steroids. At three-month follow-up (Fig. 19.42), there is notable improvement of the previously seen lesions into consolidated areas of subepithelial scarring. By one year (Fig. 19.43), the lesions are significantly improved, though peripheral scarring and haze remain. Interestingly, follow-up tomography images (Fig. 19.44 and 19.45) show a marked increase in astigmatism without significant anterior or posterior elevation changes. A corresponding myopic shift in refraction was noted, suggesting that consolidation of peripheral scars may have induced a myopic-astigmatism refractive effect, similar to changes induced by conductive keratoplasty. AS-OCT images of the right eye and left eye at one year (Fig. 19.46 and 19.47), respectively) show further improvement of lesions and consolidation of subepithelial scarring.

IV. FUNGAL KERATITIS

Fungal keratitis (FK) is a serious and potentially sight-threatening ophthalmic condition that accounts for up to 50% of microbial keratitis cases worldwide and 6% to 20% of cases in the United States. Rates of infection vary largely depending on the geographic location with warmer climates and exposure to moist vegetable matter being significant risk factors. Filamentous fungi such as *Aspergillus, Fusarium,* and *Curvularia* and yeast fungi such as *Candida* are the most common fungal organisms associated with FK.

FK is challenging to treat, making early diagnosis and prompt initiation of antifungals paramount. Despite addressing these potential issues early on, it still has an increased likelihood to perforate and require therapeutic keratoplasty compared with bacterial keratitis. Many factors contribute to disease progression, including the pathogenicity of the organism, a delay in diagnosis, infrequent availability of diagnostic tools, uncertainty regarding optimal treatment strategies, and such. Treatment of FK is further limited by a lack of commercially available antifungal ophthalmic treatment options.

Fig. 19.48 shows slit-lamp photographs and AS-OCT images of a patient with FK secondary to *Paecilomyces lilacinus*. Slit-lamp findings demonstrate classic features of FK, including a large, central infiltrate with a fluffy appearance ("fungal ball") involving the middle and posterior stroma, feathery margins, and satellite lesions. AS-OCT shows involvement and infection of the posterior stroma with endothelial plaque.

Fig. 19.49 displays images from another patient with FK. Slit-lamp photograph highlights the paracentral deep infiltrates with feathery margins and prominent peripheral neovascularization. AS-OCT shows the stromal infiltrate with associated fungal endothelial plaque.

Fig. 19.50 shows images from a patient with FK secondary to *Fusarium* infection. Notably, the AS-OCT shows an infiltrate limited to the anterior third of the cornea without involvement of the deeper corneal layers or the presence of an endothelial plaque as seen in Figs. 19.43 and 19.44.

V. ACANTHAMOEBA KERATITIS

Acanthamoeba keratitis is a potentially sight-threatening infection of the ocular surface that is produced by several amoebas of the genus *Acanthamoeba*. They are ubiquitous, free-living protozoans that have been isolated from a variety of habitats, including air, soil, dust, water, and the nasopharyngeal mucosa of healthy individuals. They are known to thrive in ponds, swimming pools, hot tubs, and contact lens solutions and exist in either an active trophozoite or dormant cystic form.

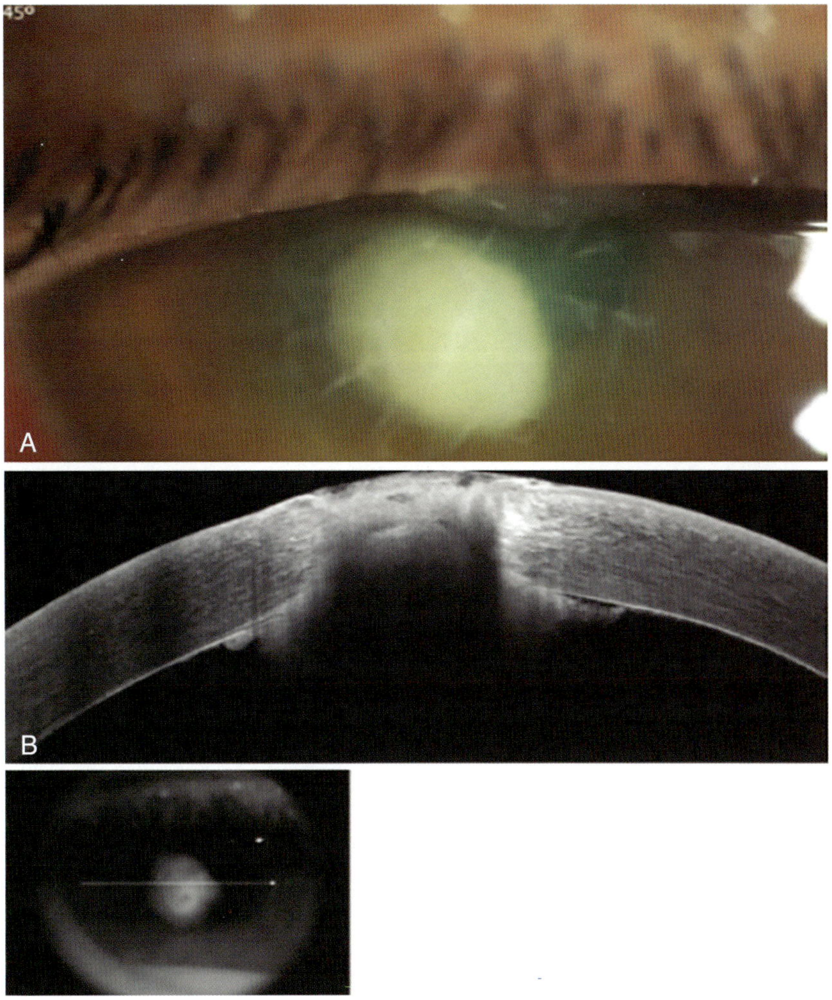

Fig. 19.48 Fungal keratitis secondary to *Paecilomyces lilacinus.* Slit-lamp photograph *(panel A)* shows a centrally located, deep fungal infiltrate ("fungal ball") with feathery margins and satellite lesions at the time of referral. AS-OCT image *(panel B)* highlights a deep corneal infiltrate and endothelial plaque. Accompanying red-free photograph taken with the AS-OCT device additionally shows presence of a hypopyon. The patient was treated with topical amphotericin, topical/oral voriconazole, and corneal glue.

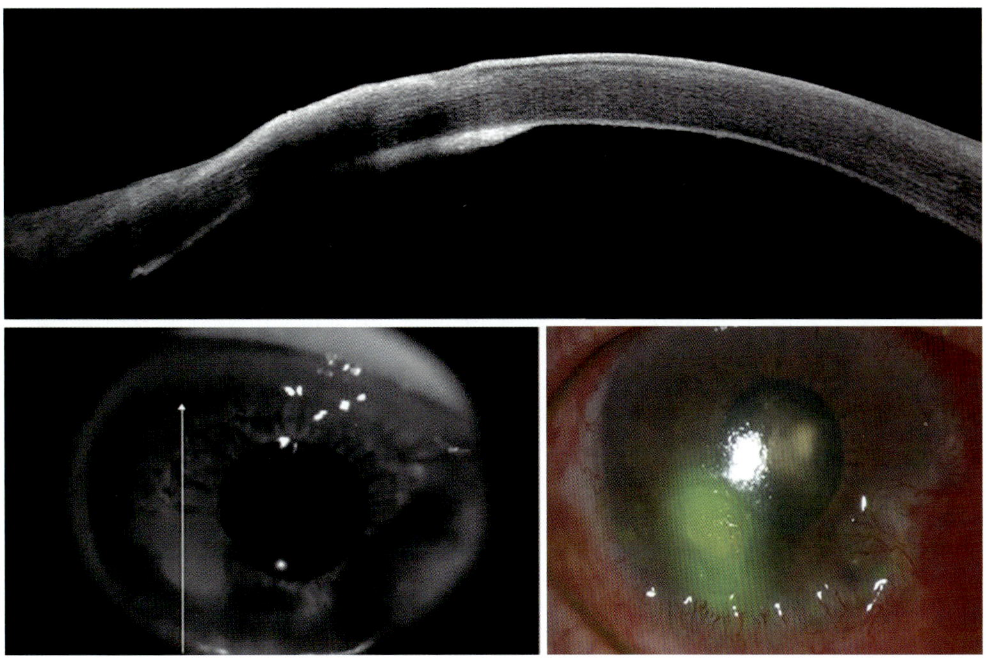

Fig. 19.49 Fungal keratitis. Slit-lamp photograph shows several deep infiltrates with feathery margins and peripheral vascularization. AS-OCT further highlights the extent of the infiltrate along with the characteristic fungal endothelial plaque.

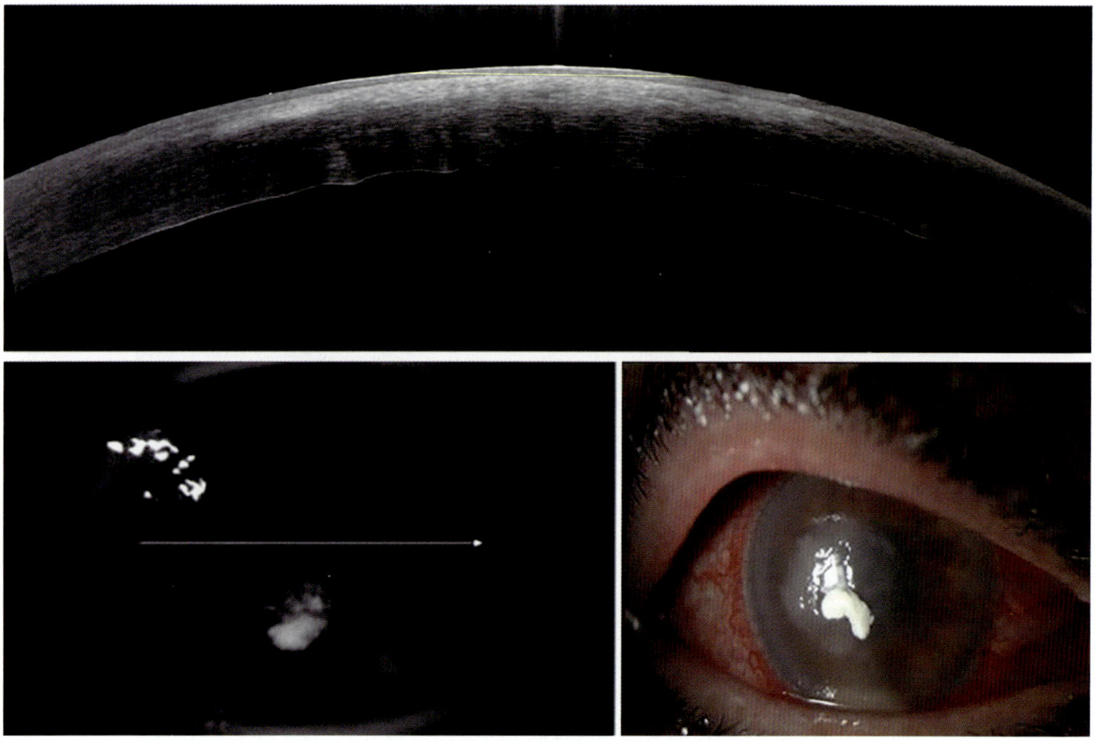

Fig. 19.50 Fungal keratitis secondary to *Fusarium* infection. Slit-lamp photograph shows a fungal infiltrate with feathery margins and hypopyon. There are also some natamycin deposits in the cornea. AS-OCT image shows a corneal infiltrate in the anterior third of the cornea without involvement of the deeper corneal layers or presence of endothelial plaque as seen in Figs. 19.43 and 19.44.

Acanthamoeba's life cycle has two stages: an active trophozoite stage that exhibits growth and a dormant cystic stage with minimal metabolic activity. The trophozoite is capable of slow locomotion by pseudopodia. It feeds on yeast, small bacteria, other protozoans, and in the cornea, keratocytes. The cyst is the dormant form and is 15 to 30 mm in size. It is important to remember and consider acanthamoeba keratitis in all cases of CLRK, especially when onset is insidious, and features are atypical because early diagnosis and treatment are essential to ensure good visual outcomes.

Clinical diagnosis may be challenging, especially in early stages of infection because features are nonspecific and often mistaken for fungal or herpes simplex infection, which may lead to a delay in diagnosis and appropriate treatment initiation. Confocal microscopy may be extremely helpful, if available, in identifying cysts, as laboratory confirmation of acanthamoeba may take several weeks.

Acanthamoeba trophozoites are sensitive to several available medications: antibiotics, antiseptics, antifungals, and antiprotozoals, including metronidazole, antivirals, and antineoplastic therapies. Diamidines and biguanides are the most effective cysticidal antiamebics, and their use has been well documented.

Fig. 19.51 shows images from a patient with acanthamoeba keratitis. Slit-lamp photograph shows a large, central infiltrate with a ring-shaped peripheral zone and central melting. AS-OCT highlights features of the central infiltrate, overlying epithelial defect, and thinning.

Fig. 19.52 shows images from a patient who was treated by an outside provider for approximately 9 months for acanthamoeba keratitis without significant improvement. Slit-lamp images show a more profound infiltrate with suppurative inflammation and prominent hypopyon. AS-OCT further highlights the areas of stromal infiltrate, associated inflammation, and epithelial irregularity. Notably, the middle and posterior corneal layers are relatively uninvolved.

Recalcitrant cases may require additional therapeutic interventions. Fig. 19.53 shows images of a patient who was treated for six months for AK without significant improvement. A deep corneal ring infiltrate was present, along with persistent hypopyon. The patient underwent rose Bengal photodynamic therapy. AS-OCT images taken one month after treatment show resolution of the infection. Follow-up AS-OCT images show marked stromal cicatrization and thinning.

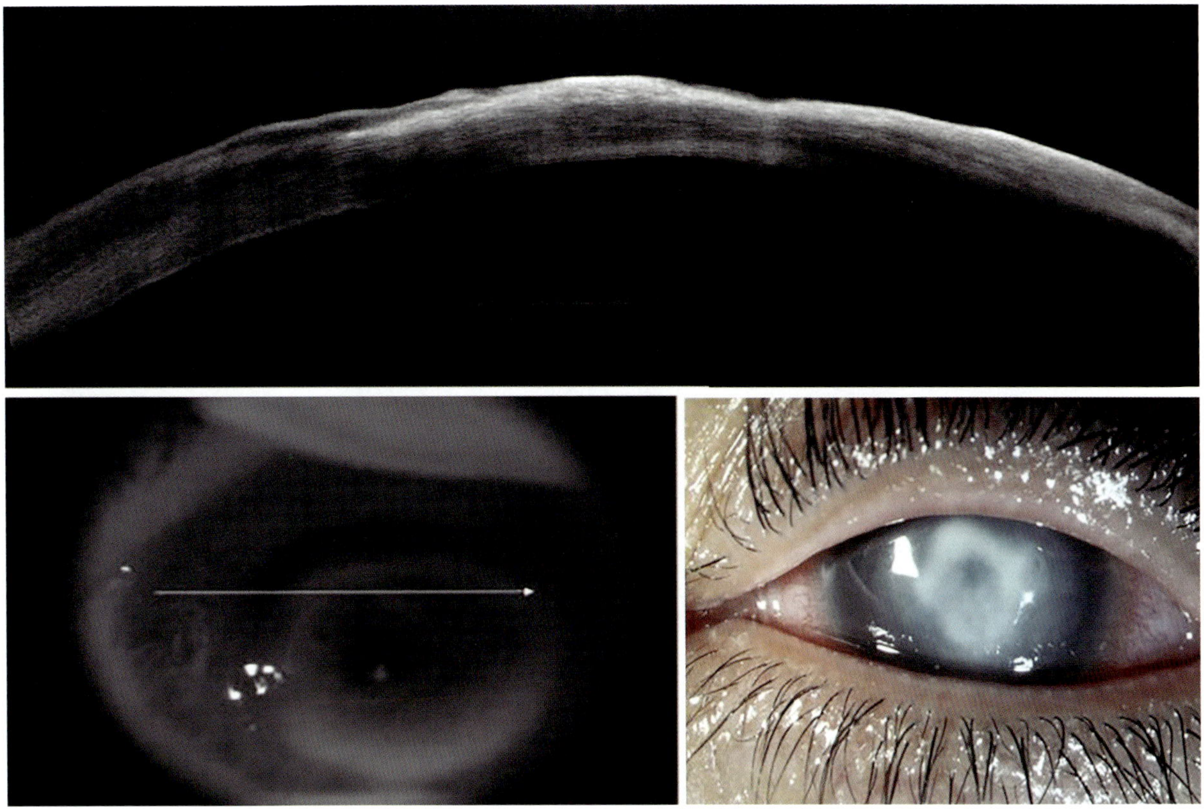

Fig. 19.51 Acanthamoeba keratitis. Slit-lamp photograph *(bottom right panel)* shows a central stromal infiltrate with an epithelial defect and central melting. AS-OCT further highlights the central stromal infiltrate, epithelial defect, and thinning in the zone of infiltrate.

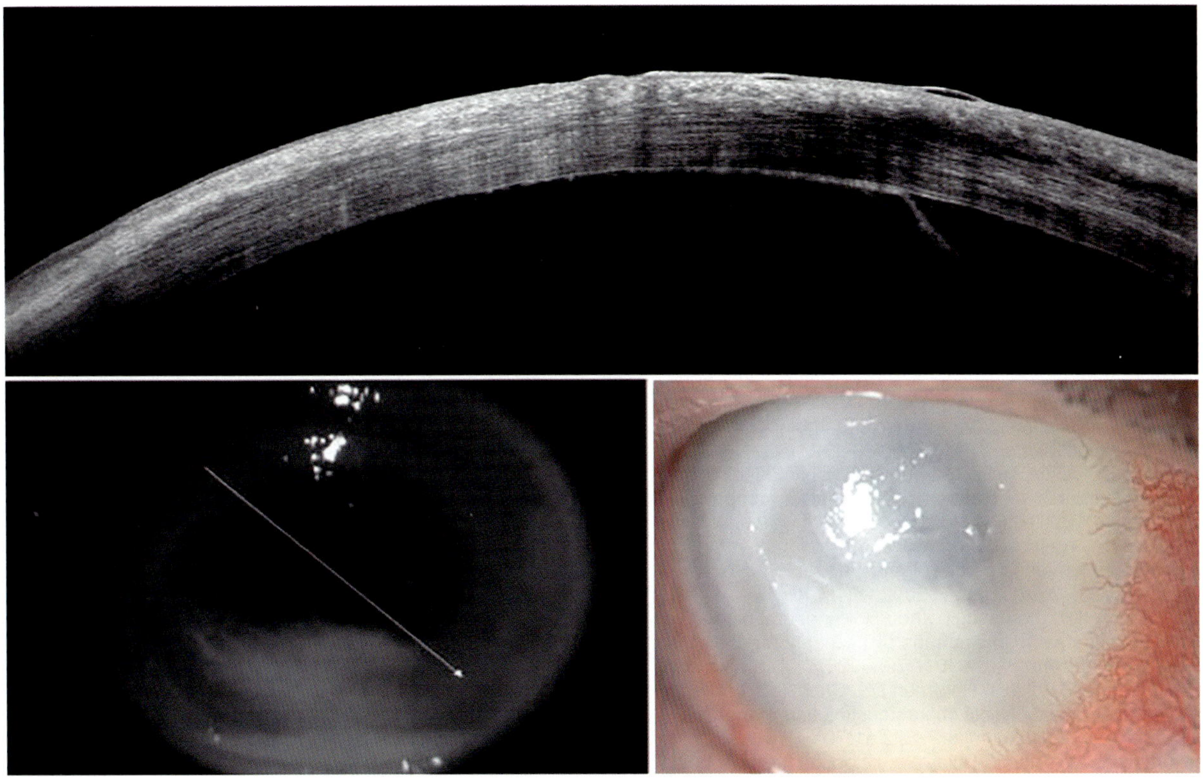

Fig. 19.52 Acanthamoeba keratitis. Images are representative of a patient who presented after being treated for nine months for acanthamoeba keratitis. Slit-lamp photograph (Panel C) shows a paracentral stromal infiltrate with opacification of entire cornea and 2-mm hypopyon. Epithelial defects are overlying the central cornea. There is 4+ conjunctival injection. AS-OCT image (Panels A and B) further delineates the stromal infiltrate with surrounding inflammation and an epithelial defect with surface irregularity.

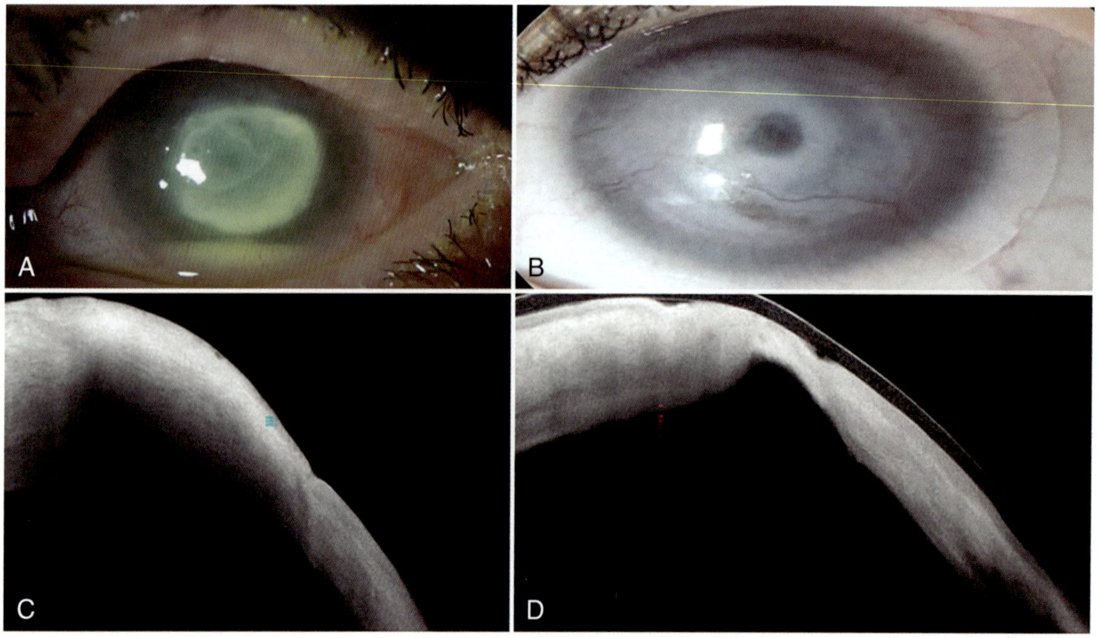

Fig. 19.53 Recalcitrant acanthamoeba keratitis. Images are representative of a patient who came to our institution after being treated for six months for acanthamoeba keratitis without resolution. Slit-lamp image *(panel A)* at the time of referral shows a large stromal ring infiltrate with a 1.5-mm hypopyon. Epithelial defects are present over the area of ring infiltrate. There is 4+ conjunctival injection. *Panel B* displays follow-up images compatible with a deep corneal infiltrate. The patient was treated with rose Bengal photodynamic therapy. AS-OCT images taken one month after treatment *(panel C)* show resolution of the infection. Follow-up AS-OCT images further demonstrate stromal cicatrization and thinning.

BIBLIOGRAPHY

1. Agrawal RV, Murthy S, Sangwan V, Biswas J. Current approach in diagnosis and management of anterior uveitis. *Indian J Ophthalmol*. 2010;58(1):11.
2. Ang M, Baskaran M, Werkmeister RM, et al. Anterior segment optical coherence tomography. *Prog Retin Eye Res*. 2018;66:132-156.
3. Ansari Z, Miller D, Galor A. Current thoughts in fungal keratitis: diagnosis and treatment. *Curr Fungal Infect Rep*. 2013;7(3):209-218.
4. Arici C, Mergen B. Late-term topical tacrolimus for subepithelial infiltrates resistant to topical steroids and ciclosporin secondary to adenoviral keratoconjunctivitis. *Br J Ophthalmol*. 2021;105(5):614-618.
5. Arici C, Sultan P, Mergen B, Buttanri B, Dogan C. The impact of bilateral subepithelial corneal infiltrates on tear film after epidemic keratoconjunctivitis. *Eye Contact Lens*. 2020;46(5):281-284.
6. Arvin AM. Varicella-zoster virus. *Clin Microbiol Rev*. 1996;9(3): 361-381.
7. Asam JS, Polzer M, Tafreshi A, Hirnschall N, Findl O. Anterior segment OCT. In: *High resolution imaging in microscopy and ophthalmology: new frontiers in biomedical optics*. 2019:285-299.
8. Aung TT, Chor WHJ, Yam JKH, Givskov M, Yang L, Beuerman RW. Discovery of novel antimycobacterial drug therapy in biofilm of pathogenic nontuberculous mycobacterial keratitis. *Ocul Surf*. 2017;15(4):770-783.
9. Austin P, Brown SI. Inflammatory Terrien's marginal corneal disease. *Am J Ophthalmol*. 1981;92(2):189-192.
10. Berisa Prado S, Riestra Ayora AC. Topical tacrolimus for corneal subepithelial infiltrates secondary to adenoviral keratoconjunctivitis reply. *Cornea*. 2018;37(7):E32-E32.
11. Brown-Elliott BA, Wallace RJ. Clinical and taxonomic status of pathogenic nonpigmented or late-pigmenting rapidly growing mycobacteria. *Clin Microbiol Rev*. 2002;15(4):716-746.
12. Cao Y, Zhang W, Wu J, Zhang H, Zhou H. Peripheral ulcerative keratitis associated with autoimmune disease: pathogenesis and treatment. *J Ophthalmol*. 2017;2017:7298026.
13. Chan AT, Ulate R, Goldich Y, Rootman DS, Chan CC. Terrien marginal degeneration: clinical characteristics and outcomes. *Am J Ophthalmol*. 2015;160(5):867-872.e1.
14. Chintakuntlawar AV, Zhou X, Rajaiya J, Chodosh J. Viral capsid is a pathogen-associated molecular pattern in adenovirus keratitis. *PLoS Pathog*. 2010;6(4):e1000841.
15. Chou TY, Adyanthaya R. Infectious crystalline keratopathy associated with Klebsiella oxytoca. *J Ophthalmic Inflamm Infect*. 2012;2(4):211-213.
16. Chu HS, Hu FR. Non-tuberculous mycobacterial keratitis. *Clin Microbiol Infect*. 2013;19(3):221-226.
17. Clarke DW, Niederkorn JY. The pathophysiology of Acanthamoeba keratitis. *Trends Parasitol*. 2006;22(4):175-180.
18. Dart JK, Saw VP, Kilvington S. Acanthamoeba keratitis: diagnosis and treatment update 2009. *Am J Ophthalmol*. 2009;148(4):487-499.e2.
19. Davis AR, Sheppard J. Herpes zoster ophthalmicus review and prevention. *Eye Contact Lens*. 2019;45(5):286-291.
20. Doors M, Berendschot TT, de Brabander J, Webers CA, Nuijts RM. Value of optical coherence tomography for anterior segment surgery. *J Cataract Refract Surg*. 2010;36(7):1213-1229.
21. Ding Y, Murri MS, Birdsong OC, Ronquillo Y, Moshirfar M. Terrien marginal degeneration. *Surv Ophthalmol*. 2019;64(2):162-174.
22. Estopinal CB, Ewald MD. Geographic disparities in the etiology of bacterial and fungal keratitis in the United States of America. *Semin Ophthalmol*. 2016;31(4):345-352.
23. Galor A, Thorne JE. Scleritis and peripheral ulcerative keratitis. *Rheum Dis Clin North Am*. 2007;33(4):835-854.
24. Garg P, Kalra P, Joseph J. Non-contact lens related Acanthamoeba keratitis. *Indian J Ophthalmol*. 2017;65(11):1079.
25. Gauthier AS, Noureddine S, Delbosc B. Interstitial keratitis diagnosis and treatment. *J Fr Ophtalmol*. 2019;42(6):e229-e237.
26. Gorovoy MS, Stern GA, Hood CI, Allen C. Intrastromal noninflammatory bacterial colonization of a corneal graft. *Arch Ophthalmol*. 1983;101(11):1749-1752.
27. Gupta Y, Kishore A, Kumari P, et al. Peripheral ulcerative keratitis. *Surv Ophthalmol*. 2021;66(6):977-998.
28. Hall-Stoodley L, Lappin-Scott H. Biofilm formation by the rapidly growing mycobacterial species Mycobacterium fortuitum. *FEMS Microbiol Lett*. 1998;168(1):77-84.
29. Han SB, Liu YC, Noriega KM, Mehta JS. Applications of anterior segment optical coherence tomography in cornea and ocular surface diseases. *J Ophthalmol*. 2016;2016:4971572.
30. Hoffman JJ, Burton MJ, Leck A. Mycotic keratitis—a global threat from the Filamentous Fungi. *J Fungi (Basel)*. 2021;7(4):273.
31. Iwamoto T, DeVoe AG, Farris RL. Electron microscopy in cases of marginal degeneration of the cornea. *Invest Ophthalmol*. 1972;11(4): 241-257.
32. Izatt JA, Hee MR, Swanson EA, et al. Micrometer-scale resolution imaging of the anterior eye in vivo with optical coherence tomography. *Arch Ophthalmol*. 1994;112(12):1584-1589.
33. Jancevski M, Foster CS. Anterior segment optical coherence tomography. *Semin Ophthalmol*. 2010;25(5-6):317-323.

34. Jeng BH, Holsclaw DS. Cyclosporine A 1% eye drops for the treatment of subepithelial infiltrates after adenoviral keratoconjunctivitis. *Cornea*. 2011;30(9):958-961.
35. Kaye S, Choudhary A. Herpes simplex keratitis. *Prog Retin Eye Res*. 2006;25(4):355-380.
36. Kilgore PE, Kruszon-Moran D, Seward JF, et al. Varicella in Americans from NHANES III: implications for control through routine immunization. *J Med Virol*. 2003;70(suppl 1):S111-S118.
37. Knickelbein JE, Hendricks RL, Charukamnoetkanok P. Management of herpes simplex virus stromal keratitis: an evidence-based review. *Surv Ophthalmol*. 2009;54(2):226-234.
38. Knox CM, Holsclaw DS. Interstitial keratitis. *Int Ophthalmol Clin*. 1998;38(4):183-195.
39. Labib BA, Minhas BK, Chigbu DI. Management of adenoviral keratoconjunctivitis: challenges and solutions. *Clin Ophthalmol*. 2020;14:837.
40. Liesegang TJ. Herpes zoster ophthalmicus: natural history, risk factors, clinical presentation, and morbidity. *Ophthalmology*. 2008;115(2):S3-S12.
41. Li JY. Herpes zoster ophthalmicus: acute keratitis. *Curr Opin Ophthalmol*. 2018;29(4):328-333.
42. Li L, Zhai H, Xie L, Cheng J, Liu W. Therapeutic effects of lamellar keratoplasty on Terrien marginal degeneration. *Cornea*. 2018;37(3):318-325.
43. Linebarger EJ, Hardten DR, Lindstrom RL. Diffuse lamellar keratitis: diagnosis and management. *J Cataract Refract Surg*. 2000;26(7):1072-1077.
44. Lobo AM, Agelidis AM, Shukla D. Pathogenesis of herpes simplex keratitis: the host cell response and ocular surface sequelae to infection and inflammation. *Ocul Surf*. 2019;17(1):40-49.
45. Lorenzo-Morales J, Khan NA, Walochnik J. An update on Acanthamoeba keratitis: diagnosis, pathogenesis and treatment. *Parasite*. 2015;22:10.
46. Maycock NJ, Jayaswal R. Update on Acanthamoeba keratitis: diagnosis, treatment, and outcomes. *Cornea*. 2016;35(5):713-720.
47. Meyer-Rüsenberg B, Loderstädt U, Richard G, Kaulfers PM, Gesser C. Epidemic keratoconjunctivitis: the current situation and recommendations for prevention and treatment. *Dtsch Arztebl Int*. 2011;108(27):475.
48. Moorthy RS, Valluri S, Rao NA. Nontuberculous mycobacterial ocular and adnexal infections. *Surv Ophthalmol*. 2012;57(3):202-235.
49. McAllum P, Bahar I, Kaiserman I, Srinivasan S, Slomovic A, Rootman D. Temporal and seasonal trends in Acanthamoeba keratitis. *Cornea*. 2009;28(1):7-10.
50. McKay KM, Jacobs DS. In vivo confocal microscopy of keratic precipitates in uveitis. *Int Ophthalmol Clin*. 2019;59(4):95-103.
51. Murray PI, Rauz S. The eye and inflammatory rheumatic diseases: the eye and rheumatoid arthritis, ankylosing spondylitis, psoriatic arthritis. *Best Pract Res Clin Rheumatol*. 2016;30(5):802-825.
52. Nakano EM, Nakano K, Oliveira MC, Portellinha W, Simonelli R, Alvarenga LS. Cleaning solutions as a cause of diffuse lamellar keratitis. *J Refract Surg*. 2002;18(suppl 3):S361-S363.
53. Neelam S, Niederkorn JY. Focus: infectious diseases: pathobiology and immunobiology of Acanthamoeba keratitis: insights from animal models. *Yale J Biol Med*. 2017;90(2):261.
54. Niederkorn JY, Alizadeh H, Leher H, McCulley JP. The pathogenesis of Acanthamoeba keratitis. *Microbes Infect*. 1999;1(6):437-443.
55. Okumus S, Coskun E, Tatar MG, et al. Cyclosporine a 0.05% eye drops for the treatment of subepithelial infiltrates after epidemic keratoconjunctivitis. *BMC Ophthalmol*. 2012;12(1):1-6.
56. Oliveira MA, Rosa A, Soares M, et al. Anterior segment optical coherence tomography in the early management of microbial keratitis: a cross-sectional study. *Acta Med Port*. 2020;33(5):318-325.
57. Pesudovs K. Terrien's marginal degeneration: case reports and literature review. *Clin Exp Optom*. 1994;77(3):97-104.
58. Porter AJ, Lee GA, Jun AS. Infectious crystalline keratopathy. *Surv Ophthalmol*. 2018;63(4):480-499.
59. Prajna NV, Krishnan T, Rajaraman R, et al. Effect of oral voriconazole on fungal keratitis in the Mycotic Ulcer Treatment Trial II (MUTT II): a randomized clinical trial. *JAMA Ophthalmol*. 2016;134(12):1365-1372.
60. Randleman JB, Shah RD. LASIK interface complications: etiology, management, and outcomes. *J Refract Surg*. 2012;28(8):575-588.
61. Robin JB, Schanzlin DJ, Verity SM, et al. Peripheral corneal disorders. *Surv Ophthalmol*. 1986;31(1):1-36.
62. Schwartz GS, Harrison AR, Holland EJ. Etiology of immune stromal (interstitial) keratitis. *Cornea*. 1998;17(3):278-281.
63. Sharma N, Vajpayee RB, Pushker N, Vajpayee M. Infectious crystalline keratopathy. *CLAO J*. 2000;26(1):40-43.
64. Shipton C, Hind J, Biagi J, Lyall D. Anterior segment optical coherence tomographic characterisation of keratic precipitates. *Cont Lens Anterior Eye*. 2020;43(5):465-468.
65. Silva BL, Cardozo JB, Marback P, Machado FC, Galvão V, Santiago MB. Peripheral ulcerative keratitis: a serious complication of rheumatoid arthritis. *Rheumatol Int*. 2010;30(9):1267.
66. Smith RJ, Maloney RK. Diffuse lamellar keratitis: a new syndrome in lamellar refractive surgery. *Ophthalmology*. 1998;105(9):1721-1726.
67. Stern GA. Infectious crystalline keratopathy. *Int Ophthalmol Clin*. 1993;33(1):1-7.
68. Stulting RD, Randleman JB, Couser JM, Thompson KP. The epidemiology of diffuse lamellar keratitis. *Cornea*. 2004;23(7):680-688.
69. Süveges I, Levai G, Alberth B. Pathology of Terrien's disease: histochemical and electron microscopic study. *Am J Ophthalmol*. 1972;74(6):1191-1200.
70. Thomas PA. Fungal infections of the cornea. *Eye (Lond)*. 2003;17(8):852-862.
71. Tsirouki T, Dastiridou A, Symeonidis C, et al. A focus on the epidemiology of uveitis. *Ocul Immunol Inflamm*. 2018;26(1):2-16.
72. Van Ingen J, Boeree M, Dekhuijzen P, Van Soolingen D. Environmental sources of rapid growing nontuberculous mycobacteria causing disease in humans. *Clin Microbiol Infect*. 2009;15(10):888-893.
73. Watanabe R, Ishii T, Yoshida M, et al. Ulcerative keratitis in patients with rheumatoid arthritis in the modern biologic era: a series of eight cases and literature review. *Int J Rheum Dis*. 2017;20(2):225-230.
74. Wilson SE, de Oliveira RC. Pathophysiology and treatment of diffuse lamellar keratitis. *J Refract Surg*. 2020;36(2):124-130.
75. Wong TY, Ng TP, Fong KS, Tan D. Risk factors and clinical outcomes between fungal and bacterial keratitis: a comparative study. *CLAO J*. 1997;23(4):275-281.
76. Yagci A. Update on peripheral ulcerative keratitis. *Clin Ophthalmol*. 2012;6:747.
77. Yawn BP, Wollan PC, St Sauver JL, Butterfield LC. Herpes zoster eye complications: rates and trends. *Mayo Clin Proc*. 2013;88(6):562-570.
78. Zghal I, Fekih O, Zgolli HM, Chargui S, Malek I, Nacef L. Cyclosporin A eye drop and subepithelial adenoviral keratoconjunctivitis infiltrates. *Tunis Med*. 2019;97(5):639-643.

20 Ocular Inflammation

Paula A. Sepulveda-Beltran | Diego S. Altamirano | Guillermo Amescua

I. INTRODUCTION

Ocular inflammation of the anterior segment is a commonly encountered pathologic condition in the clinical setting. Diagnosis of inflammatory conditions is primarily aided by clinical examination, though ancillary testing, such as laboratory workup, is often relied on by many practitioners to identify the underlying cause, especially in recalcitrant and relapsing cases. Anterior segment optical coherence tomography (AS-OCT) can be a helpful supplementary imaging modality as a result of its ability to provide the clinician with high-resolution images, especially in patients who may not be able to cooperate with prolonged examination because of extreme photophobia and other limiting factors.

Corneal scarring and neovascularization are not an infrequent result of prolonged corneal inflammation. In such cases, clinicians may be challenged with deciding between various vision rehabilitation options, including both nonsurgical and surgical interventions. In cases in which surgery is decided, preoperative AS-OCT imaging can be helpful for targeted surgical planning and postoperative monitoring of surgical success.

This chapter will primarily focus on the applicability of AS-OCT for corneal inflammation, though several instances of anterior chamber inflammation also will be discussed. Typical and variant images of these inflammatory conditions will be presented.

II. INTERSTITIAL KERATITIS

Interstitial keratitis (IK), also known as *stromal keratitis*, is defined as a nonulcerative, nonsuppurative, vascularized inflammatory reaction of the corneal stroma. Clinically, it is characterized by a cellular and neovascular infiltration of the stroma without frank involvement of the corneal epithelium or endothelium, which almost always remain intact. It usually results from an immune response to foreign antigens in the context of an infectious disease (bacterial, viral, parasitic) or a systemic disease (autoimmunity) in which the corneal stroma is affected in the absence of an active infection. Early diagnosis, workup, and intervention are important to optimize patients' visual prognosis.

Historically, IK was attributed to syphilitic or nonsyphilitic causes; however, currently a viral cause (i.e., a herpetic infection) must be considered first. The natural history of IK takes place in two phases: an acute inflammatory (active) phase and a late cicatricial (inactive) phase. Involvement may be unilateral or bilateral, localized or diffuse. In many cases, the underlying cause may never be confirmed despite repeat testing.

Clinical manifestations usually help guide the diagnosis. It may manifest in the form of a small whitish opacity, mostly as a result of the deposition of antigen-antibody complexes or secondary to cellular infiltrates. It also may be accompanied by an immune ring. Figs. 20.1 and 20.2 show images of IK of unknown cause; repeat workup was negative.

Fig. 20.3 demonstrates images of a patient with previous corneal transplant as a result of IK in the left eye that presented with decreased visual acuity because of recurrent IK. Slit-lamp images show corneal graft with central infiltrate, stromal haze temporally, stromal edema, and peripheral neovascularization with central extension. AS-OCT images show stromal edema, inflammatory changes, and neovascularization.

> **CLINICAL PEARL**
>
> AS-OCT can be used in interstitial keratitis cases to evaluate the location, depth, and extent of lesions. In addition, the clinician may assess the presence or absence of epithelial integrity or involvement of deeper layers.

In some cases, laboratory workup may reveal the underlying cause of IK. The findings on clinical examination and AS-OCT usually are nonspecific, however. In Fig. 20.4, AS-OCT of a patient with IK secondary to Lyme disease is shown. Features on imaging are similar to features seen in Figs. 20.2 and 20.3.

III. PERIPHERAL ULCERATIVE KERATITIS

Peripheral ulcerative keratitis (PUK) is a destructive and inflammatory disease of the juxtalimbal cornea. It can be classified based on its cause as infectious or noninfectious, whether associated with ocular or systemic disease or idiopathic in origin. It is often the presenting manifestation of an underlying systemic disease, particularly of autoimmune origin (53% of cases), such as rheumatoid arthritis, systemic lupus erythematosus, and granulomatosis with polyangiitis. Autoimmune causes usually indicate high severity and complicate the presentation and management; they may result in progressive ulceration with corneal perforation and vision loss.

The peripheral cornea has histologic and physiologic components that are different from the central cornea, making it prone to furrowing, ulceration, and systemic/metabolic manifestations. Histologic differences include tighter adhesion of epithelial cells to the basement membrane, higher mitogenic activity of stem cells, and looser arrangement of collagen fibrils with decreased balance between collagenases and their tissue inhibitors, which affect the corneal integrity. Physiologic differences include a well-developed capillary and lymphatic network with poor innervation, which predisposes it to injury, with deposition of circulating immune complexes and inflammation.

The clinical manifestations of PUK vary but commonly include ocular pain that is out of proportion to clinical findings, irritation, redness, photophobia, and corneal opacity. An acute, subacute, or chronic corneal ulceration may occur in either the

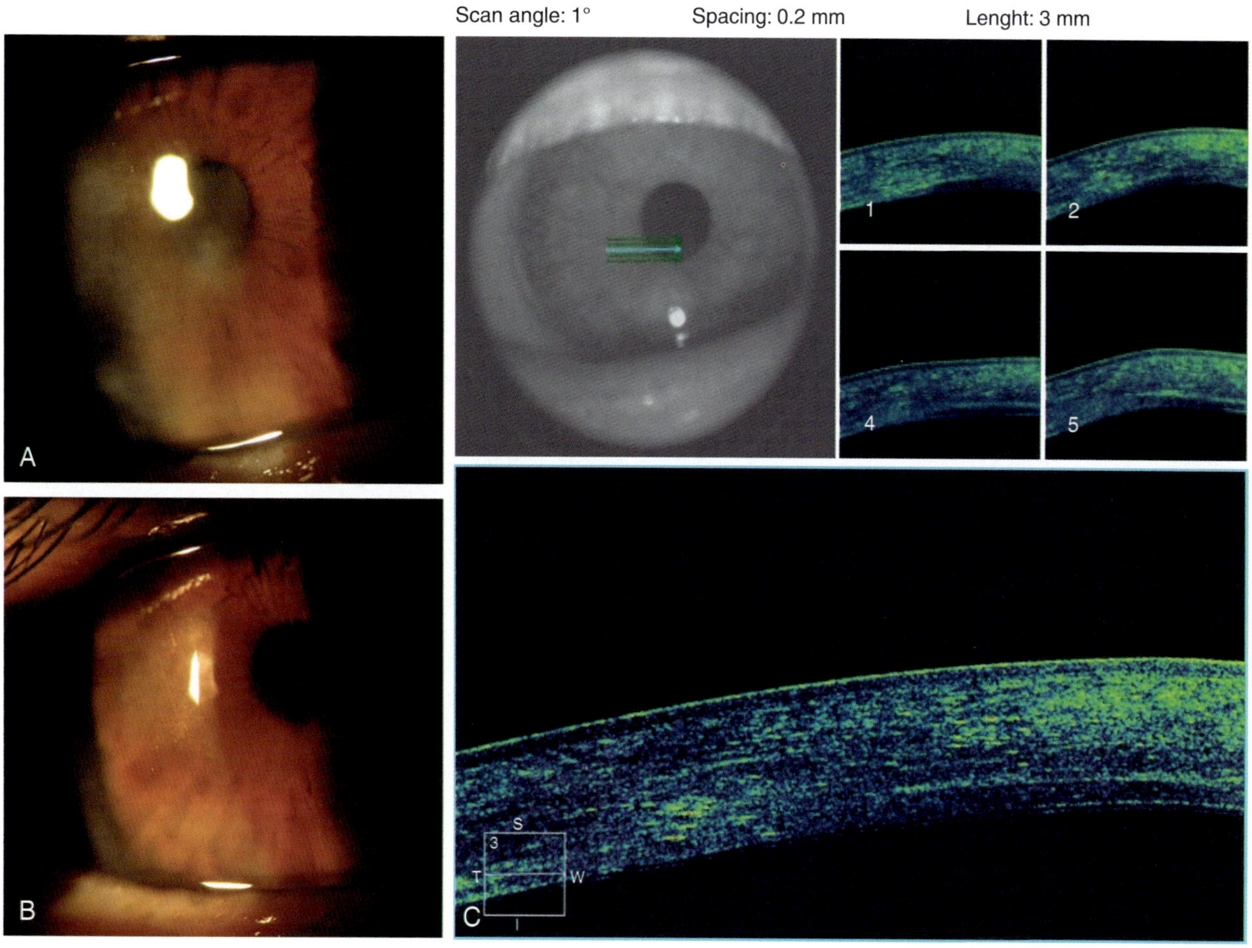

Fig. 20.1 Interstitial keratitis of unknown cause. Slit-lamp photographs *(panels A and B)* demonstrate typical findings of partial light-blocking stromal opacity and lipid deposits without overlying epithelial defect. AS-OCT raster image shows multiple focal areas of increased hyperreflectivity corresponding with areas of stromal opacity.

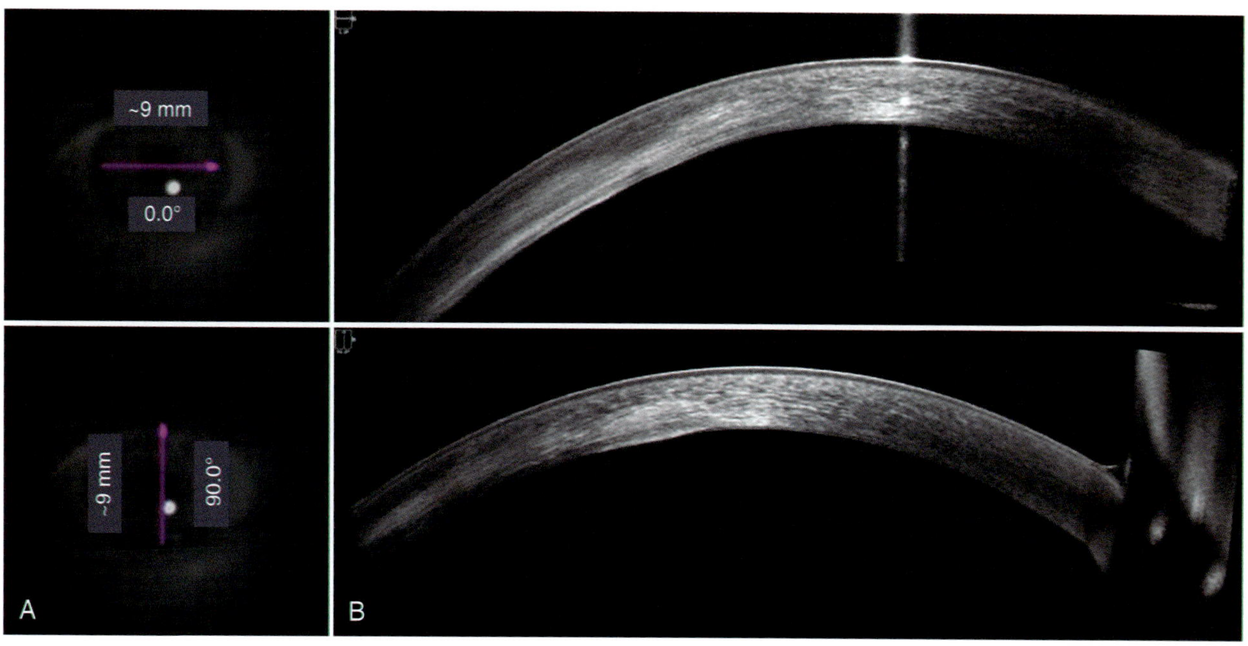

Fig. 20.2 Interstitial keratitis of unknown cause. AS-OCT images *(horizontal slice in panel A, vertical slice in panel B)* demonstrate multiple areas of increased hyperreflectivity in both the anterior and posterior stroma. The overlying epithelium and underlying endothelium are unaffected.

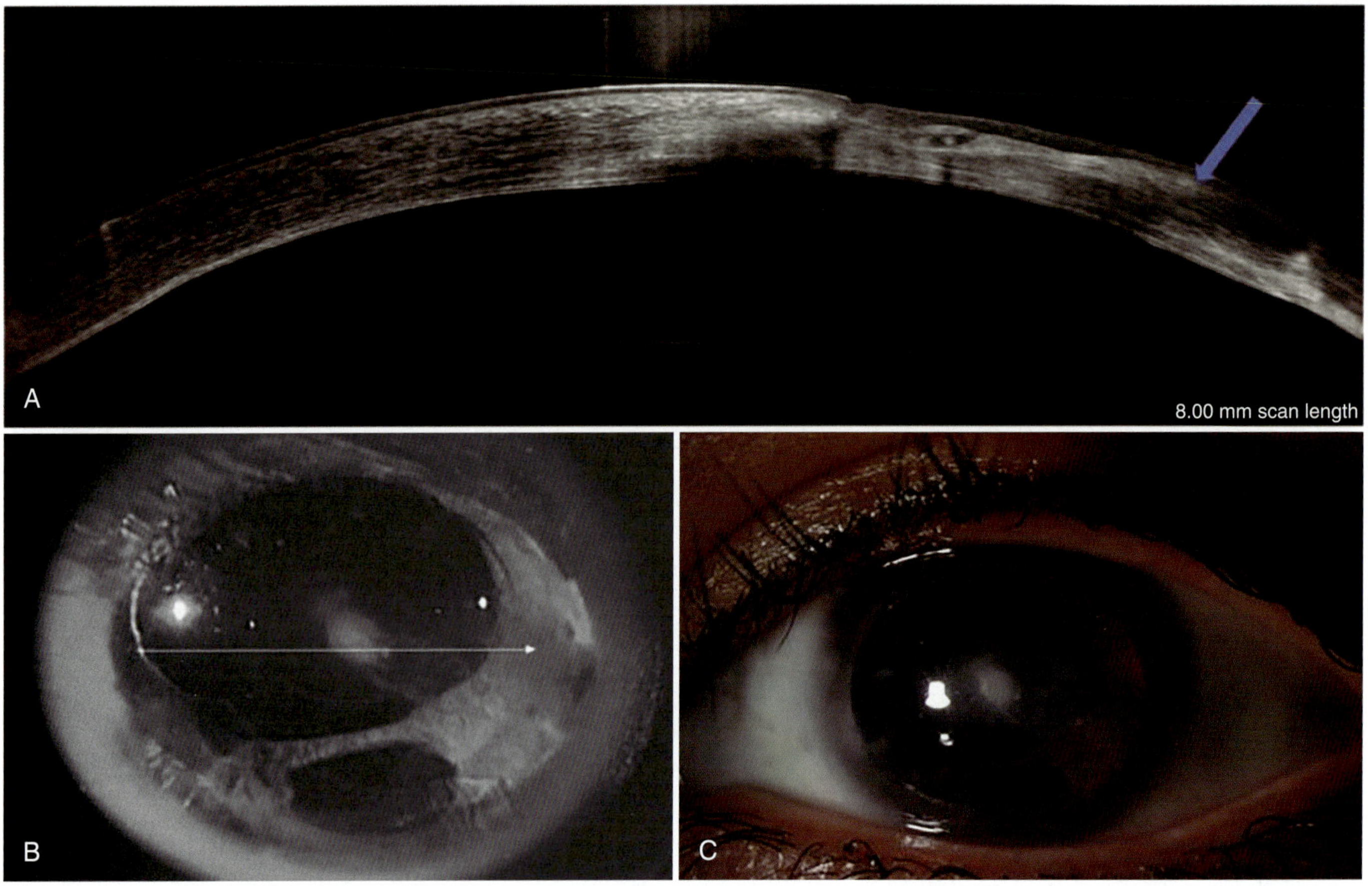

Fig. 20.3 Recurrence of interstitial keratitis in penetrating keratoplasty. AS-OCT image *(panel A)* demonstrates stromal edema, inflammatory changes, and the presence of corneal neovascularization *(arrow).* Slit-lamp image *(panel B)* shows corneal graft with central infiltrate, stromal haze temporally, stromal edema, and neovascularization to the center. Slit-lamp image *(panel C)* demonstrates stromal edema, inflammatory changes, and the presence of neovascularization.

central or paracentral regions along with crescent-shaped stromal thinning and inflammation involving the juxtalimbal cornea. The common and recommended therapeutic method for autoimmune disease patients with PUK is systemic therapy, including nonsteroidal antiinflammatory drugs (NSAIDS), corticosteroids, systemic immunosuppressive chemotherapy, and surgical therapy. Biologic therapy has become a novel therapeutic method. Topical steroids/NSAIDs should be avoided as much as possible.

Fig. 20.5 images are representative of a patient who presented with PUK. Slit-lamp photographs demonstrate inferotemporal thinning without epithelial defect and without infiltrate. AS-OCT demonstrates stromal compaction with increased stromal hyperreflectivity and corneal thinning. Fig. 20.6 shows AS-OCT images of a patient with moderate to severe PUK in which there is prominent thinning of the peripheral cornea with severe stromal compaction.

Figs. 20.7 to 20.9 show chronologic AS-OCT images of a patient who developed slowly worsening PUK that eventually

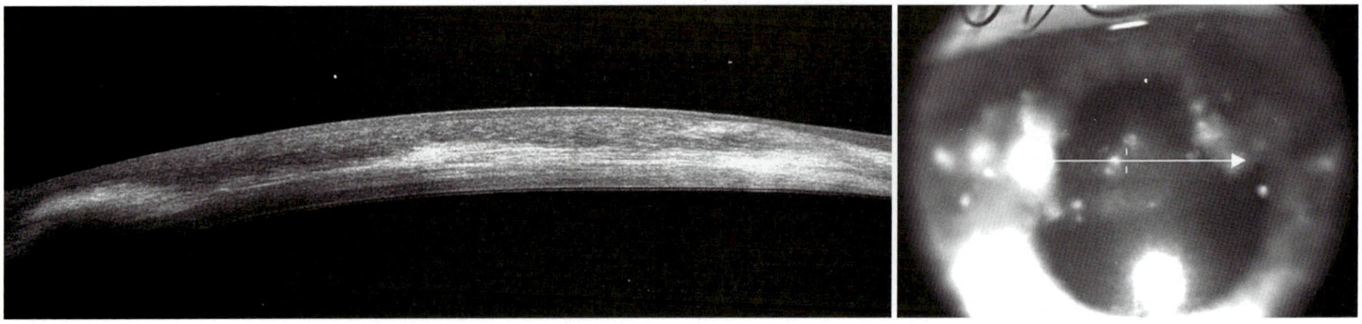

Fig. 20.4 Interstitial keratitis secondary to Lyme disease. AS-OCT images demonstrate increased stromal hyperreflectivity with additional areas of focal hyperreflectivity. The epithelium and endothelium are normal. Corneal thickness is slightly increased especially centrally.

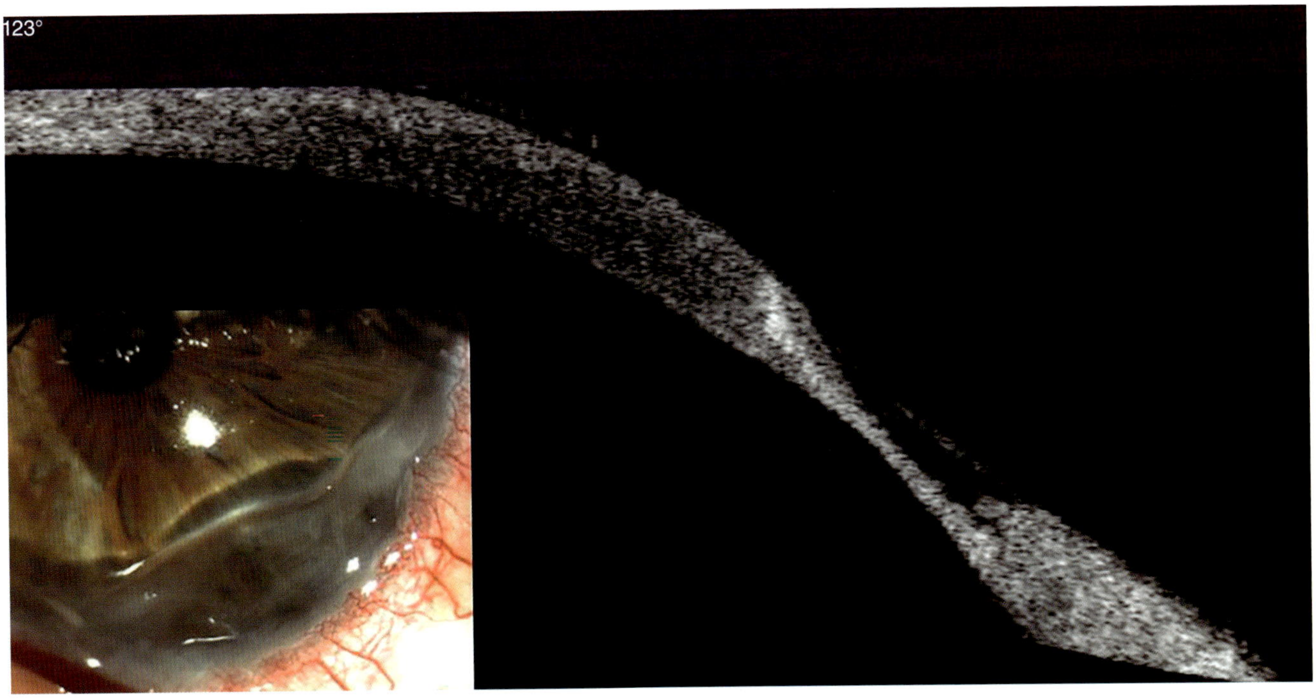

Fig. 20.5 Peripheral ulcerative keratitis. Slit-lamp photograph highlights inferotemporal thinning without epithelial defect or infiltrate. AS-OCT further highlights the stromal compaction and increased hyperreflectivity in the area of stromal thinning. (Courtesy Helena Filipe, MD, University of Lisbon, Portugal.)

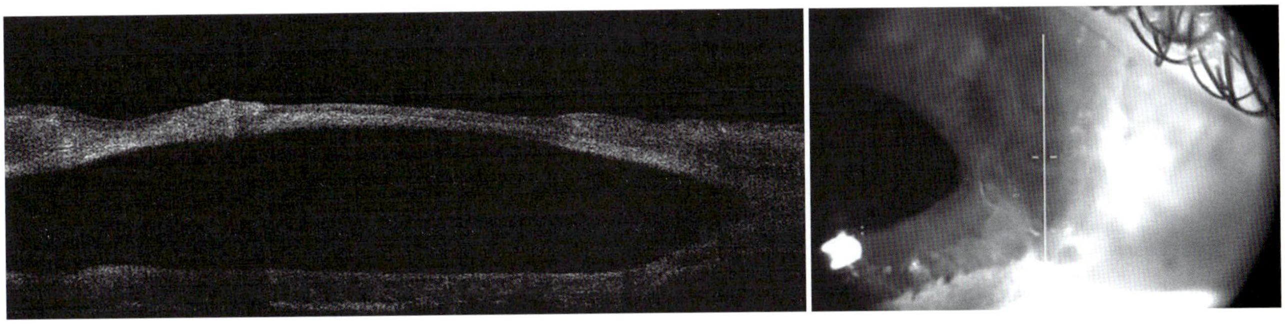

Fig. 20.6 Moderate to severe peripheral ulcerative keratitis. There is marked thinning of the peripheral cornea with significant stromal thinning.

stabilized without further ulceration. In Fig. 20.7, at the time of initial presentation, there is minimal stromal thinning with slightly increased hyperreflectivity from stromal compaction. There is some hypertrophy of the overlying epithelium. Figs. 20.8 and 20.9 show follow-up AS-OCT images in the same patient that chronologically highlight the sequences of stromal scarring, compaction, and epithelial hypertrophic remodeling to maintain a relatively smooth corneal surface at 6-month follow-up.

Fig. 20.10 and Fig. 20.11 show clinical images of a patient who developed severe PUK in the context of refractory rheumatoid arthritis. In Fig. 20.10, the slit-lamp photograph demonstrates a U-shaped ulceration of the peripheral cornea located between 1 o'clock and 10 o'clock with an associated epithelial defect and 40% stromal thinning. AS-OCT imaging further delineates the area of epithelial defect and stromal thinning. Dehydrated amniotic membrane transplant (AMT) was performed in office because of concerns of further stromal thinning and risk for perforation. Fig. 20.11 shows the interval improvement after AMT incorporation into the previously thinned area with subsequent healing.

CLINICAL PEARL

AS-OCT can be used for serial monitoring of peripheral thinning in patients with PUK and for assessing response to clinical treatments.

Fig. 20.12 shows AS-OCT images of a patient with remote history of PUK. After stabilization of the systemic autoimmune disease, no further inflammatory episodes were noted. These images represent stable, chronic changes demonstrating stromal compaction and overlying epithelial hypertrophy.

IV. DIFFUSE LAMELLAR KERATITIS

Diffuse lamellar keratitis (DLK) is a diffuse, multifocal, noninfectious inflammation formed by white blood cell infiltrates that are localized to the lamellar interface and occur within 1 to 5 days after myopic keratomileusis or laser-assisted in-situ keratomileusis (LASIK). This nonspecific interface inflammation is associated with intraoperative epithelial defects and has been linked to multiple rare potential inciting factors. Most cases, especially

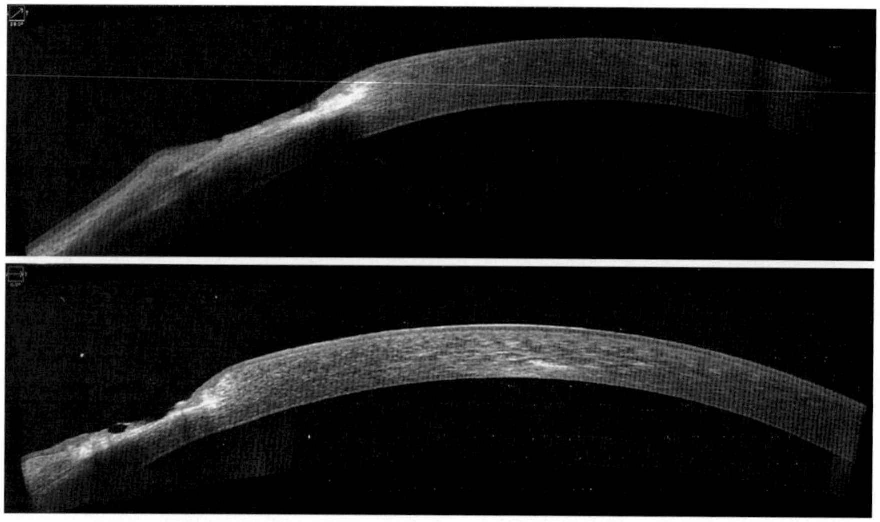

Fig. 20.7 Peripheral ulcerative keratitis initial presentation. AS-OCT images of the left eye at initial presentation reveal minimal stromal thinning with increased stromal hyperreflectivity in the area of excavation. The overlying epithelium is intact, although there are multiple areas of hypertrophic remodeling. The central cornea is unaffected.

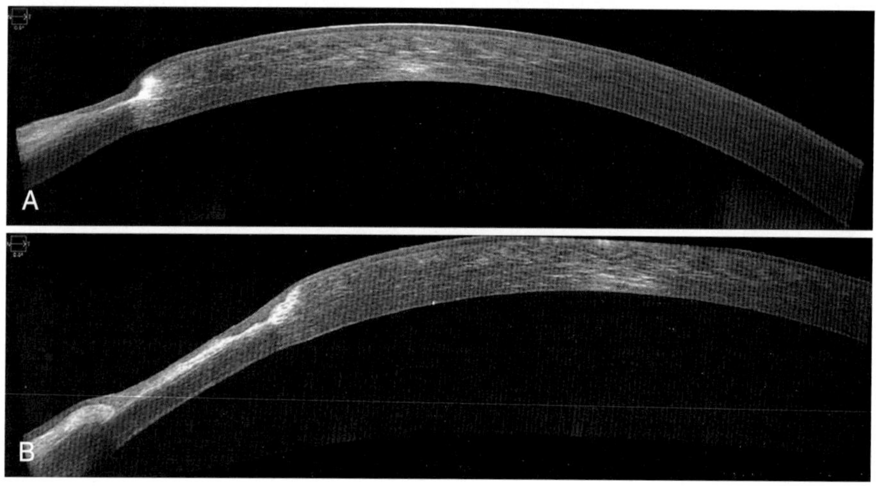

Fig. 20.8 Peripheral ulcerative keratitis follow-up images. Images of the patient from Fig. 20.7 taken at 1-month follow-up *(panel A)* demonstrate consolidation of stromal compaction with additional epithelial hypertrophic remodeling. Two months later *(panel B),* there is worsening of stromal thinning with further anterior extension. Notably, there is increased epithelial hypertrophic remodeling in this image compared with *panel A.*

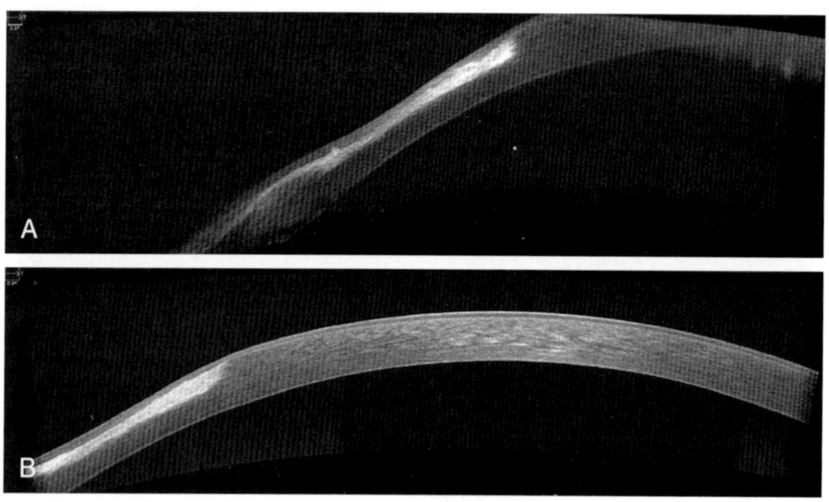

Fig. 20.9 Peripheral ulcerative keratitis follow-up images. Three months later *(panel A),* there is additional stromal compaction and scarring. The cornea has a peripheral ectatic bulge appearance in this view. Six months later, after better control of the patient's systemic disease *(panel B),* the overlying epithelium has smoothed out the peripheral area of thinning, restoring a relatively smooth outer corneal surface.

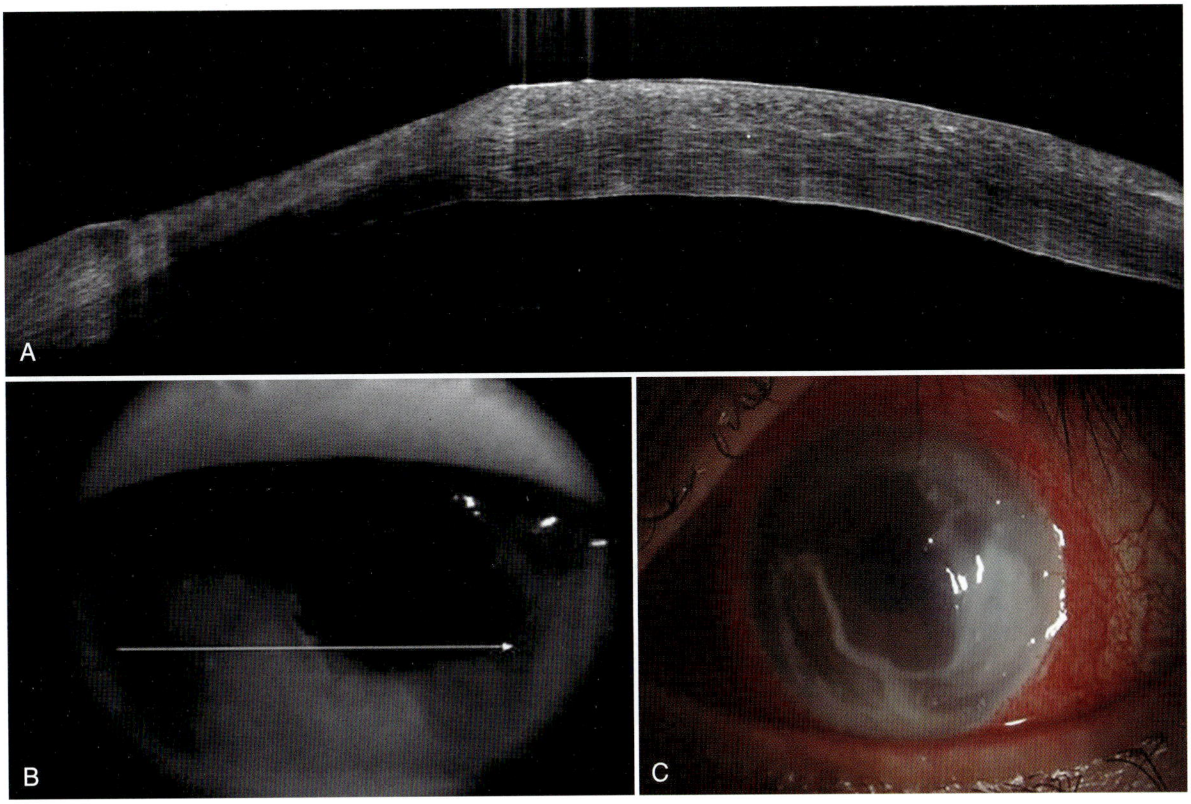

Fig. 20.10 Severe peripheral ulcerative keratitis in context of rheumatoid arthritis. Slit-lamp image *(bottom right panel)* shows a U-shaped ulceration of the peripheral cornea located between 1 o'clock and 10 o'clock with an associated epithelial defect and 40% stromal thinning. AS-OCT image further highlights the area of epithelial defect and stromal thinning.

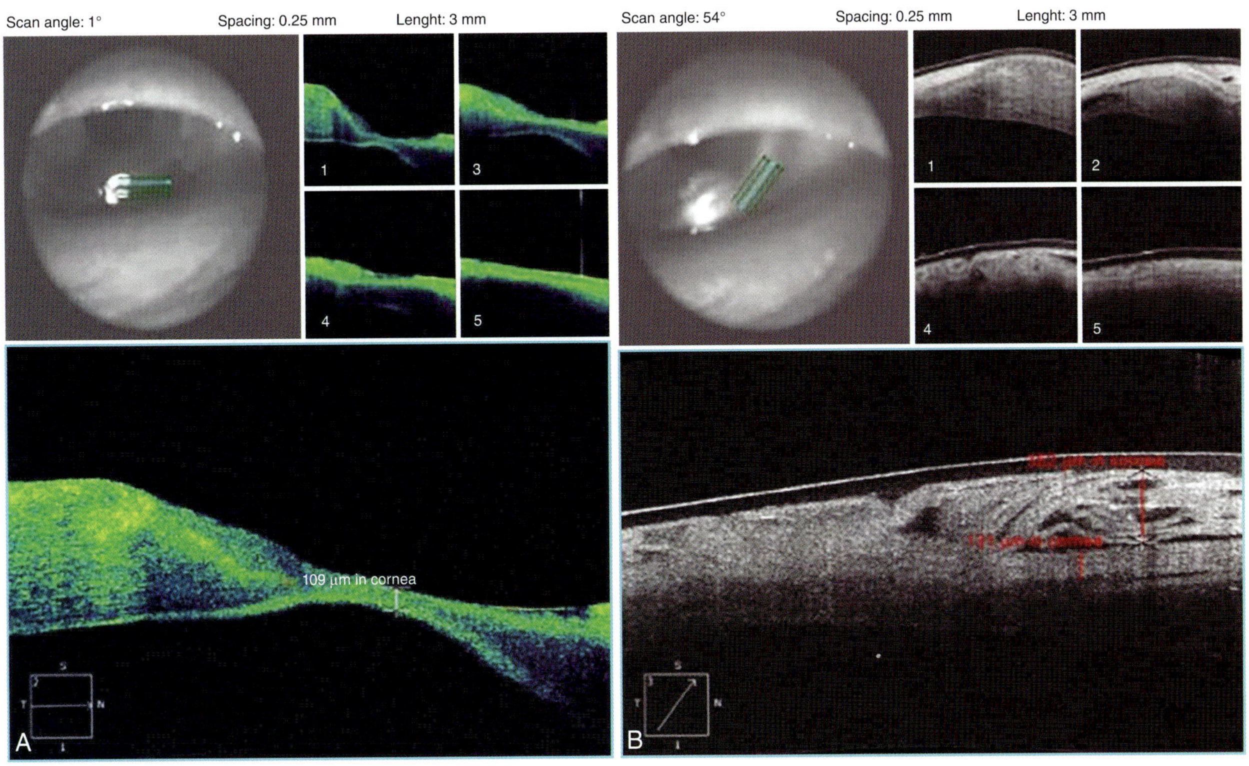

Fig. 20.11 Severe peripheral ulcerative keratitis (PUK) in context of rheumatoid arthritis. Follow-up images on AS-OCT *(panel A)* show worsening of the PUK with extreme stromal thinning, with approximately 189 microns of residual stroma remaining. The patient was treated with dehydrated amniotic membrane transplant (AMT). The amniotic membrane was folded in half and placed under a bandage contact lens. Several days later it was noted to have worked its way into the area of stromal thinning, getting folded around itself multiple times and adopting an accordion-like shape. *Panel B* shows the folded AMT, which subsequently became incorporated and allowed for epithelialization over the area of thinning. This AS-OCT image shows 352 microns of AMT incorporated over 131 microns of cornea.

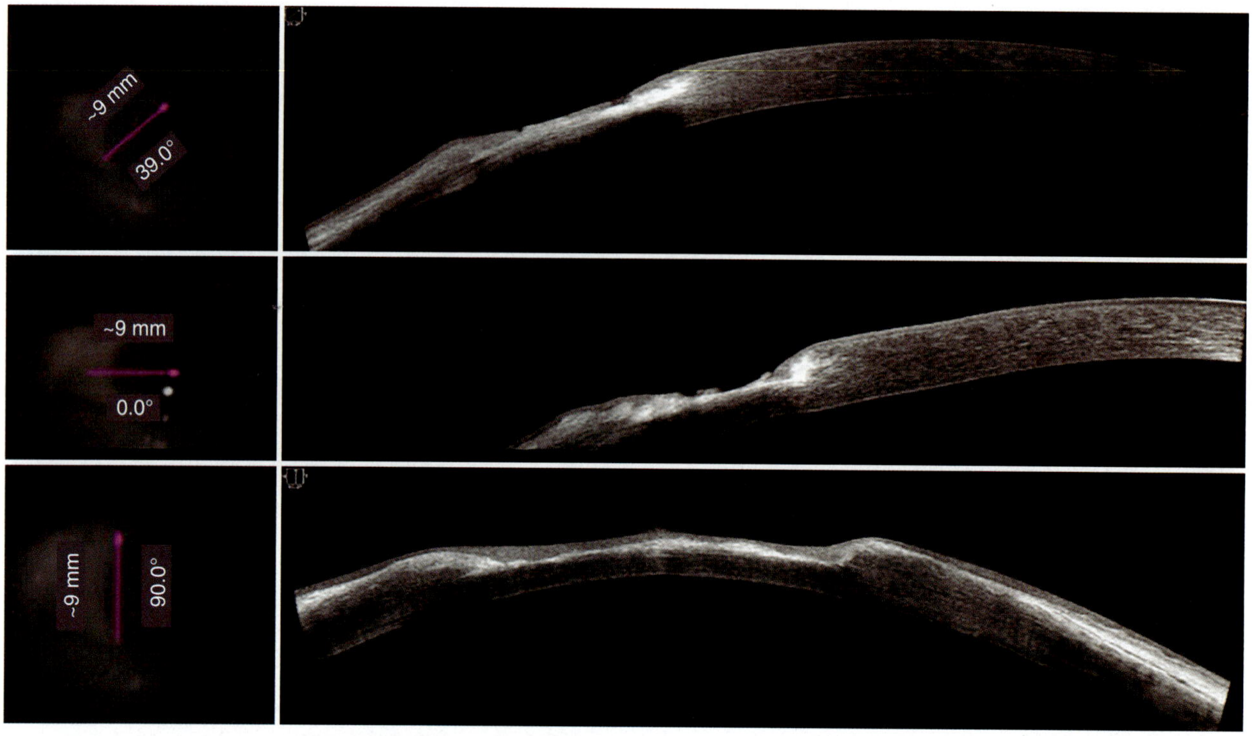

Fig. 20.12 Peripheral ulcerative keratitis (PUK) inactive. In this patient with remote history of PUK, chronic and stable changes consistent with stromal compaction and overlying epithelial hypertrophy.

DLK epidemics, have been linked to bacterial endotoxins from sterilization reservoirs or issues during the instrument sterilization process. Late-onset DLK also has been described in literature.

DLK is classified clinically in four stages as described by Linebarger and colleagues. Stage 1 consists of inflammatory cells that are present in the far periphery only. They initially manifest in the corneal stroma and then coalesce into the LASIK interface. Stage 2 consists of a diffuse infiltrate that frequently involves the paracentral and peripheral flap margins but spares the central axis. Stage 3 consists of a denser infiltrate within the flap interface, that compromises the visual axis and is frequently associated with decreased visual acuity. Stage 4 consists of a focal, coalesced dense haze associated with scarring and significant flap necrosis that usually results in permanent corneal scarring and vision loss of varying severity. DLK is highly responsive to steroids. Aggressive treatment with topical steroids is indicated for mild cases, and a combination of topical and oral steroids is indicated for moderate cases.

Fig. 20.13 shows images of a patient with DLK after LASIK procedure. Slit-lamp photographs reveal a diffuse haziness in the interface with intact epithelium and lack of infiltrate. Visual acuity was decreased compared with the first postoperative day. AS-OCT further highlights the area of stromal inflammation, epithelial edema, and fluid accumulation in the interface.

CLINICAL PEARL

When using AS-OCT for DLK assessment, it is important to obtain slices that encompass the peripheral flap interface.

Fig. 20.14 shows AS-OCT images of another patient after resolution of DLK. The cornea appears overall relatively unremarkable in the central horizontal slice view, but in peripheral slice view, some hypertrophic changes are seen in the flap as a result of healing after the initial inflammatory phase. Visual acuity was unaffected.

V. NEUROTROPHIC KERATITIS

Neurotrophic keratitis (NTK) is a degenerative corneal condition caused by impairment of trigeminal innervation that leads to refractory, episodic, and recrudescent epithelial breakdown; delayed corneal epithelial healing; secondary corneal infection; and corneal thinning and perforation. Patients with NTK have marked corneal anesthesia.

NTK may occur as a result of a variety of causes, but the most frequently encountered are herpetic infections, postneurosurgical procedures, and mechanical and chemical injuries.

Patients with NTK may present with myriad examination findings because the disease has a significant spectrum of signs and symptoms. Corneal epithelial changes, including recurrent and/or persistent epithelial defects, and associated subepithelial scarring are hallmark features in mild disease states. Fig. 20.15 displays typical slit-lamp findings of mild NTK without epithelial defect evidenced by subepithelial scarring and associated epithelial hyperplasia. Figs. 20.16 and 20.17 shows AS-OCT raster images of the right and left eye scarring, respectively. There is increased hyperreflectivity seen in the middle and posterior stroma with stromal compaction. When contrasted to PUK images, the epithelium is significantly hypertrophic over the area of scarring in both eyes, and there is a relatively smooth overlying corneal surface.

AS-OCT can be helpful to monitor progress of medical therapy (e.g., ocular surface lubrication) in NTK patients. Figs. 20.18 and 20.19 show images of a pediatric patient with bilateral, mild-stage NTK. Slit-lamp photographs show characteristic epithelial irregularity and punctate keratopathy, along with

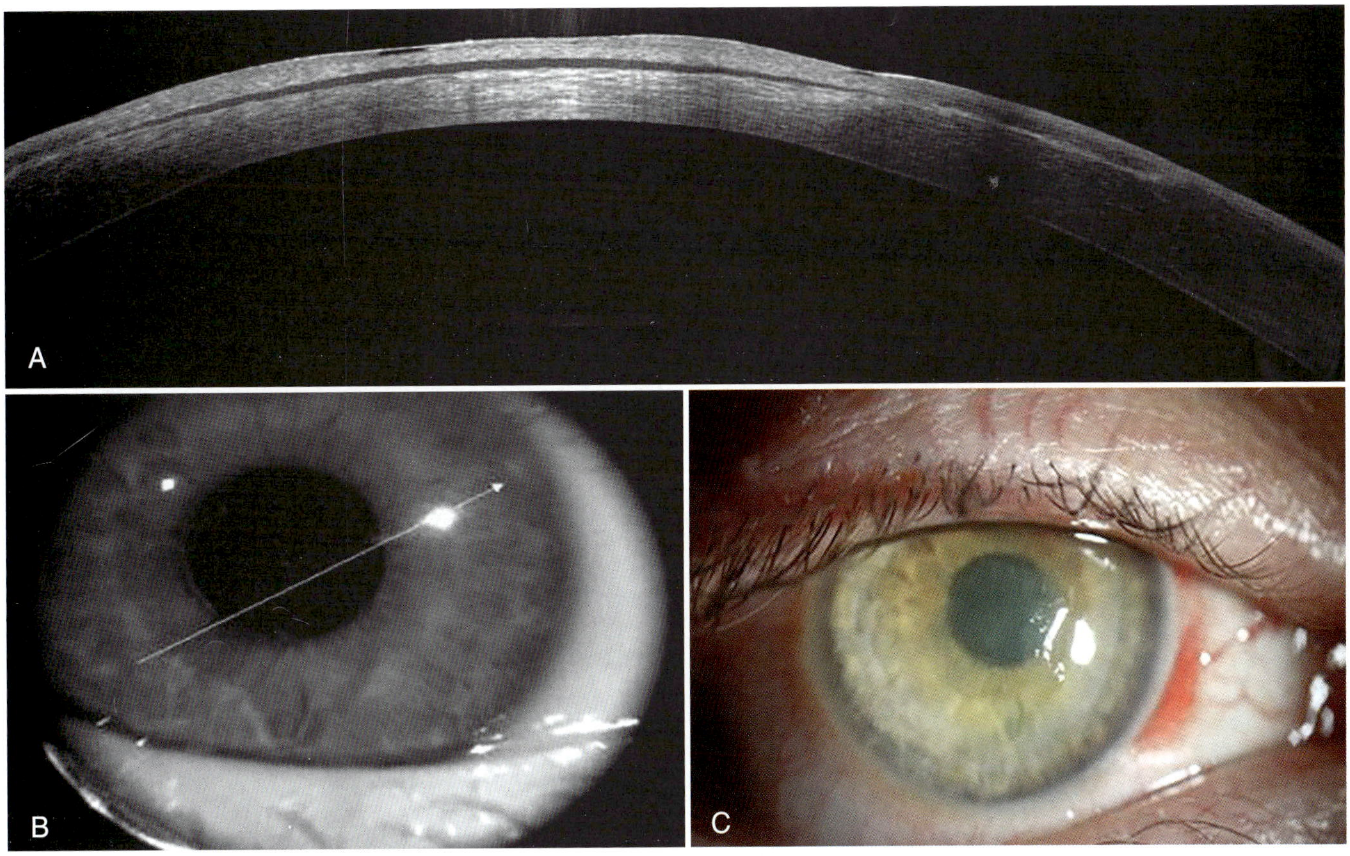

Fig. 20.13 Diffuse lamellar keratitis (DLK). Slit-lamp photograph *(bottom right panel)* shows the initial clinical presentation. There is diffuse haziness in the interface with an intact epithelium. Visual acuity was decreased compared with the first postoperative day. AS-OCT image further characterizes the central stromal inflammation, epithelial edema (seen as hyporeflective areas within the epithelium), and fluid accumulation in the interface.

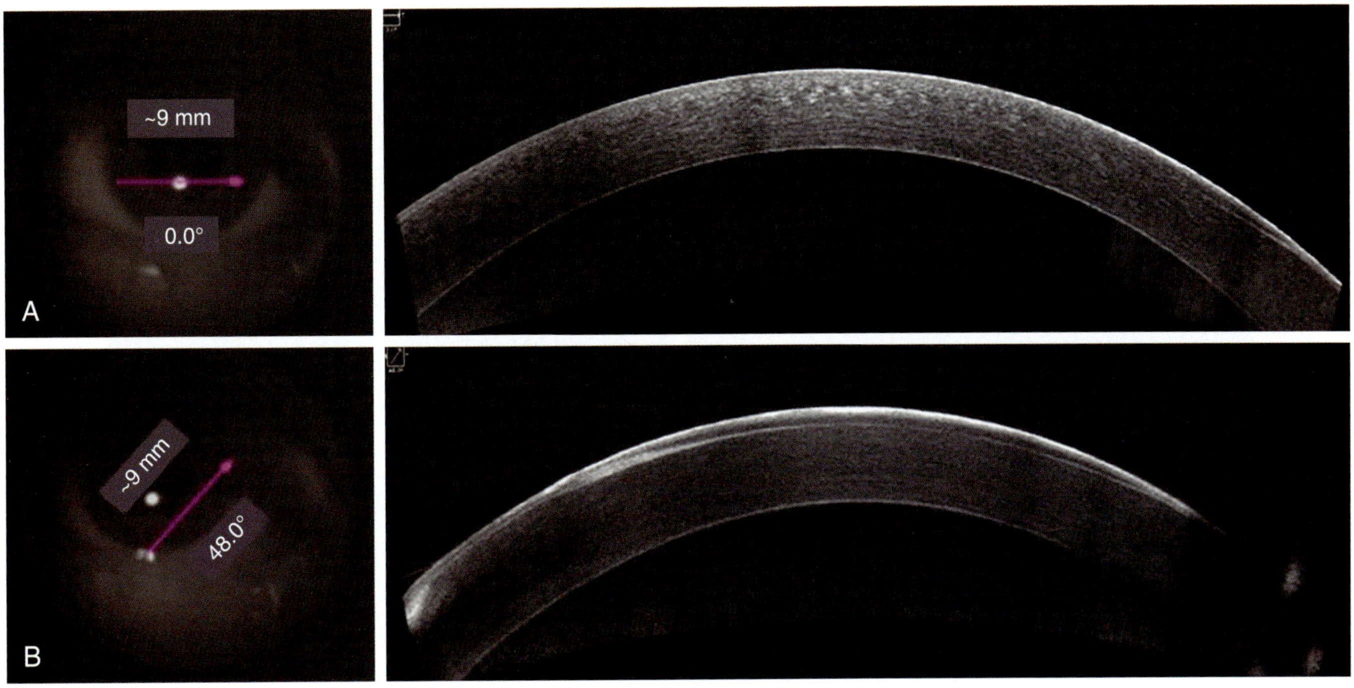

Fig. 20.14 Resolved diffuse lamellar keratitis (DLK). A patient with remote history of DLK may have an overall normal, benign-appearing cornea when central slices *(panel A)* are taken. In the mid-peripheral slice through the flap *(panel B)*, there is notable subepithelial scarring as evidenced by hyperreflective changes seen in the peripheral edge of the flap. Visual acuity was unaffected.

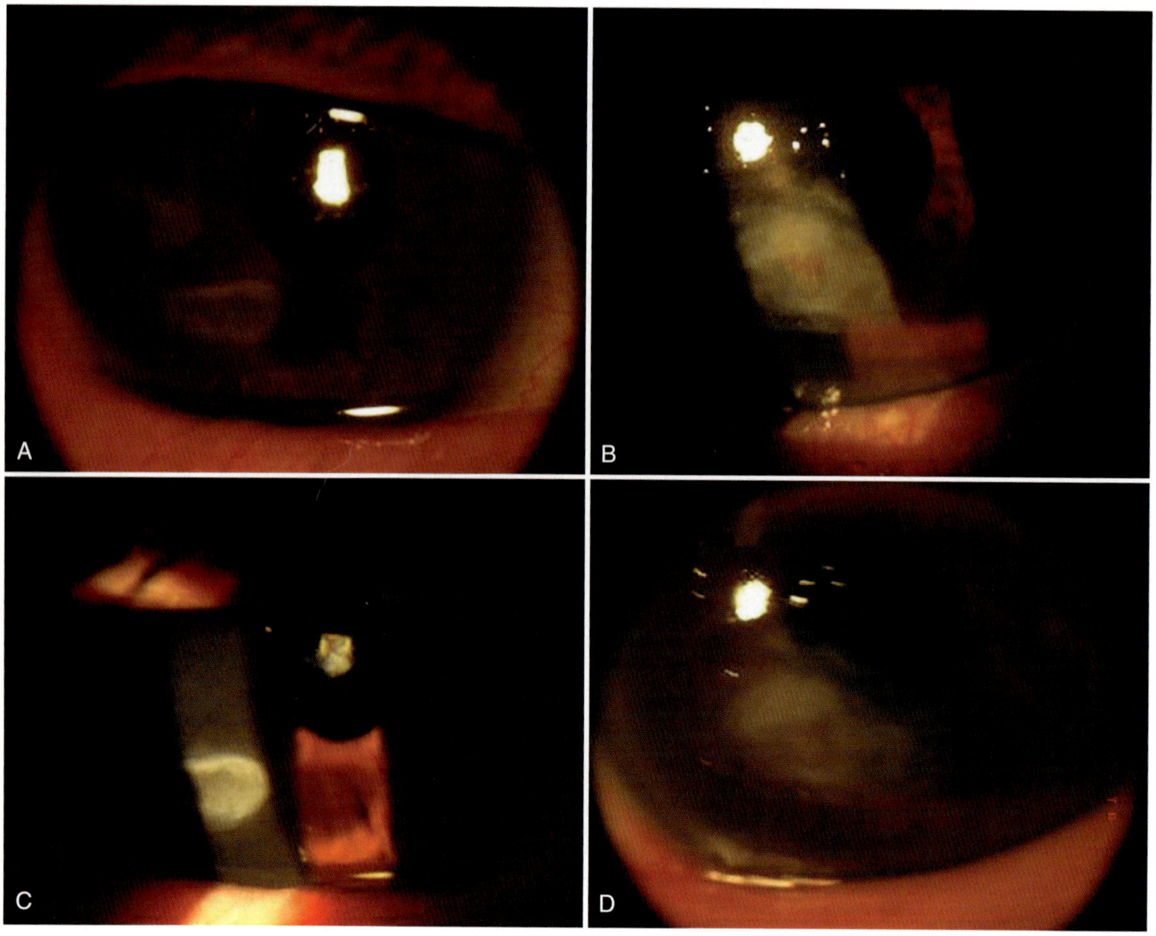

Fig. 20.15 Neurotrophic keratitis. Slit-lamp findings of the right eye *(panels A and B)* and left eye *(panels C and D)* demonstrate ovoid areas of epithelial hyperplasia and irregularity with subepithelial scarring, along with scattered small facets of dried epithelium (Gaule spots).

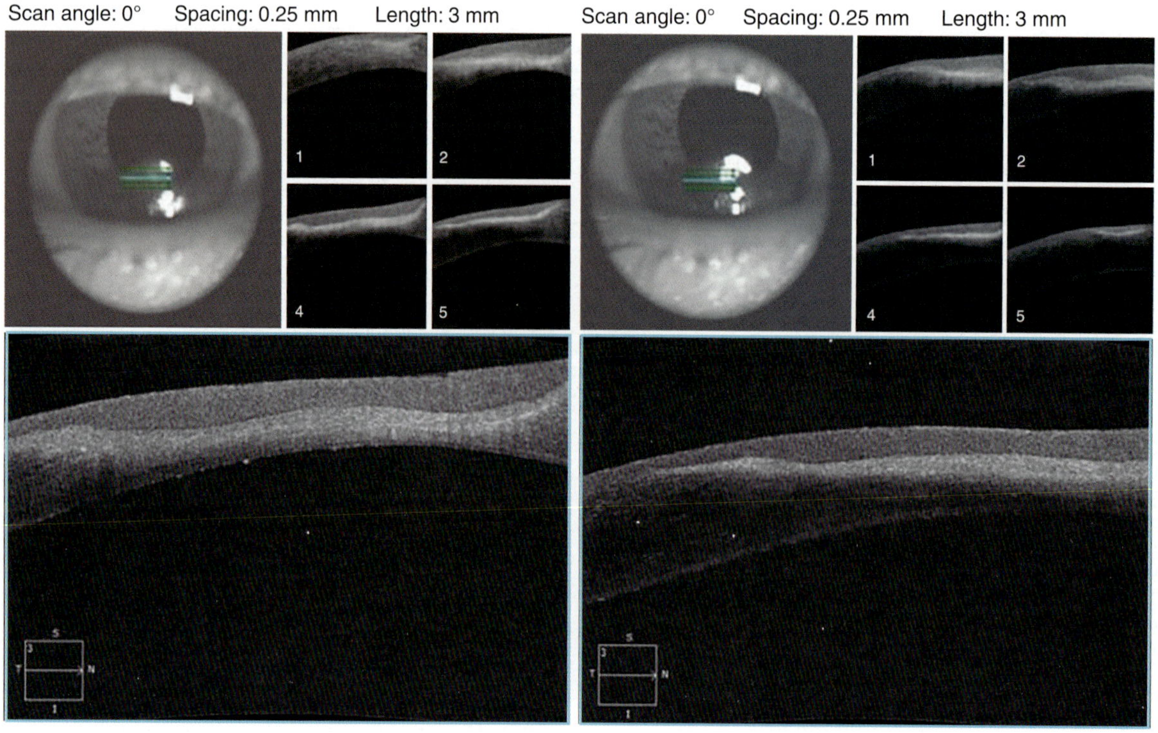

Fig. 20.16 Neurotrophic keratitis scarring. AS-OCT raster images of the right eye of the images shown in Fig. 20.15. A significant amount of stromal compaction and scarring is observed, along with compensatory overlying epithelial thickening and remodeling.

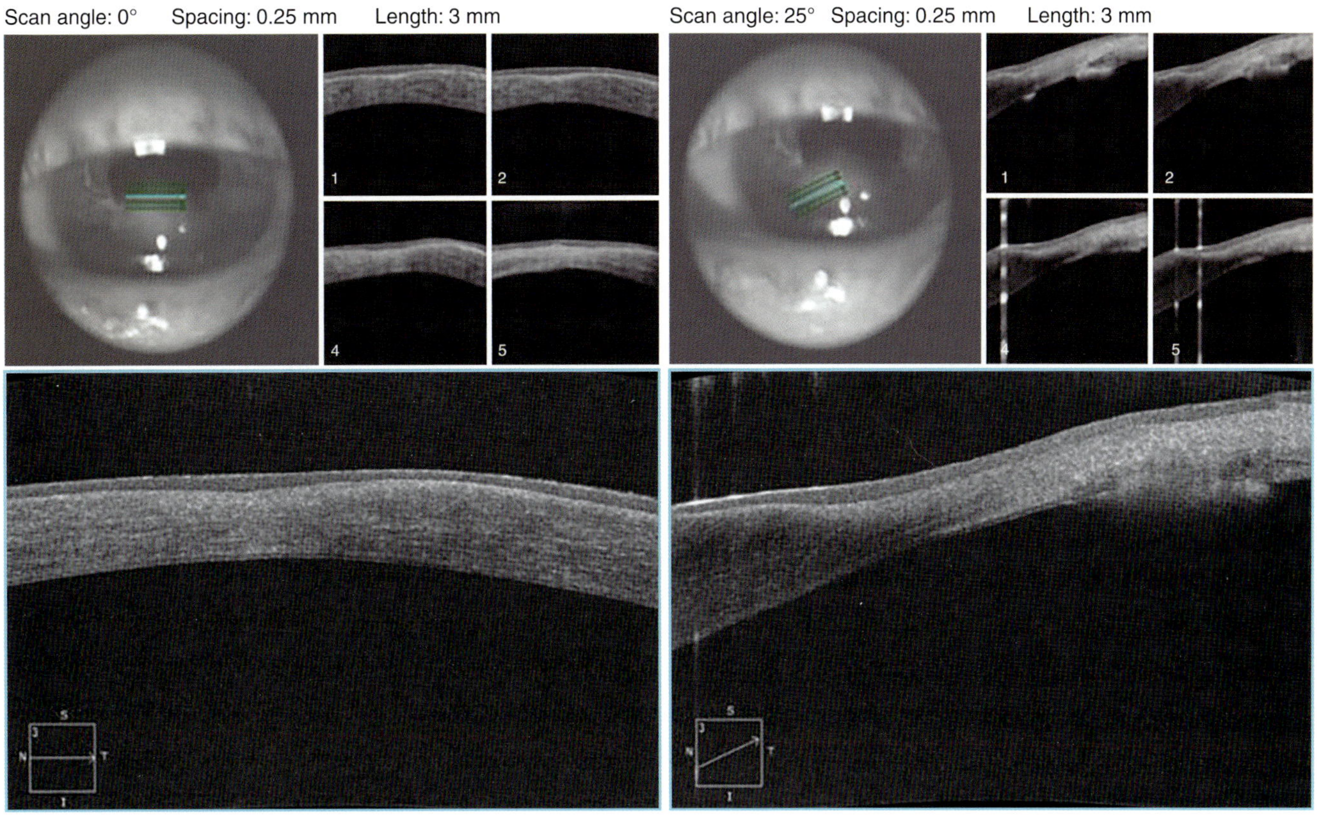

Fig. 20.17 Neurotrophic keratitis scarring. AS-OCT raster images of the left eye of the images shown in Fig. 20.15. A significant amount of stromal compaction and scarring is observed, along with compensatory overlying epithelial thickening and remodeling.

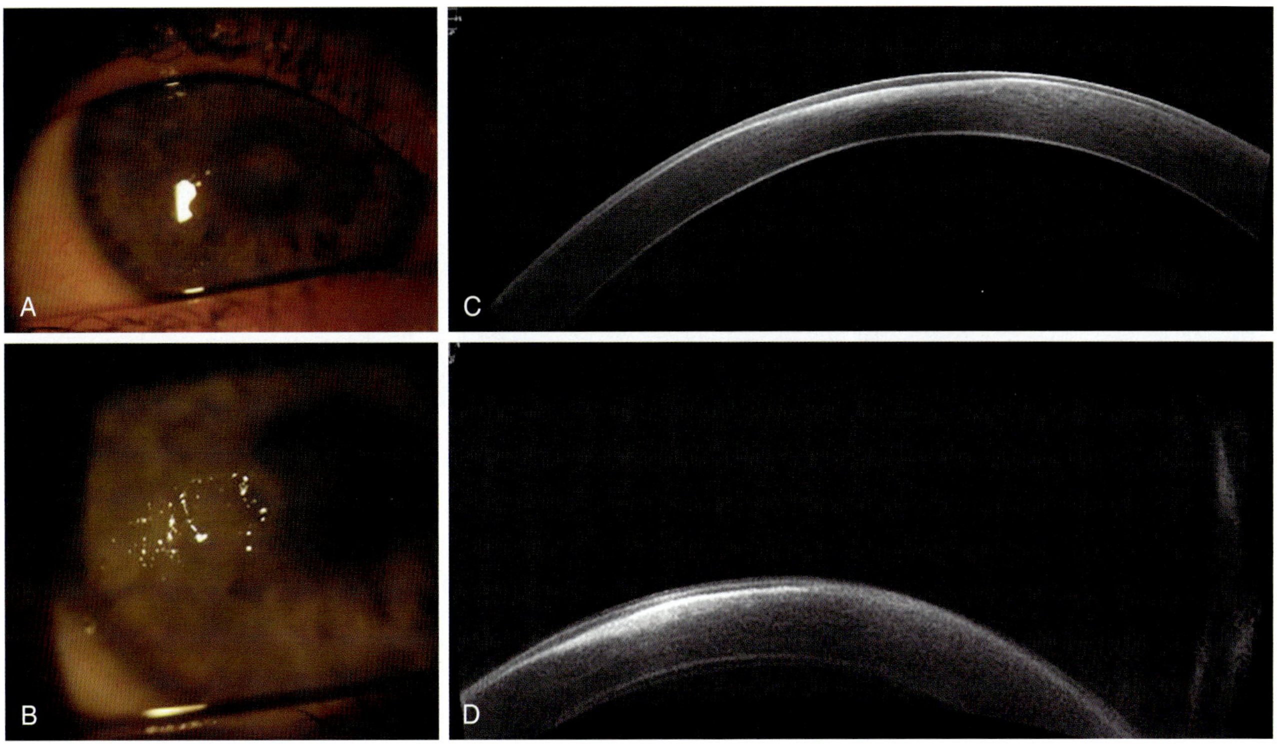

Fig. 20.18 Neurotrophic keratitis (NTK) in a pediatric patient. Slit-lamp photographs of the right eye *(panels A and B)* demonstrate features consistent with mild-stage NTK, such as epithelial irregularity, punctate keratopathy, and superficial neovascularization. Pretreatment AS-OCT images are not available. Medical therapy with frequent lubrication was initiated. Follow-up images of the right eye *(panel C, horizontal slice; panel D, vertical slice)* demonstrate stable subepithelial scarring with reestablishment of healthy corneal epithelium overlying the anterior scarring.

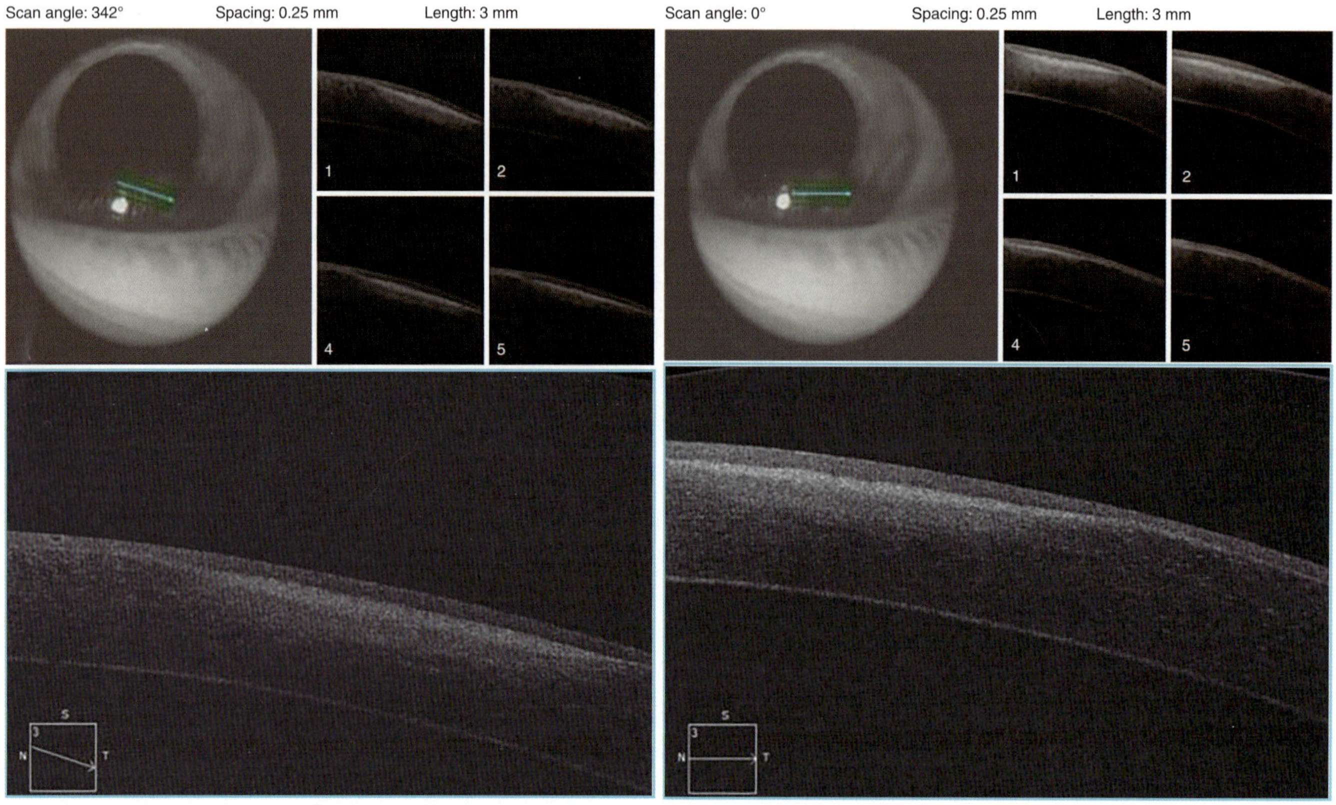

Fig. 20.19 Neurotrophic keratitis (NTK) in a pediatric patient. Follow-up images after ocular surface lubrication of the left eye show similar features to the posttreatment images seen in Fig. 20.18. There is stabilization of the subepithelial/stromal scarring with secondary epithelial hypertrophic remodeling overlying the stromal scarring. The corneal surface is overall regular and smooth.

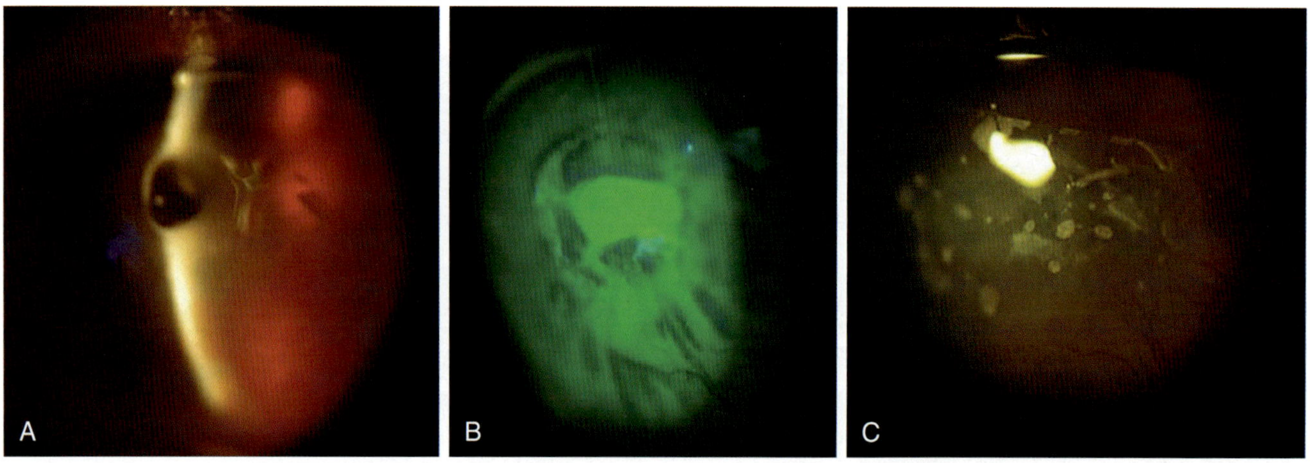

Fig. 20.20 Severe neurotrophic keratitis (NTK) with descemetocele. Slit-lamp photograph *(panel A)* shows significant thinning with descemetocele. A persistent epithelial defect is present within the area of NTK ulceration *(panel B)*. Amniotic membrane transplant placement was performed to reinforce corneal support *(panel C)*.

early peripheral, superficial neovascularization. After treatment, AS-OCT demonstrates stabilization of the subepithelial-stromal scarring with reepithelialization and secondary epithelial hypertrophic remodeling. The corneal surface is overall regular and smooth.

In severe cases, NTK can lead to persistent ulceration, thinning, stromal melting, and corneal perforation. Fig. 20.20 shows AS-OCT images and slit-lamp photographs of a patient with severe NTK with significant thinning and descemetocele requiring AMT placement. In follow-up images (Figs. 20.21 and 20.22), the inflammation persisted and the patient unfortunately rubbed his eyes, and a worsening descemetocele was seen underlying the AMT. Cyanoacrylate glue was placed, and AS-OCT images were taken after glue placement (Fig. 20.23).

Repeat episodes of NTK may cause significant scarring, even if the underlying cause of NTK is eventually treated. Options to treat subepithelial scarring are very limited, because any surface procedures (e.g., superficial keratectomy or PTK) will require epithelial removal and may risk prolonged

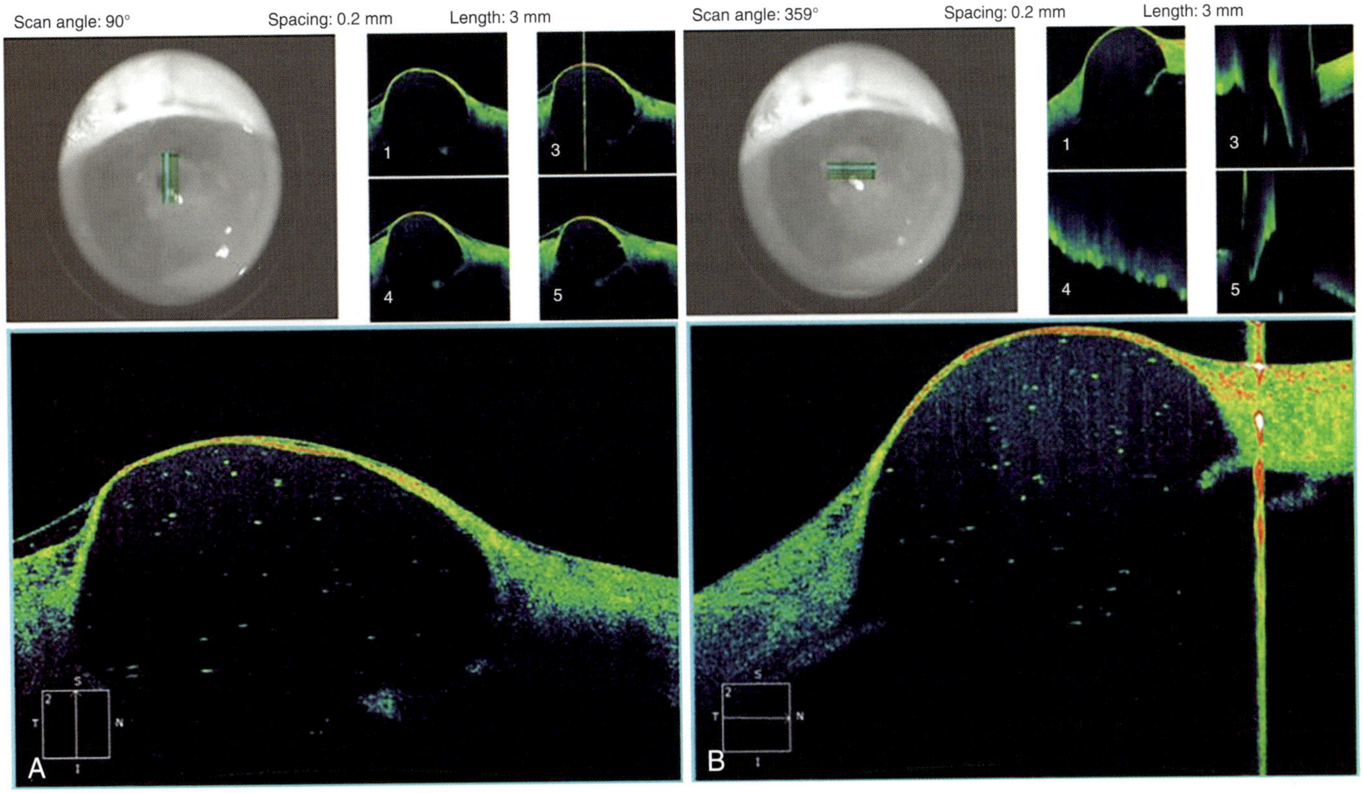

Fig. 20.21 Neurotrophic keratitis with descemetocele. Despite placement of amniotic membrane transplant (as seen in Fig. 20.20), the disease process worsened, exacerbated by eye rubbing, and the patient developed a large descemetocele. AS-OCT raster views *(left panel, vertical slice; right panel, horizontal slice)* show prominent descemetocele.

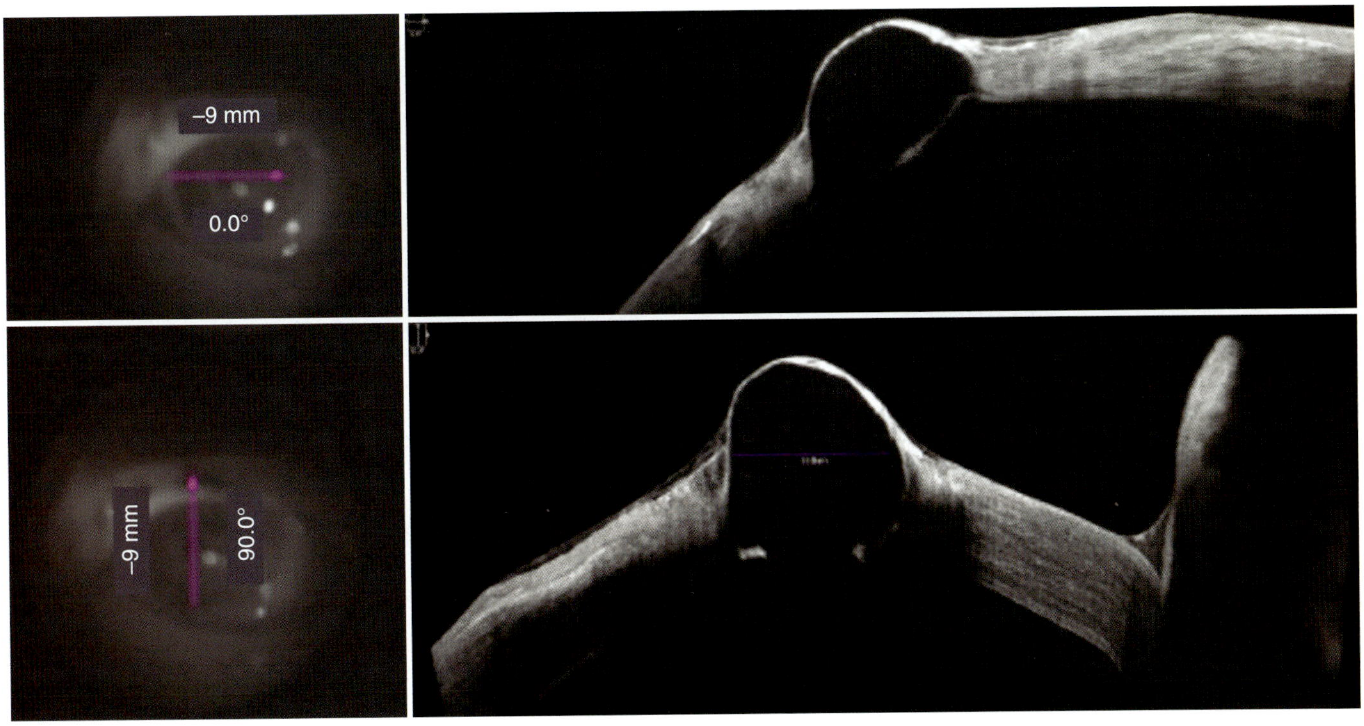

Fig. 20.22 Neurotrophic keratitis with descemetocele. Despite placement of amniotic membrane transplant (as seen in Fig. 20.21), the disease process worsened, exacerbated by eye rubbing, and the patient developed a large descemetocele. AS-OCT views *(left panel, vertical slice; right panel, horizontal slice)* show prominent descemetocele. Calipers can be used to measure the extent of the descemetocele.

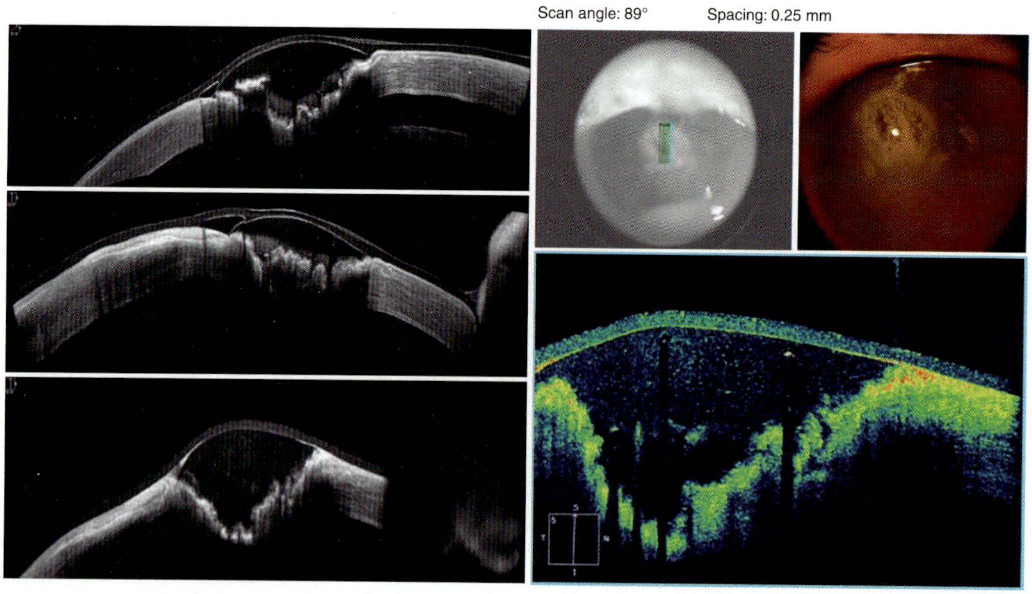

Fig. 20.23 Because of risk for impending perforation, cyanoacrylate glue was placed. AS-OCT (high definition and raster) show the appearance of the descemetocele after glue and bandage contact lens placement.

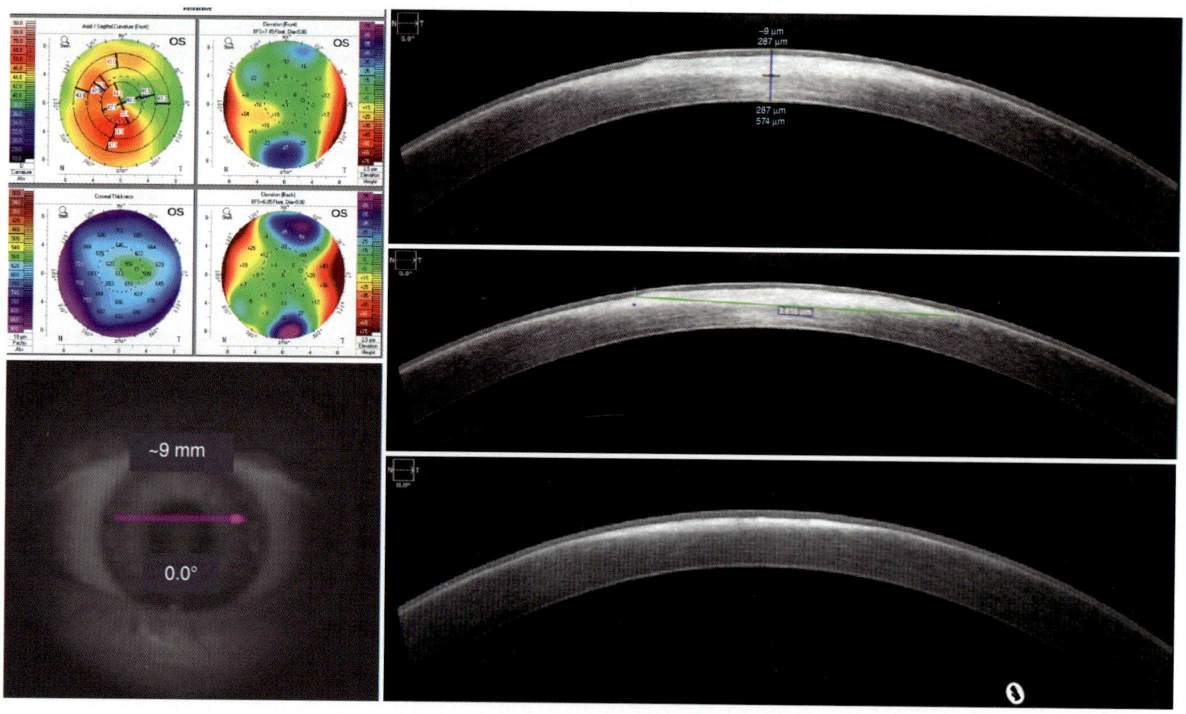

Fig. 20.24 Neurotrophic keratitis related corneal scarring in a patient with uncontrolled diabetes. Tomography images *(upper left panel)* show multiple areas of irregular astigmatism. AS-OCT images through the areas of scarring demonstrate scarring of various depths, with the deepest level of scarring extending to approximately half of the corneal thickness. In such cases, phototherapeutic keratectomy is unlikely to be successful.

deepithelialized state. In such cases, AS-OCT may be helpful to educate the patient regarding the extent of the scar and counsel the patient regarding visual rehabilitation option. For example, Fig. 20.24 shows images from a patient with NTK in the context of uncontrolled diabetes with resultant central scarring. Tomography images show prominent irregular astigmatism. AS-OCT can be used to measure the extent and depth of the scarring. In this case the scarring was approximately half of the cornea, and the patient was advised to use scleral contact lenses for vision improvement.

CLINICAL PEARL

AS-OCT can be used not only to measure the depth and extent of scarring but also to educate patients regarding clinical findings and advise them of optimal options for vision rehabilitation. If scarring occurs at significant depths, Phototherapeutic Keratectomy (PTK) and superficial keratectomy will be insufficient to noticeably improve the vision. In such cases, contact lens rehabilitation should be attempted first. If this fails, anterior lamellar keratoplasty (ALK) procedures may be next best option. If ALK is planned, measurement of the depth of the corneal scarring can help guide surgeons for appropriate amounts of partial-thickness trephination and thickness of donor lenticule.

VI. CORNEAL NEOVASCULARIZATION

Corneal neovascularization (CNV) can occur as a result of a variety of inciting factors, including infectious, inflammatory, degenerative, traumatic, and ischemic causes. Common conditions include herpetic viral infection, lipid keratopathy, corneal ulcers/scars, chemical burns, and hypoxic corneal injury from contact lens overuse. CNV and associated scarring occur when abnormal vessels invade the corneal stroma as a result of a disruption of antiangiogenic factors that normally preserve corneal transparency.

The impact of CNV on visual acuity can be minimal, especially if limited to the peripheral cornea, to sight-threatening in cases with involvement of the central visual axis.

Fig. 20.25 shows images from a patient who presented with significant CNV of the left eye with complex medical history, including recent hospitalization in the intensive care unit after complications from gastrointestinal surgery for Crohn disease requiring a nearly 3 months' stay with minimal eye care. On discharge and presentation to an ophthalmologist, the patient had 20/400 visual acuity with significant, dense, superior stromal opacification with associated CNV. There was no known history of herpetic eye disease. The patient was started on empiric systemic valacyclovir and topical prednisolone. Three weeks later, argon laser photocoagulation to feeder vessels combined with subconjunctival injection of bevacizumab and triamcinolone were given. Six weeks after this therapy, follow-up slit-lamp photographs highlight significant regression of CNV with improvement of vision acuity to 20/150. AS-OCT (Fig. 20.26) at the time of scleral fitting evaluation approximately 2 months later shows prominent area(s) of hyperreflectivity in the stroma from the regression of CNV. The patient was maintained on systemic antivirals and topical steroids once daily and maintained regression of CNV. With scleral contact lenses, the patient's visual acuity was 20/25. It is important to note that recurrence is common, and a significant number of patients may require repeat and/or chronic therapy.

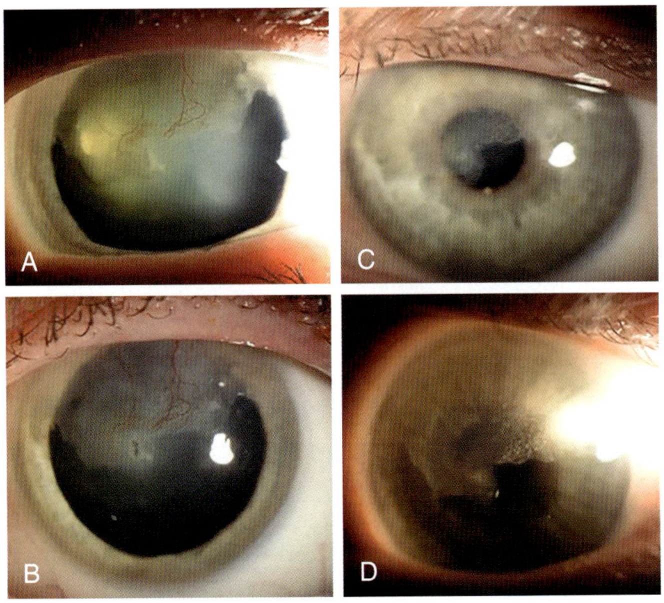

Fig. 20.25 Corneal neovascularization (CNV) from an unknown cause. At the time of presentation *(panels A and B)*, the patient's left eye was noted to have significant stromal opacification, edema, and prominent sectoral CNV with several prominent vessels encroaching on the visual axis. After treatment with systemic antivirals and topical steroids, followed by in-clinic treatment with argon laser photocoagulation to feeder vessels and subconjunctival bevacizumab/triamcinolone, significant regression of stromal opacity and CNV was noted 6 weeks later *(panels C and D)*. The patient's vision improved from 20/400 to 20/150.

Fig. 20.27 shows images from a patient with CNV associated with chronic exposure keratopathy in the context of uncontrolled diabetes complicated by cranial nerve VII palsy of the left eye. Slit-lamp photographs of the right and left eye represent minimal CNV and extensive CNV, respectively. AS-OCT taken at various depths through the CNV demonstrates the variable and prominent surface irregularity, stromal opacity, and loss of normal corneal contour.

Fig. 20.28 displays images of a patient with chemical alkali (drain cleaner) injury to the right eye. Images taken shortly after the initial injury demonstrate significant limbal ischemia and epithelial defect with associated haze (Dua classification III–IV). After medical rehabilitation, including tarsorrhaphy, lubrication, and AMT placement, significant improvement with closure of the epithelial defect was noted. A crescentic shape of sectoral CNV and associated scarring was present after healing, though without involvement of the visual axis. AS-OCT shows CNV changes primarily in the anterior stroma nasally without involvement of the central visual axis. Visual acuity was correctable to 20/30.

Fig. 20.29 shows images of a patient with CNV and lipid keratopathy secondary to topical prostaglandin analog medication use for glaucoma in the context of severe rosacea and meibomian gland dysfunction. AS-OCT highlights areas of the stromal vascularity, lipid deposition, and increased corneal thickness in the superior cornea.

Treatment of CNV can be challenging, and it includes medical therapy (systemic antiviral medications, topical steroids, topical antiinflammatory medications); laser therapy for prominent vessels; injection therapy with steroids and anti-vascular endothelial growth factor (VEGF) medications; and surgical interventions, including fine-needle monopolar diathermy, bipolar cautery, and penetrating keratoplasty.

Mitomycin intravascular chemoembolization (MICE) was introduced by Dean Ouano, MD, as an effective means to permanently treat CNV associated with lipid keratopathy using the vasodestructive properties of mitomycin-c (MMC) to both afferent and efferent vessels. Using an ultrathin, 33-gauge needle to cannulate the prominent vessel in the far peripheral cornea, 0.1 mL of 0.03% MMC is injected to achieve vessel blanching. Fig. 20.30 displays pre- and post-MICE images of a patient with lipid keratopathy and CNV. Of note, AS-OCT demonstrates stromal compaction, overlying epithelial hyperplastic remodeling, and linear scarring.

Figs. 20.31 to 20.34 represents serial images of another patient with CNV lipid keratopathy. Fig. 20.31 shows pre-MICE external photographs, slit-lamp photographs, and corneal-epithelial thickness mapping images. Fig. 20.32 shows pre-MICE AS-OCT images. Notably, there is considerable stromal hyperreflectivity and overall increased corneal thickness with areas of varying irregularity. Fig. 20.33 displays intraoperative steps of the MICE procedure. Fig. 20.34 shows the 3-week postoperative appearance after the procedure. There is notable improvement in the previously seen areas of dense lipid deposition. The iris and pupil are now visible. Short-term results of MICE are extremely promising.

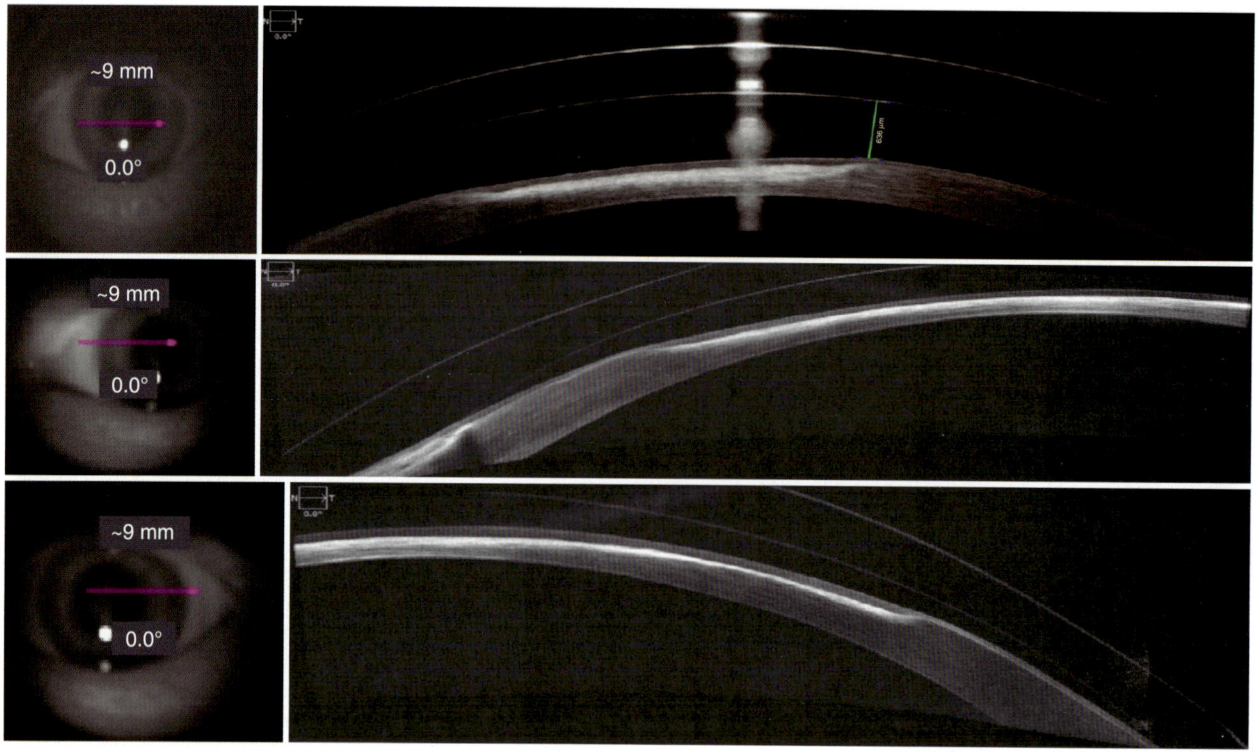

Fig. 20.26 Corneal neovascularization (CNV). Follow-up AS-OCT images of the left eye taken at the time of scleral contact lens fitting highlight the areas of regressed CNV and remaining stromal opacification. There is some thinning and compaction of the stroma in the areas of regressed CNV with some secondary epithelial hypertrophic remodeling.

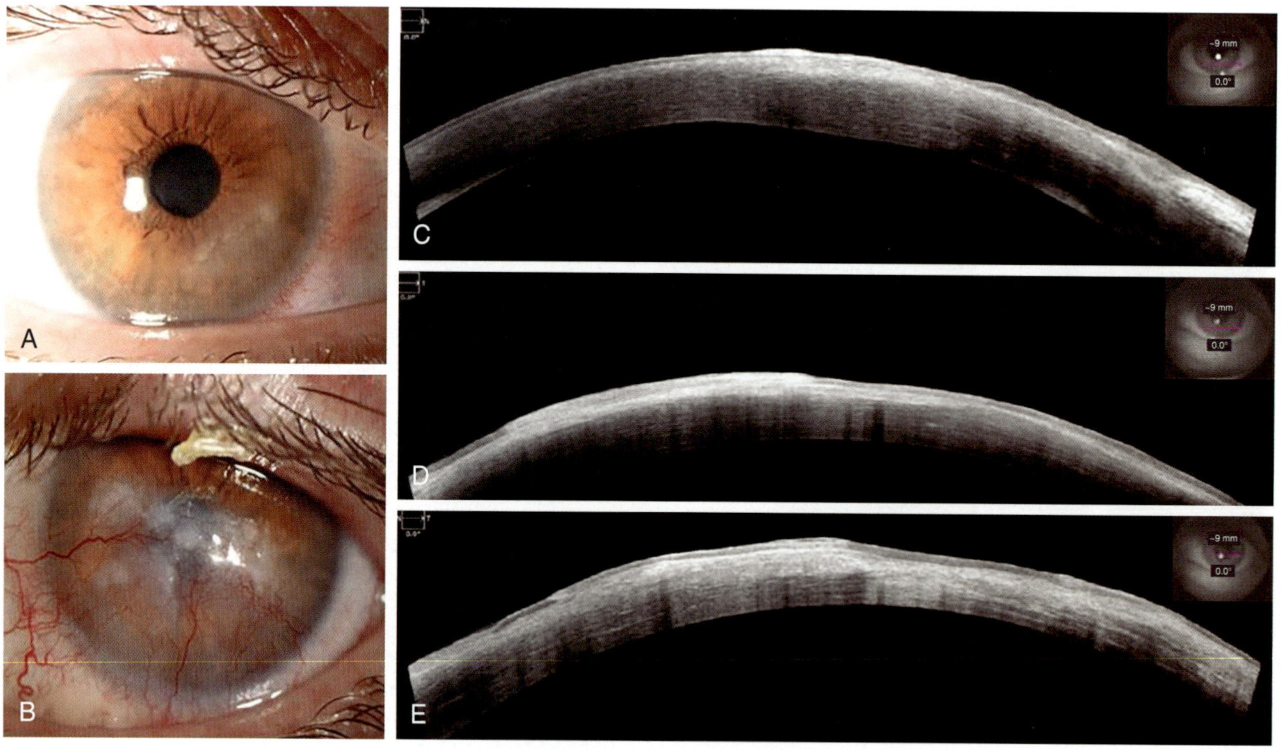

Fig. 20.27 Corneal neovascularization (CNV) associated with chronic exposure keratopathy bilaterally in the context of uncontrolled diabetes complicated by cranial nerve VII palsy of the left eye. Slit-lamp photograph of the right eye *(panel A)* displays a sectoral area of mild CNV changes inferonasally. Visual acuity was minimally affected in this eye. In the left eye *(panel B)*, there is significant CNV encompassing more than half of the cornea and involving the visual axis. Visual acuity was 20/400. AS-OCT of the right eye *(panel C)* through the area of the CNV demonstrates prominent hyperreflectivity in the anterior stroma corresponding to scarring and neovascularization with prominent irregularity of the corneal surface. Several areas of elevation and secondary epithelial remodeling changes are also observed. In the left eye *(panels D and E)*, more extensive changes involving the majority of the cornea are seen, including involvement of the central visual axis.

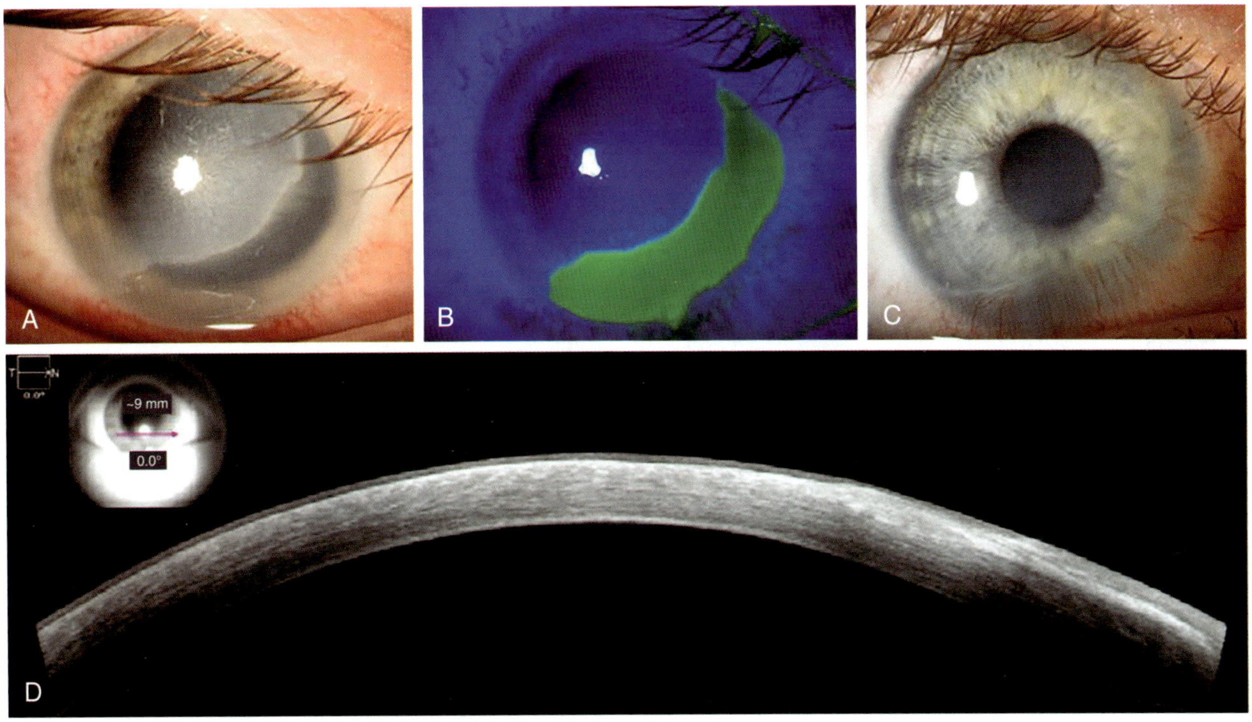

Fig. 20.28 Corneal neovascularization (CNV) secondary to chemical alkali (drain cleaner) injury to the right eye. *Panels A and B* show slit-lamp photographs after the initial injury. Notable, there is significant epithelial defect, limbal ischemia, and stromal haze, including involvement of the central visual axis. After treatment, the epithelial defect healed and a crescentic shape of sectoral CNV was present *(panel C)*. AS-OCT *(panel D)* shows prominent, linear hyperreflectivity in the anterior stroma nasally with overlying epithelial remodeling. Compared with Fig. 20.27, there is still good maintenance of corneal contour without focal irregularity and without involvement of the central visual axis. Visual acuity was correctable to 20/30.

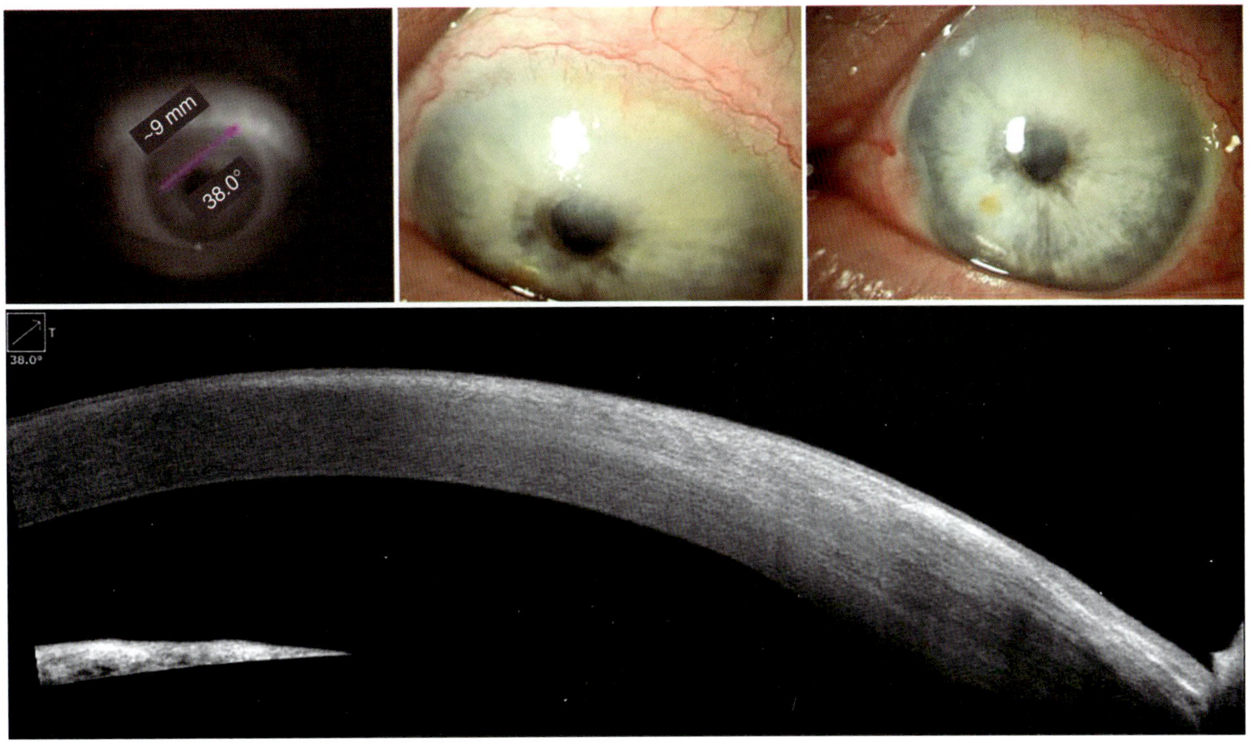

Fig. 20.29 Lipid keratopathy and corneal neovascularization secondary to prostaglandin analog medication use for glaucoma in the context of severe rosacea and meibomian gland dysfunction. AS-OCT highlights the superior area of stromal vascularity, lipid deposition, and increased corneal thickness. There is also some increased epithelial thickness overlying the vascular network. Overall, the corneal contour is maintained. (Courtesy Dean Ouano, MD, Coastal Eye Clinic, New Bern, North Carolina, United States.)

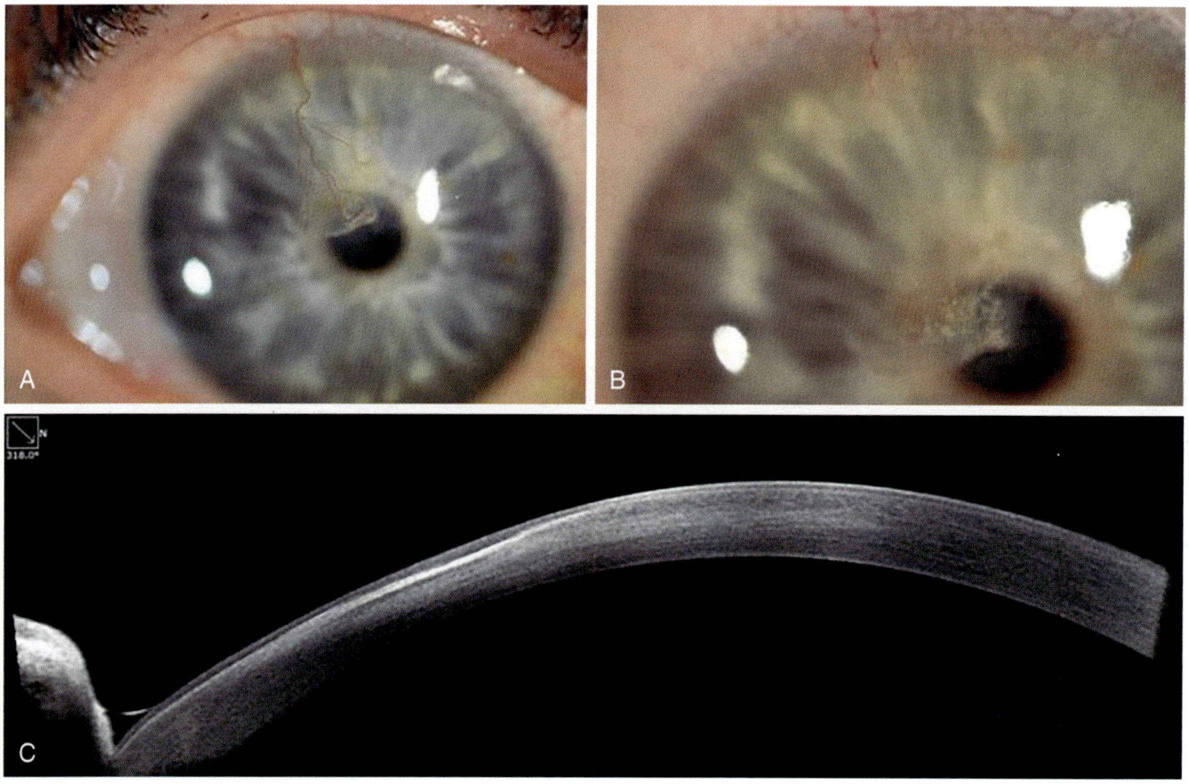

Fig. 20.30 Sectoral corneal neovascularization (CNV) with lipid keratopathy in a patient with history of herpes zoster virus stromal keratitis. In *panel A,* a prominent area of CNV with leading edge of lipid deposits encroaching on the visual axis is present. After treatment with mitomycin intravascular chemoembolization (MICE), postoperative slit-lamp image *(panel B)* demonstrates significant regression of previously observed CNV with some lipid deposits remaining. Postprocedure AS-OCT *(panel C)* demonstrates focal area of stromal compaction, overlying epithelial hyperplastic remodeling, and a prominent area of linear hyperreflectivity in the anterior stroma. Topography (not shown) showed flattening of the superior cornea with irregular astigmatism. (Courtesy Dean Ouano, MD, Coastal Eye Clinic, New Bern, North Carolina, United States.)

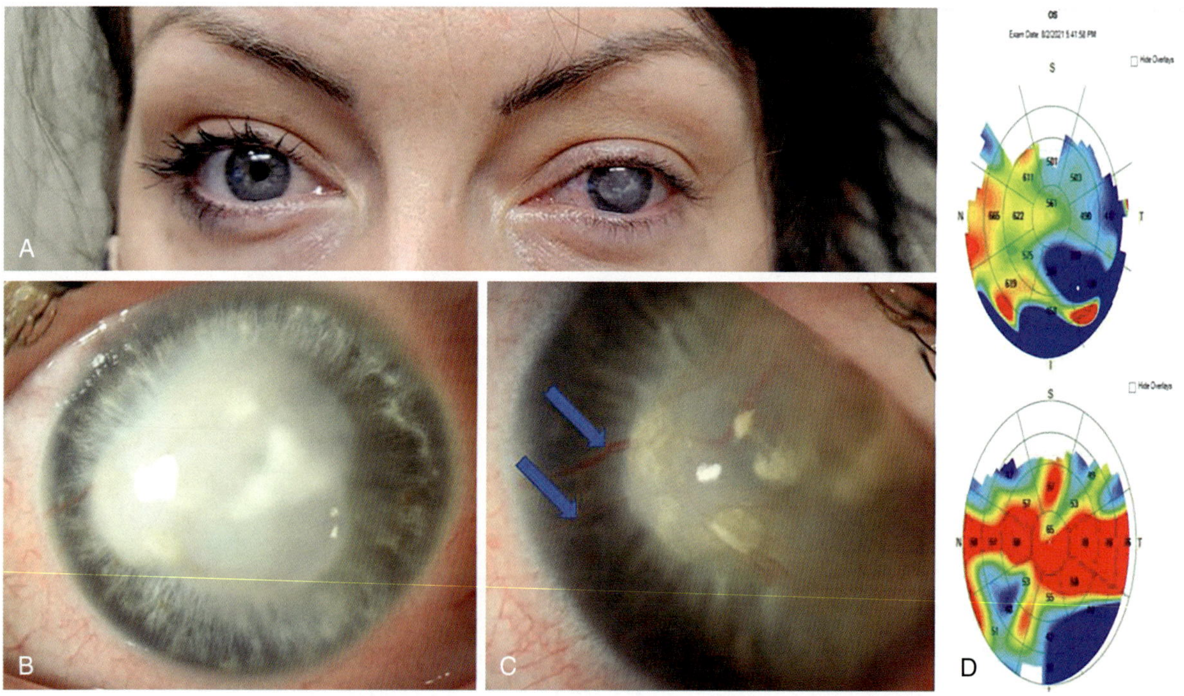

Fig. 20.31 A 37-year-old female patient presented with corneal neovascularization (CNV) secondary to herpes zoster virus–associated lipid keratopathy in the left eye. External photographs *(panel A)* demonstrate significant stromal opacity of the left eye with normal-appearing right eye. Slit-lamp photographs *(panel B)* demonstrate light-blocking stromal opacity and edema that encompass the visual axis with prominent CNV nasally. There are multiple areas of lipid deposition with varying consistency and concentration within the opacity. *Panel C* shows additional areas of denser, more compact lipid at the nasal edge of the stromal opacity. Notably, there are two prominent vessels nasally amenable for chemoembolization *(blue arrows).* Corneal-epithelial thickness mapping *(panel D)* indicates varying areas of increased corneal thickness along with thickness irregularity of overlying epithelium. (Courtesy Dean Ouano, MD, Coastal Eye Clinic, New Bern, North Carolina, United States.)

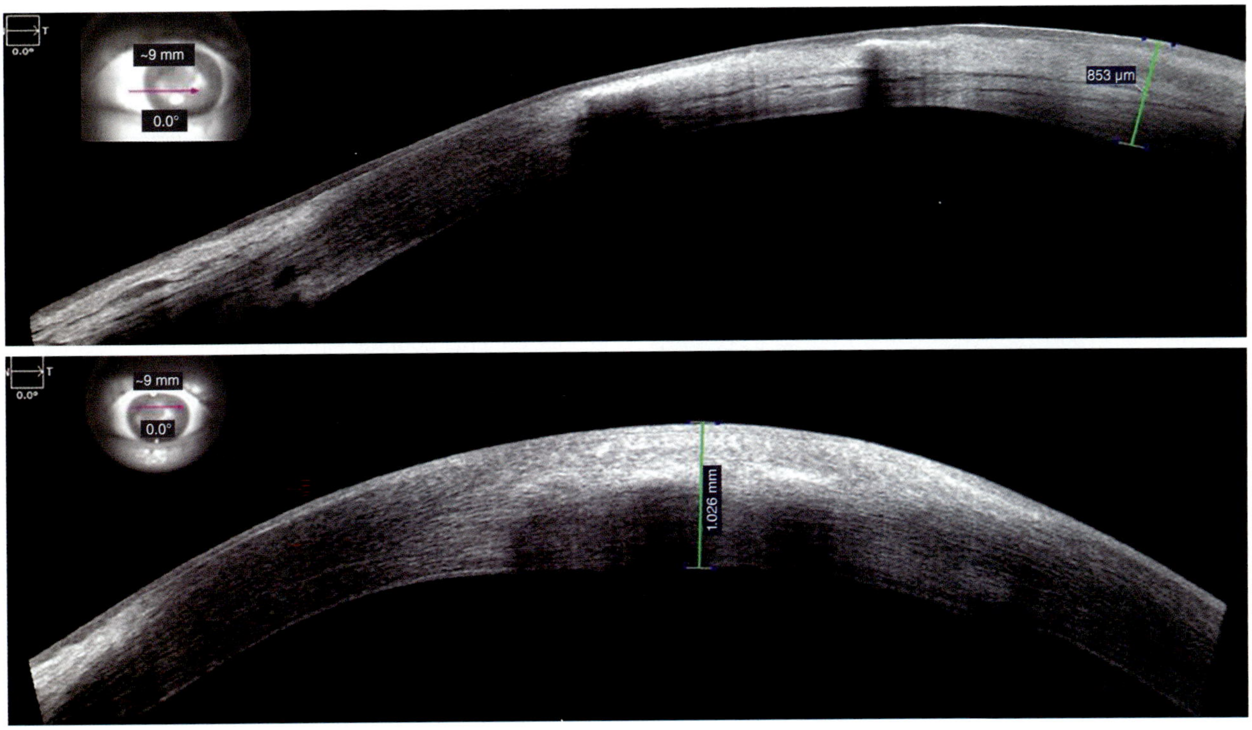

Fig. 20.32 AS-OCT images of the patient in Fig. 20.31 demonstrate variable areas of stromal hyperreflectivity. There is overall increased corneal thickness (>1000 microns) with variability and irregularity. A lucid peripheral zone *(top panel)* is seen along with a deep vascular network extending into the deep stroma. (Courtesy Dean Ouano, MD, Coastal Eye Clinic, New Bern, North Carolina, United States.)

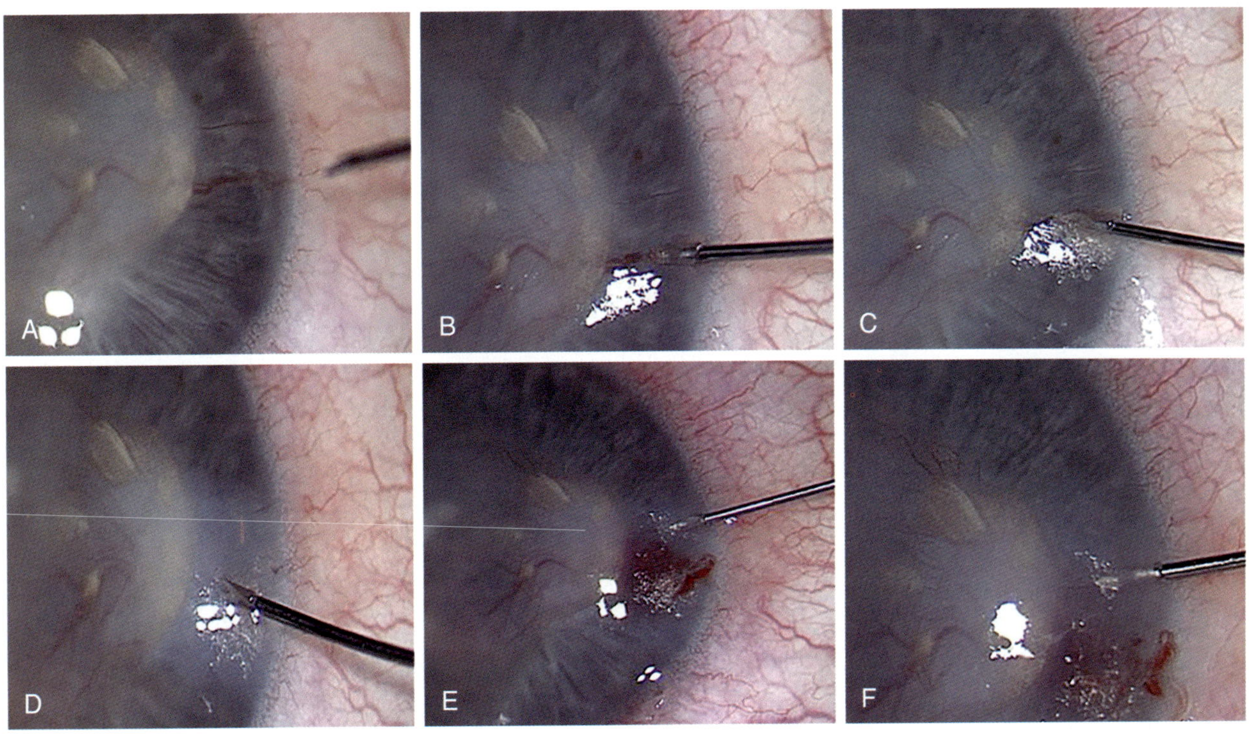

Fig. 20.33 Steps of the mitomycin intravascular chemoembolization (MICE) procedure. A feeder vessel is identified for injection of intravascular mitomycin-c (MMC) *(panel A)*. Using a 33-gauge needle, initial entry is made at an approximately 15-degree angle (relative to the conjunctiva surface) to cannulate the vessel; a flash of blood is commonly seen if the vessel is cannulized properly *(panel B)*. If the entry is too shallow, intrastromal/subepithelial air bubbles *(panel C)* may be seen. After confirmation of correct entry, 0.1 mL of MMC is injected to achieve stromal whitening *(panel D)*. Some reflux of blood is common *(panel E)*. A second vessel adjacent to the first vessel is also cannulized for intravascular MMC *(panel F)*. (Courtesy Dean Ouano, MD, Coastal Eye Clinic, New Bern, North Carolina, United States.)

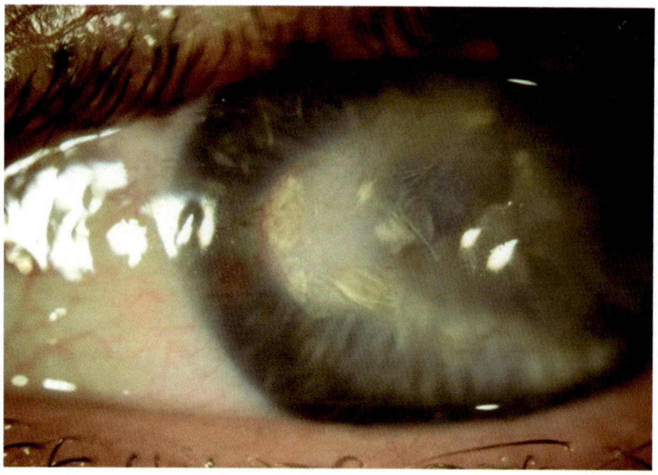

Fig. 20.34 Images of the patient in Fig. 20.33 taken 3 weeks after mitomycin intravascular chemoembolization (MICE). There is interval improvement of the previously seen stromal opacity with iris and pupil details now visible. Previously seen denser areas of lipid deposition are also resolving. Some intrastromal heme is still present nasally from the MICE procedure. (Courtesy Dean Ouano, MD, Coastal Eye Clinic, New Bern, North Carolina, United States.)

VII. MISCELLANEOUS INFLAMMATORY PATHOLOGY

A. Sterile Contact Lens–Associated Stromal Infiltrates

Peripheral, sterile stromal infiltrates may be seen in some contact lens wearers. A multifactorial mechanism is likely present, with a major component being mechanical irritation to the corneal surface triggering an inflammatory reaction and formation of peripheral infiltrates. These should be distinguished from infiltrates seen in other peripheral corneal disease, such as staphylococcal marginal keratitis. However, it may be difficult to consistently determine infectious versus inflammatory causes; sterile infiltrates are usually smaller, multiple, and bilateral and usually manifest without significant pain, epithelial defect, and/or anterior chamber reaction. Fig. 20.35 shows images from a patient with bilateral sterile contact lens–associated stromal infiltrates. AS-OCT can be helpful to identify location and number of infiltrates, and along with the clinical examination, may help guide the clinician toward appropriate management. In this patient, contact lens discontinuation, lubrication, and antibiotic-steroid drops were used.

B. Anterior Chamber Inflammation

Various clinical findings are seen in anterior chamber inflammation. Keratic precipitates (KPs) are associated with ocular inflammation and are mostly seen in patients with uveitis. They also can be found in other conditions such as infectious keratitis and corneal transplant rejection. KPs are characterized by an aggregation of inflammatory cells on the endothelial surface of the cornea. They are typically categorized as granulomatous or nongranulomatous on the basis of appearance by slit-lamp examination.

Newly formed KPs tend to be white and smoothly rounded, later transitioning to a crenated, pigmented, or glassy appearance. Large, yellowish KPs are called *"mutton-fat" KPs* and are usually associated with granulomatous types of inflammation.

Fig. 20.36 shows a slit-lamp photograph and an AS-OCT image of a patient who presented with anterior uveitis with previous history of endothelial keratoplasty. AS-OCT can help visualize KPs, which are seen as prominent, focal areas of rounded hyperreflectivity on the corneal endothelium with some protrusion into the anterior chamber.

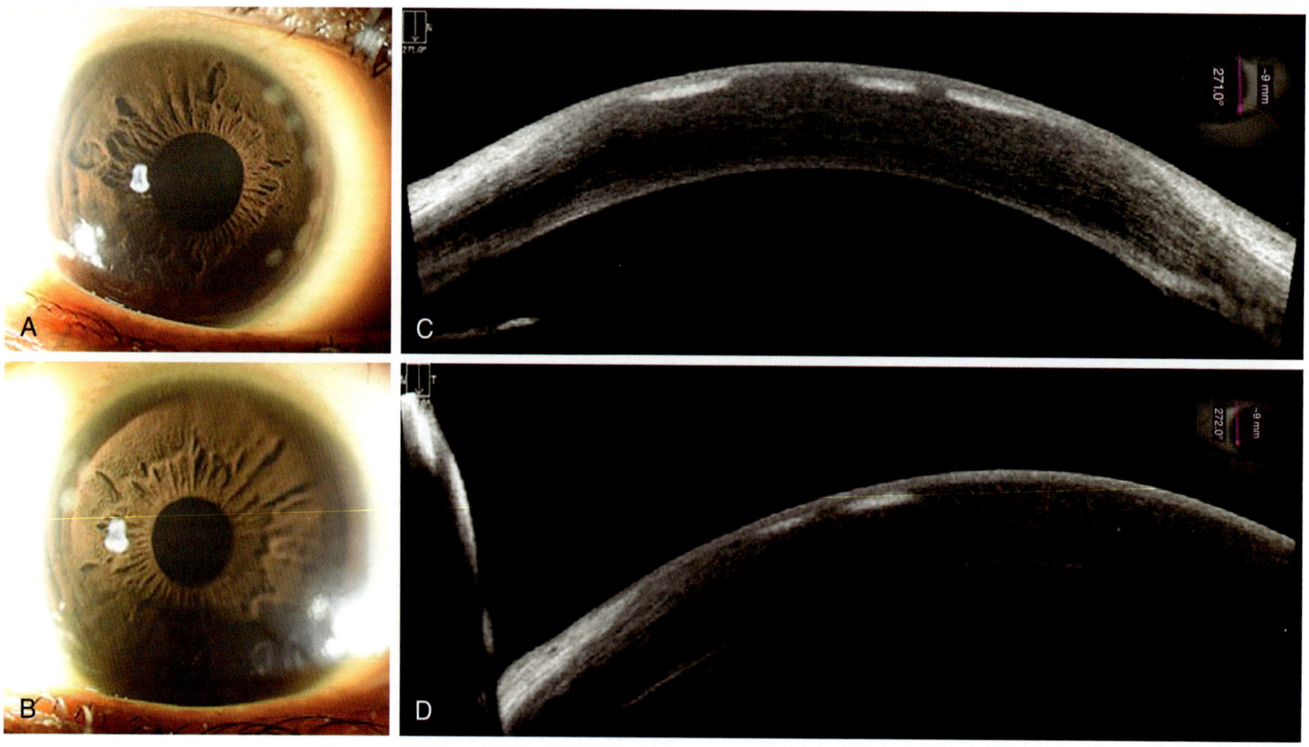

Fig. 20.35 Sterile contact lens-associated stromal infiltrates. Slit-lamp photographs demonstrate multiple peripheral infiltrates nasally in the right eye *(panel A)* and left eye *(panel B)* without involvement of the central cornea. The conjunctiva is not injected. AS-OCT of the right eye *(panel C)* and left eye *(panel D)* confirms multiple infiltrates as areas of hyperreflectivity primarily in the anterior stroma with intervening clear spaces.

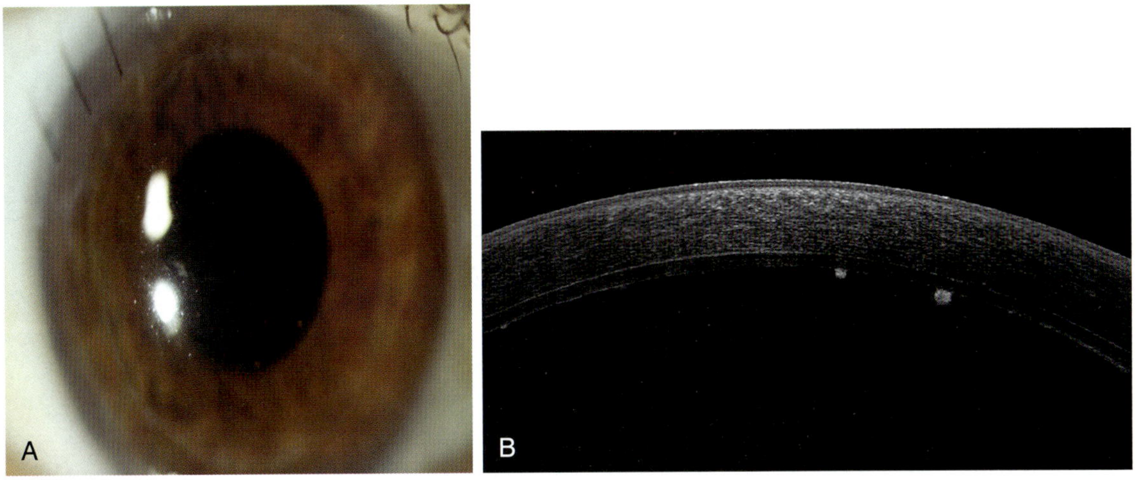

Fig. 20.36 Keratic precipitates (KPs) in a patient with anterior uveitis with previous history of endothelial keratoplasty. In the slit-lamp photograph *(panel A)*, multiple, fine, pigmented lesions can be seen on the posterior cornea inferiorly. The previous endothelial keratoplasty graft is also visible. AS-OCT *(panel B)* reveals the KPs as focal areas of hyperreflectivity on the posterior aspect of the corneal graft with protrusion into the anterior chamber. Minimal stromal edema is present.

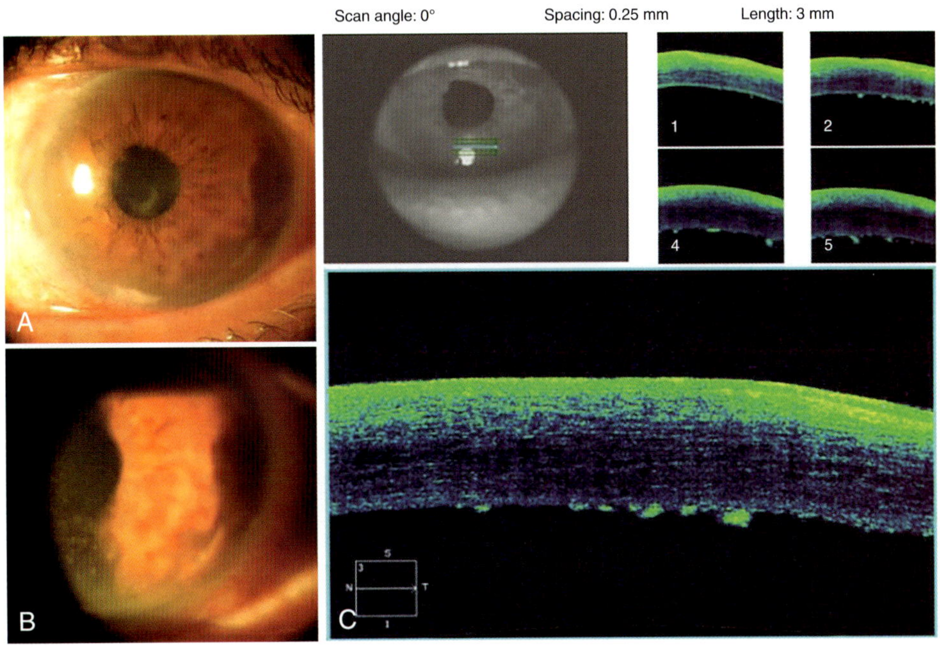

Fig. 20.37 Keratic precipitates (KPs) in a patient with human leukocyte antigen (HLA)-B27–associated uveitis. Slit-lamp photographs *(panels A and B)* demonstrate multiple KPs primarily located inferiorly. A hypopyon is present. KPs are seen on AS-OCT raster images *(panel C)* as focal, prominent areas of hyperreflectivity on the posterior endothelial surface with protrusion into the anterior chamber.

Fig. 20.37 shows images from a patient who presented with moderate to severe anterior uveitis with hypopyon of the left eye secondary to human leukocyte antigen (HLA)-B27. In this case multiple KPs are visualized on the AS-OCT images.

Figs. 20.38 and 20.39 show images of "mutton-fat" KPs, which are associated strongly with granulomatous uveitis and are clinically seen as larger, gray-white KPs that represent clusters of epithelioid cells and macrophages.

Prolonged anterior chamber inflammation can result in accumulation of inflammatory cells in multiple segments of the anterior chamber. In Figs. 20.40 and 20.41, in addition to KPs on the corneal endothelium, a significant number of inflammatory cells are clustered on the iris and anterior aspect of the intraocular lens optic. AS-OCT can be used to better visualize these KPs and identify their location in the anterior chamber.

In extreme cases of anterior chamber inflammation, especially after intraocular surgery, fibrin may be seen in the anterior chamber. This reaction can manifest on a spectrum ranging from a few fibrin strands to denser, light-blocking pupillary membranes. Fig. 20.42 shows images of a patient with significant fibrinoid reaction and pupillary membrane.

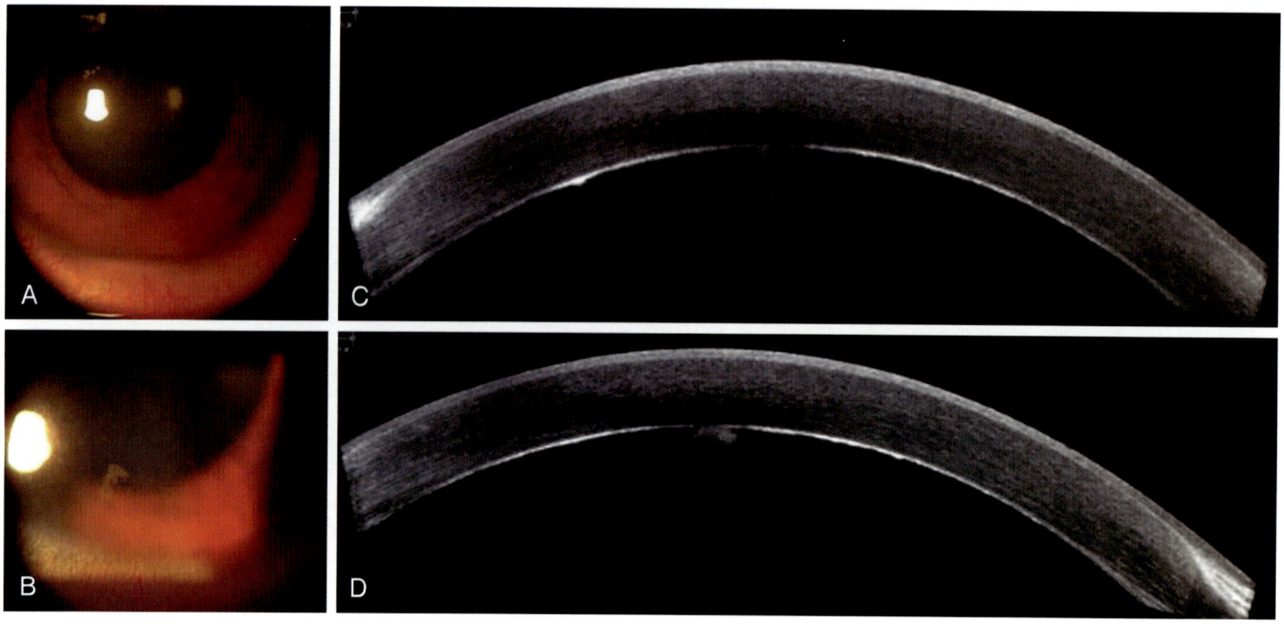

Fig. 20.38 "Mutton-fat" keratic precipitates (KPs). The large, gray-white KPs are classically associated with granulomatous uveitis and seen on slit-lamp examination *(panels A and B)* as prominent KPs within a constellation of other, smaller KPs. Mutton-fat KPs are seen on AS-OCT images with features similar to those of the KPs seen in previous figures, with notable differences in size, depth, and amount of protrusion into the anterior chamber.

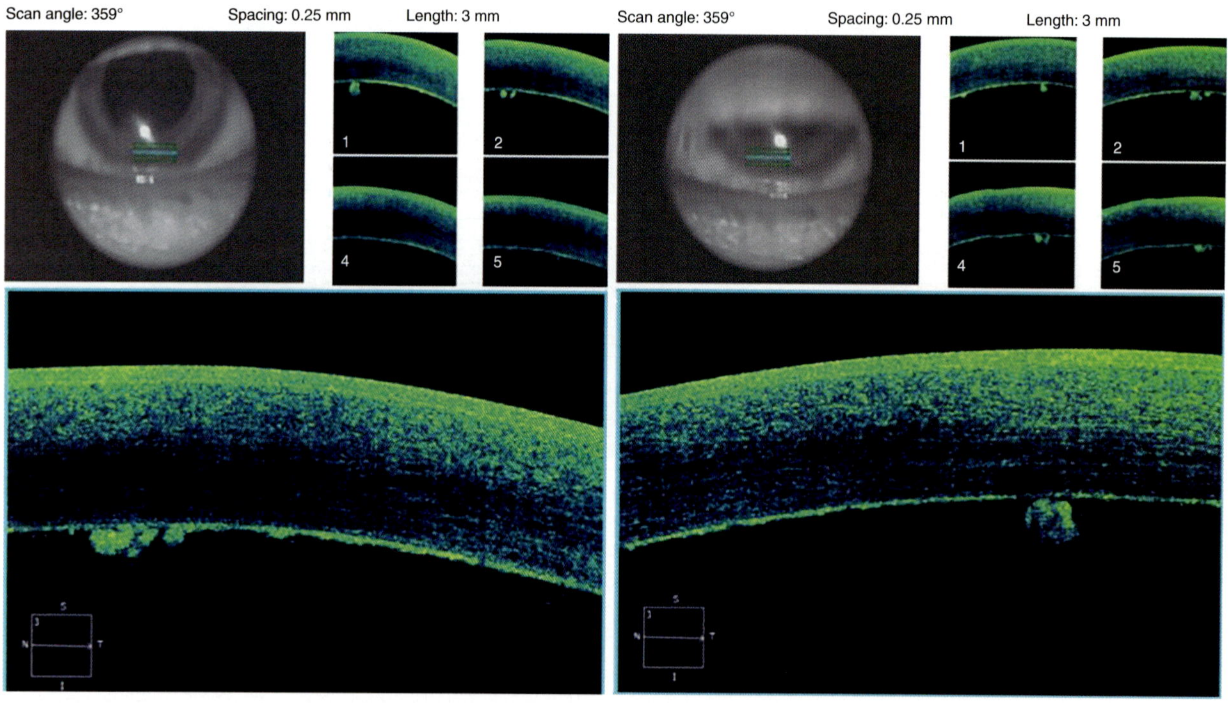

Fig. 20.39 AS-OCT raster images of the patient shown in Fig. 20.38 further highlight the prominent nature of the "mutton-fat" keratic precipitates and notable protrusion into the anterior chamber.

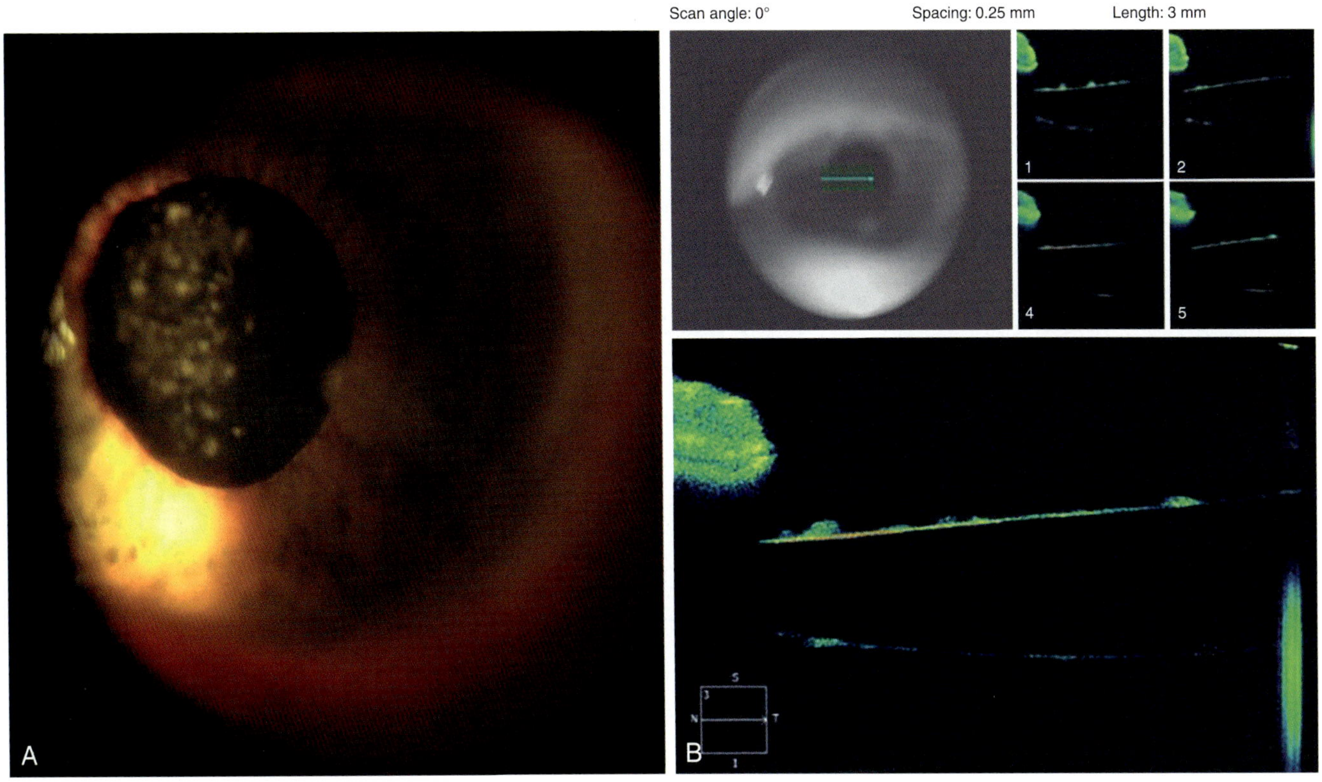

Fig. 20.40 Anterior chamber inflammation. In addition to keratic precipitates (KPs) on the corneal endothelium, prolonged and/or exuberant anterior chamber inflammation can cause deposition of inflammatory cells in multiple areas of the anterior segment. On slit-lamp examination, in addition to KPs seen on clinical examination on the corneal endothelium (though not seen in *left panel* because of the area of focus), there are significant pigmentary deposits on the anterior aspect of the interocular lens optic. AS-OCT raster image shows multiple pigmentary deposits as prominent areas of hyperreflectivity with elevation.

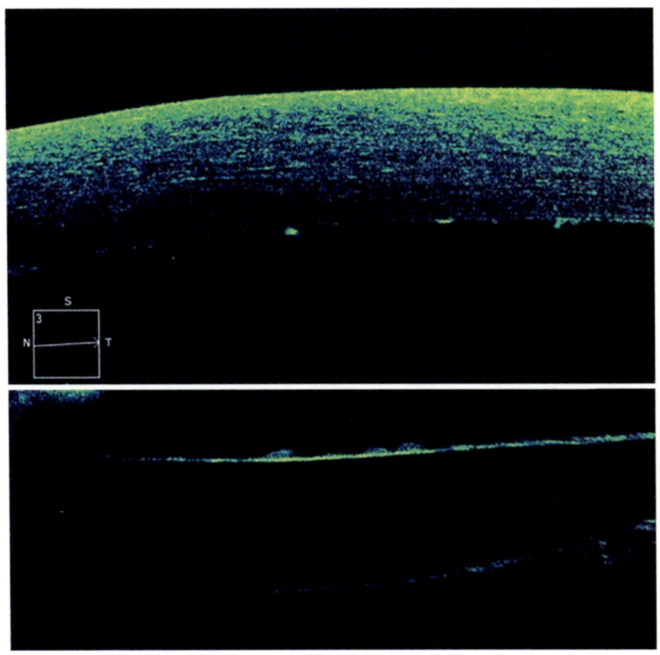

Fig. 20.41 AS-OCT image of the patient shown in Fig 20.40. Images taken through the cornea *(top panel)* and intraocular lens (IOL) *(bottom panel)* show multiple pigmentary deposits on the endothelium and anterior IOL optic, respectively.

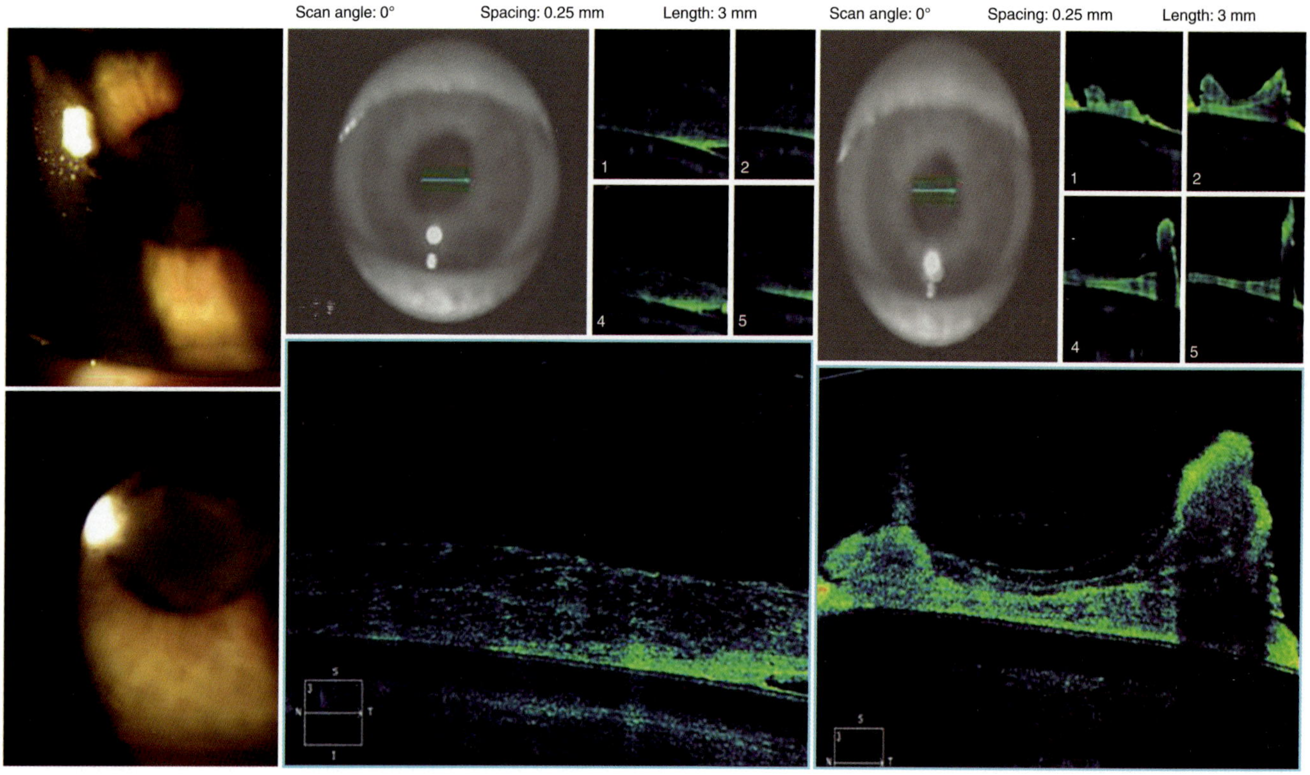

Fig. 20.42 Fibrin in anterior chamber can be seen as a thick, pigmented, celluloid-like material occupying the pupil space on slit-lamp examination. AS-OCT raster images reveal the fibrin as prominent areas of hyperreflectivity with significant elevation and extension into the anterior chamber.

BIBLIOGRAPHY

Agrawal RV, Murthy S, Sangwan V, Biswas J. Current approach in diagnosis and management of anterior uveitis. *Indian J Ophthalmol.* 2010;58(1):11.

Ang M, Baskaran M, Werkmeister RM, et al. Anterior segment optical coherence tomography. *Prog Retin Eye Res.* 2018;66:132-156.

Ansari Z, Miller D, Galor A. Current thoughts in fungal keratitis: diagnosis and treatment. *Curr Fung Infect Rep.* 2013;7(3):209-218.

Arici C, Mergen B. Late-term topical tacrolimus for subepithelial infiltrates resistant to topical steroids and ciclosporin secondary to adenoviral keratoconjunctivitis. *Br J Ophthalmol.* 2021;105(5):614-618.

Arici C, Sultan P, Mergen B, Buttanri B, Dogan C. The impact of bilateral subepithelial corneal infiltrates on tear film after epidemic keratoconjunctivitis. *Eye Contact Lens.* 2020;46(5):281-284.

Arvin AM. Varicella-zoster virus. *Clin Microbiol Rev.* 1996;9(3):361-381.

Asam JS, Polzer M, Tafreshi A, Hirnschall N, Findl O. Anterior segment OCT. In: *High Resolution Imaging in Microscopy and Ophthalmology.* Cham, CH: Springer; 2019:285-299.

Aung TT, Chor WHJ, Yam JKH, Givskov M, Yang L, Beuerman RW. Discovery of novel antimycobacterial drug therapy in biofilm of pathogenic nontuberculous mycobacterial keratitis. *Ocul Surf.* 2017;15(4):770-783.

Austin P, Brown SI. Inflammatory Terrien's marginal corneal disease. *Am J Ophthalmol.* 1981;92(2):189-192.

Berisa Prado S, Riestra Ayora AC. Topical tacrolimus for corneal subepithelial infiltrates secondary to adenoviral keratoconjunctivitis reply. *Cornea.* 2018;37(7):e32.

Brown-Elliott BA, Wallace RJ. Clinical and taxonomic status of pathogenic nonpigmented or late-pigmenting rapidly growing mycobacteria. *Clin Microbiol Rev.* 2002;15(4):716-746.

Cao Y, Zhang W, Wu J, Zhang H, Zhou H. Peripheral ulcerative keratitis associated with autoimmune disease: pathogenesis and treatment. *J Ophthalmol.* 2017;2017:7298026.

Chan AT, Ulate R, Goldich Y, Rootman DS, Chan CC. Terrien marginal degeneration: clinical characteristics and outcomes. *Am J Ophthalmol.* 2015;160(5):867-872.e1.

Chintakuntlawar AV, Zhou X, Rajaiya J, Chodosh J. Viral capsid is a pathogen-associated molecular pattern in adenovirus keratitis. *PLoS Pathog.* 2010;6(4):e1000841.

Chou TY, Adyanthaya R. Infectious crystalline keratopathy associated with *Klebsiella oxytoca. J Ophthalmic Inflamm Infect.* 2012;2(4):211-213.

Chu HS, Hu FR. Non-tuberculous mycobacterial keratitis. *Clin Microbiol Infect.* 2013;19(3):221-226.

Clarke DW, Niederkorn JY. The pathophysiology of Acanthamoeba keratitis. *Trends Parasitol.* 2006;22(4):175-180.

Dart JK, Saw VP, Kilvington S. Acanthamoeba keratitis: diagnosis and treatment update 2009. *Am J Ophthalmol.* 2009;148(4):487-499.e2.

Davis AR, Sheppard J. Herpes zoster ophthalmicus review and prevention. *Eye Contact Lens.* 2019;45(5):286-291.

Ding Y, Murri MS, Birdsong OC, Ronquillo Y, Moshirfar M. Terrien marginal degeneration. *Surv Ophthalmol.* 2019;64(2):162-174.

Doors M, Berendschot TT, de Brabander J, Webers CA, Nuijts RM. Value of optical coherence tomography for anterior segment surgery. *J Cataract Refract Surg.* 2010;36(7):1213-1229.

Estopinal CB, Ewald MD. Geographic disparities in the etiology of bacterial and fungal keratitis in the United States of America. Paper presented at: *Semin Ophthalmol.* 2016;31(4):345-352.

Galor A, Thorne JE. Scleritis and peripheral ulcerative keratitis. *Rheum Dis Clin North Am.* 2007;33(4):835-854.

Garg P, Kalra P, Joseph J. Non-contact lens related Acanthamoeba keratitis. *Indian J Ophthalmol.* 2017;65(11):1079.

Gauthier AS, Noureddine S, Delbosc B. Interstitial keratitis diagnosis and treatment. *J Fr Ophtalmol.* 2019;42(6):e229-e237.

Gorovoy MS, Stern GA, Hood CI, Allen C. Intrastromal noninflammatory bacterial colonization of a corneal graft. *Arch Ophthalmol.* 1983;101(11):1749-1752.

Gupta Y, Kishore A, Kumari P, et al. Peripheral ulcerative keratitis. *Surv Ophthalmol.* 2021;66(6):977-998.

Hall-Stoodley L, Lappin-Scott H. Biofilm formation by the rapidly growing mycobacterial species Mycobacterium fortuitum. *FEMS Microbiol Lett.* 1998;168(1):77-84.

Han SB, Liu YC, Noriega KM, Mehta JS. Applications of anterior segment optical coherence tomography in cornea and ocular surface diseases. *J Ophthalmol.* 2016;2016:4971572.
Hoffman JJ, Burton MJ, Leck A. Mycotic keratitis—a global threat from the filamentous fungi. *J Fungi.* 2021;7(4):273.
Iwamoto T, DeVoe AG, Farris RL. Electron microscopy in cases of marginal degeneration of the cornea. *Invest Ophthalmol.* 1972;11(4):241-257.
Izatt JA, Hee MR, Swanson EA, et al. Micrometer-scale resolution imaging of the anterior eye in vivo with optical coherence tomography. *Arch Ophthalmol.* 1994;112(12):1584-1589.
Jancevski M, Foster CS. Anterior segment optical coherence tomography. *Semin Ophthalmol.* 2010;25(5-6):317-323.
Jeng BH, Holsclaw DS. Cyclosporine A 1% eye drops for the treatment of subepithelial infiltrates after adenoviral keratoconjunctivitis. *Cornea.* 2011;30(9):958-961.
Kaye S, Choudhary A. Herpes simplex keratitis. *Prog Retin Eye Res.* 2006;25(4):355-380.
Kilgore PE, Kruszon-Moran D, Seward JF, et al. Varicella in Americans from NHANES III: implications for control through routine immunization. *J Med Virol.* 2003;70(suppl 1):S111-S118.
Knickelbein JE, Hendricks RL, Charukamnoetkanok P. Management of herpes simplex virus stromal keratitis: an evidence-based review. *Surv Ophthalmol.* 2009;54(2):226-234.
Knox CM, Holsclaw DS. Interstitial keratitis. *Int Ophthalmol Clin.* 1998;38(4):183-195.
Labib BA, Minhas BK, Chigbu DI. Management of adenoviral keratoconjunctivitis: challenges and solutions. *Clin Ophthalmol (Auckland, NZ).* 2020;14:837.
Li JY. Herpes zoster ophthalmicus: acute keratitis. *Curr Opin Ophthalmol.* 2018;29(4):328-333.
Li L, Zhai H, Xie L, Cheng J, Liu W. Therapeutic effects of lamellar keratoplasty on Terrien marginal degeneration. *Cornea.* 2018;37(3):318-325.
Liesegang TJ. Herpes zoster ophthalmicus: natural history, risk factors, clinical presentation, and morbidity. *Ophthalmology.* 2008;115(2):S3-S12.
Linebarger EJ, Hardten DR, Lindstrom RL. Diffuse lamellar keratitis: diagnosis and management. *J Cataract Refract Surg.* 2000;26(7):1072-1077.
Lobo AM, Agelidis AM, Shukla D. Pathogenesis of herpes simplex keratitis: The host cell response and ocular surface sequelae to infection and inflammation. *Ocul Surf.* 2019;17(1):40-49.
Lorenzo-Morales J, Khan NA, Walochnik J. An update on Acanthamoeba keratitis: diagnosis, pathogenesis and treatment. *Parasite.* 2015;22:10.
Maycock NJ, Jayaswal R. Update on Acanthamoeba keratitis: diagnosis, treatment, and outcomes. *Cornea.* 2016;35(5):713-720.
McAllum P, Bahar I, Kaiserman I, Srinivasan S, Slomovic A, Rootman D. Temporal and seasonal trends in Acanthamoeba keratitis. *Cornea.* 2009;28(1):7-10.
McKay KM, Jacobs DS. In vivo confocal microscopy of keratic precipitates in uveitis. *Int Ophthalmol Clin.* 2019;59(4):95-103.
Meyer-Rüsenberg B, Loderstädt U, Richard G, Kaulfers PM, Gesser C. Epidemic keratoconjunctivitis: the current situation and recommendations for prevention and treatment. *Dtsch Arztebl Int.* 2011;108(27):475.
Moorthy RS, Valluri S, Rao NA. Nontuberculous mycobacterial ocular and adnexal infections. *Surv Ophthalmol.* 2012;57(3):202-235.
Murray PI, Rauz S. The eye and inflammatory rheumatic diseases: the eye and rheumatoid arthritis, ankylosing spondylitis, psoriatic arthritis. *Best Pract Res Clin Rheumatol.* 2016;30(5):802-825.
Nakano EM, Nakano K, Oliveira MC, Portellinha W, Simonelli R, Alvarenga LS. Cleaning solutions as a cause of diffuse lamellar keratitis. In: Thorofare, NJ: SLACK Incorporated. *Journal of Refractive Surgery*. 2002;18(3):S361-3.
Neelam S, Niederkorn JY. Focus: infectious diseases: pathobiology and immunobiology of Acanthamoeba keratitis: insights from animal models. *Yale J Biol Med.* 2017;90(2):261.
Niederkorn JY, Alizadeh H, Leher H, McCulley JP. The pathogenesis of Acanthamoeba keratitis. *Microbes Infect.* 1999;1(6):437-443.
Okumus S, Coskun E, Tatar MG, et al. Cyclosporine a 0.05% eye drops for the treatment of subepithelial infiltrates after epidemic keratoconjunctivitis. *BMC Ophthalmol.* 2012;12(1):1-6.
Oliveira MA, Rosa A, Soares M, et al. Anterior segment optical coherence tomography in the early management of microbial keratitis: a cross-sectional study. *Acta Med Port.* 2020;33(5):318-325.
Pesudovs K. Terrien's marginal degeneration: case reports and literature review. *Clin Exp Optom.* 1994;77(3):97-104.
Porter AJ, Lee GA, Jun AS. Infectious crystalline keratopathy. *Surv Ophthalmol.* 2018;63(4):480-499.
Prajna NV, Krishnan T, Rajaraman R, et al. Effect of oral voriconazole on fungal keratitis in the Mycotic Ulcer Treatment Trial II (MUTT II): a randomized clinical trial. *JAMA Ophthalmol.* 2016;134(12):1365-1372.
Randleman JB, Shah RD. LASIK interface complications: etiology, management, and outcomes. *J Refract Surg.* 2012;28(8):575-588.
Robin JB, Schanzlin DJ, Verity SM, et al. Peripheral corneal disorders. *Surv Ophthalmol.* 1986;31(1):1-36.
Schwartz GS, Harrison AR, Holland EJ. Etiology of immune stromal (interstitial) keratitis. *Cornea.* 1998;17(3):278-281.
Sharma N, Vajpayee RB, Pushker N, Vajpayee M. Infectious crystalline keratopathy. *CLAO J.* 2000;26(1):40-43.
Shipton C, Hind J, Biagi J, Lyall D. Anterior segment optical coherence tomographic characterisation of keratic precipitates. *Cont Lens Anterior Eye.* 2020;43(5):465-468.
Silva BL, Cardozo JB, Marback P, Machado FC, Galvão V, Santiago MB. Peripheral ulcerative keratitis: a serious complication of rheumatoid arthritis. *Rheumatol Int.* 2010;30(9):1267.
Smith RJ, Maloney RK. Diffuse lamellar keratitis: a new syndrome in lamellar refractive surgery. *Ophthalmology.* 1998;105(9):1721-1726.
Stern GA. Infectious crystalline keratopathy. *Int Ophthalmol Clin.* 1993;33(1):1-7.
Stulting RD, Randleman JB, Couser JM, Thompson KP. The epidemiology of diffuse lamellar keratitis. *Cornea.* 2004;23(7):680-688.
Süveges I, Levai G, Alberth B. Pathology of Terrien's disease: histochemical and electron microscopic study. *Am J Ophthalmol.* 1972;74(6):1191-1200.
Thomas P. Fungal infections of the cornea. *Eye.* 2003;17(8):852-862.
Tsirouki T, Dastiridou A, Symeonidis C, et al. A focus on the epidemiology of uveitis. *Ocul Immunol Inflamm.* 2018;26(1):2-16.
Van Ingen J, Boeree M, Dekhuijzen P, Van Soolingen D. Environmental sources of rapid growing nontuberculous mycobacteria causing disease in humans. *Clin Microbiol Infect.* 2009;15(10):888-893.
Watanabe R, Ishii T, Yoshida M, et al. Ulcerative keratitis in patients with rheumatoid arthritis in the modern biologic era: a series of eight cases and literature review. *Int J Rheum Dis.* 2017;20(2):225-230.
Wilson SE, de Oliveira RC. Pathophysiology and treatment of diffuse lamellar keratitis. *J Refract Surg.* 2020;36(2):124-130.
Wong TY, Ng TP, Fong KS, Tan D. Risk factors and clinical outcomes between fungal and bacterial keratitis: a comparative study. *CLAO J.* 1997;23(4):275-281.
Yagci A. Update on peripheral ulcerative keratitis. *Clin Ophthalmol (Auckland, NZ).* 2012;6:747.
Yawn BP, Wollan PC, Sauver JLS, Butterfield LC. Herpes zoster eye complications: rates and trends. Paper presented at: *Mayo Clin Proc*. 2013;88(6):562-570.
Zghal I, Fekih O, Zgolli HM, Chargui S, Malek I, Nacef L. Cyclosporin A eye drop and subepithelial adenoviral keratoconjunctivitis infiltrates. *Tunis Med.* 2019;97(5):639-643.

Index

A

Acanthamoeba keratitis, 268–270, 271f, 272f
Acute primary angle closure (APAC), 135–136, 136f
Adenoviral keratoconjunctivitis (AK), 260
Adenovirus subepithelial infiltrates, corneal infections and, 260, 260b, 263f, 264f
Amantadine-associated corneal edema, 109, 110f
Amelanotic nevus, 22, 24f
Amyloidosis, 32, 32f
Angle abnormalities, 130–141
  anterior chamber angles, evaluation of, 130–131
  AS-OCT examples, 131–141, 139b
Aniridia, 126, 127f
  associated keratopathy, 216, 216f
Anterior basement membrane dystrophy (ABMD), 33–37
Anterior capsule
  debris and opacification, 154, 154f, 155f
  phimosis, 154–155, 155f
Anterior chamber, 12–13, 12f, 13f, 14f, 15f
  angles, evaluation of, 130–131
    physiologic changes, 131, 131b, 133f, 134f
    qualitative evaluation, 130–131, 131b, 131f, 132f
    quantitative evaluation, 131, 133f, 134f
  inflammation of, 292–293, 293f, 294f, 295f, 296f
  trauma in, 231, 231b
Anterior segment
  imaging, pediatric cornea and, 213–222
  lens pathologic conditions and, 219–222
    Axenfeld-Rieger syndrome, 219, 219f
    lens material proliferation, 221–222, 222b, 222f
    microspherophakia, 220, 221f
    posterior lenticonus, 220–221, 221f
    primary congenital glaucoma, 220, 220f
  quantitative analysis of, 10–20
    anterior chamber, 12–13, 12f, 13f, 14f, 15f
    conjunctiva, 12, 12f
    cornea, 10–12, 10f
    iridocorneal angle, 12–13, 12f, 13f, 14f, 15f
    iris, 12–13, 12f, 13f, 14f, 15f
    lens, 13, 15f
    techniques, 15–18, 16f, 17f, 18b, 18f, 19f, 20f
Anterior segment optical coherence tomography (AS-OCT), 1–6
  for *Acanthamoeba* keratitis, 270, 271f, 272f
  after lamellar keratoplasty, 192–195, 193b, 193f, 194b, 194f, 195b, 195f, 196f, 197f
  after penetrating keratoplasty, 192, 192f, 193f
  for angle abnormalities, 130, 131b
  for anterior chamber inflammation, 292, 293f, 294f, 295f, 296f
  for bacterial keratitis, 242–243, 243f
  brief review on, 2–3
  for capsule violation, 233, 233f
Anterior segment optical coherence tomography *(Continued)*
  changes associated with mild-moderate keratoconus, 81–83, 82f, 83b, 83f, 84f, 85f, 86f
  changes associated with severe keratoconus, 83–86, 86f, 87f
  clinical applications of, 5, 7–9
    diagnosis and evaluation of ocular pathologies, 7–8, 7f, 8b, 8f
    intraoperative guidance for, 8–9
    monitoring disease progression and severity in, 8
    postoperative monitoring in, 9, 9f
    preoperative evaluation and surgical planning for, 8, 8b
  clinical examples of, 131–141, 139b
    acute angle closure as a result of large lens vault, 135–136, 136f
    aqueous misdirection syndrome (malignant glaucoma), 139, 140f
    ciliochoroidal effusion, 135, 136f
    discernment and treatment of angle closure resulting from pupil block or phacomorphic lens, 136–137, 137f
    evaluation of peripheral anterior synechiae, 137, 137f
    glaucoma drainage devices, 141
    imaging of posttrabeculectomy bleb morphology, 139, 140f
    iridocorneal endothelial syndrome and essential iris atrophy, 137, 138f
    iris cysts, 134–135, 135f
    narrow angles and laser peripheral iridotomy, 131–134, 134f
    pigment dispersion syndrome, 137, 138f
    posterior embryotoxon, 139, 139f
    subluxated lens, 134, 135f
  for contact lens–related bacterial keratitis, 242, 242f
  for corneal abrasion, 223, 223f
  of corneal ectasias, 81
  for corneal foreign bodies, 223, 223b, 224f, 225f
  for corneal infections, 242
  for corneal neovascularization, 287, 287f, 288f, 289f, 290f, 291f, 292f
  for corneal perforation, 225, 229f
  for corneal scarring, 225, 230f
  in corneal transplant surgery, 184–191
    deep anterior lamellar keratoplasty in, 186–187, 187b, 189f, 189f, 190f, 191f
    Descemet membrane endothelial keratoplasty in, 186, 187f, 186b
    Descemet stripping automated endothelial keratoplasty in, 184, 184b, 184f, 185f, 186f
  devices, development of, 3–4, 4t
  for diffuse lamellar keratitis, 280, 280b, 281f
  for Epstein-Barr virus, 260–268, 264f, 265f, 266f, 267f, 268f
Anterior segment optical coherence tomography *(Continued)*
  for eye trauma, 223
  features and advantages of, 4–5, 5f, 5t
  for fungal keratitis, 268, 269f, 270f
  for herpes simplex virus endotheliitis, 255–256, 256f
  for herpes simplex virus-associated nummular keratitis, 251, 252f
  history of development, 2–3, 2f
  for hyphema, 231, 231f
  imaging of lens using, 142
  for infectious crystalline keratopathy, 247, 250f
  for interstitial keratitis, 274, 274b, 275f, 276f
  for iridodialysis, 231, 231b, 232f
  for iris cyst, 231, 232f
  in keratoconus interventions, 90–95
    corneal collagen cross-linking, 90, 90b, 90f, 91f, 92f
    corneal transplant surgery, 95, 96f
    intrastromal corneal ring segments, 92–95, 93f, 94f, 95f
  for LASIK flap trauma, 223–225, 225b, 226f, 227f, 228f
  for marginal keratitis, 247, 249f
  for neurotrophic keratitis, 280, 282f, 283f, 284f, 285f, 286b, 286f
  for nontuberculous mycobacteria keratitis, 251, 251f
  for ocular inflammation, 274
  for peripheral ulcerative keratitis, 276, 277b, 277f, 278f, 279f, 280f
  in postoperative management of endothelial keratoplasty, 200–212
    future directions of, 211, 211f, 212f
    other postoperative complications of, 207–208, 209f, 210f
    in post-DMEK eyes, 203–207, 204f, 205b, 205f, 206f, 207b, 207f, 208f
    in post-DSEK eyes, 200–203, 200f, 201b, 201f, 202f, 203b, 203f, 204f
  for *Pseudomonas* keratitis, 243, 244f, 245f, 246f, 247f, 248f, 249f
  in select cases of corneal transplant surgery, 195–199, 198f, 199b, 199f
  for sterile contact lens–associated stromal infiltrates, 292, 292f
  for stromal keratitis
    with herpes simplex virus, 251, 253f
    with lipid keratopathy, 251–255, 254f, 255f
    with varicella zoster virus infection, 256–260, 259f, 260f, 261f, 262f
  for stromal scarring, herpes simplex virus, 255, 257f, 258f, 259f
  for subepithelial corneal infiltrates, 260, 260b, 263f, 264f
  for traumatic cataract, 233, 234f
  for traumatic iritis, 231, 233f
Anterior staphyloma, 218, 218b, 218f
Anterior stromal puncture, 52, 53f
Aqueous misdirection syndrome (malignant glaucoma), 139, 140f

AS-OCT. *see* Anterior segment optical coherence tomography
Axenfield-Rieger syndrome, 219, 219f

B

Bacterial infections, 242–251
  bacterial keratitis, 242–243, 243f
  contact lens–related bacterial keratitis, 242, 242b, 242f
  infectious crystalline keratopathy, 247, 250f
  marginal keratitis, 245–247, 249f
  nontuberculous mycobacteria keratitis, 247–251, 251f
  Pseudomonas keratitis, 243–245, 244b, 244f, 245f, 246f, 247f, 248f, 249f
Bacterial keratitis, 242–243, 243f
Band keratopathy, 38–40, 39f, 40b, 40f, 41f
Benign lesions, 22, 22b, 22f, 23f
Blepharokeratoconjunctivitis, 214–215, 215f
Bowman layer, 10
Bullous keratopathy, 73, 74f

C

CAM. *see* Complexion-associated melanosis
Capsular block syndrome, 155–156, 156f
Capsule violation, 233, 233f
Cataracts, 142
  surgery, postoperative complications of, 151–156
    anterior capsule debris and opacification, 154, 154f, 155f
    anterior capsule phimosis, 154–155, 155f
    capsular block syndrome, 155–156, 156f
    malpositioned intraocular lens, 151f, 152f, 153, 153b
    posterior capsule opacification, 151, 153f, 154f
  types of, 142–145
    cortical cataracts, 142, 143f
    mature cataracts, 142–145, 144b, 144f, 145f
    nuclear sclerotic cataracts, 142, 143f
    posterior polar cataracts, 145, 145b, 147f, 148f
    posterior subcapsular cataracts, 142, 143f
    subluxated cataracts, 145, 146f
    traumatic cataracts, 145, 146f, 147f, 233, 234f
Central clearance, in scleral contact lenses, 236–237, 237f
Chlorpromazine (Thorazine) deposition, 71–72, 72f
Ciliochoroidal effusion, 135, 136f
CMM. *see* Conjunctival malignant melanoma
CNV. *see* Corneal neovascularization
Cogan microcystic dystrophy. *see* Epithelial basement membrane dystrophy
Coherence, 2
  spatial, 2, 2f
  temporal, 2, 2f
COL8A2-associated corneal dystrophy, 110–111, 111f, 112f
Collamer intraocular lens (ICL), 148–149, 150f
Complexion-associated melanosis (CAM), 22–25, 25f
Congenital hereditary endothelial dystrophy (CHED), 216, 216b, 216f
Congenital iris abnormalities, 126–127
Conjunctiva, 12, 12f
Conjunctival malignant melanoma (CMM), 25, 26f, 27f
Conjunctival pathologic conditions, 21–32
  amyloidosis, 32, 32f
  benign lesions, 22, 22b, 22f, 23f
  lymphoma, 30, 31f, 32f
  ocular surface squamous neoplasia, 27–30, 27b, 28f, 29f, 30b, 30f
  pigmented lesions, 22–25, 24f, 25f, 26f, 27f
Constructive interference, 2
Contact lens
  bacterial keratitis, 242, 242b, 242f
  fitting, applications in, 235–241
    hybrid, 235, 235f, 236f
    ocular pathology and, 238, 239f, 240f, 241f
    rigid gas-permeable, 235
    scleral, 236–238, 236f
    soft, 235
  overwear, 45–47, 46f, 47b, 47f, 48f
Cornea, 10–12, 10f
Corneal abrasion, 223, 223f
Corneal bullae, 52
Corneal collagen cross-linking (CXL), 90, 90b, 90f, 91f, 92f, 177, 179f
Corneal curvature, 12
Corneal dystrophy, 58
  COL8A2-associated, 110–111, 111f, 112f
  granular, 59–64, 60b, 61f, 62b, 62f, 63f
  keratoconus in conjunction with, 98, 99f, 100f, 101f
  lattice, 58–59, 58f, 59f, 60b, 60f
  macular, 64, 64b, 64f
  Schnyder, 64–66, 65f
Corneal ectasias, 81–103
  keratoconus, 81–95, 90b
  keratoglobus, 102, 103f
  pellucid marginal degeneration, 98–102, 102b, 102f
  posterior keratoconus, 102, 103f
  post-LASIK ectasia, 95–98, 96f, 97f, 98f
Corneal edema
  amantadine-associated, 109, 110f
  netarsudil-associated, 109–110, 111f
Corneal epithelium, pathology of, 33–56
  anterior stromal puncture, 52, 53f
  band keratopathy, 38–40, 39f, 40b, 40f, 41f
  contact lens overwear, hypoxia, and contact lens–associated red eye, 45–47, 46f, 47b, 47f, 48f
  corneal bullae, 52
  dellen, 47, 48f
  dendrites versus pseudodendrites, 49–50, 49f, 50f
  epithelial basement membrane dystrophy, 33–37, 33f, 34f, 35f, 36f, 37b, 37f, 38f, 39f
  epithelial defects, 50–52, 50f, 51b, 51f, 52f
  epithelial hypertrophy, 44
  Horners-Trantas dots, 53, 54f
  Lisch epithelial corneal dystrophy, 53–54, 54f
  peripheral ulcerative keratitis, 43, 43f, 44f
  punctate epithelial erosions, 45
  Reis-Bückers dystrophy, 42–43, 43f
  Salzmann nodular degeneration, 40–42, 41f, 42f, 43f
  staphylococcal marginal keratitis, 43–44, 44b, 45f
  superficial punctate keratopathy, 45, 46f
  Thygeson superficial punctate keratitis, 52–53, 53f
Corneal foreign bodies, 223, 223b, 224f, 225f
Corneal hydrops, 86–90, 87f, 88f, 89f
Corneal infections, 242–273
  Acanthamoeba keratitis, 268–270, 271f, 272f
  bacterial, 242–251
    bacterial keratitis, 242–243, 243f
    contact lens–related bacterial keratitis, 242, 242b, 242f
    infectious crystalline keratopathy, 247, 250f
    marginal keratitis, 245–247, 249f
    nontuberculous mycobacteria keratitis, 247–251, 251f
    Pseudomonas keratitis, 243–245, 244b, 244f, 245f, 246f, 247f, 248f, 249f
  fungal keratitis, 268, 269f, 270f
Corneal infections *(Continued)*
  viral, 251–268
    adenovirus subepithelial infiltrates, 260, 260b, 263f, 264f
    Epstein-Barr virus, 260–268, 264f, 265f, 266f, 267f, 268f
    herpes simplex virus, 251–256, 255b
    herpes zoster, 256–260, 259f, 260f, 261f, 262f
Corneal injuries, 223–225
  corneal abrasion, 223, 223f
  corneal foreign bodies, 223, 223b, 224f, 225f
  corneal perforation, 225, 229f
  corneal scarring, 225, 230f
  LASIK flap trauma, 223–225, 225b, 226f, 227f, 228f
Corneal inlays and onlays, 172–177
Corneal neovascularization (CNV), 287, 287f, 288f, 289f, 290f, 291f, 292f
Corneal perforation, 225, 229f
Corneal scarring, 225, 230f
Corneal transplant surgery
  AS-OCT for, 195–199, 198f, 199b, 199f
  intraoperative AS-OCT in, 184–191
    deep anterior lamellar keratoplasty in, 186–187, 187b, 189f, 189f, 190f, 191f
    Descemet membrane endothelial keratoplasty in, 186, 187f, 186b
    Descemet stripping automated endothelial keratoplasty in, 184, 184b, 184f, 185f, 186f
  postoperative management, 95, 96f
Corneolimbal dermoid, 214, 214f
Cortical cataracts, 142, 143f
Crystalline lens and intraocular lens abnormalities, 142–158
  cataracts. *see* Cataracts
  imaging using AS-OCT, 142
  implantable lenses in, 145–151
Cystic iris lesions, 118–120, 123f, 124f, 125f
Cystinosis, 70–71, 72f

D

Deep anterior lamellar keratoplasty (DALK), 186–187, 187b, 189f, 189f, 190f, 191f
Dellen, 47, 48f
Dendrites, pseudodendrites versus, 49–50, 49f, 50f
Descemet membrane, 11–12
Descemet membrane endothelial keratoplasty (DMEK), 186, 187f, 186b
  post, AS-OCT in, 203–207, 204f, 205b, 205f, 206f, 207b, 207f, 208f
Descemet membrane rupture, secondary to birth forceps trauma, 218, 218f, 219f
Descemet stripping automated endothelial keratoplasty (DSAEK), 184, 184b, 184f, 185f, 186f
  post, AS-OCT in, 200–203, 200f, 201b, 201f, 202f, 203b, 203f, 204f
Descemetocele, 75–80
Descemet's membrane detachment, after cataract surgery, 109, 110f
Destructive interference, 2
Diffuse lamellar keratitis (DLK), 162–164, 163f, 277–280, 280b, 281f
Disease progression, 8
DLK. *see* Diffuse lamellar keratitis

E

EBV. *see* Epstein-Barr virus
Ectasia, post-LASIK, 95–98, 96f, 97f, 98f
Edema, stromal, 73, 74f
Embryotoxon, posterior, 139, 139f
Endothelial debris, 113, 113f, 114f
Endothelial dystrophies, 216

Endothelial keratoplasty, postoperative management of, AS-OCT in, 200–212
future directions of, 211, 211f, 212f
other postoperative complications of, 207–208, 209f, 210f
in post-DMEK eyes, 203–207, 204f, 205b, 205f, 206f, 207b, 207f, 208f
in post-DSEK eyes, 200–203, 200f, 201b, 201f, 202f, 203b, 203f, 204f
Endotheliitis, herpes simplex virus, 255, 256f
Endothelium, 11–12
pathology of, 104–116
amantadine-associated corneal edema, 109, 110f
COL8A2-associated corneal dystrophy, 110–111, 111f, 112f
Descemet's membrane detachment after cataract surgery, 109, 110f
endothelial debris, 113, 113f, 114f
Fuchs endothelial corneal dystrophy, 104, 104b, 104f, 105f, 106f
iridocorneal endothelial syndrome, 111–112, 112f, 113f
netarsudil-associated corneal edema, 109–110, 111f
posterior polymorphous membrane/ corneal dystrophy, 105–108, 108f, 109f
pseudophakic bullous keratopathy, 104–105, 107f, 108f
Epikeratoplasty, 177, 178f
Epithelial basement membrane dystrophy (EBMD), 33–37, 33f, 34f, 35f, 36f, 37b, 37f, 38f, 39f
Epithelial defects, 50–52, 50f, 51b, 51f, 52f
Epithelial downgrowth, 125f
Epithelial hypertrophy, 44
Epithelial ingrowth, 164–166, 164f, 165f, 166f
Epithelial keratitis, herpes simplex virus, 251–255, 252f
Epithelium, 10
Epstein-Barr virus (EBV), corneal infections and, 260–268, 264f, 265f, 266f, 267f, 268f
Essential iris atrophy, 137, 138f
Extensive stromal scarring, 75

F
FD-OCT. *see* Fourier-domain optical coherence tomography
FECD. *see* Fuchs endothelial corneal dystrophy
Foreign bodies, corneal, 223, 223b, 224f, 225f
Fourier-domain optical coherence tomography (FD-OCT), 3, 4t
Free-floating cysts, 120
Fuchs endothelial corneal dystrophy (FECD), 104, 104b, 104f, 105f, 106f
Fungal keratitis (FK), 268, 269f, 270f

G
Glaucoma drainage devices, 141
intrascleral position of, 220, 220f
Granular corneal dystrophy, 59–64, 60b, 61f, 62b, 62f, 63f
type 2, 63

H
Herpes simplex virus (HSV), 251–256, 255b
endotheliitis, 255, 256f
epithelial keratitis, 251–255, 252f
stromal keratitis, 251–255, 253f
stromal scarring, 255–256, 257f, 258f, 259f
Herpes zoster, 256–260, 259f, 260f, 261f, 262f
Horners-Trantas dots, 53, 54f
HSV. *see* Herpes simplex virus
Hybrid lenses, 235, 235f, 236f
Hyphema, 231, 231f
Hypoxia, associated red eye, 45–47, 46f, 47b, 47f, 48f

I
ICK. *see* Infectious crystalline keratopathy
Implantable lenses, types of, 145–151
iris-clip intraoperative lens, 151, 152f
phakic intraocular lens, 145–149, 148f, 149b, 149f, 150f
pseudophakic intraoperative lens, 150–151, 150f, 151f, 152f
Infectious crystalline keratopathy (ICK), 247, 250f
Intacs ring segments, 174, 176f, 177f
Interface debris, 162, 163f
Interstitial keratitis (IK), 274, 274b, 275f, 276f
Intracorneal hemorrhage, 72, 73f
Intraocular lens
malpositioned, 151f, 152f, 153, 153b
phakic, 145–149, 148f, 149b, 149f, 150f
Intraoperative guidance, 8–9
Intrastromal corneal ring segments (ICRSs), 92–95, 93f, 94f, 95f
Iridocorneal angle, 12–13, 12f, 13f, 14f, 15f
Iridocorneal endothelial syndrome, 111–112, 112f, 113f, 126, 126f, 137, 138f
Iridodialysis, 231, 231b, 232f
Iris, 12–13, 12f, 13f, 14f, 15f
abnormalities, 117–129
congenital, 126–127
cystic iris lesions, 118–120, 123f, 124f, 125f
iris melanocytic tumors, 118, 119f, 121f, 122f
secondary, 126–127, 128f
solid iris lesions, 118
arteriovenous malformations (AVMs), 126, 127f
trauma in, 231, 231b
Iris bombe, 127, 128f
Iris cysts, 134–135, 135f, 231, 232f
Iris flocculi. *see* Pupillary margin cysts
Iris lesions
cystic, 118–120, 123f, 124f, 125f
solid, 118
Iris melanocytic tumors, 118, 119f, 120f, 121f, 122f
Iris nevus, 120f, 121f
Iris pigment epithelium (IPE) cysts, 118, 123f, 124f
Iris-clip intraoperative lens, 151, 152f
Iritis, traumatic, 231, 233f

K
Kamra corneal inlay, 172–174, 172f, 173f, 174f, 175f
Keratectomy
photorefractive, 166, 167f
phototherapeutic, 166–172, 170f, 171f
Keratic precipitates (KPs), 113, 292, 293f, 294f
Keratoconus (KCN), 81–95, 90b
changes on imaging, 81–90
in conjunction with other corneal dystrophies, 98, 99f, 100f, 101f
corneal hydrops, 86–90, 87f, 88f, 89f
interventions, use of AS-OCT in, 90–95
corneal collagen cross-linking, 90, 90b, 90f, 91f, 92f
corneal transplant surgery, 95, 96f
intrastromal corneal ring segments, 92–95, 93f, 94f, 95f
mild-moderate, AS-OCT changes associated with, 81–83, 82f, 83b, 83f, 84f, 85f, 86f
posterior, 102, 103f
severe, AS-OCT changes associated with, 83–86, 86f, 87f
Keratoglobus (KGB), 102, 103f
Keratopathy
bullous, 73, 74f
lipid, 67–70, 69f, 70f
Keratoplasty
lamellar, AS-OCT after, 192–195, 193b, 193f, 194b, 194f, 195b, 195f, 196f, 197f
penetrating, AS-OCT after, 192, 192f, 193f

L
Lamellar keratoplasty, AS-OCT after, 192–195, 193b, 193f, 194b, 194f, 195b, 195f, 196f, 197f
Large lens vault, acute angle closure as a result of, 135–136, 136f
Laser in-situ keratomileusis (LASIK), 160–166
complications of, 160–166
flap trauma of, 223–225, 225b, 226f, 227f, 228f
in normal flap, 160, 160f
Laser peripheral iridotomy, 131–134, 134f
LASIK. *see* Laser in-situ keratomileusis
Lattice corneal dystrophy, 58–59, 58f, 59f, 60b, 60f
Lens, 13, 15f
material proliferation, 221–222, 222b, 222f
subluxated, 134, 135f
trauma in, 233
Limbal clearance, in scleral contact lenses, 237, 237f
Limbal girdle of Vogt (LGOV), 73, 75f
Lipid keratopathy, 67–70, 69f, 70f
Lisch epithelial corneal dystrophy, 53–54, 54f
Lymphoma, 30, 31f, 32f

M
Macrostriae, 160–162, 161f, 162f
Macular corneal dystrophy, 64, 64b, 64f
Malpositioned intraocular lens, 151f, 152f, 153, 153b
Map-dot-fingerprint dystrophy (MDFD). *see* Epithelial basement membrane dystrophy
Marginal keratitis, 245–247, 249f
Mature cataracts, 142–145, 144b, 144f, 145f
Melanocytic tumors, iris, 118, 119f, 121f, 122f
MICE. *see* Mitomycin intravascular chemoembolization
Microspherophakia, 220, 221f
Mild-moderate keratoconus, AS-OCT changes associated with, 81–83, 82f, 83b, 83f, 84f, 85f, 86f
Mitomycin intravascular chemoembolization (MICE), for corneal neovascularization, 287, 290f, 291f, 292f
Monoclonal gammopathy of undetermined significance, 70, 71f

N
Netarsudil-associated corneal edema, 109–110, 111f
Neurotrophic keratitis (NTK), 280–286, 282f, 283f, 284f, 285f, 286b, 286f
Nontuberculous mycobacteria keratitis, 247–251, 251f
NTK. *see* Neurotrophic keratitis
Nuclear sclerotic cataracts, 142, 143f
Nummular keratitis, herpes simplex virus, 251, 252f

O
Ocular inflammation, 274–298
anterior chamber inflammation, 292–293, 293f, 294f, 295f, 296f
corneal neovascularization, 287, 287f, 288f, 289f, 290f, 291f, 292f
diffuse lamellar keratitis, 277–280, 280b, 281f
interstitial keratitis, 274, 274b, 275f, 276f

Ocular inflammation *(Continued)*
neurotrophic keratitis, 280–286, 282f, 283f, 284f, 285f, 286b, 286f
peripheral ulcerative keratitis, 274–277, 277b, 277f, 278f, 279f, 280f
Ocular surface squamous neoplasia (OSSN), 27–30, 27b, 28f, 29f, 30b, 30f
OSSN. *see* Ocular surface squamous neoplasia

P

PAM. *see* Primary acquired melanosis
Pediatric cornea
anterior segment imaging and, 213–222
external disease pathologic conditions and, 214–218, 215b
aniridia-associated keratopathy, 216, 216f
blepharokeratoconjunctivitis, 214–215, 215f
corneolimbal dermoid, 214, 214f
endothelial dystrophies, 216
other posterior corneal defects, 217–218
vernal keratoconjunctivitis, 215, 215f
Pellucid marginal degeneration (PMD), 98–102, 102b, 102f
Penetrating keratoplasty, AS-OCT after, 192, 192f, 193f
Peripheral anterior synechiae, evaluation of, 137, 137f
Peripheral ulcerative keratitis (PUK), 43, 43f, 44f, 274–277, 277b, 277f, 278f, 279f, 280f
Peters anomaly
type I, 217, 217f
type II, 217–218, 217f
Phacomorphic lens, discernment and treatment of angle closure resulting from, 136–137, 137f
Phakic intraocular lenses, 145–149, 148f, 149b, 149f, 150f
in refractive surgery, 177–178, 180f, 181f, 182f, 183f
Phimosis, anterior capsule, 154–155, 155f
Photorefractive keratectomy, 166, 167f
Phototherapeutic keratectomy (PTK), 166–172, 170f, 171f
corneal scar depth measurement for, 11, 11f
Pigment dispersion syndrome, 137, 138f
Pigmented lesions, 22–25, 24f, 25f, 26f, 27f
Pinguecula, 22, 22f, 23f
PMD. *see* Pellucid marginal degeneration
Polymorphic amyloid degeneration, 70, 71f
Posterior capsule opacification, 151, 153f, 154f
Posterior embryotoxon, 139, 139f
Posterior keratoconus (PKC), 102, 103f
Posterior lenticonus, 220–221, 221f
Posterior polar cataracts, 145, 145b, 147f, 148f
Posterior polymorphous corneal dystrophy (PPCD), 216, 217f
Posterior polymorphous membrane dystrophy (PPMD), 105–108, 108f, 109f
Posterior subcapsular cataracts, 142, 143f
Post-LASIK ectasia, 95–98, 96f, 97f, 98f
Postoperative monitoring, 9, 9f
Posttrabeculectomy bleb morphology, imaging of, 139, 140f
PPMD. *see* Posterior polymorphous membrane dystrophy
Preoperative evaluation, 8, 8b
Pressure-induced stromal keratitis, 166, 167f
Primary acquired melanosis (PAM), 25, 26f
Primary congenital glaucoma (PCG), 220, 220f
Pseudoexfoliation syndrome (PXF), 113, 113f
Pseudomonas keratitis, 243–245, 244b, 244f, 245f, 246f, 247f, 248f, 249f
Pseudophakic bullous keratopathy, 104–105, 107f, 108f
Pseudophakic intraoperative lens, 150–151, 150f, 151f, 152f
Pterygia, 22, 23f
PUK. *see* Peripheral ulcerative keratitis
Punctate epithelial erosions, 45
Pupil block, discernment and treatment of angle closure resulting from, 136–137, 137f
Pupillary margin cysts, 120

R

Raindrop corneal inlay, 172–174, 172f, 173f, 174f, 175f
Red eye, contact lens–associated, 45–47, 46f, 47b, 47f, 48f
Refractive surgery, 159–183
corneal collagen cross-linking, 177, 179f
corneal inlays and onlays, 172–177
laser in-situ keratomileusis (LASIK), 160–166
phakic intraocular lenses in, 177–178, 180f, 181f, 182f, 183f
photorefractive keratectomy, 166, 167f
phototherapeutic keratectomy, 166–172, 170f, 171f
Reis-Bückers dystrophy, 42–43, 43f
Rigid gas-permeable (RGP) lenses, 235

S

Salzmann nodular degeneration (SND), 40–42, 41f, 42f, 43f
Scarring
corneal, 225, 230f
stromal, 73–75, 79f, 80f
SCC. *see* Squamous cell carcinoma
SCD. *see* Schnyder corneal dystrophy
Schnyder corneal dystrophy (SCD), 64–66, 65f
Scleral contact lenses, 236–238, 236f
central clearance, 236–237, 237f
complications in, 238, 238f, 239f
landing and peripheral alignment, 238, 238f
limbal clearance, 237, 237f
Scleral spur, 13f, 130, 130f
SD-OCT. *see* Spectral domain optical coherence tomography
Secondary iris abnormalities, 126–127, 128f
Secondary iris cysts, 120
SEIs. *see* Subepithelial corneal infiltrates
Soft contact lenses, 235
Solid iris lesions, 118
Spatial coherence, 2, 2f
Spectral domain optical coherence tomography (SD-OCT), 3, 4f, 4t
Squamous cell carcinoma (SCC), 30, 30f, 31f
SS-OCT. *see* Swept-source optical coherence tomography
Staphylococcal marginal keratitis, 43–44, 44b, 45f
Sterile contact lens–associated stromal infiltrates, 292, 292f
Stroma, 10–11, 11b, 11f
Stromal cysts, 118
Stromal degenerations, 66–70
cystinosis, 70–71, 72f
lipid keratopathy, 67–70, 69f, 70f
polymorphic amyloid degeneration, 70, 71f
Terrien marginal degeneration, 66–67, 67b, 67f, 68f
Stromal depositions, 70–72
chlorpromazine (Thorazine) deposition, 71–72, 72f
intracorneal hemorrhage, 72, 73f
monoclonal gammopathy of undetermined significance, 70, 71f
Stromal dystrophies, 58–66, 64b
granular corneal dystrophy, 59–64, 60b, 61f, 62b, 62f, 63f
lattice corneal dystrophy, 58–59, 58f, 59f, 60b, 60f
macular corneal dystrophy, 64, 64b, 64f
Stromal dystrophies *(Continued)*
Schnyder corneal dystrophy, 64–66, 65f
unclassified, 66, 66f, 67f
Stromal edema, 73, 74f
Stromal infiltrates, sterile contact lens–associated, 292, 292f
Stromal keratitis, herpes simplex virus, 251–255, 253f
Stromal pathologic conditions, miscellaneous, 73–80, 73b
bullous keratopathy, 73, 74f
descemetocele, 75–80
limbal girdle of Vogt, 73, 75f
stromal edema, 73, 74f
stromal scarring, 73–75, 79f, 80f
stromal thinning and melting, 73, 75f, 76f, 77f, 78f
Stromal scarring, 73–75, 79f, 80f
herpes simplex virus, 255–256, 257f, 258f, 259f
photorefractive keratectomy for, 166, 169f
Stromal thinning and melting, 73, 75f, 76f, 77f, 78f
Subepithelial corneal infiltrates (SEIs), corneal infections and, 260, 260b, 263f, 264f
Subepithelial fibrosis, 166, 169f
Subepithelial haze, 166, 168f
Subepithelium/Bowman layer, pathology of, 33–56
anterior stromal puncture, 52, 53f
band keratopathy, 38–40, 39f, 40b, 40f, 41f
contact lens overwear, hypoxia, and contact lens–associated red eye, 45–47, 46f, 47b, 47f, 48f
corneal bullae, 52
dellen, 47, 48f
dendrites versus pseudodendrites, 49–50, 49f, 50f
epithelial basement membrane dystrophy, 33–37, 33f, 34f, 35f, 36f, 37b, 37f, 38f, 39f
epithelial defects, 50–52, 50f, 51b, 51f, 52f
epithelial hypertrophy, 44
Horners-Trantas dots, 53, 54f
Lisch epithelial corneal dystrophy, 53–54, 54f
peripheral ulcerative keratitis, 43, 43f, 44f
punctate epithelial erosions, 45
Reis-Bückers dystrophy, 42–43, 43f
Salzmann nodular degeneration, 40–42, 41f, 42f, 43f
staphylococcal marginal keratitis, 43–44, 44b, 45f
superficial punctate keratopathy, 45, 46f
Thygeson superficial punctate keratitis, 52–53, 53f
Subluxated lens, 134, 135f
Subluxated cataracts, 145, 146f
Superficial punctate keratopathy, 45, 46f
Swept-source optical coherence tomography (SS-OCT), 3, 4f, 4t

T

TD-OCT. *see* Time-domain optical coherence tomography
Temporal coherence, 2, 2f
Terrien marginal degeneration, 66–67, 67b, 67f, 68f
Thorazine (chlorpromazine) deposition, 71–72, 72f
Thygeson superficial punctate keratitis, 52–53, 53f
Time-domain optical coherence tomography (TD-OCT), 3, 4f, 4t
Tomography, 2

Trauma, of eye, 223
anterior chamber and iris, 231, 231b
corneal injuries, 223–225
corneal abrasion, 223, 223f
corneal foreign bodies, 223, 223b, 224f, 225f
corneal perforation, 225, 229f
corneal scarring, 225, 230f
LASIK flap trauma, 223–225, 225b, 226f, 227f, 228f
lens, 233
Traumatic cataracts, 145, 146f, 147f, 233, 234f
Traumatic iritis, 231, 233f

U

UBM. *see* Ultrasound biomicroscopy
Ultra-high-resolution anterior segment optical coherence tomography (AS-OCT), 4t, 7–8
Ultrasound biomicroscopy (UBM), 2, 5, 5t, 130–131

V

Vernal keratoconjunctivitis, 215, 215f
Viral infections, 251–268
adenovirus subepithelial infiltrates, 260, 260b, 263f, 264f
Epstein-Barr virus, 260–268, 264f, 265f, 266f, 267f, 268f
herpes simplex virus, 251–256, 255b
herpes zoster, 256–260, 259f, 260f, 261f, 262f